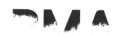

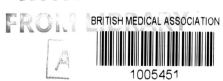

Interventional and Endovascular Tips and Tricks of the Trade

Interventional and Endovascular Tips and Tricks of the Trade

Edited by

S. Lowell Kahn, MD, MBA, FSIR

Assistant Professor of Interventional Radiology and Surgery
Tufts University School of Medicine
New England Endovascular Center
West Springfield, Massachusetts

Bulent Arslan, MD, FSIR

Associate Professor of Radiology
Director, Vascular & Interventional Radiology
Rush University Medical Center
Chicago, Illinois

Abdulrahman Masrani, MD

Radiology Resident
Mallinckrodt Institute of Radiology
Washington University in St. Louis
St. Louis, Missouri

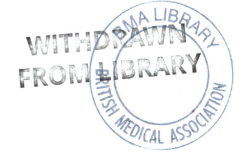

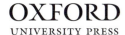

OXFORD
UNIVERSITY PRESS

OXFORD
UNIVERSITY PRESS

Oxford University Press is a department of the University of Oxford. It furthers
the University's objective of excellence in research, scholarship, and education
by publishing worldwide. Oxford is a registered trade mark of Oxford University
Press in the UK and certain other countries.

Published in the United States of America by Oxford University Press
198 Madison Avenue, New York, NY 10016, United States of America.

© Oxford University Press 2018

Library of Congress Cataloging-in-Publication Data
Names: Kahn, S. Lowell, editor. | Arslan, Bulent (Associate professor of radiology), editor. |
Masrani, Abdulrahman, editor.
Title: Interventional and endovascular tips and tricks of the trade /
edited by S. Lowell Kahn, Bulent Arslan, Abdulrahman Masrani.
Description: Oxford ; New York : Oxford University Press, [2018] |
Includes bibliographical references and index.
Identifiers: LCCN 2016036932 (print) | LCCN 2016038173 (ebook) |
ISBN 9780199986071 (alk. paper) | ISBN 9780199986095 (e-book) | ISBN 9780199390885 (online)
Subjects: | MESH: Minimally Invasive Surgical Procedures—methods
Classification: LCC RD33.53 (print) | LCC RD33.53 (ebook) | NLM WO 505 | DDC 617/.057—dc23
LC record available at https://lccn.loc.gov/2016036932

This material is not intended to be, and should not be considered, a substitute for medical or
other professional advice. Treatment for the conditions described in this material is highly
dependent on the individual circumstances. And, while this material is designed to offer
accurate information with respect to the subject matter covered and to be current as of the
time it was written, research and knowledge about medical and health issues is constantly
evolving and dose schedules for medications are being revised continually, with new side
effects recognized and accounted for regularly. Readers must therefore always check the
product information and clinical procedures with the most up-to-date published product
information and data sheets provided by the manufacturers and the most recent codes of
conduct and safety regulation. The publisher and the authors make no representations or
warranties to readers, express or implied, as to the accuracy or completeness of this material.
Without limiting the foregoing, the publisher and the authors make no representations or
warranties as to the accuracy or efficacy of the drug dosages mentioned in the material. The
authors and the publisher do not accept, and expressly disclaim, any responsibility for any
liability, loss or risk that may be claimed or incurred as a consequence of the use and/or
application of any of the contents of this material.

9 8 7 6 5 4 3 2 1
Printed by Sheridan Books, Inc., United States of America

To my loving wife, Carrie, my three amazing children, Chloe, Ella, and Kelsey, and my supportive parents—thank you for your love, patience, and encouragement in letting me pursue my dream of writing this book. You are my everything.—S.L.K.

I would like to think that, this book is written by very creative interventionalists for the curious ones. Our goal, which was sparked by Lowell, was to carry bright ideas to each other, which would help to improve patient care. Without efforts of my co-authors Lowell and Abdul, as well as all other creative interventionalists, we would not be able to learn from it. I dedicate the book to everyone who gave their time and effort for it and to their loved ones who suffered through the process including my wife Ceyda and my two sons.—B.A.

To my beloved wife, Heba and precious kid, Faisal. Your company made the journey of life much more colorful! To my devoted parents, Faisal and Faten. Your endless support is the reason I am where I am! To my mentors and friends. I am privileged to have you beside!—A.M.

Contents

Foreword

It is a great personal pleasure for me to contribute the Foreword for *Interventional and Endovascular Tips and Tricks of the Trade* edited by S. Lowell Kahn, Bulent Arslan, and Abdulrahman Masrani, three outstanding physicians. Since its early pioneering days, interventional radiology has been developed by individuals and groups of "problem-solvers." In fact, most interventionalists look forward to challenges in both the clinical and the technical arenas and are interested in providing solutions. How many of us have been approached by a colleague searching for a solution to a patient's problem and, without a solution in mind, have only his or her trust in the interventional radiologist to come up with some type of solution? The field of interventional and endovascular therapy has today grown to involve not only interventional radiologists, but also people from multiple disciplines, from varying training backgrounds, who are now called on to perform a diverse group of procedures literally involving every organ system in the body.

This book has particular resonance with me because my earliest textbook was titled *Interventional Diagnostic and Therapeutic Procedures*, the first textbook to use "Interventional" in the title, and was intended to be a "how to" manual providing a practical guide to the performance of procedures that were rapidly developing. The authors have taken the concept of technical problem-solving to a new level by recognizing how often we must confront unknown, unexpected, and undescribed events that occur during the performance of interventional procedures and, importantly, providing solutions to these problems in a practical, goal-oriented way. While we are a specialty of great improvisers, the authors have collected worldwide experience to help us confront the unknown.

A brief perusal of the table of contents confirms that regardless of what interest or practice a given interventionalist might have, there is something in this book for all. It includes vascular and nonvascular interventional techniques, pain management, and even lymphatic system interventions.

The field of interventional and endovascular therapy continues to grow rapidly as the innovations created by pioneering physicians and facilitated by evolving technology continue to broaden the scope of less-invasive therapy. As such, I'm certain that this text will be an indispensable tool to those who are performing procedures and taking care of patients on a daily basis. Importantly, I see it as an important reference source for those physicians who will be performing certain procedures less frequently than others. By sharing stories of "tips and tricks" rather than simple "how to" documentation, the authors provide their readers with practical solutions to problems that can occur every day.

My hardy congratulations to the authors for their creativity in producing a text with this innovative approach and on their hard work in accumulating valuable experiences from throughout the world, in the broadest scope of interventional and endovascular procedures, for all of us to share!

Barry T. Katzen, MD
Founder and Chief Medical Executive
Miami Cardiac and Vascular Institute
Clinical Professor of Radiology and Surgery
Associate Dean for Clinical Affairs Baptist Health
FIU Herbert Wertheim College of Medicine
Miami, Florida

Preface

In 1964, Dr. Charles Dotter performed the first successful percutaneous transluminal angioplasty, a medical milestone for which he was later nominated for the Nobel Prize. Revolutionary in its time, this simple, yet brilliant, procedure gave birth to the fields of interventional radiology (IR) and endovascular surgery. The era of minimally invasive surgery had begun, and countless patients stood to benefit.

Since its inception, IR and endovascular surgery have been defined by technological and technical innovation. The expansive growth in devices and technique is staggering and has broadened the scope of diseases amenable to treatment by minimally invasive means. Interventional radiologists and endovascular surgeons are by nature inventors, continually refining their techniques for the benefit of their patients.

As a medical student rotating through interventional radiology, I was seduced by the creativity I found in our field. While so much of medicine revolved around rote memorization and algorithm-based theory, IR appeared as much an art as the practice of science. I vividly remember watching my early mentors troubleshoot the tasks at hand with individual tricks and modifications of conventional methodology. Such techniques proved invaluable in the care of the patient.

Interventional and Endovascular Tips and Tricks of the Trade is a tribute to the spirit of innovation and represents a compilation of techniques developed and practiced by interventionalists nationwide. Inspired by the widely popular "Potpourri of Pearls" and "Extreme IR" sessions at the Society of Interventional Radiology annual meeting, the book presents unique techniques that are unlikely to be found in conventional texts. Presented in outline format with case examples, these techniques are presented in a succinct, user-friendly format. Special attention is paid to specific steps, applications, challenges, and potential pitfalls of the procedure to optimize learning, patient selection, and outcomes of the methods presented. Reference articles and suggested readings are provided for each technique.

The text is divided into 12 sections with 105 chapters covering the full gamut of vascular and nonvascular procedures. As such, it is easy to navigate and identify procedures of interest. A web-based version and forum are planned for the future.

It is the authors' vision that *Interventional and Endovascular Tips and Tricks of the Trade* will prove itself an invaluable resource in the armamentarium of the interventionalist. We seek to provide "outside-the-box" ideas and strategies for the betterment of our patients. It is our ambition to inspire ingenuity and encourage an influx of new ideas for future editions of the text. We hope you find reading this text as enjoyable as we found editing it. Cheers to a bright and innovative future for our field!

S. Lowell Kahn
Bulent Arslan
Abdulrahman Masrani

Acknowledgments

This book represents the contribution and collaboration of countless physicians, nurses, and editorial staff. As such, it has taken years to compile the information and construct a meaningful text that surely would not exist without the dedication of so many. Perhaps most importantly, we'd like to thank the mentors and role models that have shaped our careers, including Alan Matsumoto, John "Fritz" Angle, Wael Saad, Saher Sabri, Bulent Arslan, Ulku Cenk Turba, Mike Dake, Sandy Schwaner, Dot Cage, Barry Katzen, Alex Powell, Sean Samuels, Constantino Pena, James Benenati, Mark Bean, George Hartnell, and Laura Feldman. The authors would also like to thank the fabulous team at Oxford University Press, including Andrea Knobloch, Divya Vasudevan, and Rebecca Suzan. Finally, and most importantly, none of this would be possible without the unyielding support of our family and friends.

Contributors

Salim E. Abboud, MD
Department of Radiology
University Hospitals Case Medical Center
Cleveland, Ohio

Fereidoun Abtin, MD
Associate Professor of Radiological Sciences
Thoracic Imaging Section
David Geffen School of Medicine at UCLA
Los Angeles, California

Osmanuddin Ahmed, MD
Assistant Professor of Radiology
Rush University Medical Center
Chicago, Illinois

John Fritz Angle, MD
Professor of Radiology
Department of Vascular and Interventional Radiology
University of Virginia Health System
Charlottesville, Virginia

Mohammad Arabi, MD, FRCR, DABR, ABNM
Consultant Interventional Radiologist
Vascular Interventional Radiology
Medical Imaging Department
King Abdulaziz Medical City
Riyadh, Kingdom of Saudi Arabia

Anshuman Bansal, MD
Interventional Radiology Fellow
Department of Radiological Sciences
David Geffen School of Medicine at UCLA
Los Angeles, California

James F. Benenati, MD, FSIR
Miami Cardiac & Vascular Institute
Miami, Florida

Michael Brunner, MD
University of Wisconsin Madison School of Medicine and Public Health
Wm. S. Middleton VA Hospital
Madison, Wisconsin

Sabah Butty, MD
Assistant Professor of Clinical Radiology
Department of Radiology and Imaging Sciences
Indiana University School of Medicine
Indianapolis, Indiana

George Carberry, MD
Department of Radiology
University of Wisconsin Hospital and Clinics
Madison, Wisconsin

Thomas Casciani, MD
Assistant Professor of Clinical Radiology
Section Chief, Interventional Radiology
Indiana University School of Medicine
Indianapolis, Indiana

Ki Jinn Chin, MBBS, LMCC, MMed, FANZCA, FAMS, FRCPC
Associate Professor of Anesthesia
University of Toronto
Toronto Western Hospital
Toronto, Ontario, Canada

Michael D. Dake, MD
Thelma and Henry Doelger Professor of Cardiothoracic Surgery
Falk Cardiovascular Research Center
Stanford University School of Medicine
Stanford, California

William Derry, MD
Resident Physician
Department of Radiological Sciences
Thoracic Imaging and Intervention Section
Ronald Reagan UCLA Medical Center
David Geffen School of Medicine at UCLA
Los Angeles, California

Joseph Farnam, MD
Department of Diagnostic Imaging
Warren Alpert School of Medicine
Brown University
Rhode Island Hospital
Providence, Rhode Island

Hector Ferral, MD
Senior Clinician Educator
Vascular and Interventional Radiology
NorthShore Medical Group
Evanston, Illinois

Ripal T. Gandhi, MD, FSVM
Miami Cardiac & Vascular Institute
Miami, Florida

Alessandro Gasparetto, MD
Research Instructor in Radiology and Medical Imaging
University of Virginia
Charlottesville, Virginia

Scott Genshaft, MD
Assistant Professor of Radiology
Department of Radiological Sciences
Thoracic Imaging and Intervention Section
Ronald Reagan UCLA Medical Center
David Geffen School of Medicine at UCLA
Los Angeles, California

Marcelo Guimaraes, MD, FSIR
Director of Vascular & Interventional Radiology
Associate Professor of Radiology
Medical University of South Carolina
Charleston, South Carolina

John R. Haaga, MD
Department of Radiology
University Hospitals Case Medical Center
Cleveland, Ohio

Christopher Harnain, MD
Department of Radiology
New York Medical College
Westchester Medical Center
Valhalla, New York

Robert Evans Heithaus, MD
Department of Radiology
Baylor University Medical Center
Dallas, Texas

Jessica M. Ho, MD
Department of Radiology
Kaiser Permanente West Los Angeles Medical Center
Los Angeles, California

Jason Iannuccilli, MD
Department of Diagnostic Imaging
Warren Alpert School of Medicine
Brown University
Rhode Island Hospital
Providence, Rhode Island

Jonathan J. Iglesias, MD
Miami Cardiac & Vascular Institute
Miami, Florida

Zubin Irani, MBBS
Assistant Professor of Interventional Radiology
Massachusetts General Hospital
Boston, Massachusetts

Abdel Aziz A. Jaffan, MD
Department of Radiology
Division of Interventional Radiology
Aurora Healthcare
Milwaukee, Wisconsin

Harsha R. Jonna, MD
University Radiology Group
East Brunswick, New Jersey

Almamoon I. Justaniah, MD
Vascular and Interventional Radiology
Lahey Hospital & Medical Center
Tufts University School of Medicine
Burlington, Massachusetts

Michael D. Katz, MD
Associate Professor of Clinical Radiology
Chief of Interventional Radiology
University of Southern California
Los Angeles, California

Stephen Kee, MD, MMM, FSIR
Professor of Radiology
Chief of Interventional Radiology
University of California, Los Angeles
Los Angeles, California

Thomas Kinney, MD
Department of Radiology
University of California San Diego Medical Center
San Diego, California

Ganesh Krishnamurthy, MD
Department of Radiology
Children's Hospital of Philadelphia
Philadelphia, Pennsylvania

Sreekumar Madassery, MD
Assistant Professor of Radiology
Rush University Medical Center
Chicago, Illinois

Armeen Mahvash, MD
Associate Professor of Radiology
Department of Interventional Radiology
University of Texas MD Anderson Cancer Center
Houston, Texas

Sam McCabe, MD
Vascular and Interventional Radiology
New York Medical College
Westchester Medical Center
Valhalla, New York

Nikhil Mehta, MD
Vascular & Interventional Radiology Fellow
Rush University Medical Center
Chicago, Illinois

Craig Miller
Medical Student
Medical University of South Carolina
Charleston, South Carolina

Gregg A. Miller, MD
Fresenius Vascular Care
Brooklyn, New York

Peter Miller, MD
Department of Radiology and Imaging Sciences
Indiana University School of Medicine
Indianapolis, Indiana

Ravi Murthy, MD
Professor of Radiology
Department of Interventional Radiology
University of Texas MD Anderson Cancer Center
Houston, Texas

Dean A. Nakamoto, MD
Department of Radiology
University Hospitals Case Medical Center
Cleveland, Ohio

Kazim Narsinh, MD
Department of Radiology
University of California San Diego Medical Center
San Diego, California

Orhan Ozkan, MD
Department of Radiology
University of Wisconsin Hospital and Clinics
Madison, Wisconsin

Roshni A. Parikh, MD
Fellow, Vascular and Interventional Radiology
University of Michigan
Ann Arbor, Michigan

Mikin V. Patel, MD, MBA
Department of Radiology
University of Chicago Hospitals
Chicago, Illinois

Syed M. Peeran, MD, MSc
Vascular Surgery Fellow
The Mayo Clinic
Rochester, Minnesota

Constantino S. Peña, MD
Miami Cardiac & Vascular Institute
Miami, Florida

Adam N. Plotnik, MBBS, MSc, MMed, FRANZCR
Interventional Radiology Section
University of California, Los Angeles
Los Angeles, California

Dean C. Preddie, MD
Fresenius Vascular Care
Brooklyn, New York

Chet R. Rees, MD, FSIR
Department of Radiology
Baylor University Medical Center
Dallas, Texas

Steven C. Rose, MD
Department of Radiology
University of California San Diego Medical Center
San Diego, California

Grigory Rozenblit, MD
Vascular and Interventional Radiology
New York Medical College
Westchester Medical Center
Valhalla, New York

Michael Rush, MD
Interventional Radiology
Holy Cross Hospital
Fort Lauderdale, Florida

Saher S. Sabri, MD
Department of Radiology and Medical Imaging
University of Virginia Health Systems
Charlottesville, Virginia

Kyle Sanders, MD
Vascular & Interventional Radiology Fellow
Medical University of South Carolina
Charleston, South Carolina

Luke E. Sewall, MD
President, Vascular and Interventional Radiology
VIRchicago.com
Hinsdale, Illinois

Gregory Soares, MD
Department of Diagnostic Imaging
Warren Alpert School of Medicine
Brown University
Rhode Island Hospital
Providence, Rhode Island

Jayesh M. Soni, MD
Assistant Professor Radiology
Rush University Medical Center
Chicago, Illinois

David C. Stevens, MD
Radiology Resident
Department of Radiology and Imaging Sciences
Indiana University School of Medicine
Indianapolis, Indiana

Almas Syed, MD
Department of Radiology
Baylor University Medical Center
Dallas, Texas

Jordan C. Tasse, MD
Assistant Professor of Radiology
Rush University Medical Center
Chicago, Illinois

Cynthia Toot Ferguson, ARNP
Interventional Radiology
Holy Cross Hospital
Fort Lauderdale, Florida

David M. Williams, MD
Professor of Radiology
Division of Vascular and Interventional Radiology
University of Michigan
Ann Arbor, Michigan

Farrah J. Wolf, MD
Department of Diagnostic Imaging
Warren Alpert School of Medicine
Brown University
Rhode Island Hospital
Providence, Rhode Island

Ricardo Yamada, MD
Assistant Professor of Vascular & Interventional Radiology
Medical University of South Carolina
Charleston, South Carolina

Mahmoud Zahra, MD, FRCR
Department of Radiology
St. Vincent Medical Center
Bridgeport, Connecticut

Steven Zangan, MD
Department of Radiology
University of Chicago Hospitals
Chicago, Illinois

Sara Zhao, MD
Assistant Professor Radiology
Division of Vascular and Interventional Radiology
Ann Arbor, Michigan

Aortic Interventions

CHAPTER 1

Deployment Finesse of the Cook Zenith Stent Graft

John Fritz Angle

Brief Description

Although abdominal endograft placement has become a widely-performed procedure, there are still many device-specific and experience-based considerations in planning and performing these procedures safely and with good outcomes. Although not always evidence-based, reviewing some case-specific scenarios can introduce techniques or lead to standards of practice that reduce suboptimal outcomes or prevent complications in future procedures.

Applications of the Technique

This chapter focuses on the Cook Zenith Flex and Zenith LP grafts (Cook Medical Inc., Bloomington, IN), but many of the concepts presented here apply to other abdominal endografts and even thoracic endograft procedures.[1]

Challenges of the Procedure/Technique

For all abdominal aortic aneurysm endografts, the major challenge is minimizing the risk of a type I endoleak. Neck length, calcification, and angulation present an increased risk for proximal (type IA) endoleak.[2] Inadequate seal zone or poor iliac limb sizing are leading causes of distal (type IB) endoleak. Case selection and planning are the keys to reducing the incidence of a type I leak. Intraprocedural attention to the details is equally important to this goal.

Maximize Neck Length

1. As the main body of the device is advanced into position, it is rarely ever parallel to the longitudinal axis of the aorta. This device angulation can be manipulated by introducing the device on one side or the other. Advance the main body of the device from the side that will bring the device as close as possible to both renal arteries.
2. Remember that the cloth extends 2 mm above the radiopaque markers. Too aggressive device placement can lead to renal artery encroachment.
3. Deploy in the view (LAO/RAO and craniocaudal) that profiles (delineates the origin from the aorta) the lowest renal artery as determined from pre-procedure computed tomography angiography and the view that is perpendicular to the proximal end of the device (angulate the C-arm intraoperatively until the proximal marker beads come into profile without parallax).

Proximal Seal Zone

1. Most endografts are a series of Z stent segments separated by a short gap. These stent segments do not conform to an aortic neck with uneven walls or angulation. Endofixation (Aptus Endosystems Inc., Sunnyvale, CA) or balloon-expandable stents (Palmaz XL, Cordis Corp., Milpitas, CA) may address this problem.[3–5]
2. Be aware that even the suprarenal fixation can constrict the first segment of Dacron-covered Z stent, preventing wall apposition. A more proximal or distal position or using a device without suprarenal fixation may improve the seal zone apposition.

Distal Fixation

1. The next step is catheterization of the contralateral gate. Because the gate is very close to the iliac origin by design, it is important that the device orientation be assessed prior to releasing the top cap. In most cases, having the contralateral gate close to the contralateral common iliac artery origin makes for easy gate catheterization. Familiarity with reverse curve catheters (Van Schie 5, Cook Medical Inc., Bloomington, IN) and loop snare techniques is essential for placement of bifurcated endografts.
2. The author routinely deploys the top cap prior to accessing the contralateral gate. After pulling the proximal trigger wire, push the top cap slowly, pausing at the point at which the suprarenal fixation wires are still constrained but the proximal segment of the graft is nearly fully expanded to confirm the device is in the desired location. A repeat angiogram at this point is often helpful.
3. After catheterization of the contralateral gate, place a RIM catheter (Cook Medical Inc., Bloomington, IN) into the main body and pull it down to hook the ipsilateral limb. Then perform digital subtraction angiography to confirm that the device has been successfully catheterized.

4. Advance the exchange wire and rim as a unit through the device to avoid hooking the fixation struts.
5. Advance a marker pigtail (Cook Medical Inc., Bloomington, IN) over the wire, with top marker at the end of the graft. It is important to profile the internal iliac artery to measure the iliac limb length. Working in a non-orthogonal view may lead to inadequate seal zone or accidental coverage of the internal iliac artery. The interval between the 1-cm markers will appear maximized when the marker pigtail is profiled.
6. Extend the iliac graft close to the internal iliac artery. This will reduce the risk of late IB endoleak or device migration.

7. The spiral Z limb (Cook Medical Inc., Bloomington, IN) conforms better to the iliac artery than traditional Z stent-based designs.[6] In very large common iliac arteries (>21 mm), the use of an aortic cuff can be considered, but more commonly embolization of the internal iliac artery with extension of the graft to the external iliac artery or the use of a branched graft is employed.

Example
See Figures 1.1–1.4.

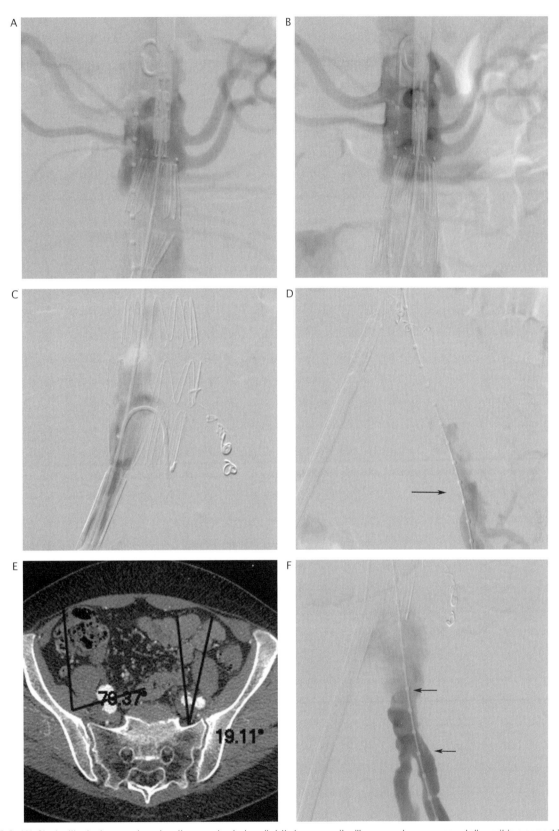

Figure 1.1 (A) Start with device overlapping the renal arteries slightly because it will appear to move caudally as it is opened. The angiographic view profiles the renal artery as evidenced by no double density of contrast over the renal origin, and the natural flair of the ostia is visible. (B) The beads have been positioned 2 mm caudal to the inferior renal artery. (C) A hand injection of a RIM catheter (Cook Medical Inc., Bloomington, IN) hooked over the flow divider confirms the gate has been successfully catheterized. (D) Projection does not profile the left internal iliac artery (arrow), which makes positioning the iliac limb difficult. (E) Computed tomography planning demonstrates the correct image detector angles to use during the procedure. (F) In the correct view, the distance between the markers appears maximized, and the length of the seal zone is revealed (arrows).

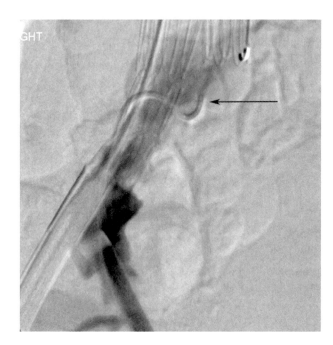

Figure 1.2 The angulation in the distal aorta makes use of an unformed reverse catheter (SOS Omni, AngioDynamics, Latham, NY) or Van Schie 5 (arrow) the best choice for catheterizing the contralateral gate.

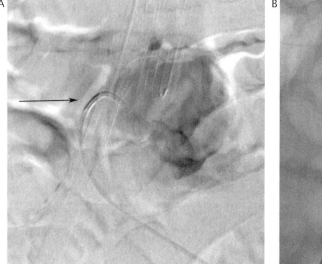

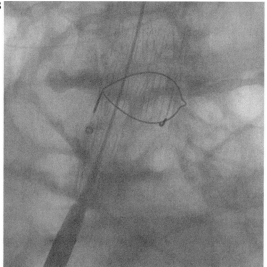

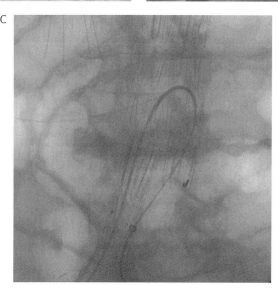

Figure 1.3 (A) Angled tip catheter (arrow) is perpendicular to gate orifice, making advancing the wire into the gate difficult. (B) An Amplatz goose neck snare (Medtronic, Inc., Minneapolis, MN) is opened with loop to the left, across the origin of the gate. (C) An up-and-over hydrophilic guidewire (Glidewire, Terumo Medical Corp., Somerset, NJ) has been snared.

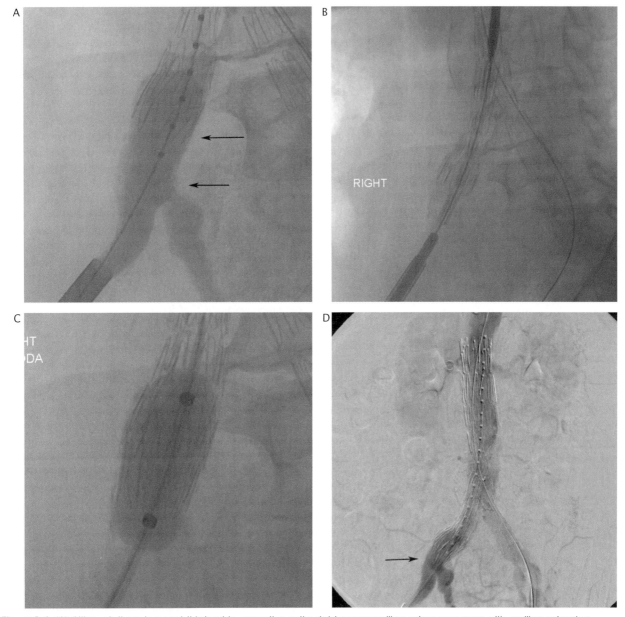

Figure 1.4 (A) Although there is a seal, it is best to cover the entire right common iliac artery aneurysm with an iliac extension (arrows). (B) Extension being inserted (Zenith). (C) A conformable balloon (Coda, Cook Medical Inc.) molds the limb to the iliac artery. Avoid dilating the native artery distal to the limb. (D) The limb now extends to the internal iliac artery (arrow), and there is no endoleak.

References and Suggested Readings

1. Sobocinski J, Briffa F, Holt PJ, et al. Evaluation of the Zenith low-profile abdominal aortic aneurysm stent graft. *J Vasc Surg.* 2015;62(4):841–847.
2. Stanley BM, Semmens JB, Mai Q, et al. Evaluation of patient selection guidelines for endoluminal AAA repair with the Zenith stent-graft: The Australasian experience. *J Endovasc Ther.* 2001;8(5):457–464.
3. Byrne J, Mehta M, Dominguez I, et al. Does Palmaz XL stent deployment for type 1 endoleak during elective or emergency endovascular aneurysm repair predict poor outcome? A multivariate analysis of 1470 patients. *Ann Vasc Surg.* 2013;27(4):401–411.
4. Jordan WD Jr, Mehta M, Varnagy D, et al. Results of the ANCHOR prospective, multicenter registry of EndoAnchors for type Ia endoleaks and endograft migration in patients with challenging anatomy. *J Vasc Surg.* 2014;60(4):885–892.e2.
5. Katada Y, Kondo S, Kondo T, Yamabe T. Endovascular treatment for type Ia major endoleak after endovascular aneurysm repair. *J Vasc Surg.* 2014;59(5):1430–1431.
6. Demanget N, Latil P, Orgeas L, et al. Finite element analysis of the mechanical performances of 8 marketed aortic stent-grafts. *J Endovasc Ther.* 2013;20(4):523–535.

CHAPTER 2

Deployment Finesse of the Gore Excluder Stent Graft

S. Lowell Kahn and Sergio Rojas

Brief Description

The Excluder, manufactured by W.L. Gore & Associates Inc. (Flagstaff, AZ), was approved for use in the United States by the US Food and Drug Administration (FDA) in 2002. The Excluder is a modular, bifurcated endoprosthesis utilized in the treatment of abdominal aortic aneurysms (AAAs). The Excluder endoprosthesis is constructed from an expanded polytetrafluoroethylene film and an incorporated "weldless" nickel–titanium stent skeleton for support. The device features no sutures, infrarenal fixation, and is made to be inserted through 12–18 Fr introducer sheaths. Since its approval by the FDA, the Excluder has undergone multiple changes, including profile reductions, the addition of an impermeable membrane (due to early graft material design associated with type IV endoleaks), and, most notably, a repositioning mechanism labeled the C3 Excluder. The C3 is the latest version and allows the operator to reposition the body of the device before deployment of the ipsilateral and contralateral limbs. The techniques described in this chapter are based on this latest C3 version.

The C3 is repositionable, facilitating optimal gate cannulation and aggressive infrarenal stent graft placement. This chapter presents three techniques that are designed to improve aneurysm exclusion with accurate deployment, decreased gate cannulation times, reduced contrast, and lower radiation exposure during complex endovascular aneurysm repair (EVAR) procedures. This is achieved in part by optimizing contralateral gate caliber and position, optimizing gate vectors, and exploiting the Excluder's unique endoprosthesis flexibility.

The temporary suprarenal deployment (TSD) technique is designed to facilitate rapid gate cannulation in challenging infrarenal aortic anatomy by temporarily placing the graft in a more favorable position during gate cannulation. The C-curve technique optimizes graft apposition in severely angled anatomy and prevents "bird-beaking" with consequent type Ia endoleaks. Finally, the renal buddy wire technique involves placement of a wire (and balloon) into the lowest renal artery from a brachial or femoral access. Placement of the balloon (± stent) protects the renal lumen during aggressive positioning of the graft when there is a suboptimal proximal seal zone. With all

these techniques, a careful review of the anatomy, ideally with reconstruction software (e.g., TeraRecon Inc., Foster City, CA), is imperative for planning and optimal success.

Applications of the Technique

Temporary Suprarenal Deployment Technique

1. Facilitate rapid gate cannulation when there is challenging infrarenal anatomy, including narrowing, entrapment (bilobed aneurysms), angulation, or thrombus impeding cannulation of the gate in a standard position.
2. Optimize graft placement at the desired location after gate cannulation: With the gate precannulated, there is a reduced likelihood of inadvertent graft migration/manipulation during gate cannulation.

C-Curve Technique

1. Optimizes graft apposition of the Excluder in severely angulated infrarenal aortas. Exploits the flexible engineering properties of the graft to minimize bird-beaking and consequent type Ia endoleaks.

Renal Buddy Wire Technique

1. Optimizes proximal seal when the neck is short, angled, or has a reverse taper. It allows aggressive positioning of the graft without compromising the renal arteries.
2. The technique is ideally used when use of a fenestrated graft or snorkeling is not feasible secondary to anatomic considerations of the neck and/or the renal and mesenteric vessels.

Challenges of the Procedure

Temporary Suprarenal Deployment Technique

1. Reconstraining of the C3 Excluder reduces the diameter of the device by approximately 30% of its

indicated diameter. In general, this allows great versatility in repositioning the graft in a cranial or caudal manner. However, in tight or tortuous anatomy, repositioning the graft after stage 1 deployment may prove difficult because the graft may encounter resistance upon its withdrawal to an infrarenal position.

2. Preprocedural planning to anticipate gate position is essential for this procedure. In addition to centerline reconstruction from a computed tomography angiography (CTA) study, digital subtraction angiography (DSA) with a marker flush catheter verifies the measurements.

C-Curve Technique

1. Determination of the access site for the main body of the graft is fundamental to the technique. However, there are times when the favored access for the technique is contrary to the optimal side from an arterial diameter/conduit standpoint.

Renal Buddy Wire Technique

1. Catheterization and delivery of a balloon (and possibly a stent) to a severely diseased renal artery can be challenging (and potentially risky).

2. The technique involves aggressive delivery of the device through difficult (e.g., narrow, calcified, irregular, and tortuous) anatomy that may make delivery of the graft problematic and prone to migration. The repositionable property of the C3 platform allows for more than one attempt to achieve the desired placement.

Potential Pitfalls/Complications

Temporary Suprarenal Deployment Technique

1. Embolization, or plaque shift of thrombus into branch vessels, can occur with this technique. The reconstrained device is still substantially larger than the undeployed device, and its manipulation within a diseased aorta may have untoward consequences. The renal arteries are the most at risk, but embolization to the mesenteric, hypogastric, and lower extremity arteries is possible. When greater than 30% of the total infrarenal aortic lumen is thrombus, the risk of distal embolization increases considerably.

2. One must be vigilant of contralateral "gate kinking" during distal repositioning as the graft is cannulated and then repositioned to its permanent, infrarenal placement. In a tortuous or plaque-/thrombus-laden aorta, the deployed gate may kink or "catch" on the wall during retraction.

3. Although repositioning is usually accomplished with little difficulty, repositioning problems are reported

in the literature.[1] This could compromise renal or mesenteric flow if the graft is positioned over the ostia of these vessels.

C-Curve Technique

1. There are times when employing the C-curve technique may not be justified by the required access. Specifically, the side required to perform the technique may be unacceptably small/diseased, and consequent vessel dissection, rupture, or thrombosis may occur with advancement of the required 16 or 18 Fr sheath in this scenario.

Renal Buddy Wire Technique

1. Catheterization and subsequent delivery of a balloon or stent to the diseased renal artery has inherent risks to the renal arteries, including dissection, rupture, thrombosis, and embolization.

2. Care must be taken when aggressively positioning the graft in a diseased neck to avoid plaque shift/ embolization. Specifically, this technique involves forward pressure on the graft to obtain positioning immediately adjacent to or slightly encroaching upon the lowest renal artery.

3. There are sharp hooks on the top of the C3 Excluder. As the graft is deployed with a balloon inflated in the renal artery, it is possible for the hooks to engage/ rupture or become trapped on the balloon. Careful monitoring with fluoroscopy is prudent to avoid this complication.

Steps of the Procedure

Temporary Suprarenal Deployment Technique

1. Preoperative planning consists of a CTA EVAR/ AAA protocol to assess length, diameter, and angle calculations of the infrarenal aorta and iliac arteries. It is also used to evaluate the access vessels and identify any plaque, thrombus, or morphologic characteristics of the aorta that may present a challenge. Patency of the superior mesenteric artery and hypogastrics is evaluated to ensure exclusion of the inferior mesenteric artery is safe. Measurements are obtained to determine the expected location at which the gate will open.

   a. The distance between the top of the Excluder and the distal edge of the gate varies as follows: 23–28 mm, 7 cm; 31 mm, 8 cm; and 35 mm, 9 cm. The Excluder endoprosthesis was engineered in this manner to create lateral stability in large-diameter necks.

2. Factors that pose a challenge for gate cannulation are assessed on the CTA:

   a. Large aortic sacs present a challenge for gate cannulation. The larger the sac size, the greater the potential space within which one must identify and successfully catheterize the gate.

    b. A broad (obtuse) angulation of the aortic bifurcation makes gate cannulation more difficult. Specifically, with a broad angle, the contralateral sheath will be naturally oriented toward the contralateral side of the aortic sac and possibly at an angle that is quite unfavorable for gate cannulation. In addition to the TSD technique, a buddy wire advanced through the contralateral sheath can help maintain the sheath along the centerline and thus closer to the gate. This technique is discussed later in chapter 5 because it is applicable to all modular grafts.

    c. Extensive plaque/thrombus, narrowing, or a bi-lobed infrarenal aneurysm can result in extrinsic compression of the graft and suboptimal gate deployment, making cannulation difficult.

3. Perioperative aortography is used to confirm the CTA findings, mark landing zones, and verify measurements.

4. If difficult gate cannulation is anticipated based on the factors discussed in list entry number 2, the graft is advanced above the renal arteries as necessary to select a location that allows the gate to open optimally for cannulation. The minimum distance required is employed to minimize unnecessary caudal repositioning after gate cannulation.

5. The graft is positioned and rotated as needed to bring the contralateral gate in close proximity to the sheath, and the catheter is advanced from the contralateral access. Stage 1 of the Excluder graft is deployed via contralateral rotation and retraction of the outer knob. Stage 1 deployment fully deploys the Excluder endoprosthesis from its proximal tip, including the fixation hooks, to the distal end of the contralateral gate while still maintaining a constrained trunk-ipsilateral limb. This maintains the graft's ability to reconstrain and move without deployment.

6. The gate is then cannulated with standard catheter and wire technique.

7. Once cannulation of the gate has been achieved, the hockey-stick catheter and wire (typically Glidewire; Terumo Medical Corp., Somerset, NJ) are exchanged for a stiff wire before reconstraining the endoprosthesis. Reconstraining is achieved via clockwise rotation of the outer knob.

8. With continuous fluoroscopy, the graft is repositioned to its intended infrarenal landing zone, and the procedure is completed per the manufacturer's instructions for use (IFU).

9. Once the graft is in place, the contralateral sheath and introducer can be advanced over the stiff wire into the gate to allow protected passage of the contralimb component.

10. If there is extrinsic compression on the graft from factors as listed previously, it is recommended to perform a "kissing balloon" technique with non-compliant balloons and/or reinforcement stenting to ensure adequate intragraft flow.

C-Curve Technique

1. Preprocedural planning utilizing coronal and sagittal CTA with three-dimensional reconstruction is performed to determine the C-curve versus the S-curve. Most aneurysms conform to this anatomy, and it is most commonly appreciated on a coronal reconstruction. The C versus the S configuration refers to the summation of angles from the lowest renal artery to the femoral access. To optimize graft apposition, placement of the main body is ideally performed on the side that offers the C-curve configuration. This minimizes the number of angles through which the graft must travel and allows for a more predictable and precise deployment that optimizes apposition.

2. Evaluate the axial and centerline reconstructions from the CTA to ensure adequate access vessel diameter for the C-curve side.

3. Perioperative DSA is performed to verify diameter, length, and angles obtained from the CTA.

4. The main body of the graft is then advanced from the chosen access and deployed per the manufacturer's IFU. Note that use of an exceedingly stiff wire (e.g., Lunderquist, Cook Medical Inc., Bloomington, IN) on one or both sides reduces the angulation of the aorta and facilitates delivery of the device to the intended location. However, the actual deployment of the graft may not be favored by this because the aorta will return to its natural configuration after withdrawal of the wire. Therefore, it is often prudent to retract the wire to the tip of the device (so that the floppy portion is within the graft) during the actual deployment. This allows the device to deploy more naturally and obtain superior apposition.

Renal Buddy Wire Technique

1. The lowest renal artery is catheterized from a brachial approach. Ideally, a long support sheath is advanced close to the ostium. Note that the contralateral femoral artery can be used as an access, but this is performed only in situations in which the brachial artery access is unavailable (e.g., subclavian occlusion) or deemed high risk for access (e.g., small).

2. A balloon sized 1:1 with the renal diameter is placed partially within the proximal renal artery and partially within the aorta.

3. The main body of the C3 Excluder is advanced to its intended position, minimally above the lowest renal artery.

4. The balloon is inflated within the renal artery.

5. The C3 is slowly deployed under magnified fluoroscopy, ensuring that the fabric falls immediately below the balloon located in the renal artery. Gentle forward

pressure on the shaft of the C3 delivery system can be applied to maintain precise approximation to the renal artery. The C3 is repositioned as necessary to attain the desired position. Care is taken to ensure that the proximal hooks do not engage the balloon material.

6. Additional angioplasty of the proximal graft is performed with a large compliant balloon (e.g., Coda, Cook Medical Inc., Bloomington, IN) as needed.

7. DSA imaging confirms proximal exclusion and the absence of a type Ia endoleak.

8. If encroachment of the renal artery is suspected, a balloon-expandable stent can be placed to ensure renal lumen preservation.

9. The remainder of the C3 Excluder graft is deployed per the manufacturer's IFU.

Example
See Figures 2.1–2.4.

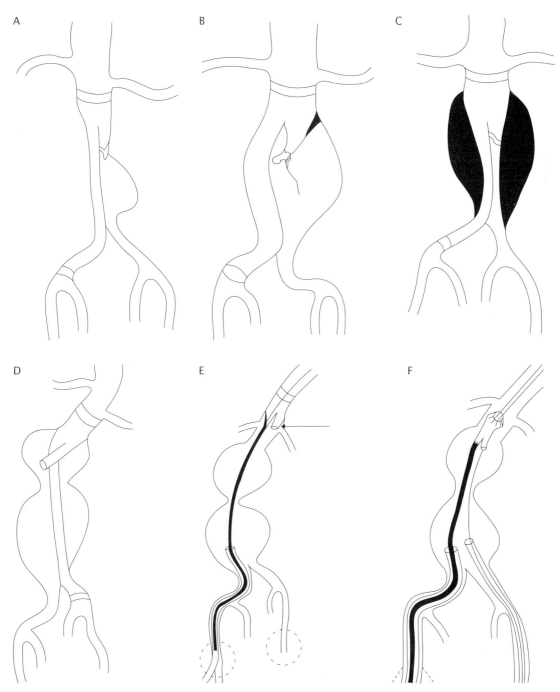

Figure 2.1 Temporary suprarenal deployment technique. A variety of factors can cause the contralateral gate to become trapped or inaccessible, rendering contralateral gate cannulation and expansion difficult. These include (A) intrinsic narrowing, (B) the presence of a calcified chronic dissection/flap, (C) mural thrombus, and (D) a bilobed aneurysm. (E) In these situations, the Gore C3 Excluder can be brought to a suprarenal position and stage 1 deployment performed to allow the gate to open (arrow) in a more favorable location. (F) After gate cannulation, the graft is reconstrained and brought to an infrarenal location for standard deployment.

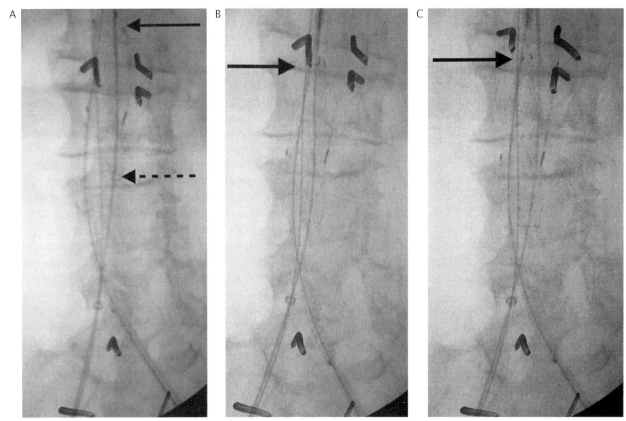

Figure 2.2 Temporary suprarenal deployment technique. Single anteroposterior projection of the abdomen with the bilateral renal arteries marked at the top of the images in black ink. (A) Note that stage 1 deployment of the graft has been performed with the top of the graft (solid arrow) lying superior to the level of the renal arteries. The contralateral gate (dashed arrow) is in an ideal position for catheterization. After catheterization, the top of the graft is reconstrained (B, arrow) and brought just below the renal arteries, before it is again deployed (C, arrow) just below the renal arteries.

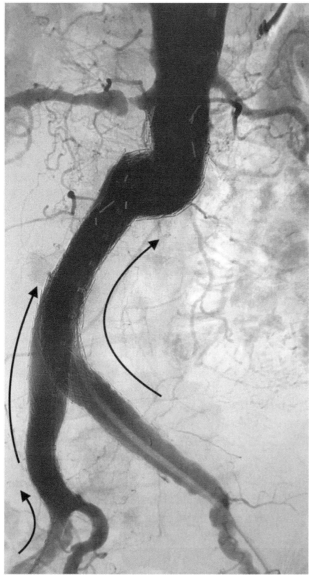

Figure 2.3 C-curve technique. Coronal DSA aortogram shows a tortuous aorta. The summation of the angles (arrows) of the tortuous aorta shows the right side to have more of an "S" configuration, whereas the left side has more of a "C" configuration. Based on the angles, a more accurate deployment was obtained by placing the main body from the left side access.

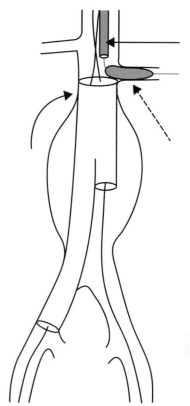

Figure 2.4 Renal buddy wire technique. Schematic demonstrates advancement of a sheath (solid arrow) from a left brachial approach with the tip lying just above the lower left renal artery. A balloon (dashed arrow) is placed into the left renal artery and extends a short distance into the aorta. The balloon protects the left renal artery while the C3 Excluder (curved arrow) is positioned immediately adjacent to the left renal artery to maximize seal in a short, reverse taper neck.

References and Suggested Readings

1. Katsargyris A, Oikonomou K, Bracale UM, Verhoeven EL. Unexpected complication with the new C3 excluder: Cause and treatment. *Cardiovasc Intervent Radiol.* 2013;36(2):536–539.
2. Maudet A, Daoudal A, Cardon A, et al. Endovascular treatment of infrarenal aneurysms: Comparison of the results of 2nd and 3rd generation stentgrafts. *Ann Vasc Surg.* 2016;May 9 [Epub ahead of print].
3. Katsargyris A, Mufty H, Wojs R, Utech G, Verhoeven EL. Single-centre experience with the Gore C3 Excluder stent-graft in 200 consecutive patients. *J Cardiovasc Surg.* 2016;57(4):485–490.
4. Verhoeven EL, Katsargyris A, Bachoo P, et al.; GREAT European C3 Module Investigators. Real-world performance of the new C3 Gore Excluder stent-graft: 1-year results from the European C3 module of the Global Registry for Endovascular Aortic Treatment (GREAT). *Eur J Vasc Endovasc Surg.* 2014;48(2):131–137.
5. Katsargyris A, Botos B, Oikonomou K, Pedraza de Leistl M, Ritter W, Verhoeven EL. The new C3 Gore Excluder stent-graft: Single-center experience with 100 patients. *Eur J Vasc Endovasc Surg.* 2014;47(4):342–348.
6. Krajcer Z. The Gore Excluder AAA endoprosthesis with C3 delivery system: Results in high-volume centers. *J Cardiovasc Surg.* 2014;55(1):41–49.

CHAPTER 3

The Turret Technique for Contralateral Gate Access

S. Lowell Kahn

Brief Description

The use of modular two- and three-piece aortic stent grafts requires catheterization of the contralateral gate on the main body of the stent graft. After catheterization of the contralateral gate, the contralateral limb(s) is deployed.

Typically, this step is readily accomplished in a short amount of time. With planning based on pre- and intraprocedural imaging, the gate can be positioned near the contralateral sheath to facilitate rapid catheterization. In fact, the newer-generation Gore Excluder AAA endoprosthesis with the C3 delivery system (W. L. Gore & Associates, Flagstaff, AZ) allows repositioning, a property that can be used to change the location of the contralateral gate for catheterization. If desired, the C3 delivery system allows further repositioning after gate cannulation.

Despite these techniques and technical advancements, occasionally, the catheterization of the gate can be challenging. A Glidewire (Terumo Medical Corp., Somerset, NJ) together with a variety of catheters are employed, most commonly either a hockey stick (e.g., Kumpe (Cook Medical Inc., Bloomington, IN) and Berenstein (AngioDynamics Inc., Latham, NY) or reverse curve (e.g., Sos 1/2, Cook Medical Inc., Bloomington, IN) configuration. Other catheters, such as a Van Schie (Cook Medical Inc., Bloomington, IN), may be useful when the gate is located away from the end of the contralateral sheath.

This chapter describes the use of the "Turret technique" for rapid gate catheterization. This technique employs a modified use of a reverse curve catheter together with the end of the sheath to allow 360-degree wire steering toward the gate.

Applications of the Technique

1. Primarily used for gate catheterization in the author's experience, but in theory, the technique could be employed to direct a wire directionally for any difficult vessel catheterizations in which the sheath can be delivered close to the intended target.

Challenges of the Procedure

1. None specifically encountered. Requires practice on the amount of catheter retraction into the sheath to obtain the desired angle of cranial wire deflection. The more the catheter is retracted into the sheath, the smaller the radius of the 360-degree arc of wire deflection. Conversely, less retraction of the catheter into the sheath will increase the radius.

Potential Pitfalls/Complications

1. None specifically encountered beyond standard wire and catheter risks.

Steps of the Procedure

1. Over a wire, advance the sheath as close as possible to the contralateral gate, ideally within 1 or 2 cm.
2. Advance a reverse curve catheter over a wire into the sac of the aortic aneurysm and allow the catheter to form. At our institution, we typically use a Sos 1/2, Sidewinder, or Simmons 1 (Cook Medical Inc., Bloomington, IN).
3. Pull the primary (proximal) curve of the reverse curve catheter into the end of the sheath to obtain the desired deflection of the tip of the catheter. This forms the Turret, and it can be rotated in any direction and at any deflection to obtain the desired wire location. Pulling the catheter further into the sheath deflects the catheter tip in a more cranial direction.
4. Once the catheter is pointing in the desired direction, advance the straight or angled Glidewire through the gate and exchange the Glidewire for a stiffer wire after confirming proper catheterization within the gate.
5. Complete deployment of the contralateral limb of the aortic stent graft per the manufacturer's instructions for use.

Example

See Figure 3.1.

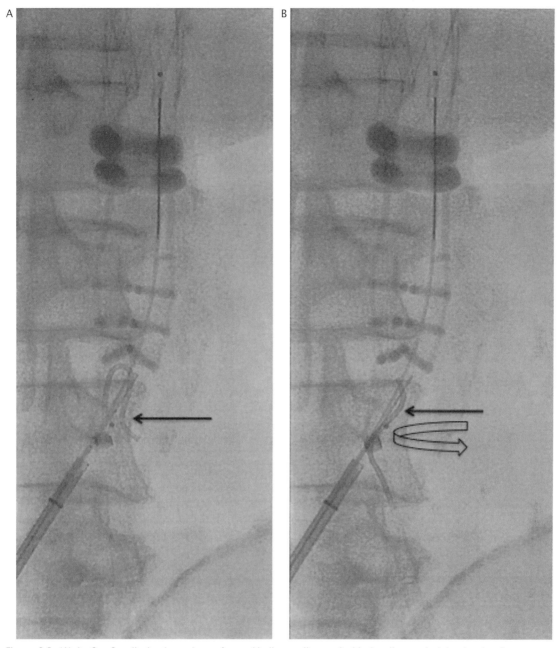

Figure 3.1 (A) An Sos 2 catheter (arrow) was formed in the aortic sac, just below the contralateral gate of a TriVascular Ovation (Endologix, Inc., Irvine, CA) graft. The gate on this graft is small and failed to expand completely, rendering catheterization by standard technique somewhat difficult. (B) The Sos 2 catheter (arrow) was partially retracted into the sheath. This allowed the tip of the catheter to be steered in a 360-degree arc (curved arrow) and ultimately allowed catheterization of the gate in a very short time period.

References and Suggested Readings

1. Verhoeven EL, Katsargyris A, Bachoo P, et al.; GREAT European C3 Module Investigators. Real-world performance of the new C3 Gore Excluder stent-graft: 1-year results from the European C3 module of the Global Registry for Endovascular Aortic Treatment (GREAT). *Eur J Vasc Endovasc Surg.* 2014;48(2):131–137.
2. Krajcer Z. The Gore Excluder AAA endoprosthesis with C3 delivery system: Results in high-volume centers. *J Cardiovasc Surg (Torino).* 2014;55(1):41–49.
3. Shie R, Hao S, Chu S, Shie F. A novel method to cannulate the contralateral limb of aortic stent graft during endovascular aneurysm repair. *Exp Clin Cardiol.* 2014;20(9):1–5.
4. Trellopoulos G, Georgiadis GS, Nikolopoulos ES, Lazarides MK. Current tips for ensuring successful transfemoral short limb cannulation in modular aortic endografts: A new method for incorporation in practice. *Perspect Vasc Surg Endovasc Ther.* 2009;21(4):232–236.

CHAPTER 4

Up-and-Over Snare Technique for the Difficult Contralateral Gate Access

S. Lowell Kahn

Brief Description

As described elsewhere in this text, the use of two- and three-piece modular aortic stent grafts requires proper catheterization of the contralateral gate. This step is typically accomplished with little difficulty, but it can be more challenging in large, angulated aneurysms in which the position of the contralateral sheath is distant from the gate of the main body of the device.

The technique described here is a bailout technique when the conventional use of a catheter and wire fails or is unlikely to succeed within a timely interval. As described in detail here, an Amplatz Gooseneck snare (ev3 Endovascular Inc., Plymouth, MN) or EN Snare (Merit Medical Systems, Inc., South Jordan, UT) may be employed to grasp a Glidewire (Terumo Medical Corp., Somerset, NJ) that is threaded through a reverse curve catheter (e.g., Sos 1/2) over the bifurcation and brought below the contralateral gate. In so doing, cannulation of the contralateral gate is readily achieved.

Applications of the Technique

1. Bailout technique utilized for obtaining catheterization of the contralateral gate when conventional methods fail.

Challenges of the Procedure

1. None specifically encountered. Requires minimal practice to understand the amount of wire that can be advanced down the contralateral gate without inadvertently straightening the reverse curve catheter and losing access to the contralateral gate.
2. Basic familiarity with the use of a snare is required.

Potential Pitfalls/Complications

1. In theory, application of too much traction on both ends of the wire could displace the main body of the graft. Therefore, a "push–pull" technique is advised (described next) to avoid this occurrence.

Steps of the Procedure

1. Advance a reverse curve catheter through the ipsilateral gate of the stent graft and form it above the bifurcation. A 5 Fr Sos 2 catheter (Angiodynamics Inc., Latham, NY) is the preferred catheter at the author's institution. The author has found that the 5 Fr catheters retain their shape and allow a deeper threading of the wire down the contralateral gate compared to their 4 Fr counterparts. The Sos 2 is only one such catheter; most reverse curve catheters are acceptable for this purpose.
2. Carefully withdraw the catheter, and seat it on the bifurcation so that the tip is directed into the contralateral gate from above.
3. Carefully spin and advance a straight or angled hydrophilic wire (e.g., angled or straight Glidewire, Terumo Medical). Ideally, the wire should be advanced 2 cm or more beyond the distal end of the contralateral gate.
4. Advance a snare from the contralateral access, and use the snare to grasp the wire that has been passed. A large (~20 mm) Amplatz Gooseneck snare (ev3 Endovascular Inc., Plymouth, MN) is usually sufficient, but some operators prefer a multiloop snare such as the EN Snare (Merit Medical Systems Inc., South Jordan, UT).
5. Once the wire has been grasped, carefully advance (push) the snare and snare catheter through the gate while the co-operator retracts (pulls) the reverse curve catheter and wire from the ipsilateral access.
6. Once the snare catheter is through the contralateral gate and at the level of the graft bifurcation, release the wire from the ipsilateral access. Remove the snare and advance a stiff support wire through the snare catheter. Remove the snare catheter.
7. Complete deployment of the contralateral limb of the aortic stent graft per the manufacturer's instructions for use.

Example

See Figure 4.1.

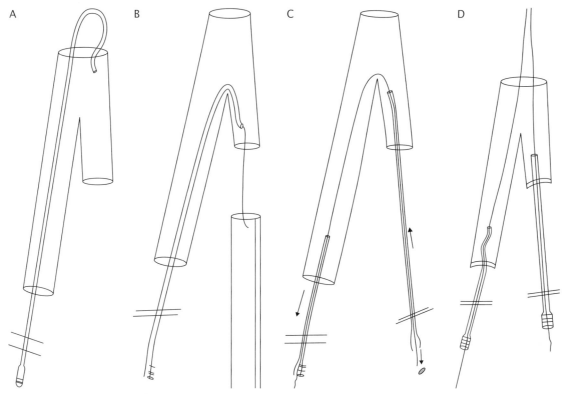

Figure 4.1 (A) A reverse curve catheter is formed above the contralateral gate. (B) The reverse curve catheter is retracted (seated) onto the bifurcation of the main body of the graft. A snare is then advanced from the contralateral side and used to grasp a threaded Glidewire. (C) The operator on the ipsilateral side retracts on the reverse curve catheter and wire. Simultaneously, the operator on the contralateral side maintains traction on the snare while advancing the snare catheter into the contralateral gate. (D) Once the snare catheter enters the contralateral gate, the wire from the ipsilateral side is released, and the snare is removed. The Glidewire is advanced above the main body and exchanged for a stiff support wire. A stiff support wire is advanced through the snare catheter. With bilateral wire access now obtained through both limbs of the graft, the procedure is completed per the manufacturer's instructions for use.

References and Suggested Readings

1. Phade SV, Garcia-Toca M, Kibbe M. Techniques in endovascular repair. *Int J Vasc Med.* 2011;2011:964250.
2. Kruse M, Khoynezhad A. Endovascular repair of abdominal aortic aneurysm (EVAR). http://www.ctsnet.org. Published January 18, 2011.
3. Kaneko K, Kanaoka Y, Ohki T. Endovascular management of abdominal aortic aneurysms. In: Casserly IP, Sachar R, Jay Yadav JS, eds. *Practical Peripheral Vascular Intervention.* 2nd ed. Philadelphia: Lippincott Williams & Wilkins; 2011: 289–290.

CHAPTER 5

Use of a Buddy Wire to Facilitate Contralateral Gate Catheterization During Endovascular Aortic Aneurysm Repair

S. Lowell Kahn

Brief Description

Catheterization of the contralateral gate is an important step during endovascular aortic aneurysm repair procedures. Except for grafts such as Nellix (Endologix Inc., Irvine, CA), which utilizes parallel stents with polymer endobags, and those that employ a unibody concept, such as the AFX (Endologix Inc., Irvine, CA), all modular grafts require this step. In experienced hands, catheterization of the gate is straightforward and readily accomplished using angled catheters (e.g., Kumpe (Cook Medical Inc., Bloomington, IN) and Berenstein [AngioDynamics Inc., Latham, NY]) in conjunction with a hydrophilic wire.

Unfortunately, there are circumstances in which catheterization of the gate can be difficult, typically because of the orientation and location of the gate relative to the catheter position. This typically occurs in larger aneurysms in which there is a significantly greater potential space for the gate or when the angulation (bias) of the contralateral iliac artery is such that any sheath and catheter arising from this vessel is oriented so that the distance between the gate and the catheter is substantial. In general, operators attempt to deploy the graft so that the gate is oriented toward the contralateral sheath/catheter, but a graft can occasionally deploy in a suboptimal orientation. Although newer designs such as the Excluder with the C3 delivery system (W.L. Gore & Associates Inc., Flagstaff, AZ) allow repositioning, most grafts allow a single deployment.

A difficult catheterization is often facilitated by using different catheters, such as the Cobra, Van Schie (Cook Medical Inc., Bloomington, IN), or Sos (AngioDynamics Inc., Latham, NY) designs. Alternatively, a wire can be advanced up and over through the contralateral gate from the ipsilateral side using a reverse curve catheter and wire. This wire can then be easily snared from the contralateral side, allowing catheterization of the gate.

This chapter describes a simple alternative buddy wire technique that facilitates rapid contralateral gate catheterization.

Applications of the Technique

1. Larger saccular aneurysms in which the gate deploys in the widest portion of the aneurysm. This larger potential space allows greater separation between the gate and the sheath/catheter from the contralateral side.
2. Iliac tortuosity in which the axis of the contralateral common iliac artery is oriented far from the position of the contralateral gate.
3. Poor gate deployment or position relative to the contralateral access.
4. Devices with small contralateral gates, such as the Ovation Prime (TriVascular, Endologix Inc., Irvine, CA), may benefit from this technique given the more difficult gate cannulation inherent with these devices.

Potential Pitfalls/Complications

1. Occasionally, the buddy wire can compress the gate. In such cases, abandonment of the technique and use of conventional methods is advised.
2. After gate cannulation, care must be taken in removing the buddy wire to ensure that it does not disrupt the position of the main body of the graft. This should be done slowly under fluoroscopy.

Steps of the Procedure

1. From both femoral access sites, stiff delivery wires (e.g., Lunderquist [Cook Medical Inc., Bloomington, IN] and Meier [Boston Scientific Inc., Marlborough, MA]) are advanced to the thoracic aorta. On the contralateral side, this will serve as the actual buddy wire.
2. On the contralateral side, an appropriately sized sheath for the contralateral limb is advanced to the aneurysm sac, just below the expected deployment site of the contralateral gate.
3. Adjacent to the buddy wire, a flush catheter (e.g., pigtail) is advanced through the contralateral sheath and

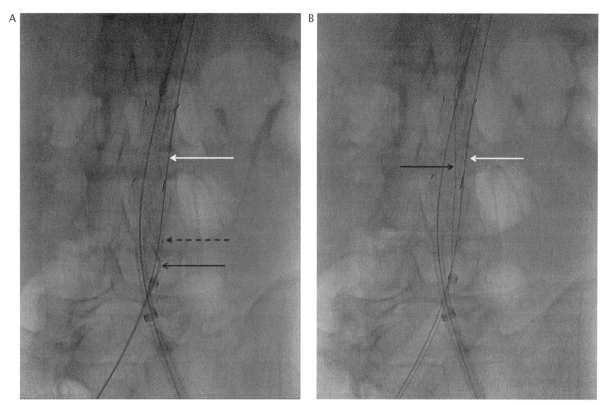

Figure 5.1 (A) Catheterizing the contralateral gate using the buddy wire technique on a Gore C3 Excluder (W.L. Gore & Associates, Inc.) graft. Immediately prior to catheterizing the contralateral gate (dashed arrow), a Kumpe catheter (black arrow) has been positioned side by side a buddy wire (white arrow) that ascends into the thoracic aorta (not shown). Note that the stiff buddy wire (in this case, a Lunderquist, Cook Medical Inc.) ensures that the 12-Fr sheath is closely approximated to the contralateral gate. (B) Successful gate catheterization. Immediately after catheterizing the gate successfully, the hydrophilic Glidewire (Terumo Medical Corp.) is seen within the gate (black arrow). The buddy wire (white arrow) remains unchanged in its position and will be removed after gate catheterization is confirmed.

placed just above the expected location of the renal arteries.

4. The main body of the device is advanced to the abdominal aorta, ideally with the contralateral gate oriented toward the contralateral sheath.
5. Additional imaging of the renal arteries is obtained as needed.
6. Final adjustment and deployment of the main body of the endograft are performed per the manufacturer's instructions for use (IFU).
7. The flush catheter in the contralateral sheath is exchanged for an angled catheter and hydrophilic wire. The presence of the buddy wire centers the contralateral sheath and ensures that the sheath and catheter remain in close approximation to the contralateral gate.

8. The gate is catheterized with a standard technique using an angled catheter and hydrophilic wire.
9. After confirming that the contralateral catheterization is within the lumen of the graft, the buddy wire is carefully removed under fluoroscopy, and deployment of the contralateral limb is conducted per the manufacturer's IFU.

Example
See Figure 5.1.

Reference and Suggested Reading
1. Murphy EH, Arko FR. Technical tips for abdominal endografting. *Semin Vasc Surg.* 2008;21(2):25–30.

CHAPTER 6

Tips for Accurate Palmaz Stent Deployment

S. Lowell Kahn

Brief Description

The Palmaz XL stent (Cordis Corp., Milpitas, CA) is a stainless-steel, closed-cell stent designed to be manually mounted on a balloon by the operator. The construction of this stent confers the ability to expand it to a large diameter, a property that makes it an essential tool for aortic interventions. The Palmaz XL is rated for diameters between 14 and 25 mm, but the stent is not uncommonly pushed beyond its intended diameter. Due to the nature of its design, the stent foreshortens as its diameter is increased, and deploying it beyond 25 mm could compromise the integrity of the stent. The use of the Palmaz stent is well described for both thoracic and abdominal aortic interventions. Most commonly, it is used for type IA and IB endoleaks, but it is commonly used for narrowing of the aortic lumen by either atheromatous plaque or coarctation.

Manual crimping of a stent onto a delivery balloon requires a degree of practice, but even in seasoned hands, it carries the risk of dislodgement during deployment. Such a complication could result in a retained intravascular undeployed stent or a maldeployed stent at a location other than that intended.

This chapter describes three simple techniques designed to ensure accurate deployment of the Palmaz XL stent for aortic interventions. The Dual Balloon Technique involves using a second balloon from the contralateral femoral arterial access to prevent distal migration of the Palmaz stent during deployment. The Elongated Balloon Technique involves using a balloon longer than the stent to take advantage of the natural hourglass effect of the balloon during inflation. The Asymmetric Mounting Technique involves asymmetric mounting of the stent on a balloon coupled with partial deployment within a delivery sheath to ensure that the proximal end of the stent deploys first, thereby preventing distal migration of the stent.

Applications of the Technique

All Techniques

1. All three techniques can be used with most Palmaz stent deployments. As stated previously, these techniques are useful for both thoracic and abdominal aortic interventions.

Challenges of the Procedure

All Techniques

1. Mounting of the stent with effective crimping is imperative. Loose crimping predisposes the stent to dislodgement either intravascularly or within the sheath. Applying circumferential pressure segmentally to the stent is ideal, and some operators also use a slight twisting motion to optimally affix the stent to the balloon. Although unproven, it may be beneficial to coat the stent with undiluted contrast prior to mounting it on the balloon because of the natural viscid/adherent nature of the contrast.

2. At least one side requires adequate femoral and iliac arterial diameter and patency to facilitate the placement of the large sheath (typically 16 Fr or greater).

Dual Balloon Technique

3. The use of a second balloon requires that the contralateral femoral and iliac arteries be of sufficient diameter to accommodate placement of a 12 Fr sheath.

Dual Balloon and Elongated Balloon Techniques

4. The use of a long balloon and/or a second balloon mandates that there is adequate space within the aorta (and possibly stent graft) to allow placement of these devices.

Potential Pitfalls/Complications

All Techniques

1. The use of large-diameter balloons/stents in a large vessel carries an increased risk of injury with

hemorrhage. This is further compounded by the fact that the Palmaz stent is frequently mounted on a compliant balloon that lacks a fixed diameter and hourglasses on either end of the stent. Therefore, it is imperative that the operator be cognizant of these properties and monitor the patient carefully for any indication of bleeding.

2. As stated previously, a 16 Fr (~6 mm outside diameter) or greater size sheath is required for these interventions, and the patient's access vessels must be able to accommodate this size to prevent iliac or femoral injury.

3. Despite these techniques, a maldeployed or undeployed stent may be encountered. "Bailout" methods are described in the literature, and the operator should be familiar with these.[1-4] It is advised to maintain wire access through a mal- or undeployed stent because maintaining access confers more options to remedy the situation.

Dual Balloon and Elongated Balloon Techniques

4. The use of two balloons or an elongated balloon requires considerable distance in the longitudinal axis to perform these techniques properly. It is conceivable that aortic tortuosity or the intended stent location relative to the aortic bifurcation or a graft bifurcation could preclude utilization of one or both techniques.

Asymmetric Mounting Technique

5. Partial deployment of a stent within a sheath carries a risk of the undeployed portion of the stent becoming stuck within the sheath. In practice, however, this is unlikely to occur.

Steps of the Procedure

Dual Balloon Technique

1. The Palmaz XL stent is carefully mounted on the balloon and subsequently inserted into the sheath. Fluoroscopy is performed to confirm that the stent did not move relative to the balloon during insertion into the sheath. In the author's experience, the use of a long sheath (e.g., 45 cm for abdominal aortic interventions) is beneficial to minimize the risk of dislodgment associated with advancing the stent in an unsheathed configuration. Typically, a 16 Fr or larger sheath is required, depending on the balloon diameter selected.

2. The sheath is advanced under fluoroscopic guidance to a location at or beyond the intended stent location.

3. The stent is advanced to its intended location, and the sheath is withdrawn to expose the Palmaz.

4. From the contralateral femoral access, a 12 Fr sheath is advanced under fluoroscopic guidance to a point located approximately 5 cm below the balloon on which the Palmaz is mounted.

5. Over a wire, a compliant aortic occlusion balloon (e.g., Reliant [Medtronic Inc., Minneapolis, MN] or Coda [Cook Medical Inc., Bloomington, IN]) is advanced through the contralateral sheath and positioned immediately below the Palmaz.

6. The contralateral balloon is inflated and supported by its sheath to prevent distal migration. With the balloon inflated, the Palmaz is deployed with inflation of the balloon on which it is mounted. Both balloons are quickly deflated after deployment of the Palmaz at the intended location.

Elongated Balloon Technique

1. The Palmaz XL stent is loaded on a balloon considerably longer than the stent. For example, the author routinely mounts the Palmaz XL 4010 (undeployed length of 39.8 mm) on a 60-mm length Z-MED II (B Braun Interventional Systems Inc., Bethlehem, PA) balloon (available diameters at this length include 15, 20, 22, 23, 25, and 30 mm).

2. The mounted stent is inserted into a long (e.g., 45 cm) 16 Fr or greater (depending on balloon diameter chosen) sheath that is advanced at or above the intended stent location. Fluoroscopy is performed to confirm that the stent did not move relative to the balloon during insertion into the sheath.

3. The sheath is withdrawn to unsheathe the stent at its intended location.

4. The stent is deployed carefully with inflation of the balloon. As it deploys, the balloon will naturally "hourglass" proximal and distal to the stent. This ensures that the stent cannot herniate proximally or distally during deployment.

5. During deployment, the stent is further supported by the sheath (positioned with its tip immediately below the distal end of the balloon) as well as gentle forward pressure on the balloon catheter to ensure there is no distal migration of the stent.

Asymmetric Mounting Technique

This technique is provided courtesy of Kim et al.[2]

1. The Palmaz XL stent is carefully loaded onto the balloon, where it is intentionally not centered on the balloon. Instead, it is mounted closer to the distal end of the balloon, leaving a considerable amount of the balloon bare on the proximal end.

2. A long (e.g., 45 cm) 16 Fr or greater (depending on balloon diameter chosen) sheath is advanced to a location beyond the intended location of the stent.

3. The mounted stent is inserted into the sheath and advanced to the intended site of deployment. Fluoroscopy is performed to confirm that the stent did not move relative to the balloon during insertion into the sheath.

4. The sheath is withdrawn approximately halfway to expose the proximal end of the balloon and stent.

5. The balloon is then inflated. The asymmetric loading of the stent allows the proximal end of the balloon to rapidly appose the aortic wall. This flaring results in fixation of the proximal end of the stent. With the support of the sheath and the asymmetric loading of the stent on the balloon, the stent is unable to migrate. The radial force of the inflated balloon within the sheath against the stent further prevents migration.

6. After the proximal portion of the stent is well apposed to the aortic wall, the distal end of the balloon and stent are unsheathed, and deployment of the stent is completed with inflation of the balloon.

Example
See Figures 6.1–6.3.

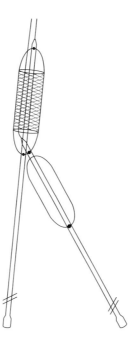

Figure 6.1 Dual Balloon Technique: Deployment of the stent occurs while there is simultaneous placement and inflation of an aortic occlusion balloon from the contralateral access. The second balloon ensures that there is no substantial distal migration of the Palmaz stent.

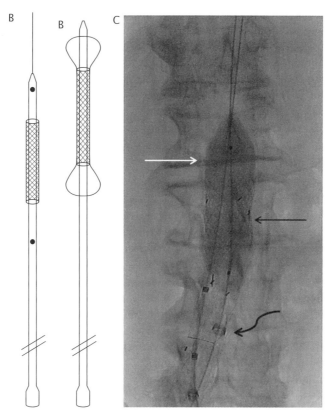

Figure 6.2 Elongated Balloon Technique: (A) The Palmaz stent is mounted on a balloon considerably longer than the undeployed length of the Palmaz stent. (B) As the stent deploys, the balloon assumes an hourglass configuration, expanding on either side of the stent. This prevents migration of the stent during deployment. (C) The stent then deploys as desired and remains centered on the balloon. (D) Example: A 25-mm Z-MED II balloon (white arrow) is mounted in a Palmaz XL 4010 stent (black arrow). The balloon measures 6 cm in length and is considerably longer than the Palmaz stent. Prior to the acquisition of this image, the balloon flared in an hourglass configuration, thereby preventing migration of the stent. Note the added support of the long sheath positioned immediately distal to the balloon (curved black arrow).

A   B   C

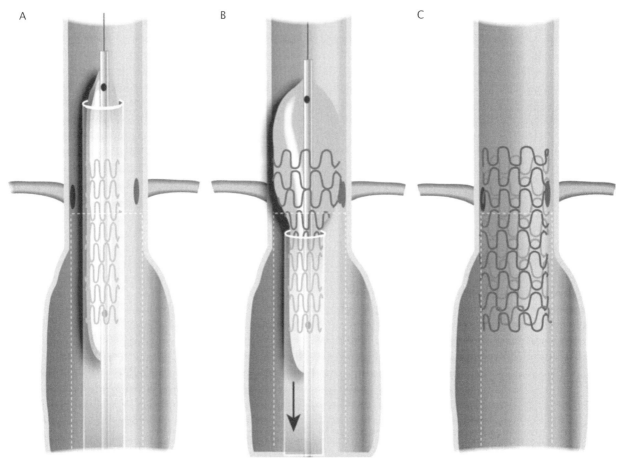

Figure 6.3 Asymmetric Mounting Technique: (A) A Palmaz stent has been loaded onto a balloon in an asymmetric manner whereby the stent is "off center" with the stent positioned toward the more distal end of the balloon. (B) The stent is partially unsheathed to its mid portion, and the balloon is inflated. The position of the sheath and the radial force of the balloon on the stent that is constrained by the sheath prevent movement of the stent while the proximal end of the balloon flares, causing the proximal end of the stent to obtain apposition to the aortic wall. (C) The stent is then fully unsheathed, and deployment is completed.

Source: From Kim JK, et al. A technique for increased accuracy in the placement of the "giant" Palmaz stent for treatment of type IA endoleak after endovascular abdominal aneurysm repair. *J Vasc Surg.* 2008;48(3):755–757. Courtesy Elsevier.

References and Suggested Readings

1. Hartnell GG, Jordan SJ. Percutaneous removal of a misplaced Palmaz stent with a coaxial snare technique. *J Vasc Intervent Radiol.* 1995;6:799–801.
2. Kim JK, Noll RE Jr, Tonnessen BH, Sternbergh WC III. A technique for increased accuracy in the placement of the "giant" Palmaz stent for treatment of type IA endoleak after endovascular abdominal aneurysm repair. *J Vasc Surg.* 2008; 48(3):755–757.
3. Slonim SM, Dake MD, Razavi MK, Kee ST, Samuels SL, Rhee JS. Management of misplaced or migrated endovascular stents. *J Vasc Intervent Radiol.* 1999;10:851–889.
4. Gabelmann A, Kramer SC, Tomczak R, Gorich J. Percutaneous techniques for managing maldeployed or migrated stents. *J Endovasc Ther.* 2001;8:291–302.

CHAPTER 7

Managing Unilateral or Bilateral Common Iliac Artery Aneurysms with Preservation of the Hypogastric Artery

S. Lowell Kahn

Brief Description

Isolated common iliac artery aneurysms are relatively infrequent, occurring in 0.03% of the population, and are responsible for less than 2% of clinically significant aneurysm disease.[1] Interestingly, however, the incidence of iliac artery aneurysms is much higher in patients with abdominal aortic aneurysms (AAAs), with an incidence close to 40% in this population.[1] The presence of bilateral iliac aneurysms in this population is common.

The Ad Hoc Committee on Reporting Standards of the Society for Vascular Surgery and International Society for Cardiovascular Surgery defines iliac aneurysms by a diameter greater than or equal to 15 mm, but rupture of aneurysms less than 3–3.5 cm is quite rare.[1,2] The rates of growth are highly variable as reported in the literature, but most investigators agree that the rate of growth increases with aneurysm size. Consensus recommendations for intervention are limited given the infrequency of this disease, but intervention is typically recommended when the size of the aneurysm exceeds 3–3.5 cm.[1,2]

The invasive nature of open surgical repair with an associated mortality rate of ≤11%[3–5] is alarming and makes endovascular options attractive. Unfortunately, endovascular options often involve sacrifice of blood flow to the hypogastric arteries on one or both sides. Given that aneurysmal disease occurs most commonly in patients with atherosclerosis, the flow in the hypogastric arteries is frequently compromised at baseline. Conventional endovascular management of iliac aneurysms frequently involves embolization of the hypogastric artery and placement of a covered stent graft in the common and external iliac arteries (either as an extension of a conventional AAA graft or as an iliac limb). When both common iliac arteries are involved with or without the presence of an AAA, an extended aorto-uni-iliac graft with ipsilateral hypogastric embolization, contralateral common iliac occlusion, placement of a femoral–femoral bypass, and contralateral reverse stent grafting to the hypogastric artery is described.[6] Unfortunately, ischemic complications after hypogastric artery embolization are quite common, including buttock claudication, colonic ischemia, gluteal necrosis, impotence, and rare spinal ischemia. Similarly, the reported 65–70% 5-year patency of a femoral–femoral bypass may be of concern, particularly for younger patients.[7]

The simplest way to repair a common iliac artery aneurysm endovascularly involves the placement of a covered stent graft in the common iliac artery to exclude it. In reality, however, this rarely works because most of these aneurysms either abut or extend into the abdominal aorta or hypogastric artery. Therefore, to adequately exclude the aneurysm, extension proximally and distally into the aorta and external iliac artery, respectively, is typically required.

This chapter describes two techniques for the management of common iliac artery aneurysms that are either isolated or found in conjunction with abdominal aortic aneurysmal disease. Both techniques involve placement of a hypogastric "snorkel" that preserves blood flow to the hypogastric artery.

The Endologix AFX Snorkel Technique involves inserting an Endologix AFX stent graft (Endologix Inc., Irvine, CA) into the abdominal aorta with or without proximal cuff extension depending on the presence or absence of coexistent abdominal aortic aneurysmal disease. After the Endologix AFX re-lines the aortic bifurcation, one or both iliac limbs (depending on whether there is unilateral or bilateral iliac aneurysmal disease) are extended with a bell-bottom extension(s). Within the bell-bottom extension, side-by-side grafts are placed with good overlap, with one graft extending into the external iliac artery and the second snorkel extending into the hypogastric artery. Unlike the other modular stent grafts, the AFX has the unique property of allowing up-and-over contralateral iliac catheterization because the graft sits on and therefore mimics the natural aortic bifurcation. This property allows the entire repair to be performed with bilateral femoral access alone.

The Dual Gore Excluder Technique has two similar, but different, methods (herein referenced as Methods A and B). Method A was first described by Arslan et al. in

2010.[8] A Gore Excluder bifurcated stent graft (W.L. Gore & Associates Inc., Flagstaff, AZ) is deployed within the aneurysmal common iliac artery such that the ipsilateral limb extends into the external iliac artery and the contralateral gate is positioned immediately above the hypogastric artery. This is followed by up-and-over catheterization of the deployed graft with placement of a 12 Fr sheath. The hypogastric artery is catheterized through the up-and-over 12 Fr sheath, and an appropriately sized limb is deployed through the contralateral gate into the hypogastric artery. This is followed by placement of a Cook Zenith bifurcated stent graft (Cook Medical Inc., Bloomington, IN) immediately below the renal arteries. On the aneurysmal iliac side, the Cook Zenith graft is bridged to the Gore Excluder stent graft with a bell-bottom limb. The remainder of the deployment of the Cook limb on the uninvolved side is performed with conventional technique.

There are times when placement of a bifurcated graft as an initial deployment in the iliac artery is not possible. For example, if the iliac artery is highly aneurysmal, the graft might be too small to obtain stable positioning. Therefore, Method B involves placement of a Gore Excluder stent graft in a conventional manner. The contralateral limb is extended with a bell-bottom limb. Within the bell-bottom limb, a second bifurcated Gore Excluder stent graft is placed and positioned such that the ipsilateral limb extends well into the external iliac artery on the affected (aneurysmal) side, and the contralateral gate of the second bifurcated device is positioned immediately above the hypogastric artery on the affected side. From the patient's brachial or axillary artery (typically left because of decreased stroke risk), a 12 Fr sheath is placed, through which a Viabahn stent (W.L. Gore & Associates Inc., Flagstaff, AR) is advanced and used as a snorkel extending from the contralateral gate of the second Excluder into the hypogastric artery to provide the seal. On the unaffected side, the ipsilateral limb of the first Excluder is deployed (and extended if necessary) per the manufacturer's instructions for use (IFU) with standard technique.

The use of two bifurcated grafts may allow a more physiologic (i.e., no snorkel) repair compared to the first technique, but many patients are not candidates for this repair because of inadequate longitudinal (i.e., renal to hypogastric artery) distance to allow placement of two bifurcated devices.

Both techniques merit consideration of cost and time, and they should be considered in the context of overall risk and other available options. With newer branched iliac grafts arriving on the market (Cook Medical Inc., Bloomington, IN and W.L. Gore & Associates Inc., Flagstaff, AZ), the need for these alternative techniques may decrease in the future.

Applications of the Technique

All Techniques
1. Unilateral common iliac artery aneurysmal disease.
2. Bilateral common iliac artery aneurysmal disease.

3. Iliac aneurysmal disease that extends slightly into the hypogastric artery (must be adequate ≥1-cm distal seal zone).
4. Iliac aneurysmal disease that has comorbid abdominal aortic aneurysmal disease.

Challenges of the Procedure

Endologix AFX Snorkel Technique and Dual Gore Excluder Technique Method A
1. Advancement of a 12 Fr sheath up and over the bifurcation can be challenging for delivery of the hypogastric snorkel.

Endologix AFX Snorkel Technique
2. Deploying the external iliac artery extension simultaneously and accurately adjacent to the hypogastric snorkel is imperative. Ideally, the proximal ends of both stent grafts should be aligned with one another. If one of the two grafts is located more proximally, it may predispose the more distal graft to thrombosis.
3. Appropriate sizing of the external iliac extension stent graft and the snorkel is imperative. The author's method of sizing is discussed later.

Dual Gore Excluder Technique Method B
4. Placement of a 12 Fr sheath in the brachial or axillary artery requires a vessel of suitable size and has an inherent risk of stroke as the sheath passes the origin of the vertebral (and carotid if right side access) artery.

Dual Gore Excluder Technique Methods A and B
5. The longitudinal distance required for placement of two bifurcated grafts is considerable, and placement requires adequate distance from the lowest renal artery to the hypogastric artery on the affected side.

Potential Pitfalls/Complications

Endologix AFX Snorkel Technique and Dual Gore Excluder Technique Method B
1. Advancing the up-and-over 12 Fr sheath can be challenging. At our institution, the Cook Flexor sheath (Cook Medical Inc., Bloomington, IN) is typically employed given its flexibility, resistance to kinking, and hydrophilic coating. Nonetheless, it is possible that a sheath of this size may not pass over the bifurcation.

Endologix AFX Snorkel Technique
2. The Endologix AFX graft is unique in that the fabric is on the outside of the metal scaffolding.

Consequently, care must be taken to ensure that the operator does not advance a wire under one of the metallic struts during this procedure.

3. The use of a side-by-side snorkel is a relatively new technique, and there is a paucity of long-term data. This type of snorkeling is a non-anatomic repair and carries an inherent risk of a gutter leak (type IIIa) or limb thrombosis. Again, the importance of appropriate sizing and positioning cannot be overstated to prevent these complications.

Dual Gore Excluder Technique Method B

4. Placing a 12 Fr sheath in the brachial or axillary artery is challenging and requires surgical exposure and closure of the vessel. Nonetheless, there is an inherent risk of injury to the artery, hematoma, or other complication. In addition, there is an increased risk of stroke, and this needs to be discussed with the patient as part of the informed consent.

Dual Gore Excluder Technique Methods A and B

5. This technique often cannot be employed because of an inadequate renal-to-hypogastric distance. If it is marginal, extreme care needs to be taken to ensure accurate graft placement. This may not be possible, particularly in tapered, angled, or heavily calcified necks.

Steps of the Procedure

Endologix AFX Snorkel Technique

1. Deploy the Endologix AFX stent graft with sizing and placement per the manufacturer's IFU. The graft should deploy at the native aortic bifurcation. The Endologix AFX system has 13-mm (available in 40-mm length only), 16-mm (available in 30-, 40-, and 55-mm lengths), and 20-mm (available in 30- and 40-mm lengths) limbs. At our institution, we typically advise use of the 20-mm limbs unless use of a bell-bottom extension is planned.

2. Extend the Endologix AFX stent graft with a proximal cuff extension per the manufacturer's IFU if there is comorbid infrarenal abdominal aortic aneurysmal disease. If there is only iliac disease, a proximal cuff may not be required.

3. On the affected side, deploy an Endologix AFX bell bottom if required for length extension or a tight proximal but large distal common iliac artery. The Endologix AFX bell bottom is available with a 25-mm diameter.

4. Plan the sizes of the ipsilateral external iliac extension and the hypogastric snorkel.
   a. The importance of this step cannot be overstated. If the two limbs (snorkel + external iliac limb) are too large relative to one another, there exists a risk of compression with turbulent flow and possible thrombosis of one or both limbs. If the two limbs are too small, a gutter endoleak (type IIIa) can develop.
   b. The limbs selected should be of similar architecture/radial strength. At our institution, we typically use a Gore Excluder ipsi- or contralateral limb for extension to the external iliac artery and a Gore Viabahn stent graft as our hypogastric snorkel. This is important because it is undesirable to have asymmetric radial force whereby one stent is disproportionately compressed.
   c. If appropriately sized and of similar radial strength, the two stent grafts should conform to one another within the common iliac limb such that they obtain a "yin–yang" or semi-lunate configuration to one another when viewed in cross-section profile.
   d. It is desirable to have the cross-sectional area of the external iliac extension limb and the hypogastric snorkel to be approximately 10% oversized relative to the cross-sectional area of the limb within which the two stent grafts are being placed.
   e. As an example, let us assume that we use a bifurcated Endologix AFX graft with 20-mm common iliac limbs. The radius of this limb is 10 mm. The cross-sectional area of this limb can be calculated using πr^2 such that the value is 3.14×10^2 or 314 mm². If we assume a 10% oversize, this means that the aggregate cross-sectional area of our two limbs should be approximately 345.4 mm². A hypogastric snorkel measuring 13 mm in diameter has a 6.5-mm radius and therefore a cross-sectional area of 132.7 mm². Subtracting this from 345.4 mm², we obtain a value of 212.7 mm². If $\pi r^2 = 212.7$ mm², $r^2 = 212.7/3.14$ or 67.8 mm². Therefore, $r = \sqrt{67.8}$ mm² or 8.2 mm. This corresponds to an external iliac limb diameter of approximately 16 mm. Therefore, a 13-mm Viabahn snorkel to the hypogastric artery adjacent to a 16-mm Gore Excluder ipsi- or contralateral limb will appropriately fill a 20-mm Endologix AFX limb.

5. Obtain up-and-over catheterization of the contralateral iliac artery with a 12 Fr sheath.
   a. This is challenging given the sheath size. At our institution, we use a Cook Flexor sheath given its hydrophilic coating, flexibility, and resistance to kinking. To facilitate this, a snare is advanced from the contralateral side (the side to which we are ultimately snorkeling) to the upper abdominal aorta.
   b. Through the 12 Fr sheath, a stiff Glidewire (Terumo Medical Corp., Somerset, NJ) is also

advanced to the upper abdominal aorta. Ensuring that this wire is not under one of the metal struts is imperative. The Glidewire is ideal because of its resistance to kinking.

c. The Glidewire is then snared and pulled through the contralateral sheath.

d. Tension is placed on the Glidewire, and this retraction is employed to facilitate up-and-over advancement of the 12 Fr sheath.

6. The hypogastric artery is catheterized through the up-and-over 12 Fr sheath, and a stiff support wire is placed.

7. The external iliac artery extension limb and the hypogastric stent graft are then deployed simultaneously within the Endologix AFX common iliac artery limb.

a. Care should be taken to ensure that both stent grafts are lined up proximally so that flow is not favored to one limb over the other.

b. Maximal overlap between the two stent grafts (the external iliac extension limb and the hypogastric snorkel) should be obtained within the Endologix AFX common iliac limb to decrease the risk of a type IIIa endoleak.

Dual Gore Excluder Technique Method A

1. A Gore Excluder stent graft is deployed within the aneurysmal common iliac artery, ideally in a location where the diameter of the common iliac artery is less than that of the Excluder so that the deployed graft remains stable during the procedure.

2. An up-and-over 12 Fr sheath is advanced from the contralateral side, and the tip of the sheath is brought within the newly deployed Excluder. For added stability, a 0.014 wire can be used as a "buddy wire" and advanced through the 12 Fr sheath into the external iliac artery. From here, it is snared and externalized to be used for traction to stabilize the 12 Fr sheath.

3. Through the 12 Fr sheath (and adjacent to a buddy wire if used), the contralateral gate and subsequently the hypogastric artery are catheterized. A stiff support wire is placed.

4. An appropriately sized hypogastric stent graft limb is then advanced through the 12 Fr sheath and deployed from the contralateral gate to the hypogastric artery.

5. The 12 Fr sheath is removed from the uninvolved side and replaced with a Cook Zenith stent graft, which is placed immediately below the renal arteries per the manufacturer's IFU.

6. On the side containing the common iliac artery Excluder stent graft, the contralateral gate of the Cook Zenith graft is catheterized via standard technique.

7. A bell-bottom limb is then deployed to connect the contralateral gate of the abdominal Cook Zenith stent graft with the iliac Gore Excluder graft. Adequate overlap is obtained to ensure seal.

8. The ipsilateral limb of the Cook Zenith stent graft is then deployed per the manufacturer's IFU.

Dual Gore Excluder Technique Method B

1. The main body of a Gore Excluder stent graft is deployed at an infrarenal location per the manufacturer's IFU. Care is made to obtain a position as close to the renal arteries as possible. The contralateral gate should correspond to the side on which the iliac aneurysm is present.

2. The contralateral gate is catheterized with standard technique.

3. A bell-bottom Gore Excluder contralateral limb is deployed per the manufacturer's IFU.

a. A 23-mm proximal diameter main body is typically chosen as our second bifurcated device with this technique.

b. To allow a modest oversizing and prevent leakage, a 20-mm-diameter bell-bottom is ideal. This allows the second 23-mm bifurcated device to be placed within the 20-mm limb.

4. The second Gore Excluder bifurcated device is then deployed with appropriate overlap (roughly 3 cm) within the bell-bottom limb.

a. The second bifurcated device should be positioned such that the contralateral gate opens immediately above the hypogastric artery.

b. A surgical cutdown is performed to expose the brachial or axillary artery (left side preferred).

c. A 12 Fr sheath is advanced from the brachial or axillary artery to the abdominal aorta.

d. From the 12 Fr sheath, the first bifurcated device and the contralateral bell-bottom limb are catheterized with subsequent catheterization of the contralateral limb of the second bifurcated device. From here, the hypogastric artery is catheterized distally, and a stiff support wire is placed.

e. The hypogastric snorkel is placed using a 13-mm Viabahn stent graft (5- or 10-cm length as needed).

f. The ipsilateral limb of the second bifurcated device is extended if necessary per the manufacturer's IFU.

g. Deployment of the first bifurcated device is completed with or without ipsilateral limb extension per the manufacturer's IFU.

Example
See Figures 7.1–7.3.

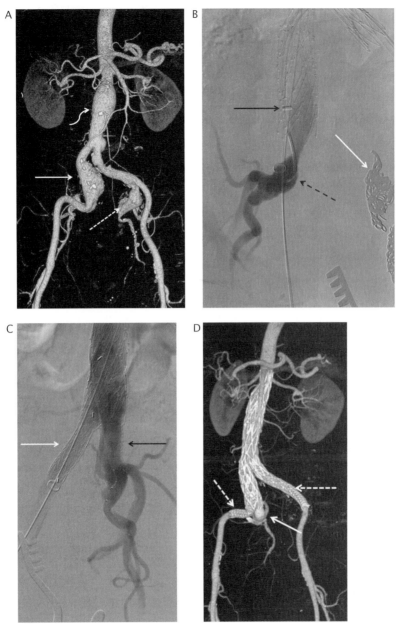

Figure 7.1 (A) Endologix AFX Snorkel Technique: Three-dimensional reconstruction obtained prior to repair. Note mild aneurysmal disease in the abdominal aorta (curved arrow). Larger aneurysms are present in the right common iliac artery (solid arrow) and the left hypogastric artery (dashed arrow). (B) Endologix AFX Snorkel Technique: Digital subtraction angiography (DSA) image with injection in the right hypogastric artery. An Endologix AFX stent graft is present within the aorta and extended on the right with a bell-bottom limb. Note the presence of an up-and-over 12-Fr Cook Flexor sheath (black arrow) within the bell bottom positioned immediately above the iliac bifurcation. A 4-Fr hockey-stick catheter is advanced through the up-and-over sheath and used to catheterize the right hypogastric artery (dashed arrow). The anterior and posterior divisions of the left hypogastric artery have been embolized (white arrow). (C) Endologix AFX Snorkel Technique: DSA image with injection in the right common iliac artery. Note that a Gore Viabahn stent graft has been deployed as the hypogastric limb (black arrow). A Gore Excluder limb has been extended into the right external iliac artery (white arrow), and the common iliac artery aneurysm is completely excluded. (D) Endologix AFX Snorkel Technique: Three-dimensional reconstruction from a computed tomography scan performed 6 weeks after repair. A Gore Viabahn stent graft is present in the right hypogastric artery, which is patent (arrow). Gore Excluder limbs have been extended into the external iliac arteries bilaterally (dashed arrows). The left hypogastric artery is embolized, and all three aneurysms are successfully excluded.

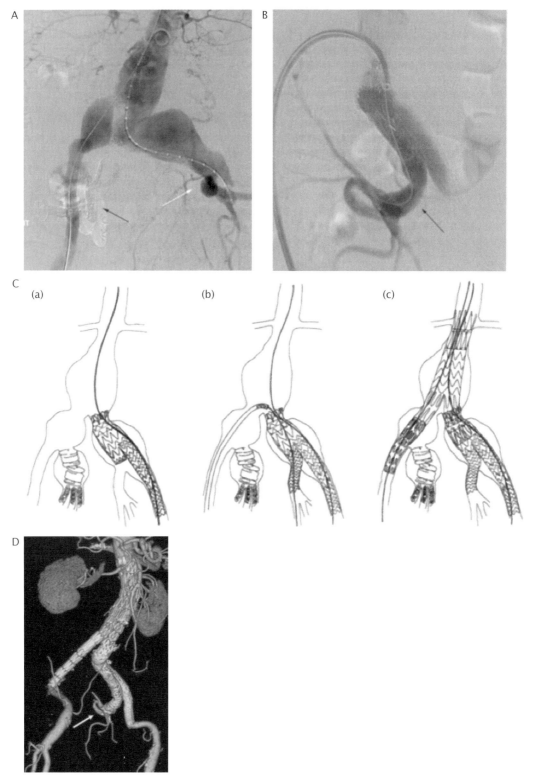

Figure 7.2 (A) Dual Gore Excluder Technique Method A: Preliminary abdominal aortogram demonstrates an abdominal aortic aneurysm and bilateral common iliac aneurysms. Note that the right internal iliac artery has been embolized (black arrow). The left common iliac aneurysm extends to the origin of the left hypogastric artery (white arrow). (B) Dual Gore Excluder Technique Method A: An up-and-over sheath has been advanced into the body of a Gore Excluder stent graft placed in the aneurysmal left common iliac artery. Note that the ipsilateral limb of the Excluder extends into the left external iliac artery. From the up-and-over sheath, the hypogastric artery has been catheterized through the contralateral gate and a hypogastric stent graft limb has been deployed (black arrow). (C) Dual Gore Excluder Technique Method A: Schematic showing deployment of the Gore Excluder stent graft in the left common iliac artery and embolization of the right internal iliac artery (a). Up-and-over catheterization of the newly deployed Excluder stent graft using a 12-Fr sheath placed in the right femoral artery. A hypogastric stent graft limb has been deployed (b). At completion, a Cook Zenith bifurcated stent graft is deployed in the abdominal aorta and bridged to the Gore Excluder using a bell-bottom limb deployed in the contralateral gate of the Cook Zenith graft (c). (D) Dual Gore Excluder Technique Method A: Three-dimensional reconstruction obtained on follow-up computed tomography angiography (CTA) shows complete exclusion of the aneurysms and preserved blood flow to the left hypogastric artery (white arrow).

Source: From Arslan B, et al. Endovascular repair of bilateral common iliac aneurysms with two bifurcated stent grafts. *J Vasc Interv Radiol.* 2010 Jun;21(6):950–952. Courtesy Elsevier.

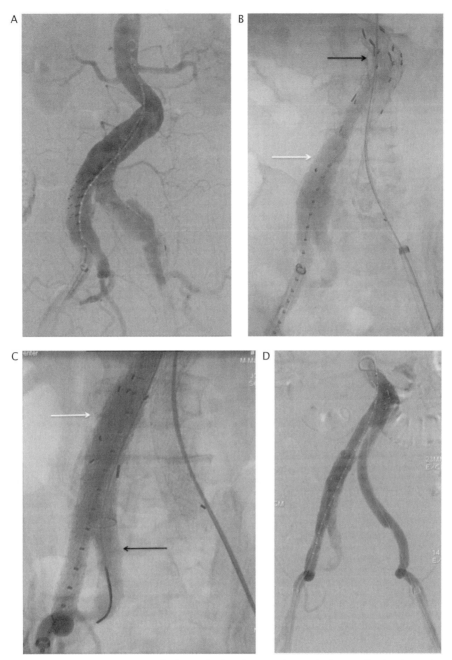

Figure 7.3 (A) Dual Gore Excluder Technique Method B: Abdominal aortogram demonstrates a patient with an infrarenal abdominal aortic aneurysm as well as bilateral iliac artery aneurysms and a left internal iliac artery aneurysm. The degree of aneurysmal dilatation is understated by the angiogram because considerable mural thrombus limited the flow lumen of all the aneurysms. (B) Technique 2, Method 2: A Gore Excluder stent graft with a proximal cuff extension (black arrow) is deployed. The angled neck necessitated placement of a proximal extension. Note that the bell-bottom limb extension (white arrow) has been deployed through the contralateral gate. (C) Dual Gore Excluder Technique Method B: The second Gore Excluder stent graft has been deployed (white arrow) with overlapping margins to the previously deployed bell-bottom limb. Note that the contralateral gate has been catheterized, and a hypogastric artery Viabahn stent graft (black arrow) is deployed. (D) Dual Gore Excluder Technique Method B: Final aortography demonstrates exclusion of the abdominal and aortic aneurysms with preserved blood flow to the right hypogastric artery. The left hypogastric artery was embolized with Amplatzer plugs, and the graft was extended to the left external iliac artery. A slow-flow type Ia endoleak fully resolved at the 1-month follow-up CTA.

References and Suggested Readings

1. Murphy EH, Woo EY. Endovascular management of common and iliac artery aneurysms. *Endovascular Today.* 2012;25:76–81.

2. Santilli SM, Wernsing SE, Lee ES. Expansion rates and outcomes for iliac aneurysms. *J Vasc Surg.* 2000;31(1 Pt 1):114–121.

3. Chaer RA, Barbato JE, Lin SC, Zenati M, Kent KC, McKinsey JF. Isolated iliac artery aneurysms: A contemporary comparison of endovascular and open repair. *J Vasc Surg.* 47(4): 708–713.

4. Krupski WC, Selzman CH, Florida R. Contemporary management of isolated iliac artery aneurysms. *J Vasc Surg.* 1998; 28:1–11.

5. Dorigo W, Pulli R, Troisi N, et al. The treatment of isolated iliac artery aneurysm in patients with non-aneurysmal aorta. *Eur J Vasc Endovasc Surg.* 2008;35(5):585–589.

6. Mitchell R. Endovascular repair of abdominal aortic aneurysms with variations of the aortouniiliac technique. In: *Advanced Hybrid and Endovascular Aortic Surgery: A Case-Based Approach.* Cincinnati, OH: Tempus Fugit Medical; 2012:31–40.

7. Devolfe C, Adeleine P, Henrie M, Violet F, Descotes J. Ilio-femoral and femoro-femoral crossover grafting: Analysis of an 11-year experience. *J Cardiovasc Surg (Torino).* 1983;24(6): 634–640.

8. Arslan B, Sabri SS, Adams JD, Turba UC, Angle JF, Cherry KJ. Endovascular repair of bilateral common iliac aneurysms with two bifurcated stent grafts. *J Vasc Interv Radiol.* 2010;21(6): 950–952.

CHAPTER 8

In Vivo Fenestration During Endovascular Aneurysm Repair

Abdulrahman Masrani and Bulent Arslan

Brief Description

Endovascular management of abdominal aortic aneurysms has become the standard of care during the past 10–15 years. Anatomical constraints are the main limitations in our ability to treat patients endovascularly. The two most important factors are aortic neck and iliofemoral access anatomy. This chapter describes a technique to overcome a hostile neck with a renal artery originating from the aneurysm that does not allow enough proximal landing zone for stent grafting. Several techniques were developed to overcome this obstacle, including custom-made grafts with fenestrations, back table fenestration, and parallel graft placement. In this chapter, we describe an in vivo graft fenestration technique to preserve the renal artery lumen during the endovascular repair of an abdominal aortic aneurysm.

Applications of the Technique

1. Endovascular repair of abdominal aneurysms with a renal artery origin that does not allow sufficient aortic length/proximal seal zone for deployment of the stent graft.

Challenges of the Procedure

1. The technique requires utilization of several steps that are all challenging, such as creating a fenestration in the graft material with a re-entry needle, dilation of the fenestration with high-pressure and/or scoring balloons (most graft materials are very resistant to dilation), and catheterizing the renal artery through the fenestration. Failure of any of these steps may result in the loss of blood flow to the renal artery.

Potential Pitfalls/Complications

1. Loss of flow to the kidney due to inability to fenestrate.

2. Dissection and/or thrombosis of the renal artery during the fenestration process.
3. Inability to catheterize the renal artery through the fenestration, which would result in a type III endoleak and possible loss of flow to the kidney.

Steps of the Procedure

1. From a femoral access, advance an 8 Fr Flexor (Cook Medical Inc., Bloomington, IN) sheath to the level of the renal artery to be targeted for the fenestration.
2. Catheterize the renal artery, and place a 0.014-in. guidewire in the renal artery for support as well as to use as a target later in the procedure.
3. Advance an OUTBACK® LTD® Re-Entry Catheter (Cordis Corp., Milpitas, CA), and park it at the level of the renal artery origin, within the sheath.
4. Deploy the stent graft covering the renal artery orifice.
5. Perform the graft fenestration using the re-entry device that is positioned between the stent graft and the aortic wall by turning and advancing the tip of the needle medially into the lumen of the graft.
6. Capture the 0.014-in. wire that was advanced into the lumen of the stent graft via the re-entry catheter using a large-diameter snare.
7. Establish a through-and-through access from inside the lumen of the stent graft to the space between the aortic wall and stent graft.
8. Using the through-and-through guidewire, use a low-profile (3- or 4-mm diameter) balloon to dilate the graft material.
9. After dilation of the stent graft material, a 5 Fr Berenstein catheter (AngioDynamics Inc., Latham, NY) is advanced over the 0.014-in. wire from inside the stent graft lumen to the space between the graft and the aortic wall.
10. Advance a 0.018-in. V18 guidewire (Boston Scientific Inc., Marlborough, MA) through the Berenstein

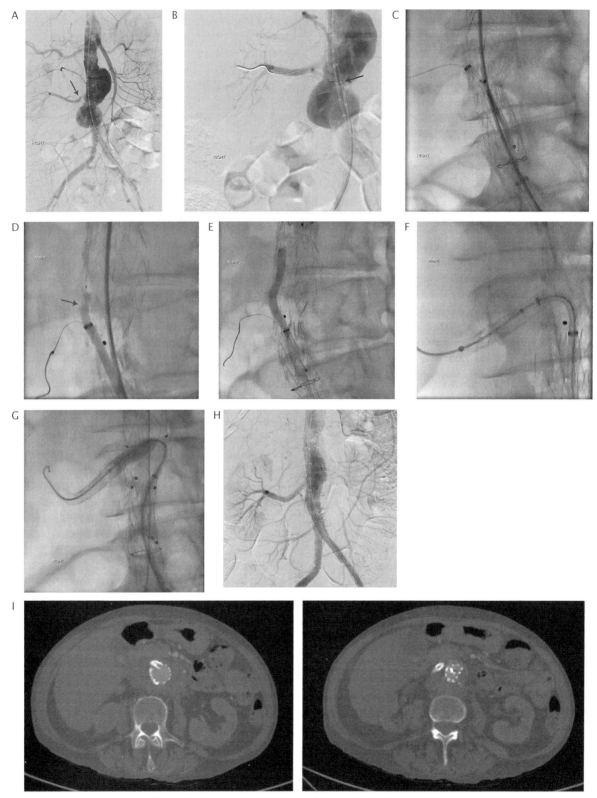

Figure 8.1 (A) Abdominal aortogram demonstrating a high origin for the left renal artery, but the right renal artery origin (arrow) is very low coming from the aneurysmal segment. (B) A 0.014-in. guidewire in the right renal artery with an 8-Fr Flexor sheath positioned at the origin of the renal artery. Over a separate 0.014-in. wire, the re-entry device (arrow) is also positioned in the sheath. (C) Bifurcated main body is deployed over the sheath, positioning the sheath between the aortic wall and the graft. (D) After puncturing through the graft wall into the lumen of the stent graft using the OUTBACK® LTD® Re-entry Catheter, the guidewire is snared from the contralateral access, and through-and-through access is achieved. A 4-mm, 0.014-in. balloon (arrow) is advanced over the 0.014-in. wire, and the graft material is dilated. (E) After initial dilation, a larger high-pressure balloon is utilized to further dilate the fenestration to accommodate the covered stents. (F) A 6-mm Viabahn and two 6-mm covered balloon-expandable stents are placed and angioplastied bridging the right renal artery with the stent graft lumen. (G) A larger 8-mm balloon is used to flair the proximal end of the covered stent graft to seal the fenestration. (H) Completion aortogram shows no evidence of endoleak and good flow to the right kidney through the in vivo fenestration. (I) Three-month CT angiogram showing patent right renal artery without any flow limitation to the right kidney.

catheter next to the through-and-through 0.014-in. wire to select the renal artery.

11. Once the V18 wire selectively catheterizes the renal artery, remove the 0.014-in. wire and advance the 5 Fr catheter into the renal artery over the V18 guidewire.

12. Exchange the V18 wire to a 0.035-in. Rosen wire.

13. If necessary, further dilate the graft fenestration up to 5- or 6-mm diameter.

14. Place a covered balloon expandable stent from the renal artery to the lumen of the stent graft through the fenestration, providing flow to the kidney and sealing the aneurysm sac.

Example

A 70-year-old female with a past medical history of chronic obstructive pulmonary disease, hypertension, and abdominal aortic aneurysm was found to have a bilobed abdominal aortic aneurysm measuring 5.1 cm in largest diameter with interval growth. Due to the low origin of the right renal artery, in vivo fenestration was performed to maintain perfusion of the right kidney (Figure 8.1).

References and Suggested Readings

1. Deng GY, Zhou J, Lu QS, et al. A novel pressure difference-induced perforation aortic stent-grafts system: An experimental study. *Chin Med J (Engl)*. 2013;126(7):1264–1268.

2. Ahanchi SS, Almaroof B, Stout CL, Panneton JM. In situ laser fenestration for revascularization of the left subclavian artery during emergent thoracic endovascular aortic repair. *J Endovasc Ther*. 2012;19(2):226–230.

3. Kolbel T, Carpenter SW, Diener H, Wipper S, Debus ES, Larena-Avellaneda A. Antegrade in situ stent-graft fenestration for the renal artery following inadvertent coverage during EVAR. *J Endovasc Ther*. 2013;20(3):289–294.

4. McWilliams RG, Murphy M, Hartley D, Lawrence-Brown MM, Harris PL. In situ stent-graft fenestration to preserve the left subclavian artery. *J Endovasc Ther*. 2004;11(2):170–174.

5. Wheatley GH 3rd. In situ fenestration of the internal iliac artery as a bailout technique associated with endovascular repair of an abdominal aortic aneurysm: Long-term follow-up. *J Endovasc Ther*. 2012;19(6):716–720.

Reverse Deployment of the Gore Excluder Contralateral Iliac Limbs for Aortoiliac Interventions

S. Lowell Kahn

Brief Description

Aortoiliac occlusive disease and aneurysmal disease are common pathologies encountered by the interventionalist.[1] There are a multitude of commercially available bifurcated grafts for use in aortoiliac disease, but these devices are costly and require at least a 14 Fr femoral access for deployment. The indications for these devices are predominantly for aneurysmal disease, but these devices are employed occasionally for occlusive disease as well.

It is not uncommon to encounter occlusive or aneurysmal disease of the aortoiliac vasculature in which the use of a single stent or stent graft is preferable to the use of a bifurcated device. In certain situations, the use of a conventional aorto-uni-iliac device (Cook Zenith Renu AAA Ancillary Graft Converter, Cook Medical Inc., Bloomington, IN; Medtronic Excluder II aorto-uni-iliac stent graft, Medtronic Inc., Minneapolis, MN) is desirable. However, these devices are not only costly but also require a large femoral access. The Zenith device requires an 18–22 Fr access, and the Excluder II device requires an 18 Fr access.

In addition to access and cost considerations, these aorto-uni-iliac (AUI) devices are not available at all institutions. Outside of the AUI devices, there are few options for commercially available stents that have an adequate diameter for aortic interventions. The largest bare-metal and covered balloon-expandable stents outside of the manually mounted Palmaz stent (Cordis Corp., Milpitas, CA) domestically are 10 mm (e.g., Express LD [Boston Scientific Inc., Marlborough, MA] and iCAST [Atrium Medical Corp., Hudson, NH]). Larger bare-metal self-expanding stents are available (e.g., E-Luminexx [14 mm; C.R. Bard Inc., Murray Hill, NJ] and Wallstent [24 mm; Boston Scientific Inc., Marlborough, MA]), but these stents may lack the accuracy, radial strength, and protection from bleeding desired for aortoiliac interventions. A covered stent is often desirable for aortic interventions given the increased risks of bleeding inherent with angioplasty of larger vessels secondary to Laplace's law. In Europe, the Advanta V12 stent graft (Atrium Medical

Corp., Hudson, NH) is available as a covered balloon-expandable stent up to 16 mm, but this is not approved in the United States.

The Gore Excluder contralateral limb (W.L. Gore & Associates Inc., Flagstaff, AZ) is a flexible self-expanding stent graft available in lengths ranging from 9.5 to 14 cm. The proximal diameter of all grafts is 16 mm, and the distal diameter ranges between 12 and 27 mm. Depending on the size selected, these grafts require a femoral access between 12 and 15 Fr. Occasionally, these grafts deployed with conventional technique may be suitable for aortoiliac interventions. However, the proximal diameter of 16 mm is commonly inadequate given that the normal infrarenal diameter of the aorta is ≤21 mm. A diseased and ectatic aorta may be considerably larger.

This chapter describes a simple and safe method for reversing deployment of the Excluder contralateral limb. This has great utility not only for aortoiliac interventions but also for central venous stenoses/occlusions. Reversal of the limb allows a proximal diameter of 12–27 mm with a fixed distal diameter of 16 mm. The technique requires use of a 12–15 Fr sheath, most commonly a 12 Fr sheath.

Applications of the Technique

1. Aortoiliac interventions for occlusive and/or aneurysmal disease as discussed previously.
2. Central venous stenoses/occlusions, particularly in the setting of failing dialysis access or superior vena cava syndrome.
3. Bailout technique for type I or type III endoleaks during conventional endovascular aneurysm repair.

Challenges of the Procedure

1. Removing the graft from its delivery system can be challenging, and it is advisable to have an assistant as described later in the chapter.
2. As described later, the sheath must be modified in that the dilator is cut to a blunt end to create the push

rod necessary for deployment of the graft. The wire lumen is often compromised during this process, preventing the dilator from being loaded on the wire. This situation is remedied by passing the back end of an Amplatz Super Stiff Guidewire (Boston Scientific Inc., Marlborough, MA) through the hub end of the dilator and forcing it through the compromised lumen on the other end.

3. After the graft is removed from its manufactured delivery system, it is reversed and then placed in a 12 Fr sheath, where it is deployed. After deployment in the sheath, the actual graft deployment is a simple pin-pull system with unsheathing of the graft. With practice, this is highly accurate, but it is advised that the operator attempt this technique outside of the patient prior to their first clinical use.

Potential Pitfalls/Complications

1. Several steps are required to remove the graft from its delivery system. These must be adhered to carefully for the technique to work. Most important, the string of the Gore Excluder delivery system must be cut very close to the knob with care taken not to pull the string to prevent inadvertent deployment of the graft.

2. It is advised that the ends of the Gore Excluder be marked with a marker to ensure that the graft is deployed in the desired orientation within the patient. Once the graft is removed from its delivery system, the ends of the undeployed graft look identical even though their diameters are different.

Steps of the Procedure

1. Over a guidewire, advance a 12 or 15 Fr sheath (depending on the size of the bell-bottom Gore Excluder limb selected) beyond the intended location for the graft deployment. Remove the dilator.

2. With heavy scissors, cut the tip of the dilator off near the transition point between the taper and shaft of the dilator. It is common for the wire lumen to become compromised where the dilator is cut. This is easily repaired by passing the back end of an Amplatz guidewire through the hub end of the dilator and pushing it though forcefully. It is imperative that the lumen be intact because the cut dilator is necessary for graft deployment.

3. Carefully unscrew the deployment knob of the Gore Excluder. With caution, the knob should be barely pulled to expose the white string to which it is attached. Once exposed, cut it with a thin blade. It is imperative that the string is not pulled any further han necessary to visualize the back of the knob where the string is attached. Pulling it further than required will result in inadvertent deployment of the graft.

4. The graft is now ready to be removed from its delivery shaft. For this step, it is useful to have an assistant. The assistant should place one hand on the graft and should pull on the tip (olive) of the deployment catheter with the other hand. When this is performed properly, the metal stylet of the delivery system is exposed. With heavy-duty (e.g., sternal) wire cutters, the stylet is cut. Be careful not to damage the graft during this process.

5. The graft should now slide easily off the distal end of the delivery system. At this point, the graft should be in its constrained configuration with the white string attached. Mark the end(s) of the graft with a marker so that the proximal and distal ends are not confused.

6. With the distal end of the graft loaded first, the undeployed graft should be advanced into the sheath over the guidewire. The blunt back end of the dilator should be used to push the graft a short distance into the sheath. The string of the graft will be hanging out of the back end of the sheath.

7. With forward pressure on the blunt dilator (acting as a push rod at this point), the string should be pulled to deploy the graft within the sheath. The blunt dilator ensures that the graft does not come back out of the sheath during deployment. The string is discarded.

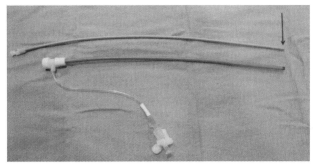

Figure 9.1 The tip of the dilator is cut with heavy scissors near the transition between the taper and the shaft of the dilator (black arrow). The blunt dilator will be used later to deploy the graft with a pin-pull technique.

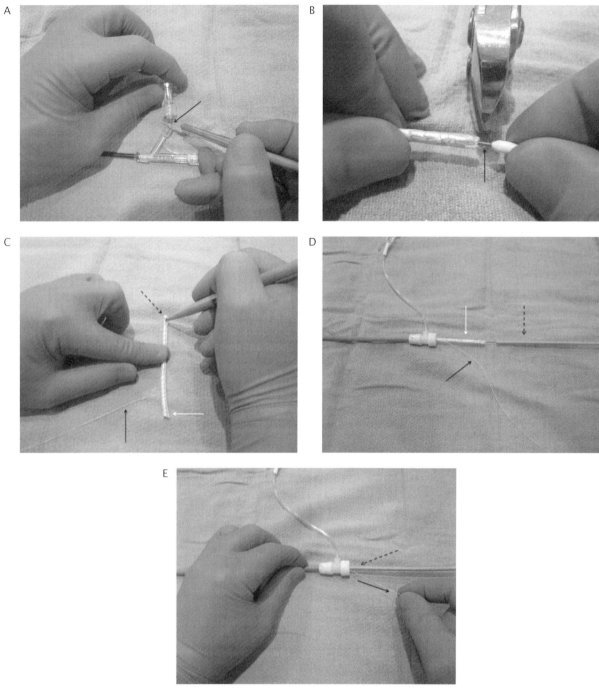

Figure 9.2 (A) The knob of the delivery system is unscrewed and pulled back minimally to expose the back end of the knob where the string is attached (black arrow). The string is cut with a thin blade. (B) With an assistant pulling on the graft and the tip (olive) of the delivery system in opposite directions, the inner metal stylet (black arrow) is exposed and cut with sternal wire cutters. (C) The end(s) of the graft is marked with a marker so that the proximal and distal ends are distinct. Note that the proximal end (dashed arrow) is marked, representing the 16-mm end. The distal end (white arrow) represents the bell-bottom end (in this case, 20 mm) and is closer to where the retention string (black arrow) exits the graft. (D) The constrained but free graft (white arrow) has been placed over a wire. It has been flipped such that the distal end (bell bottom) is inserted into the sheath first. Note the retention string (black arrow) will remain external to the sheath. The graft is loaded into the sheath using the blunt end dilator (dashed arrow) advanced over the wire. (E) The blunt tip dilator is used to push the graft a short distance into the sheath. After loading the graft fully into the sheath, the graft can be deployed in a constrained state within the sheath. To accomplish this, forward pressure is maintained on the blunt tip dilator (dashed arrow) while the string is pulled (solid arrow) and discarded. The graft is constrained within the sheath and ready for deployment using an unsheathing technique whereby the position of the graft is maintained with the blunt tip dilator and the graft is unsheathed for deployment.

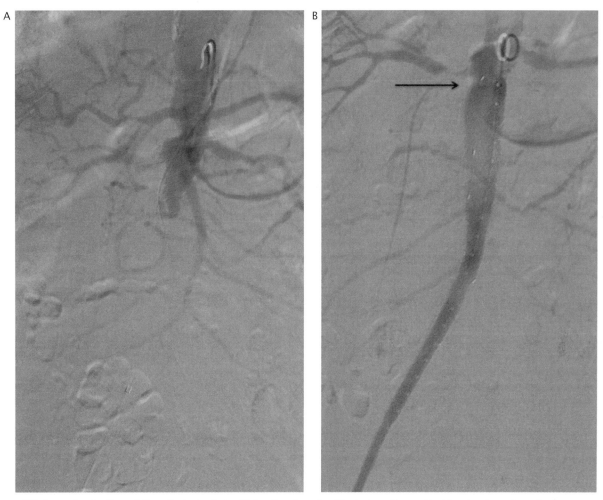

Figure 9.3 Example of a flipped Gore Excluder limb utilizing the described technique. The patient has had an above-knee amputation on the left and now has progressive critical limb ischemia of the right leg. (A) Digital subtraction angiography revealed occlusion of the aorta just below the renal arteries. The aorta just below the renal arteries measured 18 mm in diameter. (B) Using the described technique, a reversed 20-mm bell-bottom Gore Excluder limb was deployed within a 12-Fr sheath and subsequently advanced to the desired position using the blunt-tip dilator. The dilator was then used to maintain the position of the graft while the sheath was retracted. The graft deployed at its desired location with the bell-bottom end (arrow) located just below the renal arteries. The 16-mm end was deployed within a 13-mm Viabahn (W. L. Gore & Associates) that was deployed within an overdilated 10-mm iCAST stent to allow for a tapered transition to a smaller iliac diameter.

8. Push the graft with the blunt tip cut dilator to its desired place of deployment under fluoroscopic guidance. In our experience, we usually advance it just proximal to the intended site of delivery because the system can be retracted slightly early during deployment.

9. With a pin (blunt dilator) pull (sheath) method, deploy the graft at its intended location. When the graft first begins to deploy, slight adjustments in the cranial or caudal position can be made. As mentioned previously, we usually position the graft slightly proximal (cranial) to the desired position and adjust it distally by retracting the entire system slightly. We have found that the deployment of this technique is remarkably accurate, arguably more so than when the graft is deployed per instructions for use with pulling of the string.

10. Complete the procedure by removing the blunt dilator and ballooning the graft as necessary.

11. A femoral-femoral bypass is performed if needed.

Example

See Figures 9.1–9.3.

References and Suggested Readings

1. Niesen MJ. Endovascular management of aortoiliac occlusive disease. *Semin Intervent Radiol.* 2009;26(4):296–302.
2. van der Steenhoven TJ, Heyligers JM, Tielliu IF, Zeebregts CJ. The upside down Gore Excluder contralateral leg without extracorporeal predeployment for aortic or iliac aneurysm exclusion. *J Vasc Surg.* 2011;53(6):1738–1741.

CHAPTER 10

Use of Two Bifurcated Stent Grafts for Creation of an Aorto-Uni-Iliac Endograft

S. Lowell Kahn

Brief Description

Abdominal aortic aneurysms (AAAs) represent a common pathology encountered by the interventionalist. A large study conducted across Veterans Administration hospitals in the United States found an incidence of 1.4% on screening.[1] Of these AAAs, approximately 10–20% have comorbid involvement of the iliac arteries, whereas <2% of aneurysmal disease cases involve only the iliac arteries.[2,3] As of 2010, roughly 80% of AAAs repaired in the United States were performed endovascularly.[4] The overwhelming majority of endovascular repairs are performed with conventional bifurcated devices. However, there are situations in which use of a bifurcated graft is not feasible, and the use of an aorto-uni-iliac (AUI) device is required. Standard indications for use of an AUI include a narrow aortic segment precluding delivery and adequate expansion of a bifurcated graft, unilateral iliac occlusion, tortuosity, severe stenosis, and the presence of iliac aneurysmal disease. Occasionally, an AUI may be used for aortoiliac occlusive disease or as a bailout technique with conventional endografting.

Currently, there are two commercially available AUI devices available: the Cook Zenith Renu AAA Ancillary Graft Converter (Cook Medical Inc., Bloomington, IN) and the Medtronic Excluder II aorto-uni-iliac stent graft (Medtronic Inc., Minneapolis, MN). The Zenith device requires an 18–22 Fr access, and the Excluder II device requires an 18 Fr access. Although there are differences between these devices in terms of cost, profile, access requirements, stent/crown structure, fabric, flexibility, radial strength, deployment, and configurations, most pathologies requiring an AUI can be treated safely by either of these devices.

In reality, however, AUI devices are not available at all institutions, and there are times when their use may not have been planned. This chapter describes a simple technique involving the use of two bifurcated stent grafts to create an AUI. The technique involves placing a second bifurcated device slightly lower within the primary bifurcated device and rotating it such that the contralateral limb of the second device is 180 degrees away from the contralateral limb of the primary bifurcated device. In so doing, the contralateral limbs of both devices are excluded, and blood flow is diverted solely down the ipsilateral limbs

of the primary and secondary devices within one another. At our institution, this has been performed with the Gore Excluder (W. L. Gore & Associates Inc., Flagstaff, AZ) with 100% procedural success. The Excluder is rather amenable to this technique given its absence of suprarenal crowns; in practice, however, this technique can be employed by other modular bifurcated endografts as well.

Although this technique has great utility, the added expense and potential for complications mandate that this should be used only in the absence of one of the aforementioned dedicated AUI devices.

Applications of the Technique

1. Anatomic considerations requiring use of an AUI:
   a. Unilateral iliac artery occlusion or severe stenosis.
   b. Narrow aortic segment precluding passage or deployment of a bifurcated graft. A narrow segment predisposes the graft to limb thrombosis.
   c. Severe iliac tortuosity preventing gate cannulation or delivery of the contralateral limb.
   d. The presence of iliac aneurysms may require the use of an AUI depending on repair strategy.
2. Bailout technique employed during conventional bifurcated graft deployment:
   a. Unplanned inability to cannulate the contralateral gate or inability to deliver the contralateral limb.
   b. Graft failure (e.g., type III endoleak).

Challenges of the Procedure

1. Aligning the graft in optimal position is imperative. If the secondary graft is aligned improperly, a type IIIa endoleak can occur. If the secondary graft is positioned too high and/or if the contralateral gate of the secondary bifurcated device is aligned with the contralateral gate of the primary device, a type IIIa endoleak from the contralateral gate of the secondary device can occur. Similarly, if the secondary graft is positioned too low, a type IIIa endoleak from the contralateral limb of the primary device can occur.

2. Narrow iliac or aortic segments can be problematic given that the sheath and/or secondary device must be advanced through the primary deployed bifurcated device. It is advised that the primary graft undergo angioplasty as needed prior to advancing the secondary graft.

3. Visualization of the secondary graft can be challenging because both the primary and secondary bifurcated grafts have markers, and it is important that the markers of each graft are distinguished from one another to ensure proper positioning. In the case of the Excluder, radiopaque markers are present at the top of the graft, bilaterally at the level of the gate, and at the lower end of the ipsilateral limb. A radiopaque ring is present circumferentially at the contralateral gate.

4. It is important to remain mindful of the shortest renal artery-to-internal iliac artery distance because two grafts are being deployed. Given that the contralateral internal iliac artery is frequently compromised in the setting of an AUI, compromise of the internal iliac artery on the ipsilateral side may have an adverse outcome.

Potential Pitfalls/Complications

1. A type IIIa endoleak is possible with this technique, as described previously. Proper positioning of the secondary graft and angioplasty is imperative. If an endoleak occurs, more aggressive angioplasty with a 14-mm noncompliant balloon should be considered.

2. Inability to deliver the secondary bifurcated device through the primary device.

3. In theory, the crowding of both ipsilateral and contralateral limbs into the ipsilateral limb of the primary bifurcated device carries a risk of early or late graft thrombosis.

Steps of the Procedure

1. A bifurcated endograft is deployed per the manufacturer's instructions for use at an infrarenal location. We typically position the contralateral limb of the primary device toward the contralateral side. Ideally, the primary device should be located immediately below the renal arteries. Attention to the shortest renal artery-to-ipsilateral internal iliac artery distance is imperative, and the length of the primary device should fall well short of this to allow for the approximately 5-mm extension that occurs with placement of the secondary device.

2. Balloon angioplasty of the primary device is performed with a large-diameter compliant balloon (e.g., Reliant [Medtronic Inc., Minneapolis, MN] or Coda [Cook Medical Inc., Bloomington, IN]).

3. The secondary bifurcated device is now deployed. The secondary device should have a proximal diameter that is equal to or one size larger than the primary device. The device should be advanced to a position approximately 5 mm below the primary device. The contralateral limb should be oriented 180 degrees away from the contralateral limb of the primary device. In our example, if the contralateral limb of the primary device is positioned toward the contralateral iliac artery, the contralateral limb of the secondary device should be oriented toward the ipsilateral side.

4. After deployment of the secondary device, balloon angioplasty should be performed again along the length of the endograft using a large-diameter compliant balloon.

5. Completion abdominal aortography should be performed. If a residual type IIIa endoleak is present, additional angioplasty with a noncompliant 14-mm balloon should be performed. In rare circumstances, use of a balloon-expandable bare-metal stent may be necessary.

6. A femoral-femoral bypass is performed if needed.

Example

See Figures 10.1 and 10.2.

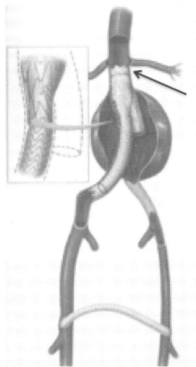

Figure 10.1 Schematic demonstration of the conversion of a bifurcated graft to an AUI endograft in a patient with an occluded left common iliac artery. The primary (outer) bifurcated Gore Excluder main body is positioned immediately below the renal arteries (arrow). Note that the contralateral gate of the primary device is oriented toward the contralateral (left) side. The secondary (inner) bifurcated Gore Excluder main body is deployed 5 mm below the primary device and oriented such that its contralateral gate is directed toward the ipsilateral (right) side (see inset). Blood flow is diverted away from the contralateral gate of the primary graft by the placement of the secondary graft. Similarly, blood flow is diverted away from the contralateral gate of the secondary graft as the gate is compressed within the ipsilateral limb of the primary graft.

Source: From Mitchell RO, editor. *Advanced Hybrid and Endovascular Aortic Surgery,* 2012. Courtesy Tempus Fugit Medical.[5]

References and Suggested Readings

1. Lederle FA, Johnson GR, Wilson SE, et al.; Aneurysm Detection and Management (ADAM) Veterans Affairs Cooperative Study Group. Prevalence and associations of abdominal aortic aneurysm detected through screening. *Ann Intern Med.* 1997:126(6):441–449.

2. Uberoi R, Tsetis D, Shrivastava V, et al. Standard of practice for the interventional management of isolated iliac artery aneurysms. *Cardiovasc Intervent Radiol.* 2011;34(1):3–13.

3. Sakamoto I, Sueyoshi E, Hazama S, et al. Endovascular treatment of iliac artery aneurysms. *Radiographics.* 2005;25 (Suppl 1):S213–S227.

4. Dua A, Kuy S, Lee CJ, Upchurch GR Jr, Desai SS. Epidemiology of aortic aneurysm repair in the United States from 2000 to 2010. *J Vasc Surg.* 2014; 59(6):1512–1517.

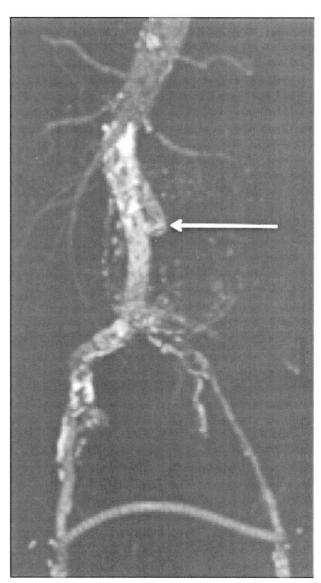

Figure 10.2 Three-dimensional reconstruction of an AUI constructed with two bifurcated Gore Excluder main body grafts. Both devices measure 23 mm proximally by 12 mm distally with a 14-cm length. Note the absence of flow within the contralateral gate (arrow) of the primary (outer) endograft as flow is excluded from it by placement of the secondary (inner) graft. Blood flow is diverted exclusively to the right femoral artery. The left common iliac artery is chronically occluded. Blood flow to the left extremity is provided via a femoral–femoral bypass.

Source: From Mitchell RO, editor. *Advanced Hybrid and Endovascular Aortic Surgery,* 2012. Courtesy Tempus Fugit Medical.[5]

5. Mitchell RO. Endovascular repair of abdominal aortic aneurysms with variations of the aortouniiliac technique. In: Mitchell RO, ed. *Advanced Hybrid and Endovascular Aortic Surgery. A Case-Based Approach.* Cincinnati, OH: Tempus Fugit Medical, 2012:312–336.

CHAPTER 11

Creation of a Flow-Modulating Stent Using Multilayered Wallstents for Aneurysm Exclusion

S. Lowell Kahn

Brief Description

Abdominal aortic aneurysms (AAAs) are a common pathology that is found in 4–9% of patients in the developed world.[1–6] Risk factors for AAAs include age, male sex, family history, comorbid cardiovascular disease, and smoking.[4,7,8] Despite the male predominance of the disease, rupture occurs at a smaller diameter in females, and the outcomes are poorer in this subgroup.[9–12] Although most are clinically silent, there are approximately 12,000–15,000 ruptures annually in the United States, and approximately 15,000 deaths are attributable to the disease.[1,13] As of 2000, AAAs were the 10th leading cause of death among men aged 65–74 years.[13] The mortality risk from rupture alone approaches 90%, but the outcome is considerably better for those patients who survive to the hospital.[14] In the 1980s and 1990s, an increase in AAA mortality was reported, but since the early 2000s, the reported incidence has been declining, largely secondary to improved screening, decreased smoking, risk factor reduction, and improved endovascular and surgical options available to patients.[9,15–22]

The risk of rupture increases with the diameter of the aneurysm, with a reported rupture rate of 9% for aneurysms between 5.5 and 6 cm in size, 10% for aneurysms between 6 and 6.9 cm, and 33% for aneurysms greater than 7 cm.[23] Although there is some variation in guidelines, treatment is typically indicated for aneurysms greater than 5 to 5.5 cm.[23,24]

Historically, open elective surgical repair has been the mainstay of therapy, but the morbidity of the procedure is considerable and many patients are poor operative candidates. The concept of a minimally invasive endovascular aneurysm repair (EVAR) was first introduced by a Russian physician named Volodos in 1986 and subsequently verified by Parodi et al. in 1991.[25,26] Although initially reserved for nonsurgical candidates, the favorable safety profile, rapid recovery, and proven track record have made EVAR the favored treatment modality as it now accounts for approximately 77% of elective AAA repairs.[27] The explosive growth of new devices and technologies has vastly expanded the scope of patients appropriate for endovascular repair. Endostaples, fenestrated grafts, and polymer-based grafts are a few of the newer technologies that allow operators to treat a broad range of challenging anatomy.

Flow-modulating stents (FDSs) are a relatively new development and consist of multilayered bare-metal self-expanding stents. Despite the inherent porosity of the stents, the interconnected stent matrix features flow-diverting properties that preserve luminal and branch vessel flow while simultaneously depressurizing the aneurysm sac, resulting in shrinkage and thrombosis. Computational fluid dynamics studies by Wailliez et al. demonstrated that stents with a porosity of 50–70% significantly dampen aneurysmal sac blood flow, thus promoting thrombosis outside of the stent.[28,29] Augsburger et al. evaluated the effects of the FDS with particle image velocimetry and found improved laminar flow within the stent lumen when the stent is placed across an aneurysm.[29,30] Although data are limited with this new technology, the early results are promising, with successful use reported in aneurysms and pseudoaneurysms of the aorta and visceral vasculature.[31–38] A review of the literature by Sfyroeras et al. in 2012 reported an overall 90.6% aneurysm thrombosis rate and an 81% aneurysm volume reduction.[31]

Use of an FDS differs considerably from use of a conventional aortic graft in that thrombosis and reduction of the aortic sac occurs at a slower rate. Despite this, the FDS may have benefits that are not conferred by an open surgical repair nor a conventional endograft. The sheath size for an FDS is less than that required for a conventional endograft, and it similarly has the minimally invasive properties of conventional EVAR. The FDS does not rely on the "seal zones" of a conventional endograft and therefore may allow treatment of more complex anatomy. The simplicity of deploying a single stent allows for a shorter procedure time with less contrast, radiation, and anesthesia time. Perhaps the greatest benefit is the preservation of branch vessel flow, which allows the stent to be safely placed over the ostia of renal and visceral vessels.

An unproven but potential benefit of the FDS is in the treatment of mycotic aneurysms. Multiple investigators have described its use in this scenario.[36–39] Mycotic aneurysms account for 2.6%[40] of all abdominal aortic aneurysms and are particularly challenging to treat given the morbidity of this patient population and the ongoing risks of rupture, septic emboli, and recurrent local infection. Surgical debridement with long-term antibiotics is the mainstay of therapy, but the reported perioperative mortality is as high as 40%.[41] For this reason, conventional stent grafts have been used successfully to treat these pseudoaneurysms with suppressive antibiotics. Nonetheless, stent grafts have been shown to have higher rates of infection compared to their bare-metal counterparts.[42] Lacking fabric as a nidus for infection, the FDS may be beneficial in these patients.

Unfortunately, FDS technology is unavailable in the United States, and currently the only commercially available FDS in Europe is the Cardiatis Multilayer Flow Modulator (Cardiatis, Isnes, Belgium). This chapter describes in vivo construction of an FDS using concentric bare-metal stents. This technique was first described by Zhang et al.[35] in 2013 for the treatment of visceral artery aneurysms and by Kahn et al.[39] in 2015 for an aortic mycotic pseudoaneurysm. The technique is simple to perform and potentially beneficial in a variety of clinical scenarios.

Applications of the Technique

1. Treatment of visceral, renal, and aortic aneurysms.
2. Treatment of mycotic visceral, renal, and aortic pseudoaneurysms.

Challenges of the Procedure

1. For renal and visceral vessels, a multitude of self-expanding stents suitable for this technique exist. However, there are limited self-expanding stents large enough to treat an adult aorta. The largest bare-metal self-expanding stent is the Wallstent (Boston Scientific Inc., Marlborough, MA). The Wallstent is notoriously difficult to deploy accurately because it foreshortens as it expands from its delivery catheter. In addition, the stent can elongate and lose radial strength if it is overly sized relative to its target vessel. If layering multiple Wallstents, 1:1 sizing or minimal oversizing is advised to prevent this complication. In addition, it may be prudent to choose a slightly smaller diameter (and shorter) stent for the inner stent(s) because the lumen decreases modestly with each stent deployed.
2. There is no definitive number of stents that should be layered. In our experience, the layering of three concentric stents most closely mimics the design of the Cardiatis stent. This has not been validated with bench testing, and judgment on a case-by-case basis for more or fewer stents is warranted.

Potential Pitfalls/Complications

1. Inaccurate stent deployment could result in jailing or thrombosis of a nontarget vessel.
2. If the aneurysm fails to thrombose, the presence of multiple bare-metal self-expanding stents may limit other surgical or endovascular options.
3. The reduction in size/thrombosis of the aneurysm after stent deployment is not immediate. Therefore, the technique is not advised for aneurysms or pseudoaneurysms with an imminent risk of rupture.
4. Layering of concentric stents in a small vessel may narrow the vessel with consequent thrombosis. Consideration of the vessel size and the thickness of the deployed stents should be made.

Steps of the Procedure

1. Fluoroscopic-guided catheterization of the target vessel is obtained, and diagnostic arteriography is performed to obtain appropriate stent planning.
2. The first bare-metal stent is deployed over a support guidewire. The initial stent size chosen should be 1:1 or minimally oversized with respect to the target vessel diameter. If using Wallstents in larger vessels, care must be taken to ensure the stent deploys at its target location. The Wallstent foreshortens as it is deployed from its delivery catheter. Conversely, vessel narrowing or the presence of plaque can cause the stent to elongate more than expected. A radiopaque marker on the delivery catheter of the Wallstent shows the point to which the stent can still be resheathed. This property of the Wallstent should be exploited to optimize stent placement.
3. Second and third stents should then be deployed within the original stent. We recommend repeating arteriography after each stent deployment to evaluate for response. The additional stents should be the same or one size smaller in diameter to accommodate the reduced lumen with each stent placement. The angiogram will show persistent flow into the aneurysm, but the filling and washout from the sac should be delayed. *Optional*: In some situations, it may be feasible and desirable to place a catheter or pressure wire (from the same or another access) in the sac to evaluate sac pressure during stent deployment. Obviously, care must be taken to ensure the catheter or wire does not become trapped behind the stent(s).
4. Completion arteriography is performed to evaluate sac flow and stent placement. As stated previously, we have performed this technique using three stents only, but the decision to place fewer or more stents should be made on an individual basis.

Example

See Figures 11.1–11.5.

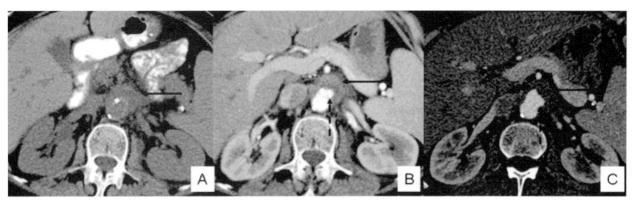

Figure 11.1 A 64-year-old female with bacteremia secondary to recurrent urinary tract infections developed abdominal and back pain and was subsequently diagnosed with an infrarenal aortic pseudoaneurysm that grew out *Escherichia coli*. Her severe chronic obstructive pulmonary disease made her a poor operative candidate. Axial computed tomography (CT) scans obtained on hospital days 5 (A), 6 (B), and 8 (C) demonstrate progressive interval enlargement of the aorta (solid arrow) as well as the development of a pseudoaneurysm with a wide neck (dashed arrow). This correlated with progressive worsening back pain experienced by the patient.

Source: From Kahn SL, et al. In vivo construction of a multilayer bare-metal stent for the treatment of an aortic mycotic pseudoaneurysm. *J Vasc Surg.* 2015;62(3):744–746. Courtesy Elsevier.

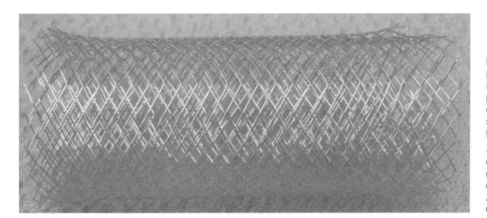

Figure 11.2 Sample of a physician-created multilayer stent using three concentrically placed Wallstents. Note the slight elongation of the innermost stent secondary to constriction by the first two stents.

Source: From Kahn SL, et al. In vivo construction of a multilayer bare-metal stent for the treatment of an aortic mycotic pseudoaneurysm. *J Vasc Surg.* 2015;62(3):744–746. Courtesy Elsevier.

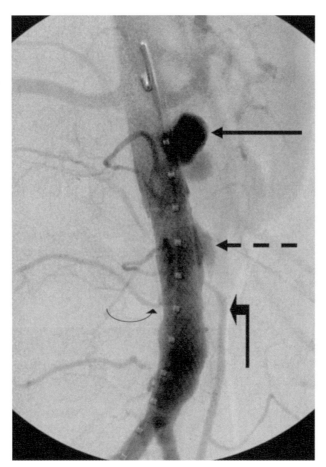

Figure 11.3 Same patient as shown in Figure 11.1. Oblique coronal digital subtraction angiography obtained immediately after the placement of three concentric 16 × 60-mm Wallstents. Note the main pseudoaneurysm located below the renal arteries (solid arrow) as demonstrated in Figure 11.1 and the smaller pseudoaneurysm developing more inferiorly (dashed arrow). Immediately after deployment of the concentric stents, the multilayer stent produced sluggish flow in both pseudoaneurysms appreciated on real-time imaging. It is hypothesized that this represents a depressurization effect on the pseudoaneurysms as laminar flow within the stent lumen is facilitated. Also note the preservation of blood flow into the inferior mesenteric artery (right-angle arrow) and a lumbar artery (curved arrow).

Source: From Kahn SL, et al. In vivo construction of a multilayer bare-metal stent for the treatment of an aortic mycotic pseudoaneurysm. *J Vasc Surg.* 2015;62(3):744–746. Courtesy Elsevier.

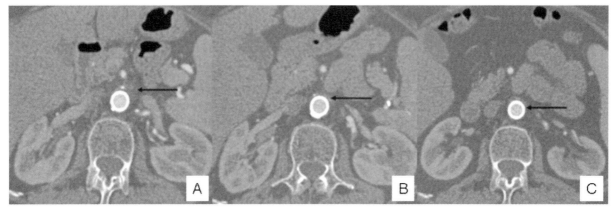

Figure 11.4 Same patient as shown in Figures 11.1 and 11.3. Axial CTs obtained at 3 (A), 6 (B), and 16 (C) months post procedure. Note the progressive resolution of the mycotic pseudoaneurysm until there is complete resolution by 16 months.

Source: From Kahn SL, et al. In vivo construction of a multilayer bare-metal stent for the treatment of an aortic mycotic pseudoaneurysm. *J Vasc Surg.* 2015;62(3):744–746. Courtesy Elsevier.

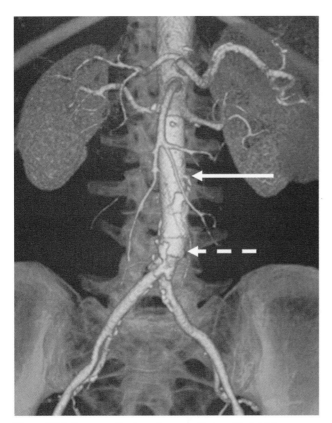

Figure 11.5 Same patient as shown in Figures 11.1, 11.3, and 11.4. Coronal three-dimensional maximal intensity projection (MIP) constructed from a CT acquired 16 months post procedure. Note the complete resolution of the main and smaller pseudoaneurysms within the infrarenal aorta. Interestingly, there continues to be perfusion within the lumbar arteries and the inferior mesenteric artery (solid arrow) demonstrating branch vessel preservation as has been reported for the Cardiatis stent. Also demonstrated is the final stent extending below (dashed arrow) the other two Wallstents. Although of no consequence for this patient, it is well known that Wallstents elongate when confined, and this property should be considered when attempting to create an in vivo multilayer stent using concentric Wallstents.

Source: From Kahn SL, et al. In vivo construction of a multilayer bare-metal stent for the treatment of an aortic mycotic pseudoaneurysm. *J Vasc Surg.* 2015;62(3):744–746. Courtesy Elsevier.

References and Suggested Readings

1. Collins KA. Overview of abdominal aortic aneurysm. From http://www.uptodate.com. Published 2016.
2. Scott RA, Ashton HA, Kay DN. Abdominal aortic aneurysm in 4237 screened patients: Prevalence, development and management over 6 years. *Br J Surg.* 1991;78:1122.
3. Wilmink AB, Quick CR. Epidemiology and potential for prevention of abdominal aortic aneurysm. *Br J Surg.* 1998;85:155.
4. Lederle FA, Johnson GR, Wilson SE, et al.; Aneurysm Detection and Management Veterans Affairs Cooperative Study Investigators. The aneurysm detection and management study screening program: Validation cohort and final results. *Arch Intern Med.* 2000;160:1425.
5. Newman AB, Arnold AM, Burke GL, O'Leary DH, Manolio TA. Cardiovascular disease and mortality in older adults with small abdominal aortic aneurysms detected by ultrasonography: The Cardiovascular Health Study. *Ann Intern Med.* 2001;134:182.
6. Collin J, Araujo L, Walton J, Lindsell D. Oxford screening programme for abdominal aortic aneurysm in men aged 65 to 74 years. *Lancet.* 1988;2:613.
7. Powell JT, Greenhalgh RM. Clinical practice: Small abdominal aortic aneurysms. *N Engl J Med.* 2003;348:1895–1901.
8. Cornuz J, Sidoti Pinto C, Tevaearai H, Egger M. Risk factors for asymptomatic abdominal aortic aneurysm: Systematic review and meta-analysis of population-based screening studies. *Eur J Public Health.* 2004;14:343–349.
9. Buck DB, van Herwaarden, JA, Schermerhorn ML, Moll FL. Endovascular treatment of abdominal aortic aneurysms. *Nat Rev Cardiol.* 2014;11(2):112–113.
10. Mofidi R, Goldie VJ, Kelman J, Dawson AR, Murie JA, Chalmers RT. Influence of sex on expansion rate of abdominal aortic aneurysms. *Br J Surg.* 2007;94:310–314.
11. Lo RC, Bensley RP, Hamdan AD, Wyers M, Adams JE, Schermerhorn ML; Vascular Study Group of New England. Gender differences in abdominal aortic aneurysm presentation, repair, and mortality in the Vascular Study Group of New England. *J Vasc Surg.* 2013;57:1261–1268.
12. Egorova NN, Vouyouka AG, McKinsey JF, et al. Effect of gender on long-term survival after abdominal aortic aneurysm repair based on results from the Medicare national database. *J Vasc Surg.* 2011;54:1–12.
13. Anderson RN. Deaths: Leading causes for 2000. *Natl Vital Stat Rep.* 2002;50:1–85.
14. Pearce WH, Zarins CK, Bacharach JM; AHA Writing Group 6. Atherosclerotic peripheral vascular disease symposium II: Controversies in abdominal aortic aneurysm repair. *Circulation.* 2008;118:2860–2863.
15. Acosta S, Ogren M, Bengtsson H, Bergqvist D, Lindblad B, Zdanowski Z. Increasing incidence of ruptured abdominal aortic aneurysm: A population-based study. *J Vasc Surg.* 2006; 44:237–243.
16. Sandiford P, Mosquera D, Bramley D. Trends in incidence and mortality from abdominal aortic aneurysm in New Zealand. *Br J Surg.* 2011;98:645–651.
17. Norman PE, Spilsbury K, Semmens JB. Falling rates of hospitalization and mortality from abdominal aortic aneurysms in Australia. *J Vasc Surg.* 2011;53:274–277.
18. Semmens JB, Norman PE, Lawrence-Brown MM, Bass AJ, Holman CD. Population-based record linkage study of the incidence of abdominal aortic aneurysm in Western Australia in 1985–1994. *Br J Surg.* 1998;85:648–652.
19. Fowkes FG, Macintyre CC, Ruckley CV. Increasing incidence of aortic aneurysms in England and Wales. *Br Med J.* 1989;298:33–35.
20. Filipovic M, Goldacre MJ, Roberts SE, Yeates D, Duncan ME, Cook-Mozaffari P. Trends in mortality and hospital admission rates for abdominal aortic aneurysm in England and Wales, 1979–1999. *Br J Surg.* 2005;92:968–975.
21. Anjum A, Powell JT. Is the incidence of abdominal aortic aneurysm declining in the 21st century? Mortality and hospital admissions for England & Wales and Scotland. *Eur J Vasc Endovasc Surg.* 2012;43:161–166.
22. Anjum A, von Allman R, Greenhalgh R, Powell JT. Explaining the decrease in mortality from abdominal aortic aneurysm rupture. *Br J Surg.* 2012;99:637–645.

23. US Preventive Services Task Force. Screening for abdominal aortic aneurysm: Recommendation statement. *Ann Intern Med.* 2005;142:198–202.

24. Moll FL, Powell JT, Fraedrich G, et al.; European Society for Vascular Surgery. Management of abdominal aortic aneurysms clinical practice guidelines of the European Society for Vascular Surgery. *Eur J Vasc Endovasc Surg.* 2011;41(Suppl 1):S1–S58.

25. Volodos NL, Shekhanin VE, Karpovich IP, Troian VI, Gur'ev IA. A self-fixing synthetic blood vessel endoprosthesis [in Russian]. *Vestn Khir Im I I Grek.* 1986;137:123–125.

26. Parodi JC, Palmaz JC, Barone HD. Transfemoral intraluminal graft implantation for abdominal aortic aneurysms. *Ann Vasc Surg.* 1991;5:491–499.

27. Schermerhorn ML, Bensley RP, Giles KA, et al. Changes in abdominal aortic aneurysm rupture and short-term mortality, 1995–2008: A retrospective observational study. *Ann Surg.* 2012;256:651–658.

28. Wailliez C, Coussement G. CFD study of multilayer stent haemodynamics effects in abdominal aortic aneurysms. http://www.cardiatis.com.

29. Augsburger L, Farhat M, Asakura F, Ouared R, Stergiopulos N, Rüfenacht D. Hemodynamical effects of Cardiatis braided stents in sidewall aneurysms silicone models using PIV. http://www.cardiatis.com.

30. Liou TM, Li YC. Effects of stent porosity on hemodynamics in sidewall aneurysm model. *J Biomech.* 2008;41:1174–1183.

31. Sfyroeras GS, Dalainas I, Giannakopoulos TG, Antonopoulos K, Kakisis JD, Liapis CD. Flow-diverting stents for the treatment of arterial aneurysms. *J Vasc Surg.* 2012;56:839–846.

32. Ferrero E, Ferri M, Viazzo A, et al. Visceral artery aneurysms, an experience on 32 cases in a single center: Treatment from surgery to multilayer stent. *Ann Vasc Surg.* 2011;25:923–935.

33. Ruffino M, Rabbia C; Italian Cardiatis Registry Investigators Group. Endovascular treatment of visceral artery aneurysms with Cardiatis multilayer flow modulator: Preliminary results at six-month follow-up. *J Cardiovasc Surg.* 2011;52:311–321.

34. Henry M, Polydorou A, Frid N, et al. Treatment of renal artery aneurysm with the multilayer stent. *J Endovasc Ther.* 2008;15:231–236.

35. Zhang L, Yin CP, Li HY, et al. Multiple overlapping bare stents for the endovascular visceral aneurysm repair: A potential alternative endovascular strategy to multilayer stents. *Ann Vasc Surg.* 2013;27(5):606–612.

36. Reijen MM, van Sterkenburg SM. Treatment of a Salmonella-induced rapidly expanding aortic pseudoaneurysm involving the visceral arteries using the Cardiatis multilayer stent. *J Vasc Surg.* 2014;60(4):1056–1058.

37. Euringer W, Südkamp M, Rylski B, Blanke P. Endovascular treatment of multiple HIV-related aneurysms using multilayer stents. *Cardiovasc Intervent Radiol.* 2012;35(4):945–949.

38. Benjelloun A, Henry M, Ghannam A, et al. Endovascular treatment of a tuberculous thoracoabdominal aneurysm with the multilayer stent. *J Endo Ther.* 2012;19:115–120.

39. Kahn SL, Peeran S, Smolinski S, Norris M, Rhee SW, Kaufman J. In vivo construction of a multilayer bare-metal stent for the treatment of an aortic mycotic pseudoaneurysm. *J Vasc Surg.* 2015;62(3):744–746.

40. Bayer AS, Scheld WM. Endocarditis and intravascular infections. In: Mandell GL, Bennett JE, Dolin R, eds. *Principles and Practice of Infectious Diseases.* 5th ed. Philadelphia: Churchill Livingstone; 2000:888–892.

41. Fillmore AJ, Valentine RJ. Surgical mortality in patients with infected aortic aneurysms. *J Am Coll Surg.* 2003;196:435–441.

42. Kim CY, Guevara CJ, Engstrom BI, et al. Analysis of infection risk following covered stent exclusion of pseudoaneurysms in prosthetic arteriovenous hemodialysis access grafts. *J Vasc Interv Radiol.* 2012;23(1):69–74.

CHAPTER 12

Obtaining True Lumen Access in Aortic Dissections with Iliac Extension

Roshni A. Parikh and David M. Williams

Brief Description

Aortic dissection resulting in lower extremity ischemia is an emergent condition requiring urgent endovascular treatment of the aorta and iliofemoral arteries to restore blood flow to the lower extremities. Most interventions require retrograde access to the true lumen of the common femoral arteries. If the common femoral artery is dissected, retrograde access to the true lumen can be challenging. This chapter describes several effective methods of obtaining access to the true lumen of a dissected common femoral artery.

It is rare for the dissection to extend into bilateral common femoral arteries. A key first step for this technique involves obtaining retrograde true lumen access to the uninvolved common femoral artery and crossing the aortic bifurcation into the true lumen of the dissected common iliac artery. A wire is passed across the bifurcation down the true lumen of the dissected common femoral artery. Wire position in the desired common femoral artery true lumen can easily be confirmed by intravascular ultrasound (IVUS) or by contrast injection from the contralateral access. A 6- or 8-mm balloon is then advanced over the wire from the puncture site down to the common femoral artery. The balloon is inflated and then punctured under fluoroscopic guidance, ideally through one wall. A guidewire is then inserted through the needle into the collapsing balloon. The balloon is deflated, and as the balloon is retracted from the opposite side, the wire is advanced from the new puncture site. Again, true lumen location of the wire is confirmed from the puncture site to the abdominal aorta by IVUS.

A variation on this technique can be used when the dissection ends at the common femoral bifurcation and spares the superficial femoral artery (SFA). The SFA is punctured under ultrasound guidance, and a 0.018-in. wire is placed and advanced into the true lumen of the external iliac artery. A 6-mm balloon is then advanced over the 0.018-in. wire to the common femoral artery, where it is inflated, punctured, and a guidewire is similarly fed into the deflating balloon as before. As the balloon deflates, it is pushed further into the ipsilateral iliac artery and the wire is advanced from the common femoral artery.

This technique can also be used when the dissection extends to the femoral bifurcation and the false lumen is thrombosed. In all cases, confirmation of true lumen access is necessary before proceeding with endovascular treatment.

Applications of the Technique

1. Access to the true lumen during endovascular intervention.
2. Retrograde access for endovascular intervention of the common femoral artery.

Challenges of the Procedure

1. Confirmation of access into the true lumen is vital prior to advancement and insufflation of the balloon. Knowledge and skill in the use and interpretation of IVUS will aid substantially with this procedure.
2. Advancement of the 0.018-in. Cope wire (Cook Medical Inc., Bloomington, IN) during balloon deflation can be difficult, but only a few centimeters is sufficient to allow conversion to a retrograde access and upsizing to a 0.035-in. system.

Potential Pitfalls/Complications

1. Femoral artery thrombosis: If the false lumen is thrombosed, access proceeds as discussed previously. If the true lumen is thrombosed, generally it is limited to the common iliac or to the internal and external iliac arteries, sparing the common femoral artery. In these cases, we perform mechanical thrombolysis (AngioJet Ultra Peripheral Thrombectomy System, Boston Scientific Inc. Marlborough, MA) in evacuation mode. Occasionally, a thrombosed false lumen extending to the common femoral artery bifurcation is encountered. In these cases, we first address all the malperfusion problems. Then, following reperfusion, we perform a femoral artery cut down with local false lumen thrombectomy. Bilateral femoral artery true lumen thrombosis is rare.

2. Vessel perforation/rupture: In these cases, the arterial wall is already disrupted and weakened by the dissection; therefore, manipulation of these vessels with balloon insufflation and guidewire movement can cause further wall injury. Careful fluoroscopic monitoring, IVUS, contrast injections, and hemodynamic monitoring will help identify vessel injury. We have not encountered this complication.

Steps of the Procedure

1. Obtain retrograde access to the uninvolved femoral artery (or the left brachial artery; however, in more than 500 cases, brachial artery access has not been required).
2. Insert the desired sheath into the true lumen of the aorta. This may require verification with IVUS.
3. Cross the aortic bifurcation within the true lumen to access the target common femoral artery antegrade from the aortic bifurcation.
4. Verify that the true lumen was selected using IVUS or contrast injection into the common femoral artery.
5. Insert a 6 × 40-mm or 8 × 40-mm semi-compliant balloon through the contralateral access, and place the balloon at the site of desired access in the true lumen of the target common femoral artery.
6. Inflate the balloon to expand the true lumen, collapsing the false lumen.
7. Using a 21 gauge micropuncture needle, under direct fluoroscopic guidance, puncture the inflated balloon, situated in the true lumen of the common femoral artery.
8. Advance a 0.018-in. Cope wire through the micropuncture needle into the balloon.
9. Deflate the balloon.
10. Withdraw the deflating balloon from the contralateral access while simultaneously advancing the wire to secure access to the true lumen of the common femoral artery.
11. Upsize to a 0.035-in. system with the transitional dilator.
12. Insert the desired sheath through the true lumen of the common femoral artery.
13. Now that true lumen access is obtained bilaterally, the desired endovascular arterial repair can begin.

Example
See Figure 12.1.

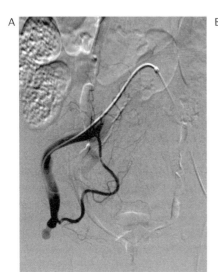 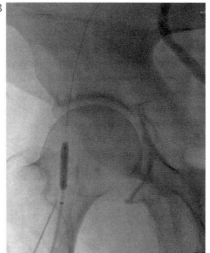 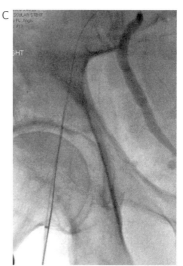

Figure 12.1 (A) Retrograde left common femoral arterial access is obtained and a catheter is seen after crossing the aortic bifurcation within the true lumen. Right pelvic angiogram shows dissection of the right common femoral artery. (B) From the left common femoral access, a 6- or 8–mm balloon is advanced to the right common femoral arterial access site and the balloon is insufflated. A 21 gauge micropuncture needle is seen being advanced toward the balloon to obtain retrograde true lumen access to the right common femoral artery. (C) During balloon deflation, a wire is advanced into the true lumen of the right common femoral artery. Bilateral true lumen access is obtained.

CHAPTER 13

The Endoconduit for Small Iliac Access

Ripal T. Gandhi, Jonathan J. Iglesias, Constantino S. Peña, and James F. Benenati

Brief Description

Advances in minimally invasive technology have led to the pioneering of novel endovascular interventions to address aortic pathology. Despite the advancement of both technique and technology, the utility of endovascular aneurysm repair (EVAR), thoracic endovascular aneurysm repair (TEVAR), and transcatheter aortic valve replacement (TAVR) remains directly correlated to the operator's ability to obtain permissible remote arterial access.

Published data demonstrate that up to 21% of patients undergoing TEVAR require the use of conduit or graft-based access techniques to combat unfavorable iliofemoral anatomy.[1,2] The presence of small-caliber, torturous, or extensively calcified diseased vessels precludes the use of standard femoral access techniques for large-profile device introduction. Thorough examination of the anatomy, beyond the aortic pathology, with computed tomography angiography (CTA) imaging extending distally through the femoral heads allows for the assessment of the distal vasculature and proper pre-procedural planning. The precise assessment of the morphology and diameter of the iliac vessels is critical for establishing a patient-specific plan for intervention, determining device selection, and avoiding potential access-related complications. In one series, iliac access-related complications were seen in 12% of patients and were significantly associated with Asian ethnicity, age older than 80 years, and external iliac diameters smaller than 7.5 mm.[3] Interpretation of the data across all ethnic backgrounds revealed female patients were twice as likely to be deemed unsuitable for standard EVAR compared to male patients (62.3% vs. 33.6%). Female patients also exhibited a statistically significant difference in external iliac artery diameter (7.29 mm vs. 8.62 mm).[4]

Many techniques exist to circumvent the challenges imposed by suboptimal iliac anatomy. Hybrid procedures implementing open surgical techniques as an adjunct to endovascular therapy employ the use of conduits for the successful passage of larger devices. The most common of these procedures involves the placement of an open surgical conduit through a retroperitoneal exposure of the common iliac artery or distal aorta. Direct iliac or aortic access via arteriotomy can also be achieved with retroperitoneal exposure. This technique does not necessitate the use of prosthesis, thus eliminating the concern for potential graft infection. Finally, transapical access is an alternative in the setting of hostile access such as aortic occlusion.

Retroperitoneal exposure and its associated morbidities can be avoided completely by using a variety of endovascular techniques that allow for successful femoral access. Balloon angioplasty and sequential dilatation may be helpful in some cases; however, they may not be adequate, and they carry a risk of arterial rupture and dissection in very diseased access vessels. A novel technique first described by Peterson and Matsumura in 2008 involves the controlled rupture of the external iliac artery.[5] This technique utilizes an endoconduit that is deployed across the diseased iliac segment from a femoral approach. Following deployment, the endoconduit is aggressively balloon-angioplastied. This creates a proximal and distal seal while rupturing the diseased iliac segment, and it allows passage of large-profile sheaths and devices.

Applications of the Technique

1. Introduction of large sheaths or large-profile devices in the presence of stenotic iliac artery disease for the following applications:
   a. EVAR
   b. TEVAR
   c. TAVR

Challenges of the Procedure

1. Distal external iliac or common femoral artery stenosis preventing advancement of large sheath: If a large sheath cannot be introduced after endoconduit placement, there may be persistent stenosis in the intervening segment between the distal end of the endoconduit and the femoral artery access site. One option is to extend the endoconduit distally; however, this may not be sufficient to introduce a large sheath/device. An approach we have utilized in the presence of a surgical cutdown is to extend a Viabahn (W.L. Gore & Associates Inc., Flagstaff, AZ) outside of the common femoral artery. We have coined the term "endoexoconduit" to describe the graft utilized in this manner. After the procedure is completed, the Viabahn is cut at the arterial access site and pushed into the artery. Alternatively, the endoexoconduit may be anastomosed to the femoral artery.

2. Inability to advance sheath after endoconduit placement secondary to compliant iliac vessel: Following

endoconduit placement, the goal is to rupture the native iliac artery to facilitate delivery of a large sheath/device. However, some patients have compliant arteries that will recoil following balloon dilatation of endoconduit, preventing advancement of a sheath/device with a large profile. In such a setting, the SoloPath sheath (Terumo Medical Corp., Somerset, NJ) may be valuable because it is a balloon-expandable sheath that is introduced as a smaller sheath and is subsequently expanded via an internal noncompliant balloon. A 15 Fr SoloPath sheath can be expanded to a 24 Fr sheath following expansion.

Potential Pitfalls/Complications

1. Ischemic complications from hypogastric artery occlusion: Avoiding sacrifice of the hypogastric artery is ideal; however, this is not always possible. Ischemic complications following coverage and/or embolization of the hypogastric artery include buttock claudication and impotence. More severe complications, such as bowel ischemia, paraplegia, and gluteal necrosis, have also been described.[6] Evaluation of the patency of the contralateral hypogastric artery is important because contralateral hypogastric stenosis or occlusion may increase the risk of ischemic complications. In the presence of inferior mesenteric artery occlusion and contralateral hypogastric occlusion, there is increased risk of colonic ischemia from ipsilateral hypogastric occlusion. Maintaining patency of the ipsilateral deep circumflex iliac and inferior epigastric arteries, whenever possible, is recommended to allow for collateral perfusion of the pelvis.

2. Hemorrhage from rupture at patent hypogastric artery: During controlled rupture of the iliac artery after placement of a covered stent across the hypogastric artery, rupture at the hypogastric artery may occur with potential for retrograde hemorrhage. Embolization of the hypogastric artery prior to endoconduit placement would preclude this complication, and this strategy should be considered when there is significant stenosis adjacent to the hypogastric artery.[7] If hypogastric embolization has not been performed and there is hemorrhage related to hypogastric artery back bleeding after endoconduit placement, one may consider embolization of the contralateral hypogastric artery with gelfoam to stop the hemorrhage. Gelfoam is preferred over other embolic agents because it is temporary.

3. Endoconduit enfolding or collapse: Meticulous sizing of the proximal and distal landing zone is mandatory, and the endoconduit should be appropriately sized. Covered stents should not be oversized because there is risk of device infolding and collapse, resulting in technical failure and the need for additional interventions.[8]

Steps of the Procedure/Technique

1. Evaluate preprocedural imaging (i.e., CTA) for the presence of stenotic iliac arteries, which may prevent delivery of a large-profile sheath or device. Significant calcification and tortuosity may also present a challenge.

2. Based on anticipated delivery sheath French size, determine the diameter of endoconduit necessary (Table 13.1). Experience has shown that at least 10-mm balloon angioplasty is necessary for passage of sheaths up to 22 Fr and 12-mm angioplasty for 24 Fr sheaths.[9]

3. Obtain femoral artery access and perform a pelvic angiogram to further delineate the degree of iliac artery disease. There must be relatively normal proximal and distal landing zones into which the endoconduit is placed to allow for adequate seal and prevention of endoleak.

4. After placement of a stiff guidewire (i.e., Amplatzer [St. Jude Medical Inc., St. Paul, MN], Meier [Boston Scientific Inc., Marlborough, MA], or Lunderquist [Cook Medical Inc., Bloomington, IN]), an initial attempt with serial dilatation of the iliac arteries may be made if there is a possibility of advancing the sheath without placing an endoconduit. If there is resistance, one should not force the device because rupture may occur.

5. If covering the hypogastric artery with endoconduit, consider hypogastric embolization, especially if there is significant narrowing and calcification adjacent to this vessel.

6. Advance and deploy a covered stent in the common and external iliac artery, typically across the hypogastric artery. If the disease is limited to the external iliac artery, the hypogastric may be spared. The distal end of the endoconduit should be extended to at

Table 13.1 Determining Endoconduit Diameter

FRENCH SIZE	SHEATH OUTER DIAMETER (MM)	ENDOCONDUIT DIAMETER (MM)	ANGIOPLASTY BALLOON (MM)
20	7.6	10	10
22	8.3	10	10
24	9.2	11–13	12

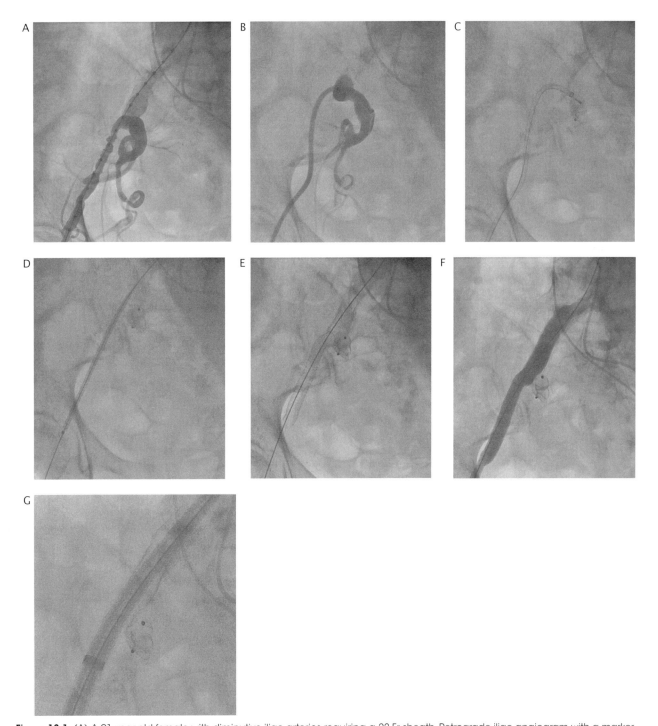

Figure 13.1 (A) A 91-year-old female with diminutive iliac arteries requiring a 22-Fr sheath. Retrograde iliac angiogram with a marker straight catheter in place over a stiff Lunderquist wire highlights small vessel size. (B) Placement of a 6-Fr Destination sheath (Terumo) into the right hypogastric artery in preparation to embolize the hypogastric artery origin. (C) Embolization of the hypogastric artery origin with an Amplatzer device. This can also be performed with coils. (D) A 10-mm-diameter Viabahn stent graft was placed from the distal external iliac artery across the hypogastric into the proximal common iliac artery. (E) A 13-mm-diameter Viabahn stent graft was then placed into the right common iliac artery overlapping with the distal stent graft. Attention is focused on avoiding the aortic bifurcation and minimizing overlap with the distal stent graft. The larger common iliac stent is placed into the smaller diameter external iliac stent graft so that the smaller stent graft does not float inside the larger diameter graft. (F) Using an insufflator, the external iliac stent graft was dilated to 10 mm and the common iliac stent graft was dilated to 12 mm. The most stenotic or smaller diameter vessels will undergo a controlled rupture. Angiography confirms new diameter conduit and lack of extravasation of contrast. (G) The delivery sheath is then slowly advanced using fluoroscopy into the distal aorta for further therapy.

least the inguinal ligament. Viabahn is our covered stent of choice for endoconduits because it is a self-expandable stent that is flexible, low profile, and can handle tortuous anatomy quite well. In addition, it is available in long lengths. Iliac limb endoprosthetic limbs designed for EVAR can also be used in this manner; however, they are larger in profile. iCAST covered stent (Atrium Medical Corp., Hudson, NH) is an alternative and may be more beneficial for common iliac occlusive disease.

7. The proximal and distal ends of the endoconduit are initially balloon dilated to create a seal. This is followed by noncompliant balloon angioplasty of the covered stent for controlled dilatation and potential rupture of the native iliac arteries.[10]

8. Angiogram is performed to evaluate the endoconduit and for potential complications.

9. Introduce the sheath/delivery device under fluoroscopic guidance to ensure smooth passage through the endoconduit.

10. Anticoagulate the patient.

11. After completion of the aortic procedure, a final iliac angiogram should be considered after removal of the delivery sheath/device to exclude access complications. Guidewire access should be maintained until final angiogram is completed.

Example
See Figure 13.1.

References and Suggested Readings

1. Matsumura JS. Worldwide survey of thoracic endografts: Practical clinical application. *J Vasc Surg.* 2005;43:20-1A.

2. Matsumura JS, Cambria RP, Dake MD, Moore RD, Svensson LG, Snyder S; TX2 Clinical Trial Investigators. International controlled clinical trial of thoracic endovascular aneurysm repair with the Zenith TX2 endovascular graft: 1-year results. *J Vasc Surg.* 2008;47:247–257.

3. Masuda EM, Caps MT, Singh N, et al. Effect of ethnicity on access and device complications during endovascular aneurysm repair. *J Vasc Surg.* 2004;40:24–29.

4. Velazquez OC, Larson RA, Baum RA, et al. Gender-related differences in infrarenal aortic aneurysm morphologic features: Issues relevant to Ancure and Talent endografts. *J Vasc Surg.* 2001;33(2 Suppl):S77–S84.

5. Peterson BG, Matsumura JS. Internal endoconduit: An innovative technique to address unfavorable iliac artery anatomy encountered during thoracic endovascular aortic repair. *J Vasc Surg.* 2008;47:441–445.

6. Lee WA, O'Dorisio J, Wolf YG, et al. Outcome after unilateral hypogastric artery occlusion during endovascular aneurysm repair. *J Vasc Surg.* 2001;33(5):921–926.

7. Peterson BG, Matsumura JS. Tips and tricks for avoiding access problems when using large sheath endografts. *J Vasc Surg.* 2009;49(2):524–527.

8. Peterson BG, Matsumura JS. Creative options for large sheath access during aortic endografting. *J Vasc Interv Radiol.* 2008;19(6):S22–S26.

9. Peterson BG. Conduits and endoconduits, percutaneous access. *J Vasc Surg.* 2010;52(4):60S–64S.

10. Peterson BG, Matsumura JS. Internal endoconduit: An innovative technique to address unfavorable iliac artery anatomy encountered during thoracic endovascular aortic repair. *J Vasc Surg.* 2008;47(2):441–445.

CHAPTER 14

Transcaval Aortic Catheterization for Transcatheter Aortic Valve Replacement and Thoracic Endovascular Aortic Repair Device Delivery

Michael D. Dake

Brief Description

During the past decade, the development and wide-scale adoption of catheter-based techniques for treatment of thoracic aortic lesions and aortic valve pathology has required that interventionalists focus on the anatomic suitability of vascular access to allow safe introduction of large-device delivery systems during thoracic endovascular aortic repair (TEVAR) and transcatheter aortic valve implantation (TAVI).

The introduction of these technologies has been associated with the need for large-caliber arterial access ranging from 18 to 24 Fr that mandates relatively large femoral and iliac conduit arteries without significant disease. The adequacy of femoral arterial access is challenging in patients with advanced atherosclerotic disease or women with smaller iliofemoral arteries.

This consideration for TEVAR or TAVI is especially problematic when assessing candidates with high or prohibitive open surgical risk. Some reports estimate inadequate arterial access may exclude up to 25% of patients evaluated for TEVAR or TAVI.

In general, the use of large arterial sheaths is associated with a risk of major vascular complications, including arterial dissection, occlusion, rupture, as well as hemorrhage and death. Consistently, in published reports of endovascular abdominal aortic aneurysm repair (EVAR) and TEVAR, the most common complication detailed is vascular injury of the conduit iliofemoral arteries.[1-4] The frequency is typically more than twice that observed for the next most common reported complication.

Consequently, considerations of alternative arterial access or adjunctive femoral access techniques to increase the safety of access and reduce the overall procedural risk for patients with challenging access is critically important for the success of TEVAR or TAVI. In patients with no good options for traditional access to the aorta, a wide variety of alternative approaches have been employed, including (1) creation of surgical or endovascular conduits with open placement of a graft segment onto the femoral, iliac, axillary, or subclavian arteries and (2) an intraluminal stent graft dilated to a sufficient caliber to allow passage of the delivery system.

Alternatively, depending on the specific anatomy of the patient, direct aortic, carotid, and transapical cardiac access following surgical exposure have all been used for device introduction.[5-9] However, unfavorable anatomy and patient comorbidities may limit all these nonstandard approaches, which require more invasive exposure and have been associated with increased morbidity and mortality. Recent studies detail considerable postoperative complication rates as high as 16% and associated mortality rates ranging from 3% to 12%.[5,6]

In the treatment of type II endoleaks following EVAR, transcaval aortic access has been used as an alternative to translumbar aortic access to avoid the need for prone positioning of the patient, which is uncomfortable; the necessity of traversing multiple tissue planes via a translumbar needle trajectory with potential risk of inadvertent injury to adjacent peri-aortic structures; and general anesthesia, which is often required.[10] This approach for embolization of type II endoleaks after EVAR is now considered a complimentary strategy in selected cases when more traditional techniques have failed or are less attractive due to anatomic challenges.

Similarly, transcaval aortic access to allow TAVI and TEVAR has been described in patients in whom adequate standard femoral arterial access for device introduction was not anatomically feasible.[11-15] The technique in conjunction with TAVI was initially reported in 2014 by Greenbaum et al.[12] and Lederman et al.[13]

Technique

The procedure involves transcatheter puncture of the abdominal aorta from the inferior vena cava (IVC), with delivery of a large vascular sheath and tract closure post device delivery using a nitinol occlusion device. The feasibility of this technique was initially demonstrated in preclinical testing in swine.[11]

In a TAVI series detailed by Greenbaum et al.,[12] 19 patients with severe symptomatic aortic valvular heart disease were deemed high or prohibitive surgical risk. All were not suitable for femoral arterial or transapical TAVI due to iliofemoral arteries that were anatomically unsuitable for standard access due to small size, advanced occlusive disease, and/or heavy calcification.

In preparation for caval-aortic access, patients underwent contrast-enhanced computed tomography (CT) of the abdomen and pelvis to identify a caval-aortic crossing path designed to intersect the aorta in its least calcified segment while avoiding vital interposed structures. Ideally, this is at a level at which the IVC and abdominal aorta are adjacent to one another to limit the length of the communicating tract. The CT scan is also used to determine the ideal angiographic projections for the procedure and to landmark key soft tissue structures to specific lumbar vertebrae for the purpose of translating this registration to fluoroscopic imaging at the time of aortic access.

At the time of the procedure, the patient is placed supine on the examination table, and after standard prepping and draping, arterial and femoral venous access are obtained. After heparin administration, simultaneous aortography and iliocaval venography are performed. A 15- to 20-mm-diameter gooseneck or trilobe snare is then positioned within the aorta at the desired level of crossing via the left femoral artery approach. The preferred location is viewed in orthogonal fluoroscopic projections.

Two techniques for caval-aortic crossing have been employed. The method detailed by Greenbaum et al.[12] and Lederman et al.[13,14] involves a triaxial system consisting of an exchange, stiff 0.014-in. inside a 0.035-in. wire convertor (PiggyBack, Vascular Solutions, Minneapolis, MN) inside a 4 Fr support catheter (Navicross [Terumo, Somerset, NJ] or Minnie Support Catheter [Vascular Solutions]). The PiggyBack catheter has a 0.035-in. outer diameter and 0.014-in. inner diameter, which allow conversion from 0.014-in. guidewires to 0.035-in. inner-lumen catheters.

This system is loaded into a preshaped 6 Fr guiding catheter (RDC or RDC1) placed in the caudal IVC via the right femoral vein and selected on the basis of the caval diameter at the level of crossing. The crossing system is then directed toward the aortic snare, which serves as a target.

The proximal end of the 0.014-in. caval guidewire is connected by a clamp to an electrocautery device (Bovie Medical, Clearwater, FL) or unipolar electrosurgery pencil (Valleylab, Covidien, Mansfield, MA), and the patient is connected to a ground pad. The distal tip of the guidewire is extended 2–5 mm beyond the wire converter and energized by using the "cut" setting at 50–70 W. Short 1- to 3-second bursts of energy are administered to vaporize tissue as the wire aimed at the snare is advanced into the abdominal aorta. After initial case experience, the distal 1 cm of the guidewire was amputated to ease crossing.

Intraluminal wire position within the aorta is confirmed by its capture within the snare. The guidewire and enclosing snare are advanced into the thoracic aorta. The transitional converting catheter and the 4 Fr support catheter follow the wire into the thoracic aorta. At this point, the guidewire and converting catheter are removed, and a stiff 0.035-in. guidewire (Lunderquist, Cook Medical, Bloomington, IN) is introduced via the support catheter.

Alternatively, transcaval puncture of the aorta has been accomplished with a needle and sheath system that is directed by a stainless-steel guiding cannula. Initially, a precurved (60- to 80-degrees tip angle) cannula intended for use in transjugular intrahepatic portosystemic shunt procedures (Rosch-Uchida transjugular liver access set, Cook Medical) or, alternatively, to facilitate percutaneous creation of a gastrojejunostomy (Cope gastrojejunostomy cannula, Cook Medical) is advanced over a 0.035-in. guidewire through a sheath (9 Fr) placed in the right femoral vein. Once at the appropriate level for crossing, the guidewire is withdrawn and a needle/sheath combination composed of a 21 gauge needle within a 4 or 5 Fr catheter with 0.035-in. lumen is coaxially inserted and advanced until just below the tip of the cannula.

The cannula is then turned so its tip is directed at the aortic target based on imaging landmarks and an intra-aortic snare. The needle is positioned approximately 1 or 2 cm outside the catheter, and this combination is advanced out of the cannula through the IVC wall for a predetermined distance to ensure intraluminal communication out of the cannula. After the needle is advanced a proper distance and presumed to be within the aortic lumen, a 0.014- or 0.018-in. guidewire is introduced through the 21 gauge needle and directed into the snare in the thoracic aorta. The catheter is then advanced over the guidewire while pinning the needle in its position. Once the catheter is well above the crossing site, the guidewire and needle are withdrawn together and a hand injection of contrast media is used to confirm an intra-aortic location. The stiff 0.035-in. exchange guidewire is then introduced through the catheter to support placement of the crossing sheath.

An appropriately sized angiographic sheath to allow device introduction for TAVI or TEVAR is advanced from the right femoral vein into the IVC and then passed across the intravascular tract into the abdominal aorta in a single step without progressive dilation. In some reports, an expandable vascular sheath (eSheath [Edwards Lifesciences, Irvine, CA] or Solo-Path [Terumo]) has been used to bridge the caval-aortic tract.

Immediately following sheath placement, aortography is performed to evaluate hemostasis. Then, TAVI or TEVAR is performed in the standard manner. After successful device deployment, heparin anticoagulation is reversed fully with protamine before the caval-aortic access tract is closed using a septal closure device. This is an important step in order to enhance hemostasis because nitinol septal closure devices (Amplatzer ASD and Muscular VSD Occluders, St. Jude Medical Inc., St. Paul, MN) are not designed for this application and are commonly not immediately hemostatic.

After heparin reversal, a soft or medium-stiffness 0.014-in. buddy guidewire is advanced into the thoracic aorta through the aortocaval sheath. This wire serves as insurance to allow bailout access to the aorta in case of unintended premature withdrawal of the sheath into the cava, inadvertent pull-through of the closure device out of the aorta, or other unexpected failure of the aortocaval closure that requires retrieval of the closure device that is not deployed using an over-the-wire catheter delivery system.

In this regard, it is important to have a back table bail rescue kit ready in case of tract closure failure necessitating Amplatzer retrieval or removal. This should include a 4 or 5 Fr multipurpose shape catheter for insertion over the buddy wire, 0.035-in. Lunderquist wire to replace the buddy wire, and appropriately sized dilator for the caval-aortic sheath to allow re-advancement of the sheath over the stiff guidewire into the aorta to obturate the tract and aortic communication.

A deflectable 8.5 Fr catheter (Agilis NxT or SML curl, St. Jude Medical Inc., St. Paul, MN) is used to facilitate deployment of the Amplatzer closure device by allowing the initial disc of the device to orient perpendicular to the aortic wall during pullback and exposure. Selection of the most appropriate nitinol Amplatzer closure device requires some experience and judgment for optimal results and balances the risk of inadequate hemostasis associated with undersizing and pinching of the aorta with device malapposition related to oversizing.

In most cases, the aortocaval tract length is 7 mm or less. In the setting when the sheath for TAVI or TEVAR device introduction is greater than 18 Fr, an 8-mm Amplatzer Muscular VSD Occluder is ideal. This device is composed of two 8-mm nitinol discs connected by a 7-mm stem. One disc is placed within the aorta and the other in the IVC with the 7-mm-long stem located in the intervening tract. The discs are composed of a nitinol mesh with polyester fabric lining.

The ventricular septal defect (VSD) closure device is designed differently from the atrial septal defect (ASD) device, which incorporates asymmetric disc diameters with a disc intended for left atrial placement that is 4 mm greater in diameter than the right atrial disc. This is independent of the size of the defect. The stem connecting the discs is 3 or 4 mm long, depending on the diameter of the defect to be closed.

If the aortocaval tract is greater than 7 mm long, a 10/8 Amplatzer Duct Occluder (generation 1 type) is recommended. Like the ASD and VSD devices, the discs are made of nitinol mesh with polyester fabric lining. The device has an anchoring skirt that is 12 mm in diameter and is placed in juxtaposition to the luminal wall of the aorta. The device below the skirt tapers from 10 mm at the aortic end to 8 mm at the caval end over a length of 8 mm.

When the introducer sheath for TAVI or TEVAR is equal to or less than 18 Fr, a 6-mm Amplatzer Muscular VSD Occluder is recommended for aortocaval tracts that are 7 mm long or less; for tracts longer than 7 mm, an 8/6 Amplatzer Duct Occluder (generation 1 type) is used for closure.

Measurement of these parameters is important in selecting the most appropriate closure device. If the waist of the occluder is too short for the length of the aortocaval tract, such that the venous disc of the Amplatzer Muscular VSD Occluder is unable to reach the cava, it probably will not be effective.

After selection of the Amplatzer system for tract closure, it is flushed, prepped, and loaded into the deflectable delivery catheter. It is then advanced to the tip of the delivery catheter, which is positioned just beyond the end of the large TAVI/TEVAR introducer sheath in the aorta. This relative position of the tandem of delivery catheter outside the introducer sheath is fixed, and the two are slowly withdrawn until they are 3 or 4 cm or one-half a vertebral body above the aortic entry location.

Care is taken to not inadvertently withdraw the sheath outside the aorta prematurely. The aortic disc is then passively exposed, and the deflectable delivery catheter is flexed to orient the disc parallel with the aortic wall. There must be adequate separation of the delivery catheter outside the introducer sheath to permit the desired degree of catheter flexion.

The next maneuver is steady withdrawal of the introducer sheath until it is completely outside of the aorta and well inside the IVC. Partial or incomplete withdrawal of the sheath into the cava will cause massive retroperitoneal bleeding due to blockage of the naturally protective route of low-pressure venous return. The pressure in the IVC is lower than the pressure in the retroperitoneal tissue surrounding the aortocaval tract and thus provides a preferred direction of drainage for blood escaping the aorta.

Continued flexion of the deflectable delivery catheter after the sheath is fully withdrawn and further deployment of the aortic disc are performed using a push–pull motion to expose more of the disc while maintaining an orientation of the disc so that it is parallel to the aortic wall. Once the aortic disc is fully exposed and properly oriented, the occluder is withdrawn to snuggly abut the right aortic wall.

At this point, a pigtail aortic flush catheter previously positioned below the aortic entry site from a femoral approach is advanced above the occluder device. Catheter injections of contrast media followed by imaging are used to evaluate the disc position. Even with appropriate disc apposition, brisk aortocaval tract flow and IVC opacification is commonly seen.

While maintaining tension on the aortic disc, the deflectable delivery catheter is gradually straightened as it is further withdrawn to passively expose the stretched extra-aortic segment within the retroperitoneal tract. If the device used is an Amplatzer Muscular VSD Occluder, the goal is to reach the cava and reform the second disc within the IVC lumen. If an Amplatzer Duct Occluder is used, the aim is only to oppose the right wall of the aorta.

The final maneuver is to advance the delivery cable attached to the Amplatzer VSD Occluder to re-form the second disc of the closure device within the IVC. Occasionally, despite preprocedure CT imaging and planning measurements that indicate an adequate aortocaval distance to allow intraluminal expansion of the double disc occlude within the aorta and IVC, the venous disc of the Amplatzer Muscular VSD Occluder fails to reach the cava. This may be due to intervening retroperitoneal hematoma that develops intraprocedurally and displaces the vascular structures. Although this is not ideal, there is little recourse; fortunately, there is little clinical consequence from not achieving caval disc position.

During these maneuvers, a drop in systolic blood pressure is frequently encountered. This is usually not sustained unless there is an associated severe aortic injury or failure to fully withdraw the large venous sheath into the IVC, thus preventing venous decompression. Once the closure device is fully exposed and positioned, the blood pressure typically returns rapidly to baseline levels. If there is prolonged hemodynamic instability at this stage, urgent blood transfusion may be necessary, but this is an uncommon event.

Digital subtraction angiography via the aortic pigtail catheter positioned proximal to the closure device is performed to confirm proper device position before final release. This is carried out during patient breath-hold and using late-phase imaging to enhance detection and extravasation of contrast media. If the positioning of the closure device is adequate, the delivery cable is released by a counterclockwise rotational maneuver. The twisting motion unscrews the connection between the delivery cable and the device. At this point, the safety buddy guidewire is also removed.

If the device is not satisfactorily positioned, it may be recaptured prior to release. However, this maneuver should not be performed without clear and strong justification because recapture of the closure device may result in vascular injury to the aorta and/or IVC. If there is an obvious indication for device recapture, proper preparation for recrossing must be undertaken. This includes readying of a 0.035-in. diagnostic catheter, 0.035-in. Lunderquist stiff guidewire, and appropriately sized dilator for advancement of large delivery sheath.

Once the need for recapture is determined, the device is recaptured by a combination of coaxial advancement of the delivery catheter and withdrawal of the device until the entire implant is completely resheathed. Then, in rapid succession, the diagnostic catheter is advanced over the indwelling 0.014-in. safety buddy wire to allow rapid exchange for the Lunderquist wire. The fully constrained device and delivery catheter are then removed from the external large sheath. Next, the diagnostic catheter is withdrawn over the Lunderquist wire and the original dilator for the large sheath is introduced to allow re-advancement of the sheath from the IVC back into the aortic lumen.

Following recapture and recrossing of the sheath into the aorta, upsizing by 2 mm of a subsequent Amplatzer closure device is recommended.

Once satisfied with the outcome of the closure device placement, completion aortography is performed during breath-hold with late-phase imaging through contrast washout. In the published experience to date, four distinct angiographic patterns are noted post closure device deployment: (1) complete occlusion around the closure device with no contrast media observed outside the aorta, (2) patent fistula with residual aortocaval flow in a cylindrical pattern through the occluder, (3) patent fistula with a "cruciform" appearance extending from around the stem-like aortocaval channel but with contrast drainage to the IVC, and (4) extravasation of contrast media with persistent staining of the retroperitoneal space and minimal return to the IVC.

When using Amplatzer devices following TAVI or TEVAR performed through delivery sheaths with an outer diameter greater than 6 mm (18 Fr), a residual aortocaval fistula should be anticipated initially. Lederman et al.[14] report in their experience the most commonly encountered post-closure angiographic appearances are a patent cylindrical aortocaval fistula and a "cruciform" appearance with contrast flowing within and extending around the connecting neck of the device before draining to the IVC.

If the patient is hemodynamically stable following completion angiography and the device is satisfactorily positioned, the large-caliber delivery sheath may be removed from the femoral vein and hemostasis obtained with the use of two suture-mediated access closure devices and a preclose technique (Perclose ProGLide, Abbott Vascular, Santa Clara, CA). Alternatively, placement of a figure-of-eight suture or manual compression techniques may be used to achieve hemostasis. Once femoral vein hemostasis is obtained or approximately 10 minutes after sheath removal, it is a good idea to perform a final arteriogram from the arterial pigtail catheter.

Provided there are no complications related to the TAVI or TEVAR procedure, hemodynamic instability following removal of the venous sheath and achieving femoral hemostasis is most likely due to extravasation at the aortocaval closure site or by patient intolerance of the acute effects of a persistent arteriovenous shunt due to underlying myocardial dysfunction or pulmonary vascular disease.

If hemodynamic compromise occurs, immediate attention must be directed at excluding aortic extravasation. This is usually a straightforward diagnosis made by conventional catheter aortography. If contrast extravasation is not observed, echocardiography should be performed to evaluate acute right ventricular failure and/or sudden venous hypertension, which may indicate an inability to tolerate a persistent aortocaval fistula.

If a small volume of contrast media extravasation is identified, confirm that protamine has been administered and there is a full reversal of heparin effects. This type of mild aortic extravasation typically stops after a few minutes of observation. If it persists, it can be managed conservatively with intravenous administration of fluids and/or blood. If low blood pressure is unresponsive to volume replacement, low-dose vasopressor solutions may be initiated.

One important cause of mild persistent aortic extravasation is premature occlusion of the vena cava site of crossing by the Amplatzer Muscular VSD Occluder prior to achieving hemostasis at the aortic site. This commonly stops in short order, but occasionally the complete cessation of extravasation may be facilitated by temporary inflation of a compliant occlusion balloon at the level of the closure device.

Persistent mild leakage of contrast or more than mild aortic extravasation or any cases with hemodynamic instability unresponsive to supportive measures warrant further invasive management. A frequent initial step in these settings is inflation of a low-pressure aortic occlusion balloon (e.g., Coda [Cook Medical] and Reliant [Medtronic, Minneapolis, MN]) for approximately 5 minutes. This usually promotes successful hemostasis. In patients with small aortoiliac access vessels, the balloon catheter may be introduced without an angiographic sheath, if necessary in these situations.

After a 5-minute inflation period, aortography is repeated to check for residual extravasation. If leakage of contrast media persists, a second balloon inflation trial is performed for another 5 minutes. If this is not successful and there is continued extravasation or if the extravasation is massive, proceeding to immediate placement of an endograft of covered stent within the aorta is recommended. The diameter of the aorta at the crossing site and the length of the infrarenal abdominal aorta are important considerations that influence device selection.

Depending on these measurements and the size of the aortoiliac access for graft delivery, possible selections include self-expanding aortic extension cuffs, iliac limb extensions used in EVAR procedures, large self-expanding peripheral stent grafts (Viabahn, W. L. Gore & Associates, Flagstaff, AZ), and balloon-expandable covered stents (iCast, Maquet Medical Systems, Wayne, NJ).

Placement of an endograft to address aortic extravasation following transcaval access is estimated to be required in approximately 5% of cases. Once properly positioned and deployed in the aorta, the communication is obliterated and hemodynamic stability is restored almost immediately. To date, there are no reports of worsening of the type of angiographic pattern post closure or deterioration of the completion aortographic appearance subsequently.

Results from the literature

In the largest series of transcaval aortic access for TAVI reported in the medical literature by Greenbaum et al.,[12] 15 of 19 patients were women, underscoring the need for development of smaller profile catheter delivery systems to meet the demands of smaller iliofemoral arteries typically encountered more commonly in women than in men.

Access to the aorta via the IVC followed by transcatheter valve introduction were successful in all cases. TAVI was successful in 17 patients, with one TAVI-related mortality caused by post-deployment embolization of the valve into the ascending aorta. Another patient required emergency surgery to retrieve a transcatheter valve that embolized into the left ventricle after a too low deployment. In addition, 6 patients had major vascular complications, including significant hemorrhage in 3 patients, the requirement of abdominal aortic stent graft placement in 2 patients, and vasopressor administration in 1 patient with a pseudoaneurysm.

In this group of patients, crossing between the IVC and the aorta required 1.4 ± 0.8 puncture attempts and took an average of 20 minutes (range, 10–75 minutes) to accomplish. The intent was to create the crossings between the right renal artery and the aortic bifurcation, typically over the third lumbar vertebral body. At this level, the caval-aortic distance of separation was 6 ± 3 mm (range, 3–12 mm), and the IVC and aortic diameters were 21 ± 3 mm and 16 ± 4 mm, respectively. During the puncture and sheath placement, there were no hemodynamic changes in any of the patients, and the sheath was confirmed hemostatic in all by abdominal aortography.

Successful closure device implantation in the caval-aortic tract was accomplished in all patients. The mean time for successful device deployment was 11 minutes (range, 3–37 minutes), and this required 1.3 ± 0.7 device deployment attempts. In 5 patients, the closure device was recaptured and redeployed because of malapposition or contrast extravasation observed after the initial positioning. In five of the cases, there was transient hypotension during tract closure, including three that required device repositioning. Upon completion of the procedure, there was residual aortocaval flow documented in all patients. In 12 patients (63%), there was persistence of extra-aortic contrast staining within the retroperitoneal tissues diagnosed by aortography (cruciform appearance, $n = 11$; frank extravasation, $n = 1$). This was accompanied by hypotension in 4 patients. In 5 of the 12 patients, the closure device was reconstrained and repositioned.

Fifteen patients (79%) required blood transfusions (mean total 3 ± 4 units), 7 during the TAVI procedure and 10 post-procedures. The most serious bleeding was observed in 3 patients with an elevated international normalized ratio during TAVI. No patient had ischemic or embolic complications related to the transcaval aortic access. One patient experienced deep venous thrombosis of the femoral vein used for delivery of the transcaval large angiographic sheath.

Post-procedural care following transcaval aortic access is predicated on close surveillance of the patient's hemodynamic status. In most cases, mild to moderate anemia is tolerated without the need for transfusion of blood products. However, if hemodynamic instability exists, transfusion may be necessary, especially when the hemoglobin is less than 6 or 7 g/dl. Small amounts of retroperitoneal bleeding can be managed conservatively during the first 12–24 hours with volume replacement therapy and even low-dose vasopressor administration.

Infrequently, a patient may develop thrombocytopenia that may be severe. Generally, the patients are asymptomatic. The presumed cause is mechanical platelet injury resulting from a persistent aortocaval fistula. The thrombocytopenia described in most cases is temporary and resolves with the spontaneous closure of the fistula. In such cases, other important causes of severe thrombocytopenia must be considered, especially the possibility of a heparin-induced reaction.

In most cases, the periprocedural course is uneventful, and hemodynamic stability is maintained. Upon preparation for hospital discharge, a contrast-enhanced CT angiogram of the abdomen and pelvis is obtained to evaluate the positioning of the closure devise, aortocaval fistula patency, and any iatrogenic aortic injury. This should be performed in all patients to provide a baseline study even if completion aortography fails to demonstrate an aortocaval fistula or in cases that required a supplemental endograft. If contrast administration is not advised, alternative imaging (e.g., non-contrast magnetic resonance angiography, abdominal ultrasound of the aortocaval region, or non-contrast CT) should be performed.

Post-discharge from the hospital, follow-up CT angiographic imaging of the abdomen and pelvis should be obtained in all patients 1 month and 1 year post-procedure to evaluate any vascular or nonvascular injuries related to the transcaval aortic access, diagnose any small pseudoaneurysms developing adjacent to the aortic closure site, and to search for a persistent aortocaval fistula. There are no published reports that detail any late complications or sequelae of transcaval aortic access and closure. Of note, no cases of aortic or caval thrombosis have been reported.

In the case series reported by Greenbaum et al.,[12] CT imaging of the abdomen was performed prior to hospital discharge in 16 of the 18 eligible patients. Two patients did not undergo follow-up imaging due to renal insufficiency. Extravascular blood was identified in the retroperitoneal space in 10 patients. It was graded as mild in 8 patients and moderate to severe in 2 patients. Follow-up through 111 ± 57 days (range, 36–229 days) revealed no post-discharge access-related adverse events in the 18 survivors. Of the 16 who underwent follow-up imaging after hospital discharge, 15 had completed closure of the caval-aortic tract by 42 ± 50 days (range, 7–189 days) after TAVI.

Of note, Lederman et al.[16] published a case report describing transcaval access into a polyester abdominal aortic graft to enable TAVR. The identical technical steps described previously were employed, including the use of an Amplatzer Muscular VSD Occluder for closure, and there were no complications. The patient did well and was discharged home after 3 days.

Prior benchtop testing by Eadie et al.[17] demonstrated only minor changes in graft resistance to tearing after radio frequency perforation and dilatation of polyester and expanded polytetrafluoroethylene material used in commercial endografts. Riga et al.[18] performed benchtop fenestration and found that graft tears were unlikely when grafts were penetrated at an orthogonal angle and dilated using standard angioplasty balloons. Graft tears were more likely when the grafts were entered at an oblique angle or when dilated with a cutting balloon.

Limitations

Procedural warnings that should be considered include the increased risks of complications in the patient with a heavily calcified ("porcelain") abdominal aorta or graft. Transcaval aortic access in this setting should be avoided because the rigidity of the aortic wall may make creation of the aortotomy and subsequent passage of catheters and sheaths more difficult or impossible. The presence of heavy calcification within the aortic wall may also prevent proper closure with the occluding device due to catching or hanging up of the aortic luminal disc on an irregular and/or eccentric rigid plaque. This may prevent the necessary disc apposition and conformability required to seal.

Similarly, heavy aortic calcification may be an impediment to successful stent graft bailout in cases of brisk extravasation due to the sealing challenge it poses. Likewise, patients with near occlusion of aortoiliac arterial access, in whom bailout endovascular graft or covered stent placement in the abdominal aorta cannot be performed, should be approached cautiously.

Indeed, there are potential pitfalls associated with the transcaval approach for aortic access, and this technique should be reserved for patients with suitable anatomic features. Preferred candidates include patients with close proximity between the abdominal aorta and the IVC, a calcium-free window at the intended level of caval-aortic crossing, aortic luminal diameter sufficient to allow deployment of a closure device, and the absence of important interposed structures (i.e., duodenum and lumbar arteries) in the crossing path. Finally, the target zone should be at least 1 cm proximal to the aortic bifurcation, lowest renal artery, or lower renal vein to avoid encroachment by the occluder device.

Alternatives

The transcaval aortic access technique can be a valuable part of the endovascular interventional armamentarium to allow TAVI and TEVAR in patients without traditional or alternative options for access to the aorta. Careful patient selection based on preoperative imaging is mandatory. Although this technique has proven useful, a number of developments have enabled procedures to be performed now via access vessels that were previously deemed insufficient.

The unrelenting trend of reducing the profile of device delivery systems for TAVI and TEVAR will continue to

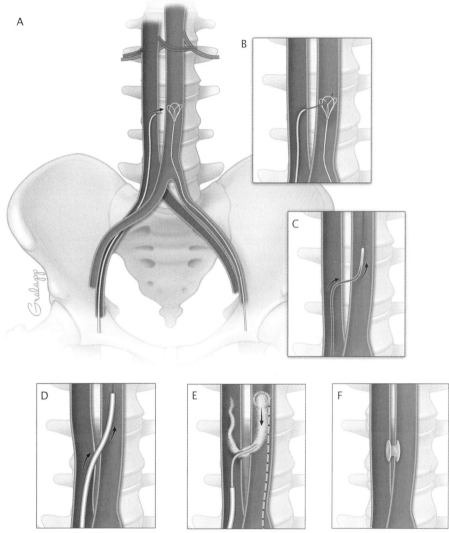

Figure 14.1 Key steps of the transcaval aortic access procedure. (A) Intra-aortic snare used as target for transcaval puncture using needle or radio-frequency and guidewire combination advanced though guiding catheter or cannula at the level of the L3 vertebral body. (B) Guidewire advanced with aid of snare into more proximal aorta. (C) 5-Fr catheter advanced over guidewire to establish transcaval aortic access. Guidewire exchange via transcaval aortic catheter to establish Lunderquist or equivalent stiff guidewire for large sheath and device introduction. (D) Large delivery sheath and dilator advanced via femoral vein access over transcaval aortic exchange guidewire. (E) Post-delivery of TAVI or TEVAR device, large delivery sheath is withdrawn into inferior vena cava (IVC) and delivery catheter positioned for implantation of tract closure device. Injection of contrast media from aortic catheter flows through tract and drains preferentially via fistula to IVC. (F) Appearance following deployment of double disc occlusion device in tract between aorta and IVC.

enable increasingly more patients to be approached via traditional femoral arterial access. TAVI and TEVAR delivery catheters in the 16–18 Fr outer diameter range are now available, and further reductions are possible in the future. Patients with diseased and/or calcified iliofemoral arteries that are too small for newer TAVI and TEVAR devices are now routinely approached with newer expandable (and compressible upon removal) sheaths in sizes that can pass unexpanded through smaller vessels because they do not require expansion to the larger sizes needed for the early higher profile TAVI and TEVAR devices. Once in place, they are temporarily dilated along with the artery to allow device passage.

Alternatively, some interventionalists prefer the so-called "pave and crack" technique to initially prepare diseased iliofemoral arteries before EVAR, TEVAR, or TAVI device introduction and passage into the aorta.[19,20] This procedure is intended to enlarge small and/or diseased conduit vessels by initially placing a generously long self-expanding peripheral stent graft (Viabahn) or iliac limb from an EVAR system before balloon dilating throughout the length of the graft. In most cases, the Viabahn is the preferred device because EVAR iliac limb delivery systems have a larger profile and may be difficult to introduce into extensively diseased iliac arteries. Once the graft is deployed, it is post-dilated with a high-pressure angioplasty balloon to its nominal diameter or to a diameter sufficient to permit TAVI or TEVAR device delivery. In some patients with heavily calcified lesions, this may result in vessel overdilation and even rupture. In these cases, the graft provides a protective luminal lining to prevent hemorrhage.

In addition to the pave and crack technique designed to be used as a preplanned procedure antecedent to TAVI or TEVAR, the use of self-expanding stent grafts, balloon-expandable stent grafts, or a combination has proven invaluable as a rescue maneuver to address rupture of an iliac artery that may occur as an unintended consequence of balloon angioplasty, bare stent placement, angiographic sheath passage, device delivery, or aborted attempts at sheath or device introduction.[21] Judgment and experience are valuable in deciding when supplemental maneuvers are necessary and likely to succeed and which techniques should be selected to optimally address the challenge of an individual patient's iliac anatomy.

The judicious use of these techniques can provide a benefit to patients because the prudent application of traditional access routes prevents exposure to the higher risks and significant complications that accompany the more invasive and complicated transcaval approach. Thus, it is unlikely that transcaval aortic access will have an expanding role. More likely, its use in conjunction with TAVI and TEVAR will be limited to highly selected cases.

Example

See Figure 14.1.

References and Suggested Readings

1. Aljabri B, Obrand DI, Montreuil B, Mackenzie KS, Steinmetz OK. Early vascular complications after endovascular repair of aortoiliac aneurysms. *Ann Vasc Surg.* 2001;6:608–614.
2. Pratesi C, Piffaretti G, Pratesi G, Castelli P; the Italian Excluder Registry (ITER) Investigators. Italian Excluder Registry and results of Gore Excluder endograft for the treatment of elective infrarenal abdominal aortic aneurysms. *J Vasc Surg.* 2014;59:52–57.
3. Fairman RM, Criado F, Farber M, et al.; the VALOR Investigators. Pivotal results of the Medtronic Vascular Talent Thoracic Stent Graft System: The VALOR Trial. *J Vasc Surg.* 2008;48:546–554.
4. Makaroun MS, Dillavou ED, Wheatley GH, Cambria RP; the Gore TAG Investigators. Five-year results of endovascular treatment with the Gore TAG device compared with open repair of thoracic aortic aneurysms. *J Vasc Surg.* 2008;47:912–918.
5. Gupta PK, Sundaram A, Kent KC. Morbidity and mortality after use of iliac conduits for endovascular aortic aneurysm repair. *J Vasc Surg.* 2015;62:22–26.
6. Tsilimparis N, Dayama A, Perez S, Ricotta J. Iliac conduits for endovascular repair of aortic pathologies. *Eur J Vasc Endovasc Surg.* 2013;45:443–448.
7. Ramponi F, Stephen MS, Wilson MK, Vallely MP. Think differently; transapical platform for TEVAR. *Ann Cardiothorac Surg.* 2012;1:412–416.
8. Lichtenstein SV, Cheung A, Ye J, et al. Transapical transcatheter aortic valve implantation in humans: Initial clinical experience. *Circulation.* 2006;114:591–596.
9. Cheung A, Lichtenstein KM. Illustrated techniques for transapical aortic valve implantation. *Ann Cardiothorac Surg.* 2012;2:231–239.
10. Scali ST, Vlada A, Chang CK, Beck AW. Transcaval embolization as an alternative technique for the treatment of type II endoleak after endovascular aortic aneurysm repair. *J Vasc Surg.* 2013;57:869–874.
11. Halabi M, Ratnayaka K, Faranesh AZ, Chen MY, Schenke WH, Lederman RJ. *J Am Coll Cardiol* 2013;61:1745–1746.
12. Greenbaum AB, O'Neill WW, Paone G, et al. Caval-aortic access to allow transcatheter aortic valve replacement in patients otherwise ineligible: Initial human experience. *J Am Coll Cardiol.* 2014;63:2795–2804.
13. Lederman RJ, Chen MY, Rogers T, et al. Planning transcaval access using CT for large transcatheter implants. *J Am Coll Cardiol Cardiovasc Imaging.* 2014;7:1167–1171.
14. Lederman RJ, Babaliaros VC, Greenbaum AB. How to perform transcaval access and closure for transcatheter aortic valve implantation. *Catheter Cardiovasc Interv.* 2015;86:1242–1254.
15. Uflacker A, Lim S, Ragosta M, et al. Transcaval aortic access for percutaneous thoracic aortic aneurysm repair: Initial human experience. *J Vasc Interv Radiol.* 2015;26:1437–1441.
16. Lederman RJ, O'Neill WW, Greenbaum AB. Transcaval access for TAVR across a polyester aortic graft. *Catheter Cardiovasc Interv.* 2015;85:1270–1273.
17. Eadie LA, Soulez G, King MW, Tse LW. Graft durability and fatigue after in situ fenestration of endovascular stent grafts using radiofrequency puncture and balloon dilatation. *Eur J Vasc Endovasc Surg.* 2014;47:501–508.
18. Riga CV, Bicknell CD, Basra M, Hamady M, Chesire NJ. In vitro fenestration of aortic stent-grafts: Implications of puncture methods for in situ fenestration durability. *J Endovasc Ther.* 2013;20:536–543.
19. Hinchliffe RJ, Ivancev K, Sonesson B, Malina M. "Paving and cracking": An endovascular technique to facilitate the introduction of aortic stent-grafts through stenosed iliac arteries. *J Endovasc Ther.* 2007;14:630–633.
20. Weinkauf C, Montero-Baker M, Mills JL. Dynamic tailoring of the "pave and crack" technique in EVAR cases with prohibitive iliac artery anatomy: Lessons from a small case series. *J Vasc Surg.* 2013;58:555–556.
21. Fernandez JD, Craig JM, Garrett HE, Burgar SR, Bush AJ. Endovascular management of iliac rupture during endovascular aneurysm repair. *J Vasc Surg.* 2009;50:1293–1299.

Section II

Peripheral Vascular Interventions

CHAPTER 15

Subintimal Arterial Recanalization Using the Bull's-Eye Technique

S. Lowell Kahn

Brief Description

Originally described in 1989 by Bolia et al.,[1] subintimal recanalization remains one of the most common methods for lower extremity revascularization. Traversal of chronic total occlusions (CTOs) in the false lumen is readily achieved with standard catheter and wire technique in most cases. Reported technical success rates for subintimal recanalization range between 67% and 98%.[2]

The most common cause of technical failure is the inability to re-enter the true lumen beyond the occlusion. This is particularly the case in the tibial vasculature, in which re-entry is known to be difficult. Refinements of the subintimal technique, including the use of retrograde access, have further improved technical and clinical outcomes. In 2005, Spinosa et al.[3] described the SAFARI technique (subintimal arterial flossing with antegrade–retrograde intervention to treat CTOs in patients with critical limb ischemia). The authors reported 100% technical success and 90% limb salvage utilizing this method, which involves obtaining bidirectional access to the subintimal space and snaring the retrograde-placed wire.

Beyond technical refinements, a variety of true lumen re-entry devices have entered the market. Although subtle variations exist among the devices, they each advance within the false lumen and employ use of a small needle or wire that is directed toward the true lumen. Early devices such as the Outback® LTD® Re-Entry Catheter (Cordis Corp., Milpitas, CA) and the Pioneer Catheter (Volcano, San Diego, CA) expanded options for re-entry with a steerable needle platform. Directing the needle of the Outback® is based on proper alignment of the "T" and "L" markers relative to contrast opacified digital subtraction angiography (DSA) images of the true lumen acquired 90 degrees apart. In contrast, the Pioneer needle offers a longer needle and incorporates built-in intravascular ultrasound (IVUS) technology so that the needle is manually steered toward the vessel true lumen based on IVUS imaging. This of course comes with added expense and the need for the Volcano IVUS platform.

Relatively recently, the Enteer Re-entry system (Covidien LTD, Dublin, Ireland) and the OffRoad Re-entry Catheter system (Boston Scientific Inc., Marlborough, MA) were introduced to the market. These devices employ use of a self-centering balloon that is designed to automatically steer a needle or wire toward the true lumen of the vessel once advanced in the subintimal space beyond the occlusion. The Enteer catheter is the lowest profile system, allowing above- and below-knee re-entry indications, a property unique to this device. The catheter has a flat balloon with two 180-degree opposed and offset ports allowing selective guidewire re-entry. The system is 0.014- and 0.018-in. guidewire compatible and utilizes the blunt end of a wire rather than a needle for re-entry.

The OffRoad catheter features a bell-shaped balloon that orients the catheter lumen toward the true lumen. A microcatheter lancet is then advanced through the lumen of the balloon catheter and is used to penetrate the intima and regain luminal access. As with the Enteer system, the OffRoad is designed to improve the technical success of the procedure by eliminating the manual steering of the device toward the true lumen.

Although both the Enteer and OffRoad devices represent advancements, there are times when maintaining the ability to steer the needle 360 degrees is beneficial. Specifically, success with the balloon-based devices may not be possible if the subintimal space is irregular or violated (e.g., stretched and vessel perforation). Therefore, maintaining the ability to direct the needle toward a specific target is a valuable property.

This chapter describes the "bull's-eye" technique with use of the Outback® LTD® Re-Entry Catheter steered toward a specific target, most commonly a snare to guide true lumen re-entry. Although a snare is our most commonly used target, we have employed this technique using a balloon or catheter as the target for the Outback®.

The described technique is not unique to our institution and has been described by others.[4] We have found this technique to be widely applicable from large (aortic) to small (tibial) vessel revascularizations. We have also employed this technique successfully with challenging chronic central and peripheral venous occlusions. This is a powerful tool that with little practice is easily mastered.

Applications of the Technique

1. Any subintimal arterial or venous recanalization where access to the true lumen distally is possible via a separate access to facilitate placement of the target.

2. Extravascular revascularization: Revascularization of an occluded vessel can be performed when both antegrade and retrograde accesses leave the confines of the vessel. This method requires use of a covered stent and is described in chapter 18.

Challenges of the Procedure

1. Heavy calcium at the point of re-entry: The needle of the Outback® catheter may be unable to penetrate a heavily calcified intima and instead deflect away from the lumen.[5-7] Selecting a site with less calcium and firm/rapid firing of the needle may prevent failure.

2. Failure of the Outback® catheter to advance in the subintimal space of a heavily calcified vessel:[5] This is not uncommon. At our institution, we typically overcome this by advancing the sheath into the subintimal space for support and pre-dilating the subintimal tract prior to advancing the Outback® catheter.

3. Advancing the Outback® catheter over a steeply angled aortic bifurcation: Advancement of the Outback® over the aortic bifurcation can be challenging despite use of a kink-resistant sheath and upsizing the sheath beyond the required 6 Fr.[5] This is sometimes overcome by rotating and pushing the Outback® catheter while placing back traction on the sheath. Also, because we perform most our interventions on the ipsilateral side, this is rarely a problem.

4. Excessive distance between the Outback® catheter and the intended target (snare): The short needle throw of the Outback® catheter necessitates that the Outback® and snare be near one another. Also, if the subintimal plane is overdistended, the Outback® can fail to penetrate the intima and instead kick away within the distended subintimal space when fired. Maintaining a tight subintimal space is imperative to ensure optimal performance of the Outback®.

5. Advancing the snare to the intended site can be challenging. The passage of a snare retrograde through small diseased tibials may result in injury to these vessels. In some cases, use of a microsnare (Amplatz GooseNeck Microsnare, ev3 Endovascular Inc., Plymouth, MN) may be beneficial.

6. Occasionally, the 0.014-in. wire will bind to the Outback® catheter, making removal of the Outback® over the wire after successful use difficult. This can result in loss of access. This is rare, but avoidance of kinking of the wire and repeat flushes through the side port of the Outback® may help.[5]

Potential Pitfalls/Complications

1. Arteriovenous fistulae creation is reported with use of the Outback® LTD® catheter.[5] Fortunately, this is uncommon and usually of little clinical consequence.

2. Inadvertent extravascular revascularization can occur with use of this device.[5,8] This is acceptable practice if not intentional and the use of a covered stent is employed. However, if not recognized, there is a risk of bleeding or delayed pseudoaneurysm formation.

3. Dissection/injury to small vessels (e.g., tibial) with consequent occlusion is possible given the advancement of the 6 Fr Outback® catheter as well as a snare into this limited space.

4. Bleeding: In theory, this is of greatest risk in large vessels, such as the common iliac arteries or aorta. However, the needle on the Outback® catheter is quite small, and in the author's experience, this risk is very low.

Steps of the Procedure

1. Catheterization of the subintimal space at the proximal end of the occlusion is obtained with standard catheter and wire technique.

2. A tight loop is formed with the wire in the subintimal plane and advanced distally through the entirety of the CTO. Subintimal extension is extended to a point where retrograde flow into the true lumen via collaterals has been re-established. This point is verified by DSA fluoroscopy or ultrasound guidance.

3. After obtaining the desired catheterization of the subintimal space beyond the CTO, a stiff 0.035-in. guidewire is placed, over which the sheath is advanced, ideally into the subintimal space to provide further support for delivery of the Outback® LTD® catheter.

4. The stiff 0.035-in. wire is exchanged for one of the compatible 0.014-in. wires for the Outback® (see the instructions for use for the device). At our institution, the SpartaCore guidewire (Abbott Vascular Inc., Santa Clara, CA) is used for most cases.

5. The Outback® catheter is advanced over the 0.014-in. wire to the desired site for actuation. If the Outback® fails to deliver secondary to a tight or tortuous subintimal space, balloon angioplasty with a 0.014-in. balloon is advised. If possible, further advancement of the sheath may be beneficial as well.

6. Retrograde access is obtained. For femoropopliteal and tibial occlusions, this is performed in the distal tibial vasculature under ultrasound guidance. For aortic occlusions, contralateral femoral or brachial access is obtained. As mentioned previously, this technique can be employed in a similar manner for venous occlusions, but this is not elaborated on further in this chapter.

7. Using the retrograde access, the snare catheter is advanced over a wire within the true lumen to the desired point of re-entry of the antegrade access. Depending on the vessel used for the retrograde access, this can be performed with or without a sheath. For most cases, a 10-mm or smaller snare is sufficient. As noted previously, a microsnare may be safer when advanced retrograde through small tibial vessels.

8. The snare is positioned and opened as an ovoid target at the intended site of re-entry.

9. The Outback® catheter needle exit site is directed toward the snare. The C-arm is rotated to optimally profile the Outback® in the "T" configuration over the snare. A 90-degree rotation to the "L" configuration is then used to ensure proper direction of the Outback® catheter toward the snare.
10. The needle of the Outback® catheter is actuated.
11. The snare is tightened, ideally grasping the needle of the Outback® catheter. If successful, the 0.014-in. wire is threaded through the snare approximately 3 or 4 cm.
12. The needle is retracted, leaving the snare grasping the wire alone.

13. The wire is withdrawn through the retrograde access site while the wire is slowly pushed through the Outback® catheter.
14. Once the end of the 0.014-in. wire has been externalized through the retrograde sheath, the Outback® catheter is carefully removed over the wire.
15. The procedure is completed with additional interventions (angioplasty, stenting, etc.) as necessary to obtain successful revascularization.

Example
See Figures 15.1–15.3.

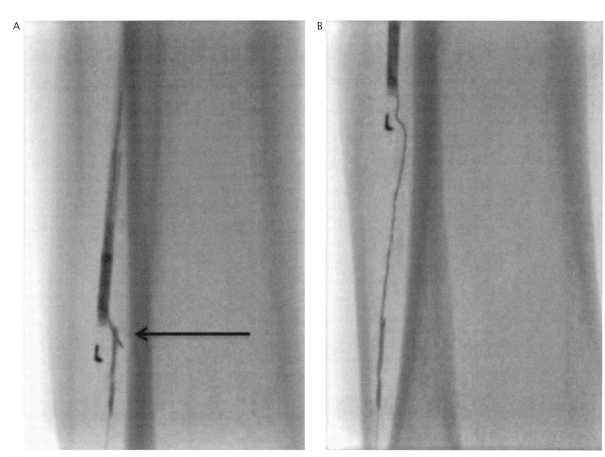

Figure 15.1 Subintimal recanalization of an occluded posterior tibial artery using the bull's-eye technique. (A) The Outback catheter has been advanced in the subintimal plane of the posterior tibial artery from an antegrade approach, and a snare has been advanced in the subintimal plane from a distal retrograde approach. The needle of the Outback has been deployed through the snare and grasped (arrow); the wire will be subsequently fed through the snare. (B) The wire has now been grasped by the snare and is retracted through the retrograde tibial access. Wire access has been obtained across the occlusion, facilitating additional interventions as necessary.

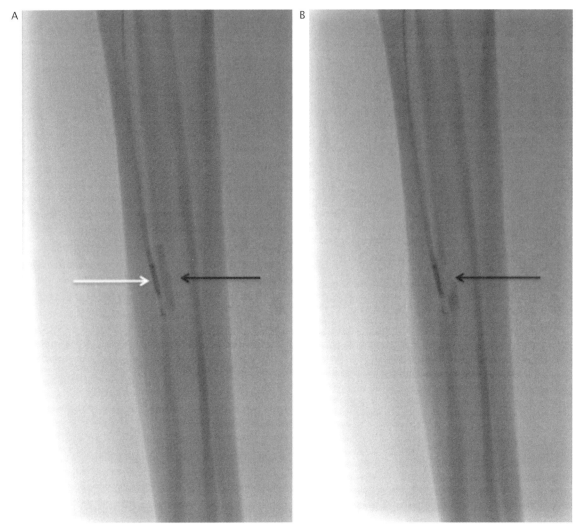

Figure 15.2 Alternative bull's-eye technique using a balloon as a target. (A) From the antegrade approach in a peroneal artery, the Outback catheter has been advanced within the subintimal plane (white arrow). From a retrograde peroneal access, a 2.5-mm balloon (black arrow) has been advanced within the subintimal plane. (B) The balloon is penetrated (black arrow) by the needle of the Outback device. Immediately, a 0.014-in. wire is threaded into the collapsed balloon. The wire is pushed while the balloon is carefully withdrawn to obtain through-and-through access. This allowed subsequent revascularization of the occluded peroneal artery. In the author's experience, a balloon offers a larger target than a snare, but advancing a wire into the collapsed balloon can be difficult and therefore use of a snare is preferred.

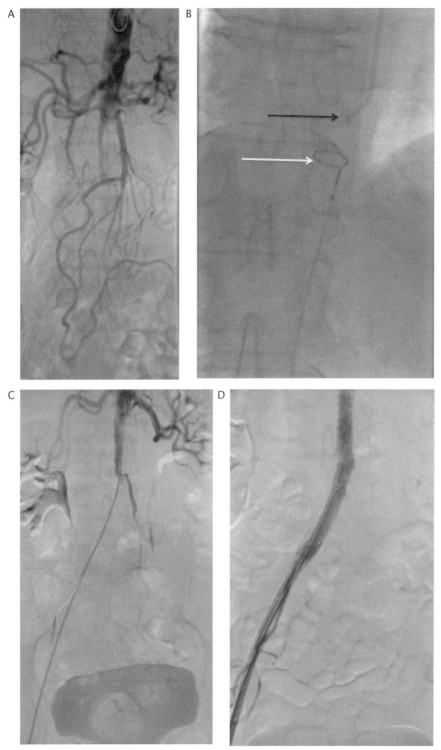

Figure 15.3 Bull's-eye technique employed with simple catheter and wire use. (A) The patient presented with severe lower extremity claudication, and fulminant infrarenal aortic occlusion was demonstrated by aortography. Difficulty was encountered with a retrograde-placed wire, which easily traversed the subintimal space but was unable to re-enter the true lumen of the aorta. (B) A brachial access was obtained through which a long hockey-stick catheter (black arrow) was advanced to the occlusion. A retrograde snare (white arrow) was advanced in the subintimal plane. With forward pressure on the catheter, wire access to the subintimal plane was obtained from the brachial access, and the wire was easily threaded through and grasped by the snare. This facilitated wire access across the lesion (C), over which covered stents were deployed to direct flow to the right femoral artery and subsequently perform a femoral–femoral bypass (D).

References and Suggested Readings

1. Bolia A, Brennan J, Bell PR. Recanalization of femoro-popliteal occlusions: Improving success rate by subintimal recanalisation. *Clin Radiol.* 1989;40:325.

2. Bown MJ, Bolia A, Sutton AJ. Subintimal angioplasty: Meta-analytical evidence of clinical utility. *Eur J Vasc Endovasc Surg.* 2009;38:323–337.

3. Spinosa DJ, Harthun NL, Bissonette EA, et al. Subintimal arterial flossing with antegrade–retrograde intervention (SAFARI) for subintimal recanalization to treat chronic critical limb ischemia. *J Vasc Interv Radiol.* 2005;16(1):37–44.

4. Rundback JH, Herman KC. Transpedal Interventions for Critical Limb Ischemia. *Vasc Dis Manage.* 2013;10(8):E152–E158.

5. Shin SH, Baril D, Chaer R, Rhee R, Makaroun M, Marone L. Limitations of the Outback® LTD® re-entry device in femoropopliteal chronic total occlusions. *J Vasc Surg.* 2011;53(5):1260–1264.

6. Setacci C, Chisci E, de Donato G, Setacci F, Iacoponi F, Galzerano G. Subintimal angioplasty with the aid of a re-entry device for TASC C and D lesions of the SFA. *Eur J Vasc Endovasc Surg.* 2009;38:76–87.

7. Hausegger KA, Georgieva B, Portugaller H, Tauss J, Stark G. The Outback® catheter: A new device for true lumen re-entry after dissection during recanalization of arterial occlusions. *Cardiovasc Intervent Radiol.* 2004;27:26–30.

8. Wagner JK, Chaer RA, Rhee RY, Marone LK. True lumen re-entry after extravascular recanalization of a superficial femoral artery chronic total occlusion. *J Vasc Surg.* 2010;52:216–218.

CHAPTER 16

Alternative Subintimal Entry and True Lumen Re-entry Techniques

S. Lowell Kahn

Brief Description

Chronic total occlusions (CTOs), long-segment stenoses, and heavily calcified lesions of the lower extremity vasculature are common causes of failed peripheral interventions[1-6] with resultant patient morbidity.

Since its initial description by Bolia et al. in 1989, subintimal revascularization has been a mainstay of endovascular therapy for patients with long-segment stenoses, CTOs, heavily calcified vessels, and critical limb ischemia.[1,7-11] In addition to its potential for re-establishing in-line flow in difficult lesions, employment of this technique allows for protection of potentially critical collateral vessels[1,12,13] and the isolation of thrombogenic atheromatous debris produced with conventional intraluminal angioplasty.[1,14] Moreover, the new lumen created by subintimal angioplasty is free of endothelium, and thus neo-endothelialization, offering the potential for improved long-term patency.[1,7,13]

Despite its promise, subintimal revascularization remains hampered by a technical success rate ranging from 76% to 95%.[1,10,11,15-19] The "Achilles' heel" of the procedure is the inability to gain re-entry into the true lumen of the target vessel while using conventional catheter technique.[1,17,18] Although higher rates have been reported, true lumen re-entry is reported in roughly 80% of patients.[1,7,20]

In addition, the unpredictability of lumen re-entry is a hazard with potentially serious consequences. Uncontrolled re-entry can result in compromise of critical collateral vessels, unintentional dissection, and limitation of potential future surgical anastomotic sites.[1,2,7,10,11,16,17] It is reported that 47% of distal and 26% of proximal collateral vessels may be compromised during conventional subintimal angioplasty.[1,21] Unnecessary extension of subintimal recanalization increases the risk of reocclusion given that longer subintimal courses are associated with a higher risk of occlusion.[1,5] The lack of precision re-entry conferred with traditional re-entry also results in angioplasty and stenting of the uninvolved segment of the vessel.[1,2]

Recognizing the shortcomings of conventional catheter-based true lumen re-entry, several innovative devices have entered the market, all of which employ use of a needle or wire for directional intimal penetration.

Interestingly, the use of a guided transseptal needle for luminal re-entry has been described, and these devices share this concept.[22] The earliest device developed for this application was the Re-entry Catheter (Cordis Corp., Milpitas, CA). The Outback® LTD® is a 6 Fr catheter that advances over a 0.014-in. wire. A steerable nitinol needle exits the catheter tip at an angle, allowing traversal of the intima and re-entry to the true lumen beyond an occlusion through which a 0.014-in. wire can be advanced. The Pioneer Plus Catheter (Philips, Amsterdam, Netherlands) has a similar design but features a longer needle and incorporates intravascular ultrasound (IVUS) to guide the needle toward the true lumen.[23] Relatively recently, the Enteer Re-entry System (Medtronic Inc., Minneapolis, MN) and the OffRoad Re-entry Catheter (Boston Scientific Inc., Marlborough, MA) were introduced. These devices employ use of a self-centering balloon to automatically steer a needle or wire toward the true lumen. Except for the Enteer catheter, which has above- and below-knee indications, these devices are intended for re-entry above the knee, but off-label use elsewhere in the body is described. Although the selection of these devices is largely based on preference, there are important differences that should be considered, the specifics of which are outside the scope of this chapter. The addition of these devices to the interventionalist's repertoire improves technical success rates, patient safety, and future surgical options.

Entry to the subintimal plane is usually easily obtained at the point of occlusion, frequently unintentionally because the catheter and wire will enter this plane as a path of least resistance. If a vessel terminates abruptly with a side branch collateral, this can present a challenge because the catheter and wire will have a natural bias toward the side branch. Such a scenario is typically not problematic because the interventionalist simply steers a directional catheter away from the side branch and with forward pressure is able to traverse the occlusion in either the true or the false lumen.

Once entry to the false lumen is obtained, it is advised that the wire loop be maintained in a narrow configuration throughout the occlusion to avoid making the subintimal space patulous and less efficient for re-entry.[24]

Catheter and wire advancement in the subintimal plane is usually easy, but severely calcified vessels may require intermittent balloon dilatation to facilitate delivery. Re-entry is obtained distal to the occlusion at a location free of calcium, ideally as proximal as possible to avoid unnecessary compromise of important collaterals and to preserve future bypass options.[24] Orthogonal digital subtraction angiography (DSA) images help localize the true lumen beyond the occlusion, and with the catheter directed accordingly, the wire loop enters the true lumen in the majority of cases.[24] When unsuccessful, a straight wire or the back end of a wire can be used with forward catheter support to obtain re-entry, but use of the back end should be performed cautiously and over a very limited distance to avoid vessel injury or perforation.

When re-entry fails by conventional means, a second retrograde access in the popliteal or tibiopedal vasculature may be obtained. Initially described by Spinosa et al.[25] in 2005, the subintimal arterial flossing with antegrade–retrograde intervention (SAFARI) technique employs bidirectional entry into the subintimal plane with use of a snare to obtain through-and-through wire access. With a reported technical success of up to 100%, the SAFARI procedure largely overcomes the limitations of conventional techniques with little added equipment or expense.[25]

The techniques and tools described previously are successful in the overwhelming majority of cases. However, there are times when entry and re-entry prove difficult despite these measures. This chapter describes lesser known alternative techniques for subintimal entry and re-entry when conventional measures fail. Three alternative methods for subintimal entry are described herein. The *diverting balloon technique* involves placing a 0.014-in. compatible balloon in the terminal side-branch collateral of an occlusion. Adjacent to this balloon, a catheter and wire are advanced to the occlusion and used to traverse the occlusion in either the true or the false lumen. The presence of the balloon prevents the natural bias of the catheter and wire to the side branch. The *retrograde wire technique* is essentially a variant of the SAFARI procedure and involves percutaneous retrograde puncture of an occluded vessel near the occlusion under ultrasound (US) guidance. This technique was first described by Chin H'ng and Punamiya[26] and involves threading a wire through the occlusion and into the antegrade catheter. This wire is then used to allow the catheter to enter the occluded vessel. Finally, the *reverse Outback® LTD® technique* involves use of the Outback® LTD® catheter to enter the false lumen from the true lumen.

With respect to alternative re-entry techniques, we describe four methods. The *hydrodynamic boost technique* was described by Ferraresi et al.[27] in 2016 and involves a small volume injection of contrast close to the patent lumen to create a rent in the intima and allow re-entry to the true lumen. Similarly, the *antegrade balloon technique* employs focal-directed inflation of a balloon in the subintimal space to create an intimal tear and allow re-entry. If this fails, the *confluent balloon technique* is useful for meeting antegrade and retrograde wires by advancing balloons from both directions and inflating them in a kissing manner. This was initially described in the coronary setting by Wu et al.,[28] but it has peripheral application as well. The kissing balloons create a fenestration and allow threading of a wire from one lumen to the other to obtain through-and-through access. Finally, the *targeted Outback® LTD® technique* involves retrograde advancement of a balloon or snare with antegrade advancement of the Outback® LTD® catheter. This technique has been described successfully by multiple authors whereby the retrograde balloon or snare functions as a target for the antegrade Outback® LTD® catheter.[29,30] This allows re-entry to the true lumen or communication between the antegrade and retrograde wires in noncontiguous locations of the false lumen.

These alternative entry and re-entry techniques are easy to learn and require little added inventory. Although not commonly necessary, we have found each of these techniques to be useful in our own practice when standard techniques and equipment fail to deliver the desired results.

Applications of the Techniques

Diverting Balloon Technique

1. Entry to the true or false lumen of an occluded vessel when the vessel terminates with side branch collateral.
2. Jaffan et al.[31] described a variant of this technique whereby a balloon was placed in an undesirable false lumen or extravascular tract while attempting to traverse a CTO. The balloon blocked entry to this plane and favored the catheter and wire to remain in the occluded true lumen. This technique is described in chapter 17.
3. A balloon could be used in this capacity at any location where a vessel bifurcates and catheterization of the target vessel is difficult because of an inherent bias for the catheter to track to the nontarget vessel.

Retrograde Wire Technique

1. This technique is most useful for obtaining catheter entry to the true or false lumen of an occluded vessel when there is a flush occlusion. A flush occlusion is challenging to enter because there is poor catheter support available for forward wire advancement.
2. This technique is commonly employed when obtaining access to an occluded venous or prosthetic bypass, again most commonly when there is a flush occlusion or when the occlusion is firmer secondary to being subacute in nature.

Reverse Outback® LTD® Technique

1. This technique is very rarely necessary, but the Outback® LTD® catheter can be fired in the true lumen at the level of the occlusion to obtain wire entry to the false lumen when true lumen traversal is not possible and entry to the subintimal space via conventional methods is difficult.

Hydrodynamic Boost Technique

1. Re-entrance to the true lumen distal to the occlusion. This is optimally used in small vessels (e.g., mid to distal tibial). The use of contrast reveals the presence of a tear in the intima that allows re-entry to the true lumen.

Antegrade Balloon Technique

1. Re-entry to the true lumen via the creation of a tear in the intima.
2. The technique can be applied for similar applications in the venous system.

Confluent Balloon Technique

1. This technique is most commonly employed in the setting of a failed SAFARI procedure in which wires in the subintimal plane from the antegrade and retrograde access fail to meet one another. The kissing balloons create one or more tears in the intima that allow communication between the two accesses.

Targeted Outback® LTD® Technique

1. Re-entry to the true lumen distal to an occlusion. In a small vessel, catheterization of the true lumen with the Outback® LTD® catheter alone is difficult to cannulate. Placement of a snare or balloon in the retrograde true lumen allows for an optimal target to guide re-entry.
2. As with the confluent balloon technique, the Outback® LTD® catheter can be used with a snare or balloon to not only connect the true and false lumen but also connect two wires in a noncontiguous subintimal plane.
3. As with the arterial applications, the Outback® LTD® catheter combined with a snare or balloon as a target can be employed in the venous system as well (e.g., central venous occlusions).

Challenges of the Procedure

Diverting Balloon Technique

1. The sheath must be adequately upsized to allow advancement of the catheter adjacent to the diverting balloon without excessive friction. In most cases, a 6 or 7 Fr sheath is adequate, but the size required depends on the catheter/wire combination and diverting balloon sizes chosen. In general, the diverting balloon should be on a 0.014- or 0.018-in. platform because this allows for a low profile with sufficient side-branch occlusion.

Retrograde Wire Technique

1. Depending on the location of the occlusion, catheterization of the occluded segment may not be possible. For example, at a proximal tibial location near the trifurcation, the vessel may be too small or deep to adequately visualize and catheterize. In our experience, we have reserved this technique for proximal superficial femoral artery (SFA) occlusions or femoral–popliteal bypasses.
2. Use of this technique is typically straightforward with an occluded bypass because the wire will advance without difficulty through the thrombus in most cases. However, with an occluded artery, advancement of the wire beyond the needle tip can be difficult. We find that ideally the wire is advanced retrograde through the subintimal space, but identifying the subintimal space is challenging. We typically advance the needle well into the occluded vessel and then slowly withdraw it while gently probing with the wire until the subintimal plane is found.

Reverse Outback® LTD® Technique

1. This technique is unlikely to be successful in larger parent vessels because the needle will simply buckle the entire catheter away from the vessel wall rather than penetrate the intima. In tighter spaces, success is more likely.
2. As with the retrograde wire technique, advancement of the wire can be difficult because the needle must find the subintimal plane. In a similar manner as described previously, the needle is fired and incrementally withdrawn with advancement of the wire at each location to identify the subintimal plane.

Hydrodynamic Boost Technique

1. The greatest challenge of this technique is maintaining an intact subintimal space without violation of the adventitia and extravasation of contrast. Success of this technique requires the contrast to be retained in the subintimal space such that the buildup of pressure results in spilling of contrast into the distal true lumen. The technique has a reported technical success rate of 83%.[27] Success is more likely if attention is paid to maintaining a tight subintimal space with a narrow wire loop during traversal.

Antegrade Balloon Technique

1. Again, there are no specific challenges to this technique other than advancement of the balloon. It is recommended to maintain a very tight subintimal

plane (narrow wire loop) and use a small-diameter short balloon.

Confluent Balloon Technique

1. No specific challenges other than balloon delivery from both antegrade and retrograde accesses. This technique has limited data in the literature, but in our practice, it is successful only approximately 60% of the time.

Targeted Outback® LTD® Technique

1. Some authors prefer use of a balloon with this technique. Once the balloon is ruptured, it can be challenging to advance a wire into the collapsed balloon. Furthermore, the wire must then stay in the collapsed balloon as it is withdrawn. For these reasons, we exclusively perform this procedure with a snare and have attained a very high technical success rate as a result.
2. The needle of the Outback® LTD® catheter may deflect off the balloon.
3. Opening the snare adequately to make a large target can be difficult, particularly if the snare is in the confined subintimal plane of a small vessel. Hitting the snare is challenging and may require several needle passes and different orientations of the c-arm to optimize visualization.
4. The Outback® LTD® catheter works best if it is confined in a small vessel or tight subintimal plane and is likely to deflect from the intima in a capacious subintimal space. In addition, the device may fail to penetrate a calcified intima.

Potential Pitfalls/Complications

Diverting Balloon Technique

1. It is possible that despite the presence of a diverting balloon, the catheter and wire may still fail to enter the true or false lumen of the vessel and instead enter an extravascular plane, resulting in technical failure and vessel extravasation.
2. It is important to not oversize the balloon and to make every effort to preserve the collateral being temporarily occluded. Should the traversal fail or the revascularized segment go on to occlude later, the collateral may be of critical importance to maintain adequate distal blood flow.

Retrograde Wire Technique

1. It is possible that advancement of a wire in the retrograde subintimal space could result in proximal extension of the subintimal tract, thereby decreasing patency and potentially compromising critical collaterals and branch vessels (e.g., profunda).

Reverse Outback® LTD® Technique

1. The needle can perforate the vessel, resulting in extravasation. In reality, this is likely of little consequence given the small 22 gauge size of the needle.

Hydrodynamic Boost Technique

1. If the injection fails to create a tear in the intima, it is possible that it could make the subintimal space more patulous, which would make re-entry with a catheter or re-entry device more difficult given the lack of support for penetration.

Antegrade Balloon Technique

1. As with the hydrodynamic boost technique, dilatation of the balloon can make the subintimal space more patulous, further hampering efforts to obtain true lumen re-entry.

Confluent Balloon Technique

1. As with the prior techniques, inflation of a balloon can make the subintimal space from both directions more capacious and consequently more difficult to re-enter the true lumen if this method fails.

Targeted Outback® LTD® Technique

1. Use of the Outback® LTD® catheter carries a risk of vessel injury, penetration, and extravasation. However, the risk is low given the very small 22 gauge needle of this device.
2. Rupturing a balloon intentionally can result in a transverse tear in the balloon and possibly retention of a balloon fragment.
3. Advancing a retrograde snare catheter or balloon could result in injury, dissection, or thrombosis of a small tibial vessel. This risk should be considered in the decision to use this technique.

Steps of the Procedure

Diverting Balloon Technique

1. This technique is employed when an abrupt occlusion terminates with a collateral side branch. The catheter and wire continue to enter the side branch rather than allowing traversal of the occlusion. DSA is performed to evaluate the size and course of the side branch relative to the occluded target vessel. After assessing the side branch, the sheath is upsized accordingly to allow side-by-side placement of the crossing catheter and wire and a balloon large enough to occlude the side branch. This may require back table testing, but in most cases a 6 or 7 Fr sheath is adequate.
2. A 0.014-in. wire is threaded into the side-branch collateral. A short, appropriately sized (1:1 with respect

to vessel diameter) balloon is placed into the side branch and inflated.

3. With the balloon inflated, the crossing catheter and wire are advanced side-by-side through the sheath, and traversal of the occlusion is attempted in the true or false lumen.

4. Once adequate purchase into the occluded vessel is obtained, the collateral occlusion balloon can be deflated and removed.

5. The procedure is completed in standard fashion.

Retrograde Wire Technique

1. This technique is utilized when a flush occlusion (no stump) is present and the operator is unable to catheterize the occluded vessel in either the true or false lumen. DSA is performed to study the occlusion. If the occluded vessel is visible by US, a location near the origin of the occlusion is selected for access. Under US guidance, a micropuncture 21 gauge needle is inserted into the occluded vessel in a retrograde manner.

2. As the micropuncture needle is slowly withdrawn, a 0.018-in. wire is gently advanced until it advances without resistance. Although this is possible in the occluded true lumen, more commonly the wire will advance in the subintimal plane because there is less resistance.

3. Once the 0.018-in. wire pops into the patent vessel proximally, the transitional dilator is used to exchange for a 0.035-in. Glidewire (Terumo Medical Corp., Somerset, NJ).

4. Over the Glidewire, a hockey stick catheter is advanced retrograde into the patent vessel.

5. The hockey stick catheter and Glidewire are then used to obtain antegrade access into the occluded vessel. There are multiple options for this. The retrograde hockey stick catheter and Glidewire can be steered into an antegrade sheath over which the sheath is advanced into the occluded vessel. Alternatively, the retrograde hockey stick catheter can be used to deliver a wire into an antegrade catheter that is pulled through and through, allowing for antegrade sheath or catheter advancement into the occluded vessel. Finally, a snare can be employed to grasp a retrograde wire delivered through the hockey stick catheter. This wire is then used to allow delivery of an antegrade sheath or catheter into the occlusion. Regardless of the method chosen, antegrade access into the flush occluded vessel is obtained, and the occluded vessel is traversed and revascularized with standard technique.

Reverse Outback® LTD® Technique

1. This technique should be reserved as a late effort when other methods to enter the subintimal plane from the antegrade access have failed. It is used when entry to the subintimal space proves difficult with a catheter and wire, and it should be used in relatively small vessels (i.e., <4 mm) so that the Outback® LTD® is able to penetrate the intima rather than deflect as would be expected in a larger vessel. A compatible 0.014-in. wire (see Outback® LTD® instructions for use) is advanced to the occlusion over which the Outback® LTD® is delivered.

2. The Outback® LTD® is steered toward the desired subintimal tract (typically the less calcified side of the vessel).

3. The Outback® LTD® needle is deployed in a firm, swift motion to penetrate the intima.

4. The needle is then slowly retracted with gentle probing performed with the 0.014-in. wire until the wire finds the subintimal space. Once it loops within the subintimal space, it is advanced sufficiently to provide enough purchase to allow safe removal of the Outback® LTD® without sacrificing access.

5. The Outback® LTD® catheter is exchanged over the 0.014-in. wire for a support catheter, and the subintimal recanalization is completed with standard technique.

Hydrodynamic Boost Technique

See Ferraresi et al.[27]

1. This technique is used to re-enter the true lumen, most commonly in the tibial vasculature. The catheter and wire are advanced within the subintimal tract to the desired point of re-entry. The selected point of re-entry should be as proximal as possible (to limit the subintimal tract and avoid compromise of important collaterals). The selected point of re-entry should also be relatively free of calcium.

2. The catheter is directed toward the true lumen. In some cases, we apply gentle forward pressure on the catheter so that it buckles in a more perpendicular configuration to the vessel lumen.

3. A syringe is filled with dilute contrast and is injected slowly through the catheter during continuous magnified fluoroscopy. The contrast forms a chamber around the catheter tip and typically ascends along the subintimal space proximally. As the pressure builds up, the contrast eventually spills into the distal true lumen, creating a rent in the intima.

4. A small hydrophilic guidewire is then inserted and used to gently probe until it advances into the true lumen through the newly created rent. The procedure is then completed in standard fashion.

5. *Note*: If contrast leaves the vessel with gross extravasation, no further contrast is injected and the technique is abandoned. Another strategy, such as retrograde access, is then employed.

Antegrade Balloon Technique

1. This technique is used to re-enter the true lumen, most commonly in the tibial vasculature. The catheter and wire are advanced within the subintimal tract to the desired point of re-entry. As mentioned previously, the entry point should be as proximal as possible, with mindfulness of calcification that would prevent successful re-entry.

2. A short balloon that is compatible with the wire platform being used should be advanced to the point of occlusion. The diameter chosen should be the same or less than the target vessel diameter.

3. The balloon is rapidly inflated and then deflated.

4. Contrast can be injected through the balloon to assess for a successful intimal tear with communication to the true lumen.

5. The balloon may be exchanged for a catheter if desired, but we typically advance a hydrophilic wire through the balloon and gently probe to find the intimal tear and regain wire entry to the true lumen.

6. Once access to the true lumen is successfully obtained, the procedure is completed with standard technique.

Confluent Balloon Technique

1. Antegrade and retrograde wire access to the subintimal space of the occluded vessel is obtained as if performing a standard SAFARI technique. If the two wires fail to meet, this technique can be employed.

2. From each access, a short balloon is advanced with a diameter that roughly approximates the expected diameter of the vessel undergoing revascularization. With tibial interventions, we commonly advance the balloon bareback over a 0.014- or 0.018-in. wire.

3. The balloons are advanced such that there is minimal (e.g., ~5 mm) overlap between the balloons.

4. Both balloons are rapidly inflated and deflated.

5. From both accesses, a hydrophilic guidewire is advanced to determine whether there is now communication between the two planes. If successful, through-and-through wire access is obtained, and the procedure is subsequently completed with additional intervention as needed. *Note*: We often advance the wires through the balloons themselves rather than exchanging for a catheter because this allows us to quickly repeat the maneuver at a different location without an additional exchange. Also, balloon catheters often work well as crossing/support catheters in the tibial vasculature.

Targeted Outback® LTD® Technique

1. Both antegrade and retrograde wire access to the occlusion are obtained. After failed conventional technique to obtain through-and-through wire access, this technique may be employed to connect any two tissue planes. Specifically, it works for connecting the true lumen to the subintimal plane or for connecting noncontiguous segments of the subintimal plane (false to false). In fact, we have used this technique for extravascular revascularization when the wires have traveled beyond the adventitia. Extravascular revascularization is described elsewhere in chapter 18.

2. Most commonly because of the 6 Fr sheath required, the Outback® LTD® catheter is delivered from the antegrade access over a 0.014-in. wire to the desired point of communication with the retrograde access. This can be at a point of true lumen re-entry just beyond an occlusion or at any point within the subintimal when connecting two noncontiguous subintimal planes.

3. From the retrograde access, a snare or balloon is advanced as a target. In our experience, a 5- or 10-mm Amplatz GooseNeck snare or a 4- or 7-mm Amplatz GooseNeck Microsnare (ev3 Endovascular Inc., Plymouth, MN) works well. As stated previously, we prefer use of a snare compared to the balloon given the technical issues and potential complications associated with the balloon.

4. The snare or balloon is maintained in place. Using the "T" and "L" markers with orthogonal views (up to 90 degrees), the Outback® LTD® catheter is directed toward the target and the needle is fired.

5. If a snare is used, the snare is cinched around the needle. If the capture is successful, the wire is threaded 4 or 5 cm out and the needle is retracted, leaving the wire grasped by the snare. If a balloon is used, the wire is rapidly threaded into the balloon once it has burst.

6. With use of a snare, the wire is pushed through the hub of the Outback® LTD® catheter while the snare is pulled from the retrograde access. Similarly, with use of a balloon, the wire is pushed through the hub of the Outback® LTD® catheter while the balloon is slowly pulled beyond the occlusion into a patent portion of the vessel distally. Once in good position, the wire is pinned and the balloon is removed from the retrograde access, leaving the wire tip in the true lumen beyond the occlusion.

7. With wire access obtained across the occlusion, the Outback® LTD® catheter is removed carefully, and the procedure is completed with additional interventions as necessary.

Example

See Figures 16.1–16.6.

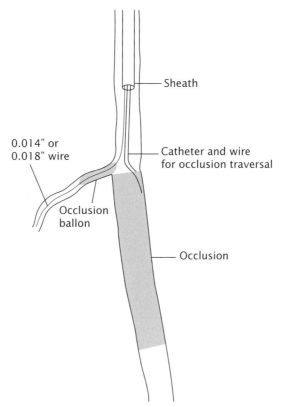

Figure 16.1 Diverting balloon technique. The sheath is positioned proximal to the occlusion. Wires advanced to the occlusion continue to pass into the terminal side branch collateral rather than engaging the occlusion. The sheath is upsized accordingly (typically 6 or 7 Fr) to accommodate this procedure. A 0.014- or 0.018-in. wire is passed into the side branch collateral. A short balloon sized 1:1 with this side branch collateral is placed at the ostium of the collateral and inflated to block entry. Adjacent to the 0.014- or 0.018-in. wire, a crossing catheter and guidewire are advanced and subsequently used to traverse the occluded vessel in the true or false lumen.

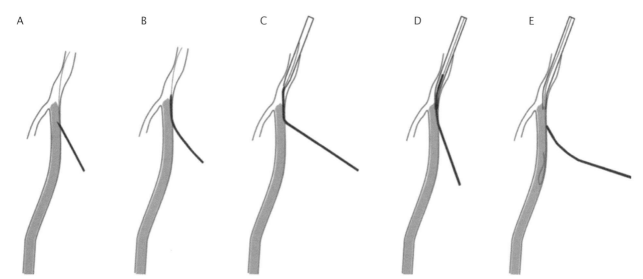

Figure 16.2 Retrograde wire technique. A flush occlusion of the SFA is present and cannot be engaged from a standard antegrade approach. (A) Under ultrasound guidance, a micropuncture needle is passed into the occluded vessel proximally, and a wire is passed into the subintimal space and ultimately into the patent common femoral artery. (B) The transitional dilator is advanced over the microwire into the common femoral artery. (C) After being exchanged for a hockey stick catheter and guidewire, it is steered into the antegrade sheath. (D) Once it is well advanced into the sheath, the sheath is advanced over the catheter and guidewire and into the occluded SFA. (E) The hockey stick catheter is then inserted into the antegrade sheath (which is engaged in the subintimal plane of the occlusion) and used with a guidewire to perform a subintimal recanalization of the SFA.

Source: From Chin H'ng, MW, Punamiya S. An innovative modification of the retrograde approach to angioplasty and recanalization of the superficial femoral artery. Diagn Interv Radiol. 2014;20(2):164–167. Courtesy the Turkish Society of Radiology.

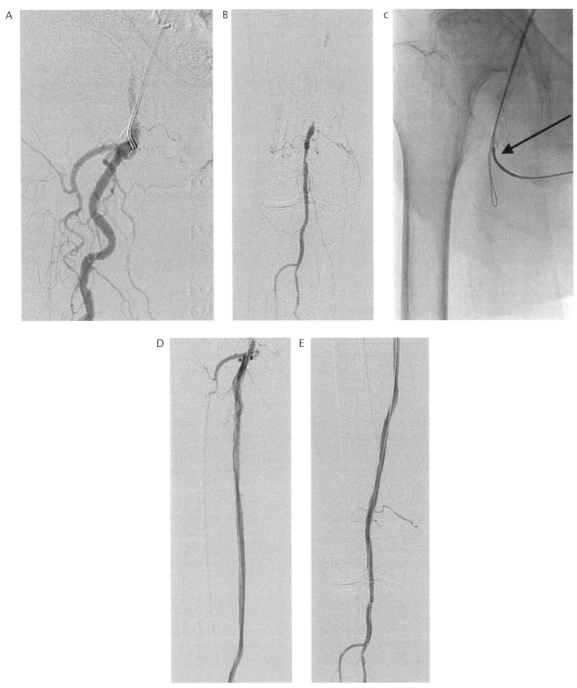

Figure 16.3 Retrograde wire technique. A flush occlusion of the SFA at its origin (A) is present with reconstitution via collaterals of the popliteal artery (B). A catheter and wire introduced into the occluded SFA in a retrograde manner (C) allow successful subintimal revascularization of the occluded SFA (D and E).

Source: From Chin H'ng, MW, Punamiya S. An innovative modification of the retrograde approach to angioplasty and recanalization of the superficial femoral artery. *Diagn Interv Radiol.* 2014;20(2):164–167. Courtesy the Turkish Society of Radiology.

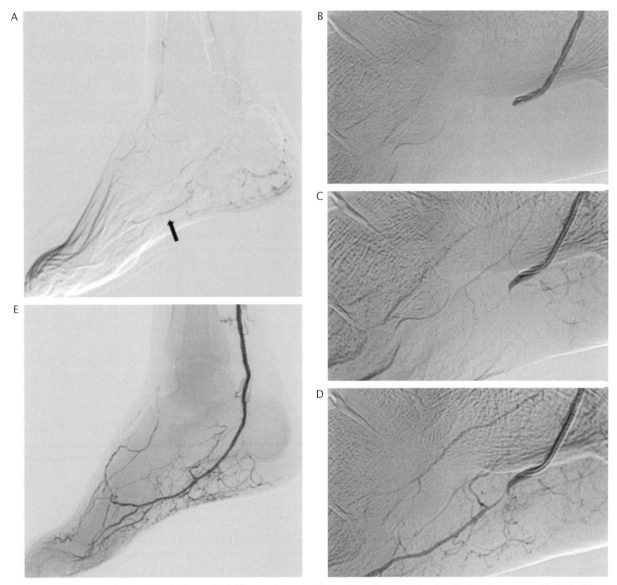

Figure 16.4 Hydrodynamic boost technique. (A) DSA reveals an occlusion from the posterior tibial artery to a reconstituted mid-plantar artery (arrow). (B and C) A catheter and wire are advanced distally into the subintimal space of the plantar artery just proximal to the point of reconstitution. Contrast is injected slowly around the catheter tip, forming a chamber of contrast that ascends along the subintimal tract proximally. (D) As pressure builds up, it ultimately creates a rent in the intima and spills into the reconstituted true lumen distally, allowing successful passage of a 0.014-in. wire into the distal plantar artery. (E) A final angiogram after angioplasty shows direct in-line flow to the plantar artery.

Source: From Ferraresi R, et al. Hydrodynamic boost: A novel re-entry technique in subintimal angioplasty of below the knee vessels. *Eur Radiol.* 2016;26(8):2419–2425. Courtesy Springer Healthcare.

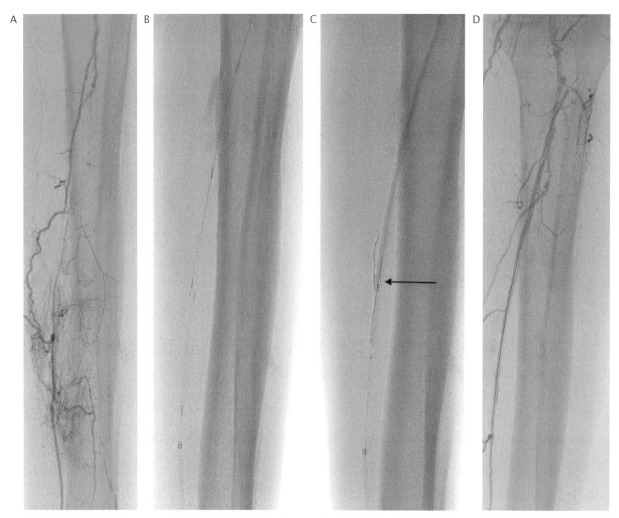

Figure 16.5 Confluent balloon technique. (A) DSA angiography reveals a mid-posterior tibial artery occlusion. (B) Access to the subintimal space of the occlusion was obtained from both anterior and retrograde accesses, but the wires failed to meet. (C) Antegrade and retrograde balloons were inserted from both accesses and overlapped (arrow) approximately 3 mm. The inflated balloons created a small rent in the intima that allowed the retrograde wire to pass into the true lumen and angioplasty was performed. (D) Subsequent DSA revealed in-line flow through the posterior tibial artery.

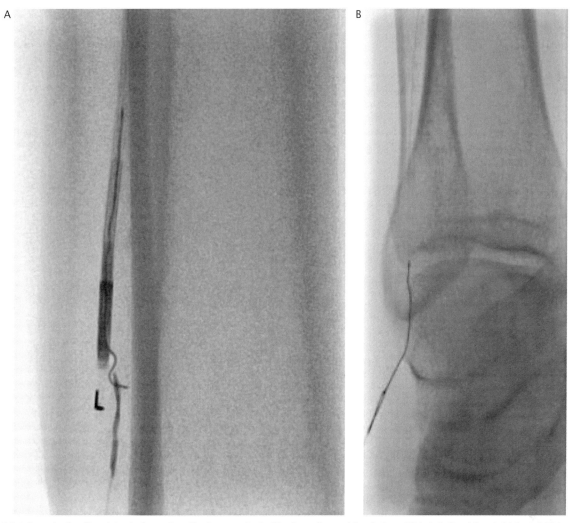

Figure 16.6 Targeted outback technique. A patient presented with ulcerations of the first and third digits of the right foot. DSA images (not shown) revealed occlusion of the anterior tibial artery. Access to the subintimal plane of the anterior tibial artery was obtained through both antegrade and retrograde accesses. A 5-mm Amplatz GooseNeck snare was inserted retrograde from the dorsalis pedis while the Outback catheter was advanced over a 0.014-in. wire from the antegrade access. (A) The Outback needle was used to penetrate the open snare and subsequently grasp the wire. (B) The grasped wire was pulled through the dorsalis pedis access and used to obtain through-and-through wire access.

References and Suggested Readings

1. Kahn SL, Angle JF, Matsumoto AH, Hagspiel KD, Turba UC. True lumen re-entry methods employed during subintimal recanalization: Proper technique, merits, and shortcomings. SIR 2007 annual meeting. e-Poster: 282.

2. Jacobs DL, Motanganahalli RL, Cox DE, Wittgen CM, Peterson, GJ. True lumen re-entry devices facilitate subintimal angioplasty and stenting of total chronic occlusions: Initial report. *J Vasc Surg.* 2006;43:1291–1296.

3. Lipsitz EC, Ohki T, Veith FJ, et al. Does subintimal angioplasty have a role in the treatment of severe lower extremity ischemia? *J Vasc Surg.* 2003;37:386–391.

4. Dormandy JA, Rutherford RB. Management of peripheral arterial disease (PAD). TransAtlantic Inter-Society Consensus (TASC). *J Vasc Surg.* 2000;31:S1–S296.

5. London NJ, Srinivasan R, Naylor AR, et al. Subintimal angioplasty of femoropopliteal artery occlusions: The long-term results. *Eur J Vasc Surg.* 1994;8:148–155.

6. Saket RR, Razavi MK, Padidar A, Kee ST, Sze DY, Dake MD. Novel intravascular ultrasound-guided method to create transintimal arterial communications: Initial experience in peripheral occlusive disease and aortic dissection. *J Endovasc Ther.* 2004;11:274–280.

7. Wiesinger B, Steinkamp H, Konig C, Tepe G, Duda SH. Technical report and preliminary clinical data of a novel catheter for luminal re-entry after subintimal dissection. *Invest Radiol.* 2005;40:725–728.

8. Reekers JA, Kromhout JG, Jacobs MJHM. Percutaneous intentional extraluminal recanalization of the femoropopliteal artery. *Eur J Vasc Surg.* 1994;8:723–728.

9. Bolia A. Subintimal angioplasty: The way forward. *Intervention.* 1998;2:47–52.

10. Reekers JA, Bolia A. Percutaneous intentional extraluminal (subintimal) recanalization: How to do it yourself. *Eur J Radiol.* 1998;28:192–198.

11. Yilmaz S, Sindel T, Ceken K, et al. Subintimal recanalization of long superficial femoral artery occlusions through the

retrograde popliteal approach. *Cardiovasc Intervent Radiol.* 2001;24:154–160.

12. Nydahl S, London NJM, Bolia A. Technical report: Recanalization of all three infrapopliteal arteries by subintimal angioplasty. *Clin Radiol.* 1996;51:366–367.

13. Bolia A, Fishwick G. Recanalization of iliac artery occlusion by subintimal dissection using the ipsilateral and contralateral approach. *Clin Radiol.* 1997;52:684–687.

14. Martin EC, Fankuchen KB, Karlson KB, et al. Angioplasty for femoral artery occlusion: Comparison with surgery. *AJR Am J Roentgenol.* 1981;137:915–919.

15. Bolia A, Nasim A, Bell PR. Percutaneous extraluminal (subintimal) recanalization of a brachial artery occlusion following cardiac catheterization. *Cardiovasc Intervent Radiol.* 1996;19:184–186.

16. Murphy TP, Marks MJ, Webb MS. Use of a curved needle for true lumen re-entry during subintimal iliac artery revascularization. *J Vasc Interv Radiol.* 1997;8(4):633–636.

17. Vorwerk D, Geunther RW, Schurmann K, Wendt G, Peters I. Primary stent placement for chronic iliac artery occlusions: Follow-up results in 103 patients. *Radiology.* 1995;194:745–749.

18. Murphy TP, Webb MS, Lambiase RE, et al. Percutaneous revascularization of complex iliac artery stenoses and occlusions with use of wallstents: Three year experience. *J Vasc Interv Radiol.* 1996;7:21–27.

19. Spinosa DJ, Leung DA, Harthun NL, et al. Simultaneous antegrade and retrograde access for subintimal recanalization of peripheral arterial occlusion. *J Vasc Interv Radiol.* 2003;14:1449–1454.

20. Lipsitz EC, Okhi T, Vieth FJ, et al. Fate of collateral vessels following subintimal angioplasty. *J Endovasc Ther.* 2004;11:269–273.

21. Hausegger KA, Geourgieva B, Portugaller H, Tauss J, Stark G. The Outback® LTD® catheter: A new device for true lumen re-entry after dissection during recanalization of arterial occlusions. *Cardiovasc Intervent Radiol.* 2004;27:26–30.

22. Gastaldo F, Tirukonda P, Yip G, Patlas M. Subintimal recanalization of peripheral chronic occlusive arterial disease with modified transseptal needle. *J Vasc Interv Radiol.* 2013;24(2):184–189.

23. Saketkhoo RR, Razavi MK, Padidar A, Kee ST, Sze DY, Dake MD. Percutaneous bypass: Subintimal recanalization of peripheral occlusive disease with IVUS guided luminal re-entry. *Techniques Vasc Interv Radiol.* 2004;7(1):23–27.

24. Schneider PA, Caps MT, Nelken N. Re-entry into the true lumen from the subintimal space. *J Vasc Surg.* 2013;58(2):529–534.

25. Spinosa DJ, Harthun NL, Bissonette EA, et al. Subintimal arterial flossing with antegrade–retrograde intervention (SAFARI) for subintimal recanalization to treat chronic critical limb ischemia. *J Vasc Interv Radiol.* 2005;16:37–44.

26. Chin H'ng, MW, Punamiya S. An innovative modification of the retrograde approach to angioplasty and recanalization of the superficial femoral artery. *Diagn Interv Radiol.* 2014;20(2):164–167.

27. Ferraresi R, Hamade M, Gallicchio V, Troisi N, Mauri G. Hydrodynamic boost: A novel re-entry technique in subintimal angioplasty of below the knee vessels. *Eur Radiol.* 2016;26(8):2419–2425.

28. Wu EB, Chan WW, Yu CM. The confluent balloon technique—Two cases illustrating a novel method to achieve rapid wire crossing of chronic total occlusion during retrograde approach percutaneous coronary intervention. *J Invasive Cardiol.* 2009;21:539–542.

29. Bozlar U, Shih MC, Harthun NL, Hagspiel KD. Outback® LTD® catheter-assisted simultaneous antegrade and retrograde access for subintimal recanalization of peripheral arterial occlusion. *Clin Imaging.* 2008;32(3):236–240.

30. Tai Z, Lee A. Reentry-catheter assisted SAFARI technique. *J Invasive Cardiol.* 2015;27(7):E146–E152.

31. Jaffan AA, Shroff KR, Murphy TP. Balloon occlusion of subintimal tract to assist distal luminal reentry into popliteal artery. *J Vasc Interv Radiol.* 2012;23(10):1389–1391.

Balloon Occlusion of Subintimal Tract to Assist Distal Luminal Re-entry During Subintimal Recanalization of Chronic Total Occlusions

Abdel Aziz A. Jaffan

Brief Description

The balloon occlusion of subintimal tract (BOST) technique may be used to assist in regaining luminal re-entry in difficult cases during subintimal recanalization of chronic total occlusions (CTOs) in the femoropopliteal artery. Subintimal recanalization or percutaneous intentional extraluminal recanalization (PIER) is an established technique used in endovascular recanalization of chronically occluded arteries of the peripheral circulation. The primary limitation of PIER is the high technical failure rate, estimated to be approximately 20%. Failure is mainly due to the inability to re-enter the patent true lumen distal to the site of the occlusion. Technical success can be increased with adjunct techniques such as the use of re-entry devices (e.g., Outback® LTD®, Cordis Corp., Milpitas, CA) or the establishment of a retrograde pedal access (subintimal arterial flossing with antegrade–retrograde intervention [SAFARI]). During challenging PIER, in which spontaneous distal luminal re-entry does not occur, and once an extraluminal tract has been created, redirecting the crossing wire to a new tract is very difficult because the wire tends to follow the path of least resistance—that is, the initially created extraluminal tract. The BOST technique can be another tool in the kit to increase the likelihood of distal luminal re-entry. With the wire in the extraluminal tract, a low-profile balloon is advanced over the wire into the proximal aspect of the extra-luminal tract, and then inflated to seal the entrance to the tract. A second wire is advanced alongside the preexisting wire. The presence of the inflated balloon prevents the second wire from entering the preexisting tract and diverts it to create a new extraluminal tract, increasing the probability of luminal re-entry. Once true lumen re-entry is achieved, the procedure is then completed using the standard technique.

Application of the Technique

1. Chronic total occlusions (CTOs) of the femoropopliteal artery.
2. PIER with inability to re-establish true lumen re-entry distal to the occlusion.
3. Alternative to re-entry devices to regain true lumen re-entry during endovascular recanalization of a CTO.

Challenges of the Procedure

1. Requires a relatively larger sheath to accommodate two wire/catheter systems comfortably.
2. Having two wires inserted through the sheath can render the sheath valve nonhemostatic with blood leakage from the sheath.
3. Advancing a wire alongside another wire can cause the wires to kink.

Potential Pitfalls/Complications

1. Increased risk of vessel perforation/soft tissue hematoma: When advancing the wire next to the inflated balloon, the wire can completely perforate the arterial wall with subsequent soft tissue hematoma.
2. Increased risk of arteriovenous fistula: When advancing the wire next to the inflated balloon, the wire can completely perforate the arterial wall into an adjacent vein and in theory increase the risk of an arteriovenous fistula.
3. Failure to achieve true lumen re-entry: The wire may create a second extraluminal space without achieving true lumen re-entry.

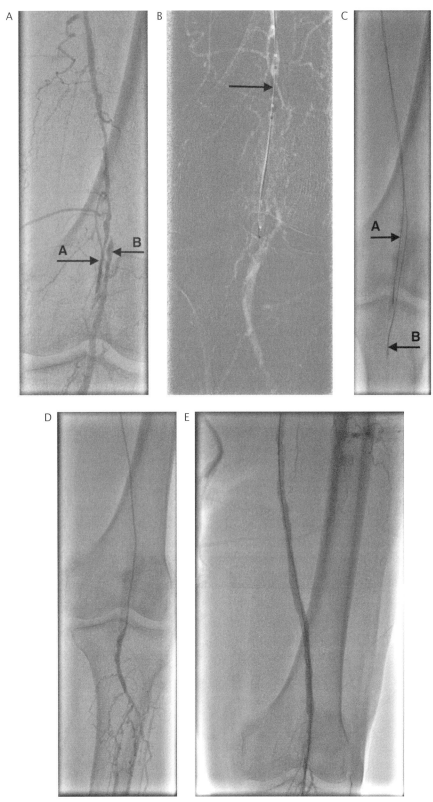

Figure 17.1 (A) Arteriogram of the left lower extremity shows the created extraluminal tract in the popliteal artery (arrow A) and the reconstituted popliteal artery (arrow B). (B) Road map image at the popliteal level showing a V-18 wire (Boston Scientific Inc., Marlborough, MA) in the extraluminal tract. A low-profile balloon (3 mm × 2 cm PowerCross [ev3 Endovascular, Inc., Plymouth, MN]) is inflated to seal the initial extraluminal tract (arrow). (C) Spot fluoroscopic image following successful distal luminal re-entry into the popliteal artery. The initial wire (V-18 wire; arrow A) ends in the initial extraluminal tract. The second wire (a Glidewire; arrow B) ends in the true lumen of the popliteal artery. The balloon catheter was removed from the extraluminal tract. (D) Following true lumen re-entry, a catheter was advanced into the true lumen of the popliteal artery, with contrast material injection confirming intraluminal position. The wire has already been removed from the extraluminal tract. (E) A stent has been deployed in the distal superficial artery/proximal popliteal artery over a Rosen wire (Cook Medical Inc., Bloomington, IN), with an arteriogram confirming patency of the deployed stent.

Steps of the Procedure

1. This technique assumes that an extraluminal tract has already been created during endovascular recanalization of a CTO of the superficial femoral/popliteal artery, with inability to re-enter the true lumen distal to the occlusion. The common femoral arterial access, whether antegrade or retrograde, is obtained and catheterization of the superficial femoral artery and initiation of PIER are done using a standard access technique.

2. The femoral access site is upsized with placement of a 7 Fr sheath to allow for simultaneous insertion of two catheter–wire systems side by side.

3. A 0.018-in. wire is advanced to the subintimal tract. A low-profile balloon catheter (~3 mm in diameter) is advanced over the wire into the subintimal tract and inflated to seal the entrance into the subintimal tract. Alternatively, a 0.014-in. wire and a compatible low-profile balloon may be utilized.

4. Through the same femoral sheath, a 0.035-in. compatible crossing catheter (Quick-Cross (Spectranetics Corp., Colorado Springs, CO) or similar catheter) is advanced over a 0.035-in. Glidewire (Terumo Medical Corp., Somerset, NJ), adjacent to the balloon catheter. Alternatively, a 0.018-in. compatible crossing catheter advanced over a 0.018-in. wire, or a 0.014-in. compatible crossing catheter advanced over a 0.014-in. wire, can be used.

5. The crossing catheter–wire combination is advanced to the level of the occlusion; the presence of the inflated balloon in the subintimal tract diverts the wire into a new subintimal channel, away from the initially created subintimal tract, increasing the probability of true lumen re-entry.

6. Once true lumen re-entry is confirmed, the balloon is deflated, and the balloon–catheter–wire combination is removed from the old subintimal tract.

7. While the other wire is in the true lumen of the patent distal superficial femoral/popliteal artery, the crossing catheter is removed. The procedure is then continued using a standard technique (angioplasty, stent placement, atherectomy, etc.).

Example

See Figure 17.1.

Reference and Suggested Reading

1. Jaffan AAA, Shroff KR, Murphy TP. Balloon occlusion of subintimal tract to assist distal luminal reentry into popliteal artery. *J Vasc Interv Radiol.* 2012;23(10):1389–1391.

CHAPTER 18

Extravascular Recanalization of Chronic Total Occlusions

S. Lowell Kahn

Brief Description

Revascularization of chronic total occlusions (CTOs) commonly involves an extraluminal approach with consequent subintimal recanalization of a vessel. Although officially described by Bolia et al. in 1989,[1] subintimal recanalization or percutaneous intentional extraluminal revascularization (PIER) was likely performed by other operators prior to this, either intentionally or unintentionally. Today, subintimal revascularization is a mainstay of therapy for lower extremity interventions. This stems from the realization that true lumen traversal is not always possible, subintimal revascularization has a high technical success rate, and the subintimal space may confer advantages over a heavily calcified true lumen.

Although the reported technical success of subintimal recanalization is between 67% and 98%,[2] the "Achilles' heel" of the procedure remains re-entry to the true lumen beyond the occlusion. The development of the subintimal arterial flossing with antegrade–retrograde intervention (SAFARI) technique by Spinosa et al.[3] overcame many of these limitations and created a paradigm shift with the widespread adoption of retrograde intervention. This technique is analogous to the controlled antegrade and retrograde subintimal tracking (CART) technique described in the cardiology literature[4] and employs bidirectional traversal of an occlusion, with substantially higher technical success than prior reports of an exclusive antegrade traversal.

As discussed previously in the text, the value of extraluminal revascularization has been recognized by industry with the introduction of multiple subintimal re-entry devices (Outback® LTD® Re-Entry Catheter, Cordis Corp., Milpitas, CA; Pioneer Catheter, Volcano Corp., San Diego, CA; Enteer Re-entry System, Covidien LTD., Dublin, Ireland; OffRoad Re-entry Catheter system, Boston Scientific Inc., Marlborough, MA) over the last decade. These devices employ use of a directionally controlled wire or needle that is either automatically or manually steered toward the true lumen beyond an occlusion. Coupled with improved technique, these devices have expanded options and success rates in the management of CTOs.

Most commonly in the tibial vasculature, there are times when subintimal recanalization is not possible because the wire and catheter may leave the subintimal plane and enter the periadventitial tissue. Although this is not intentional, exit from the vessel historically results in a technical failure because future passes of the wire and catheter are likely to follow suit, as evidenced by extravasation on contrast injection.

This chapter describes two techniques to salvage this scenario and accept an extravascular tract for revascularization. The first technique, herein referred to as the Outback® extravascular revascularization technique, employs use of the Outback® LTD Re-Entry Catheter to connect discontiguous tissue planes from the antegrade and retrograde accesses. Described in detail later, this technique involves the bidirectional steerage of a catheter and wire toward one another irrespective of the tissue plane within which they lie. The goal for revascularization is to steer the catheters close to one another, ideally within 5 mm in a three-dimensional plane. Confirmation of their proximity is performed with multiple oblique images or employment of biplane imaging if available. Once the two catheters are in close proximity, the "bull's-eye" technique is used, which involves placing a snare as a target (typically from the retrograde approach) and an Outback® (or Pioneer) catheter from the other (typically antegrade) approach. The needle on the re-entry device is used to target the open snare, allowing the pulling through of the wire from the Outback® and obtaining access across the occlusion. Although serendipitously discovered, this has proven invaluable in several cases that would otherwise have been technical failures by a standard subintimal approach. Similar success has been described with this technique by other authors.[5,6]

The percutaneous gun-sight extravascular revascularization technique is a vascular application of the gun-sight technique described in the literature for transjugular intrahepatic portosystemic shunt (TIPS) applications.[7] With this technique, bidirectionally advanced snares are aligned with one another, and a percutaneous needle is advanced under live fluoroscopy with obliquity to allow a "down-the-barrel" perspective during needle advancement. Once both snares are penetrated, the needle is used to introduce a wire that is grasped by both snares, and the needle is removed. The wire can then be pulled through the antegrade and retrograde accesses, thereby accomplishing wire access across the occlusion and facilitating additional intervention. Unlike the Outback® extravascular revascularization technique, which requires close approximation of the Outback® and snare, the percutaneous gun-sight extravascular revascularization technique can connect antegrade and retrograde catheterizations that lie a substantial distance from one another.

Although an endoluminal or subintimal approach is always the preferred revascularization strategy, extravascular recanalization of CTOs has become an important bailout technique when subintimal recanalization is not possible. Performed methodically, we believe these techniques represent safe and effective strategies in the management of critical limb ischemia. Both techniques are moderately challenging, but they can be accomplished with practice in a reasonable amount of time. Given that these techniques involve a truly extravascular (not subintimal) course, covered stents are typically required to prevent hemorrhage and complete the procedure. Due to this fact and the absence of long-term patency data, we reserve these techniques exclusively for limb salvage when traditional methods have failed.

Applications of the Technique

Outback® Extravascular Revascularization and Percutaneous Gun-Sight Extravascular Revascularization Techniques

1. Bailout techniques for failed intraluminal or subintimal traversals of chronic total occlusions in the setting of limb salvage.
2. Extravascular recanalization of venous occlusions when standard intraluminal technique has failed.

Challenges of the Procedure

Outback® Extravascular Revascularization Technique

1. Steering the catheter and wire outside of a subintimal plane is inherently challenging. Unlike the subintimal plane, where the wire and catheter are constrained in a finite space, extravascular catheter manipulation has no such guidance. Ideally, the extravascular tract is as short as possible, and every effort should be made to remain within the intraluminal or subintimal plane as far as possible from both approaches. We have found that the floppy end of a guidewire together with a catheter, although safe, is often poorly steerable in the extravascular or interstitial space. For short controlled manipulations, we have found the back end of a Glidewire (Terumo Medical Corp., Somerset, NJ) useful for bringing the antegrade and retrograde catheters together.

2. Performing the "bull's-eye" technique whereby the re-entry device needle passes through an open snare can be challenging, but with practice, it is usually accomplished in a short time interval.
3. Advancing an Outback® (or Pioneer) re-entry catheter through a calcified subintimal plane or through the extravascular space is challenging. To overcome this, we advise obtaining distal sheath support as far as possible. Furthermore, pre-dilatation of the tract with balloon angioplasty is sometimes necessary, but this must be done expeditiously and conservatively (smallest balloon diameter possible) because of the inherent risk of bleeding in the extravascular space.
4. From the retrograde access, advancement of a snare may be challenging, depending on the presence of stenotic or occlusive disease in the tibial vasculature. Ideally, a retrograde tibial sheath is placed, but small/diseased tibial vessels may not tolerate this safely. Occasionally, we have advanced a small snare "bareback" over a wire to prevent injury to the tibial vessel from a larger sheath.
5. After wire access is obtained through the occlusion, advancement of a catheter over the wire can be difficult. Judicious pre-dilatation with a small 0.014- or 0.018-in. balloon may be necessary to facilitate additional interventions and wire exchanges. As described previously, this must be performed cautiously given the risk of bleeding.

Percutaneous Gun-Sight Extravascular Revascularization Technique

1. As with the Outback® technique, advancing the catheters bidirectionally through even a short extravascular tract can be challenging and potentially hazardous to surrounding structures (e.g., other vessels, lymphatics, and nerves). Although this technique does not require the proximity necessitated with the Outback® technique, we still make every effort to keep our antegrade and retrograde catheters along a similar tissue plane.
2. Aligning the bidirectional snares mandates that there are no critical intervening structures that either cannot (i.e., bone) or should not (vessels, lymphatics, and nerves) be traversed. Knowledge of the salient anatomy and evaluation with multiple oblique images is advised to select a location where the two snares can be safely aligned.
3. Steering a needle through both snares is difficult and requires angling the image intensifier to a potentially steep angle for alignment that allows a "down-the-barrel" perspective of the needle. A long needle (e.g., ≥15 cm) may be required. Moreover, it is challenging for the operator to keep his or her hands out of the field during needle advancement.
4. After a wire is introduced through the needle and grasped by both snares, pulling it through

both accesses is difficult, and kinking of the wire is an inherent risk. We advise use of a nitinol, kink-resistant wire (e.g., Glidewire Gold, Terumo Medical Corp., Somerset, NJ) for this purpose. Care must also be taken when withdrawing the back end of the wire from one of the snares to avoid vessel trauma.

5. Advancement of the snares through tight, tortuous, or calcified anatomy can be difficult from one or both accesses (particularly a small tibial access). Judicious pre-dilatation of the tract(s) may be necessary first to facilitate snare placement.

6. After wire access is obtained, subsequent catheter passage may be difficult, and pre-dilatation may again be necessary. As with the Outback® technique, pre-dilatation can result in bleeding, and use of balloons (for tamponade effect), rapid catheter exchanges, and employment of covered stents are necessary to prevent this complication.

Potential Pitfalls/Complications

1. The major risk of extravascular revascularization is hemorrhage. Fortunately, the risk is low because typically occlusive or severely stenotic disease exists proximal to the extravascular tract. Although repaired later, proximal occlusive disease confers a measure of safety from a hemorrhage perspective. Nonetheless, particularly when pre-dilatation is involved, we advise limiting the size of the balloon used and treating the shortest possible distance. Treatment of occlusive disease proximal to the extravascular tract with angioplasty and/or stenting should be deferred until the extravascular segment has been re-lined with a covered stent.

2. Use of an Outback® (or Pioneer) catheter in the extravascular space carries a small risk of injury to adjacent vascular, lymphatic, and neural structures. Fortunately, the risk is low given the small size of the 22 (Outback®) or 24 (Pioneer) gauge needles used with these devices. Nonetheless, maintaining the shortest extravascular tract possible is advised. In addition, we commonly perform a pull-back angiogram (Check-Flo valve (Cook Medical Inc., Bloomington, IN) attached to a 0.035-in. catheter advanced over the 0.014-in. wire) to confirm that the tract does not violate critical structures.

Percutaneous Gun-Sight Extravascular Revascularization Technique

1. As with the Outback® technique, any extravascular revascularization carries a risk of bleeding. As previously mentioned, proximal occlusive disease confers an element of safety prior to the placement of a covered stent, and we typically defer repair of the proximal disease until the extravascular tract is addressed with a short covered stent. Occasionally, this is not possible because the devices will not deliver. If proximal pre-dilation is necessary, use of the smallest balloon possible to facilitate device delivery is advised. The proximal disease can be further dilated/stented later once the bleeding risk has been mitigated.

2. Akin to the Outback® technique, there is a minor risk of injury to adjacent vascular, lymphatic, or neural structures when performing this technique. As discussed previously, a pull-back arteriogram of the extravascular tract may be helpful prior to further ballooning or stenting.

3. As mentioned previously, the technique requires pulling both ends of a kink-resistant wire through the antegrade and retrograde accesses. Pulling the floppy end of the wire is usually easy, but the back end tends to be more challenging and risky. We place the wire such that the back end of the wire is pulled through the femoral (rather than the tibial) sheath. Furthermore, we advance a long femoral sheath close to the point of occlusion so that the back end is not pulled through healthy vessel.

Steps of the Procedure

Outback® Extravascular Revascularization Technique

1. The procedure is performed after a failed intraluminal or subintimal revascularization, including an attempt to revascularize the occlusion using both antegrade and retrograde accesses. As with all antegrade–retrograde interventions, every effort should be made from both accesses to remain in the intraluminal or subintimal space as far as possible to minimize the length of the extravascular tract.

2. Once an extravascular revascularization is intended, a long 6 Fr sheath should be placed from the antegrade approach. Maximal sheath support with the sheath terminating close to the point of occlusion is desirable. Pre-dilatation of the antegrade subintimal and/or intraluminal tract of the antegrade access should be performed with a small balloon that allows delivery of the sheath to its intended site.

3. If the tibial vessel of the retrograde access is of adequate size, a 4 or 5 Fr sheath should be placed so that the retrograde snare does not have to be advanced in a "bareback" manner.

4. Imaging should be performed as necessary from one or both accesses to clearly delineate the intended extravascular tract.

5. If the catheter and wire from *one or both* accesses leave the subintimal plane with extravasation demonstrated by gentle injection of contrast, an attempt at extravascular recanalization can be made.

a. From both directions, the catheters and wires should be steered as close as possible to one another.

b. It is imperative that the C-arm be frequently rotated to ensure that the catheters are approaching one another in a three-dimensional plane.

c. Because a catheter is not confined to a specific plane with extravascular advancement, it is easy to run off course. It is frequently necessary to pull the catheter back slightly and redirect it as necessary.

d. Occasionally, the floppy end of a straight or angled Glidewire may be difficult to direct in an intended direction. In this situation, we employ the back end of a Glidewire together with a hockey stick catheter to direct ourselves along a straighter tract in an intended direction. This maneuver is to be performed for short distances and with caution.

6. Proximity of the antegrade and retrograde catheters is confirmed with multiple oblique images or bi-plane as available. The goal is to have the catheters within 5 mm of one another.

7. An Outback® LTD Re-Entry catheter is advanced over a 0.014-in. wire to the point of closest proximity to the retrograde wire. As mentioned previously, occasionally, pre-dilatation with a small balloon is necessary to allow delivery of the Outback® to the intended target. Pre-dilatation should be done with the minimum balloon size necessary to decrease the risk of bleeding at the extravascular tract.

8. From the retrograde access, a 5- or 10-mm Amplatz GooseNeck Snare (Covidien LTD., Dublin, Ireland) is advanced as close as possible to the Outback® catheter. The snare is fully opened.

9. With magnification and oblique views (up to 90 degrees apart as mandated in the instructions for use [IFU]), the Outback® needle is deployed through the open snare.

10. The snare is tightened and used to grasp the needle. Once grabbed, a compatible 0.014-in. wire (see Outback® IFU) is threaded approximately 5 cm through the snare and the needle is retracted.

11. The wire is then grasped and pulled through the retrograde tibial access while the wire is gently pushed through the hub of the Outback® catheter.

12. With through-and-through wire access, the Outback® catheter is removed.

13. *Optional*: If clinical concern exists with respect to the course of the extravascular tract and possible traversal of critical structures, a pull-back angiogram can be performed. To do this, we advise advancing a 4 Fr catheter over the 0.014-in. wire with a Check-Flo valve attached to the hub of the catheter. The catheter is advanced from the antegrade sheath beyond the occlusion and extravascular tract, and a pull-back angiogram is performed. Contrast is injected through the side port of the Check-Flo valve, confirming suitability of the tract for dilatation and placement of a covered stent.

14. Appropriate measurements are obtained for angioplasty and stenting.

15. The wire is exchanged as needed for deployment of a Viabahn stent (W. L. Gore & Associates Inc., Flagstaff, AZ). At our institution, we prefer use of the V-18 ControlWire (Boston Scientific) because it offers good support for additional interventions. The tract is pre-dilated as necessary to facilitate placement of a covered Viabahn stent graft.

16. The Viabahn is deployed over the extravascular tract and angioplastied to the desired diameter.

17. Additional repair of stenotic/occlusive disease proximal and distal to the extravascular tract is performed at the operator's discretion.

Percutaneous Gun-Sight Extravascular Revascularization Technique

1. For this technique, steps 1–5 of the Outback® extravascular revascularization technique are performed as discussed previously. Although not as important, every effort is made to bring the catheters near one another.

2. Two 10-mm Amplatz GooseNeck snares are advanced from the antegrade and retrograde accesses to a location that allows alignment without interference from osseous structures. In the example presented in this chapter, this was performed high in the popliteal fossa from a medial approach with steep obliquity of the image intensifier to eliminate overlying bone. As described previously, this step may require pre-dilatation of the tract from one or both accesses. To mitigate the risk of bleeding during extravascular pre-dilatation, use of the smallest balloon possible is advised.

3. With the image intensifier obliqued to overlap the snares, a 21 gauge needle of sufficient length (e.g., Chiba, Cook Medical) is advanced through both snares. This is accomplished by orienting the needle exactly in-plane with the image intensifier such that just the hub and a central dot (needle) are seen.

4. After the needle is advanced through both snares, the snares are tightened to verify that each is gripping the needle. If successful, a nitinol, kink-resistant guidewire (e.g., Glidewire Gold) is advanced through the needle, and the needle is removed with the snares grasping the wire alone. It is very important for the wire to be oriented properly so that the back end is pulled through the femoral sheath and the atraumatic floppy end is pulled through the tibial access. If the femoral snare is deeper, the back end should be passed through the needle first; if the femoral snare is more superficial, the front end of the wire should be

passed first. Finally, the long femoral sheath should be advanced as close as possible to the occlusion so that the back end of the wire (which could be traumatic) is not dragged through healthy patent vessel.

5. Feeding the guidewire is challenging because the goal is to avoid kinking. To do this, we advise retracting the back end of the wire first. Therefore, the femoral snare is tightened first, and the wire is carefully threaded percutaneously into the patient while the other end is pulled through the sheath. We advise continuing to pull the wire out from the groin until only the floppy end of the guidewire is present at the skin (this minimizes the amount of redundant wire pulled through the tibial access). With the wire externalized through the femoral sheath, the process is repeated through the tibial sheath, again feeding the wire into the leg to assist withdrawal from below.

6. Once the wire is externalized through both femoral accesses, the guidewire is exchanged for a stiff support wire. As discussed previously, we prefer the V-18 ControlWire because angioplasty and deployment of a Viabahn stent can be performed over a single wire.

7. The tract is pre-dilated as necessary, and a short Viabahn stent is deployed over the extravascular tract. Care should be taken to avoid covering crucial collateral vessels that may be important if the stent occludes in the future.

8. Additional interventions are performed as required above and below the extravascular tract.

Example
See Figures 18.1–18.4.

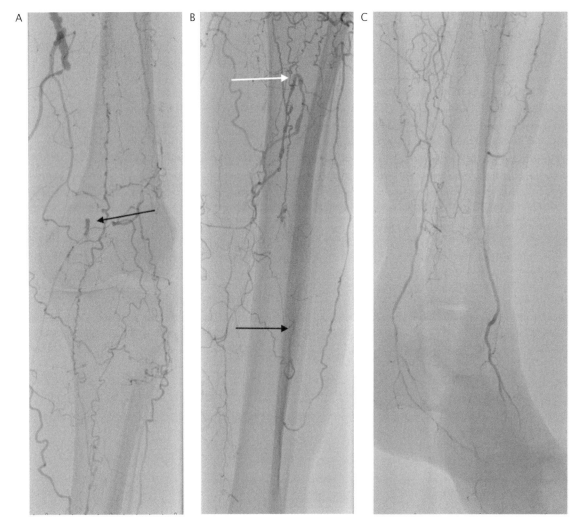

Figure 18.1 Outback extravascular revascularization technique. An 83-year-old male presented with left foot cellulitis and profound ischemia with osteomyelitis of the L4 and L5 digits. He underwent amputation of L4 and L5, but his wound failed to heal. (A) A left leg angiogram shows occlusion of the proximal popliteal artery near the adductor canal. Minimal reconstitution of a short segment of the mid-popliteal artery (arrow) is seen. (B) There is late filling of the most distal tibioperoneal trunk (white arrow) and reconstitution of the mid to distal anterior tibial artery (black arrow). (C) Distally, both anterior and posterior tibial arteries are intact.

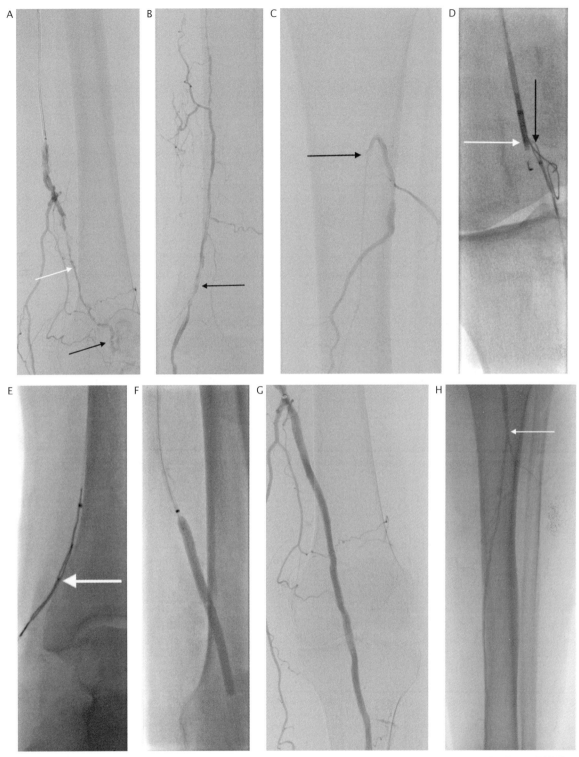

Figure 18.2 Outback extravascular revascularization technique. Images are obtained from the same patient illustrated in Figure 18.1. The patient was denied surgery based on his poor risk factors for a bypass with general anesthesia and was referred back for intervention. An attempt was made from an antegrade approach to traverse the popliteal occlusion and ultimately regain access to a tibial vessel below. (A) The wire failed to stay in the subintimal space of the occlusion and instead an extravascular tract (white arrow) was observed with contrast seen to extravasate freely more distally (black arrow). (B) Retrograde access to both the posterior tibial artery (arrow) and the anterior tibial artery (not shown) was obtained. Attempts from the anterior tibial artery to traverse the long segment occlusion were unsuccessful. (C) From the posterior tibial artery access, the catheter reached the short segment of reconstituted tibioperoneal trunk (arrow), with contrast seen in a short segment of the peroneal artery. However, as we advanced proximally beyond this, we similarly entered an extravascular plane after a short distance of ascending within the subintimal plane of the distal popliteal artery. (D) With both antegrade and retrograde accesses, we could steer two catheters near one another, as verified with multiple oblique projections. We then performed a bull's-eye maneuver whereby an Outback® LTD® Re-entry Catheter (white arrow) was advanced through the antegrade 6-Fr sheath and a 5-mm Amplatz GooseNeck snare (black arrow) was advanced through the retrograde 4-Fr posterior tibial sheath. The needle of the Outback catheter is seen passing through the snare. A 0.014-in. wire is then passed through the needle, and the needle is retracted, leaving only a grasped wire. (E) The wire is pushed through the hub of the Outback catheter and pulled with the snare (white arrow) through the retrograde tibial access. (F) After careful pre-dilatation, a 5-mm Viabahn stent graft is deployed and angioplastied. (G) Final angiogram demonstrates brisk flow into the extravascular Viabahn stent, which was deployed distally into a short 4-mm XIENCE Xpedition (Abbott Vascular, Inc., Santa Clara, CA) drug eluting stent (H; white arrow) to allow a better taper to the tibioperoneal trunk. In-line flow has been achieved to the posterior tibial artery.

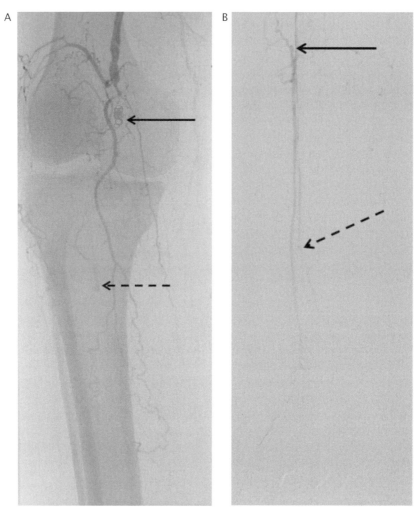

Figure 18.3 Percutaneous gun-sight extravascular revascularization technique. An 89-year-old male with right toe and heel ulceration did not have a suitable vein for bypass and was a poor operative candidate due to congestive heart failure. (A) The patient underwent an angiogram, which demonstrates acute occlusion of the proximal popliteal artery. Coils are present in the popliteal fossa (solid arrow) from a prior failed Outback extravascular revascularization attempt. The distance between the antegrade Outback and the retrograde snare prevented the Outback needle from reaching the snare. Coils were placed in the extravascular tract to prevent hemorrhage into the popliteal fossa. Note the small segment of the tibioperoneal trunk that reconstitutes (dashed arrow) but otherwise absent proximal tibial flow. (B) Distal arteriography shows reconstitution of the mid to distal anterior tibial artery (solid arrow) and a diminutive partially reconstituted peroneal artery (dashed arrow). The posterior tibial artery is completely occluded.

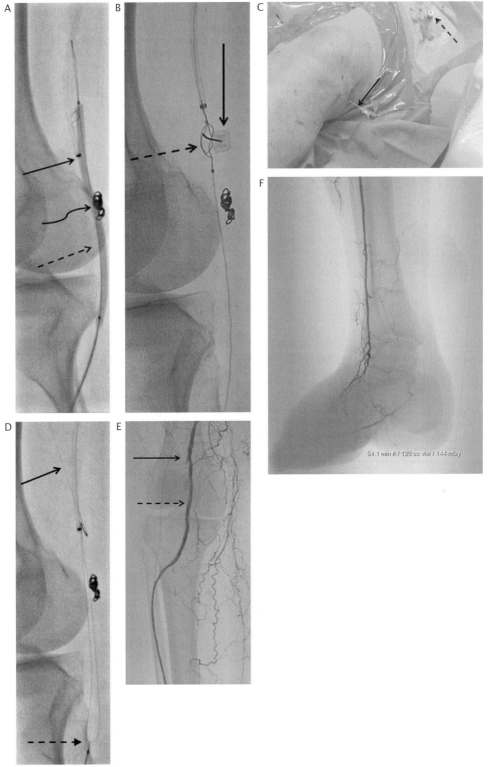

Figure 18.4 Percutaneous gun-sight extravascular revascularization technique. Images were obtained from the same patient illustrated in Figure 18.3. The decision was made to attempt the percutaneous gun-sight extravascular revascularization technique. (A) Retrograde anterior tibial artery access was obtained, but the tract had to be pre-dilated (dashed arrow) to facilitate retrograde snare advancement to the popliteal fossa. Coils are again noted (curved arrow). Note that the antegrade sheath (solid arrow) has been advanced close to the site of occlusion for optimal support and safe retraction of the back end of the wire to be placed. (B) With the image intensifier obliqued steeply in the left anterior oblique orientation, a 15-cm AccuStick needle (Boston Scientific; solid arrow) is advanced from a medial approach through overlapping antegrade and retrograde snares (dashed arrow). (C) An intraoperative photograph shows the 15-cm AccuStick needle (solid arrow) advanced into the popliteal fossa from a medial approach. A snare is seen entering the antegrade right femoral sheath (dashed arrow). (D) The back end of a Glidewire Gold wire was inserted first (because the femoral snare was deeper), and the needle was removed. The back end of the Glidewire Gold has been pulled through the femoral sheath. The retrograde snare (dashed arrow) is seen pulling the floppy end of the wire distally while the floppy end of the wire external to the patient (solid arrow) is threaded percutaneously into the patient. (E) After wire access is obtained, the extravascular tract is pre-dilated and stented (dashed arrow) with a short 5-mm Viabahn stent, and the occluded popliteal and anterior tibial arteries are angioplastied. Note that the vessel has a step-off (solid arrow) at the origin of the extravascular tract. (F) Final angiography distally shows unimpeded blood flow into the distal anterior tibial artery and dorsalis pedis with collateralized flow to the plantar artery.

References and Suggested Readings

1. Bolia A, Brennan J, Bell PR. Recanalization of femoro-popliteal occlusions: Improving success rate by subintimal recanalisation. *Clin Radiol.* 1989;40:325.

2. Bown MJ, Bolia A, Sutton AJ. Subintimal angioplasty: Meta-analytical evidence of clinical utility. *Eur J Vasc Endovasc Surg.* 2009;38:323–337.

3. Spinosa DJ, Harthun NL, Bissonette EA, et al. Subintimal arterial flossing with antegrade–retrograde intervention (SAFARI) for subintimal recanalization to treat chronic critical limb ischemia. *J Vasc Interv Radiol.* 2005;16(1):37–44.

4. Kahn JK, Hartzler GO. Retrograde coronary angioplasty of isolated arterial segments through saphenous vein bypass grafts. *Cathet Cardiovasc Diagn.* 1990;20:88–93.

5. Kirk J, Wilson R, Kovacs F, Tennant W, Braithwaite B, Habib S. Successful extra-anatomical recanalization of occluded superficial femoral arteries using the Outback® device—A report of 2 cases. *Vasc Endovasc Surg.* 2012;46(1):62–65.

6. Wagner JK, Chaer RA, Rhee RY, Marone LK. True lumen re-entry after extravascular recanalization of a superficial femoral artery chronic total occlusion. *J Vasc Surg.* 2010;52(1):216–218.

7. Haskal ZJ, Duszak R Jr, Furth EE. Transjugular intrahepatic transcaval portosystemic shunt: The gun-sight approach. *J Vasc Interv Radiol.* 1996;7(1):139–142.

CHAPTER 19

Retrograde Femoral Access for Difficult Superficial Femoral Artery Occlusions

Luke E. Sewall

Brief Description

Ultrasound-guided direct retrograde access of the superficial femoral artery can be a valuable technique to increase the success rate of treating total occlusions of the superficial femoral artery. The technique can be particularly useful in patients with a "flush" occlusion at the origin of the superficial femoral artery, where standard antegrade or around the bifurcation techniques fail to engage the origin of the vessel. The technique involves using ultrasound to identify a suitable location in the superficial femoral artery for direct puncture. This is ideally an area where flow is observed on ultrasound; however, occluded segments can also be accessed to successfully complete the procedure. Using the direct superficial femoral access, a wire is advanced in a retrograde manner into the common femoral artery. The wire is then manipulated into the up-and-over contralateral sheath or snared and pulled through the sheath. The remainder of the superficial femoral artery occlusion is then traversed in a standard fashion. This technique is extremely useful in patients who have occluded superficial femoral artery stents.[1] Standard techniques to traverse the stent are frequently frustrated by the convex proximal cap of the occlusion, which tends to force the guidewire to the periphery of the vessel and ultimately into the subintimal space outside of the stent. The benefits of the technique include the comfort level most interventionalists have with ultrasound-guided access, the decrease in fluoroscopy and contrast dose needed for prolonged crossing techniques, and the ability to complete the procedure without changing patient positioning. Previously used techniques include pedal access, which requires a very long pathway through much smaller vessels, and popliteal access, which often requires flipping the patient to the prone position.

Applications of the Technique

1. Flush occlusions of the superficial femoral artery that cannot be accessed using standard techniques.
2. Chronically occluded superficial femoral artery stents that have such fibrotic proximal caps that wires tend to go subintimally around the stents.

3. Subintimal antegrade access that fails to re-enter the true lumen.

Challenges of the Procedure

1. In morbidly obese patients, visualization of the superficial femoral artery may be difficult on ultrasound.
2. Need for pre-procedure planning of the technique to allow appropriate prepping of the patient.

Potential Pitfalls/Complications

1. Uncommon but possible bleeding from the superficial femoral artery access site, necessitating placement of a covered stent or prolonged balloon inflation.
2. Unintentional subintimal access of the superficial femoral artery, necessitating use of a subintimal arterial flossing with antegrade–retrograde intervention (SAFARI) technique.[2]

Steps of the Procedure

1. Contralateral femoral access: After a standard diagnostic angiogram, access is gained over the bifurcation. A stiff wire is advanced into the contralateral deep femoral artery, and a 6 Fr up-and-over sheath is placed.
2. Proper angiography: Ipsilateral oblique angiography is performed to identify the origin of the occluded superficial femoral artery. Often, a tiny nipple of the vessel can be identified.
3. Standard technique: If the vessel origin can be engaged, the vessel is crossed using any number of techniques, including guidewire and catheter techniques, or crossing devices such as the Ocelot (Avinger Inc., Redwood City, CA), the Crosser (C.R. Bard Inc., Murray Hill, NJ), the TruePath (Boston Scientific Inc., Marlborough, MA), the Frontrunner XP (Cordis Corp., Milpitas, CA), and the CrossBoss (BridgePoint Medical Inc., Plymouth, MN).

4. Direct superficial femoral artery access: If the origin cannot be successfully engaged or the proximal end can be engaged but a wire will not advance, the next step of the procedure is initiated.

5. Pre-procedure preparation: In chronic total occlusions of the superficial femoral artery, the entire leg is routinely prepped and draped from the groin through the knee. Using the initial angiogram, in combination with ultrasound imaging, a suitable access site is identified. This is ideally an area with flow at the site of reconstitution of flow distally or an area of "hibernating" vessel that is still patent. If neither is available, an easily visible segment of the occluded vessel is chosen.

6. Ultrasound-guided access: Using ultrasound guidance, the artery is accessed using either a micropunture needle for standard patients or a longer Chiba-type needle for larger patients or deeper vessels.

7. Retrograde crossing: A micropunture wire or V-18 wire is advanced. If necessary, a Quick-Cross-type catheter (Spectranetics Corp., Colorado Springs, CO) is added for support to allow the wire to be advanced through the superficial femoral artery origin and into the common femoral artery.

8. Capture of wire: Once in the femoral artery, the wire can be manipulated into the sheath directly, or a snare can be advanced through the contralateral sheath to pull the wire out for "through-and-through" access.

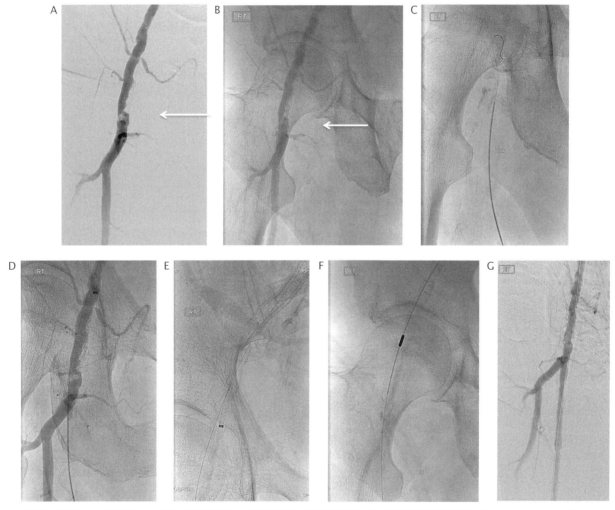

Figure 19.1 Subtracted and non-subtracted oblique angiogram of right groin. (A and B) Contralateral access and selective catheterization of the right external iliac artery showing a flush occlusion of the right superficial femoral artery (arrows). Also, there is densely calcified plaque in the distal common femoral artery, which makes attempts at standard superficial femoral artery access difficult. (C) Retrograde access of proximal superficial femoral artery. Image shows a micropuncture catheter and guidewire in the proximal superficial femoral artery after the proximal third of the vessel was accessed under ultrasound guidance. Retrograde access of the occluded superficial femoral artery. (D) A micropuncture catheter and V-18 guidewire were advanced in a retrograde fashion and manipulated into the external iliac artery. (E) The wire was later manipulated directly into the sheath and pulled out the contralateral groin access. The sheath was then advanced into the occluded superficial femoral artery. (F) Orbital atherectomy of the common femoral artery and superficial femoral artery done in a standard fashion. (G) Final angiogram. After successfully crossing the occlusion, the procedure was completed using an atherectomy catheter and standard angioplasty using a drug-eluting balloon.

9. Conversion to standard approach: A catheter is then advanced over the wire from the contralateral approach, and the remainder of the superficial femoral artery occlusion is traversed in the standard fashion.

10. Removal of direct retrograde puncture: Once a catheter is advanced to the level of the directly accessed vessel, the retrograde access is abandoned and removed.

11. Completion of procedure: Standard angioplasty and/or stenting are then completed from the contralateral approach. Completion angiography is done to ensure there is no bleeding from the direct access site.

12. Full anticoagulation and antiplatelets are used and continued after the procedure per individual preferences.

Example

See Figure 19.1.

References and Suggested Readings

1. Palena L, Cester G, Manzi M. Treatment of in-stent occlusion: New technique for recanalization of long superficial femoral artery occlusion (direct stent puncture technique). *Cardiovasc Intervent Radiol.* 2012;35(2):418–421.

2. Spinosa DJ, Harthun NL, Bissonette EA, et al. Subintimal arterial flossing with antegrade–retrograde intervention (SAFARI) for subintimal recanalization to treat chronic critical limb ischemia. *J Vasc Interv Radiol.* 2005;16(1):37–44.

CHAPTER 20

The "Poor Man's" Scoring Balloon

S. Lowell Kahn

Brief Description

Critical limb ischemia (CLI) is increasingly common, with a prevalence of 12% in the adult population.[1] The disease affects the elderly and diabetics disproportionally and is associated with a 20–30% 1-year mortality and a 25% rate of amputation in the same period.[2] Despite its prevalence and the gravity of the disease, CLI remains grossly underdiagnosed. A recent study found that more than 70% of primary care providers were unaware of the presence of critical limb ischemia in their patients.[3]

The optimal treatment for CLI has not been elucidated since there are many surgical and endovascular options for intervention. Comparing endovascular and surgical intervention has proven difficult given the high variability in the definitions of success, patency, clinical improvement, and follow-up reported in the literature.[4] Further compounding the problem is the wide variability in the disease itself (e.g., single vs. multilevel disease, ± calcium, and length/extent of stenosis or occlusion), patient comorbidities, operator experience, surgical and endovascular treatment options, and the rapid advances in endovascular technology. To date, the largest study comparing endovascular and bypass surgery is the randomized multicenter BASIL trial (Bypass Versus Angioplasty in Severe Ischemia of the Leg), which found similar outcomes for overall survival and amputation-free survival between the groups, despite a modest benefit with surgery in patients with a longer life expectancy.[5] Further data on the optimal use of surgery and endovascular therapy are forthcoming with the ongoing BASIL-2 and BEST trials. Nonetheless, the overall efficacy, reduced morbidity and mortality, and cost-effectiveness of endovascular therapy have led to more widespread adoption of an endo-first approach to critical limb ischemia.[6–8]

Although angioplasty is the foundation of endovascular intervention, it is not without limitation, particularly in heavily calcified or fibrotic lesions. Higher rates of restenosis and complications are observed when angioplasty is employed in small, diseased vessels.[9] Although estimates vary, it is likely that dissection occurs in more than 30% of cases.[10] Angioplasty produces irregular tears in the intima and stretching of the media with consequent neointimal proliferation and restenosis.[11,12] A variety of techniques and technologies exist to improve the outcomes of angioplasty. One such development was the advent of cutting and scoring balloons. Cutting balloons were introduced for coronary procedures more than 25 years ago and allow for a more controlled angioplasty of complex lesions. The microtomes mounted on the balloon concentrate the dilating force and create focal controlled disruptions in the plaque. This optimizes luminal expansion with less recoil and barotrauma to the vessel.[12,13] In addition, the cutting balloon is designed to reduce dissections and avoid slippage that might result in injury and consequent neointimal hyperplasia to the uninvolved adjacent vessel.[12–15] Although a major technological advance, cutting balloons are limited by their rigidity and short lengths, making the delivery to and the treatment of certain lesions impractical. Moreover, their use is associated with some risk, with a reported vessel rupture rate of up to 0.8%.[16]

More recently, scoring balloons entered the market as a solution to the shortcomings of cutting balloons. Like their predecessors, scoring balloons are designed to provide optimal luminal gain, decrease recoil and slippage, and minimize dissection. These balloons consist of a longer semicompliant balloon wrapped in one or more nitinol scoring elements (wires). The balloons are available in longer lengths and offer greater flexibility and deliverability—properties that make them ideal for peripheral applications. Data on these balloons are limited, but one study reported use of the AngioSculpt (Spectranetics Corp., Colorado Springs, CO) as primary therapy for infrapopliteal disease. Technical success without stenting was achieved in 89.3% of patients. The balloon had no reported slippage or vessel rupture, and dissection was observed in only 10.7% of cases.[10] These balloons are promising, but they are expensive and not universally available to all institutions.

This chapter describes bench creation of a "poor man's scoring balloon" as an alternative to commercially available scoring balloons. This is a simple procedure whereby two wires are placed side by side through the stenosis or occlusion to be treated. A standard angioplasty balloon is advanced over the working wire adjacent to the buddy wire. A minimal twisting is performed while advancing the balloon to wrap the buddy wire modestly around the balloon. The balloon is then inflated, and the spiral buddy wire acts as scoring element to produce a more effective angioplasty. Given that two or more wires are often utilized in a peripheral revascularization, this technique can be performed with little or no additional cost. In our experience, this procedure is simple to perform and works well in calcified or fibrotic lesions.

Applications of the Technique

1. Balloon angioplasty of calcified or fibrotic arterial occlusive disease.
2. Balloon angioplasty of arterial occlusive disease that demonstrates recoil.
3. Balloon angioplasty of refractory venous occlusive disease.

Challenges of the Procedure

1. Delivery of two wires through an occluded or highly stenotic lesion may be difficult.
2. Maintaining the scoring wire position during balloon advancement and withdrawal requires attention to prevent dislodgment to an undesired location.

Potential Pitfalls/Complications

1. Inadvertent movement of the scoring wire can occur while advancing or withdrawing the balloon over the adjacent wire. In theory, this could result in vessel injury or loss of access of the scoring wire.
2. Overly aggressive twisting of the balloon and scoring wire could result in entanglement requiring removal of both wires and the balloon with consequent loss of access.

Steps of the Procedure

1. The sheath is advanced immediately proximal to the lesion to be treated.
2. Diagnostic angiography with or without additional imaging (e.g., extravascular or intravascular ultrasound) is performed to delineate the nature of the stenosis or occlusion to be treated.
3. Over an appropriate support guidewire, the sheath should be upsized. Generally, the addition of an

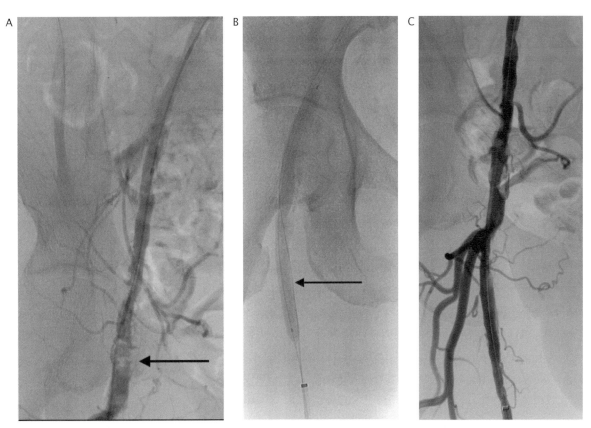

Figure 20.1 A 66-year-old female with rest pain and digital ulceration. The patient has multiple comorbidities rendering her a poor operative candidate who was declined a femoral endarterectomy by vascular surgery. Existing iliac stents necessitated a retrograde left popliteal artery access. (A) Preliminary arteriography demonstrates a heavily calcified eccentric plaque (arrow) with critical stenosis of the left common femoral artery. (B) After atherectomy with a Stealth 360 2.0 device (Cardiovascular Systems, Inc., St. Paul, MN), angioplasty was performed with a 6-mm Sterling (Boston Scientific Inc., Marlborough, MA) balloon. A 0.018-in. V-18 ControlWire (Boston Scientific Inc.) is utilized as a scoring wire and is seen wrapping helically around the balloon (solid black arrow). (C) Final retrograde angiography performed through the sheath shows persistent plaque but an improved caliber of the vessel.

adjacent scoring wire requires that the sheath be upsized 1 or 2 Fr sizes over the size required for the balloon to be used. For example, if the desired balloon requires a 5 Fr sheath, we recommend placing a 6 or 7 Fr sheath. The size required depends on the balloon used and the size of the adjacent scoring balloon. The combination should be tested on the back table prior to selecting the sheath.

4. Catheterization beyond the lesion to be treated is obtained. Ideally, the sheath should be advanced beyond the lesion because placement of the sheath allows easy placement of dual wires beyond the lesion. If the lesion is too tight, catheterization beyond the lesion can be obtained twice to facilitate the placement of two wires. In general, we prefer use of 0.014- or 0.018-in. balloons given their low profile relative to the 0.035-in. platform. The low profile is desirable with this technique given that the sheath size must be increased to accommodate the scoring wire. Adjacent to the working wire, a second wire is placed as the scoring wire. Again, we prefer use of a 0.014- or 0.018-in. wire for this purpose.

5. Over the working wire, the balloon is advanced in standard fashion to the target lesion. *Optional*: If desired, the balloon can be rotated a few times around the scoring wire during advancement to give the scoring wire a helical wrap around the balloon. This should only involve two or three turns to avoid kinking or tangling of the wire.

6. A prolonged balloon angioplasty is then conducted with a slow inflation and deflation. The scoring wire is located on the outside of the balloon.

7. Ideally, the balloon and scoring wire should be rotated between inflations, and a total of two or three inflations can be performed to score the plaque at more than one location.

8. Follow-up angiography is performed with additional interventions as needed.

Example
See Figure 20.1.

References and Suggested Readings

1. Norgren L, Hiatt WR, Dormandy JA, Nehler MR, Harris KA, Fowkes FGR. Inter-society consensus for the management of peripheral arterial disease (TASC II). *J Vasc Surg.* 2007;45(Suppl S):S5–S67.
2. Feiring AJ, Wesolowski AA, Lade S. Primary stent-supported angioplasty for treatment of below-knee critical limb ischemia and severe claudication: Early and one-year outcomes. *J Am Coll Cardiol.* 2004;44:2307–2314.
3. Hirsch AT, Criqui MH, Treat-Jacobson D, et al. Peripheral arterial disease detection, awareness, and treatment in primary care. *JAMA.* 2001;286(11):1317–1324.
4. Fu X, Zhang Z, Liang K, et al. Angioplasty versus bypass surgery in patients with critical limb ischemia—A meta-analysis. *Int J Clin Exp Med.* 2015;8(7):10595–10602.
5. Adam DJ, Beard JD, Cleveland T, et al.; BASIL trial participants. Bypass versus angioplasty in severe ischaemia of the leg (BASIL): Multicentre, randomised controlled trial. *Lancet.* 2005;366(9501):1925–1934.
6. Kudo T, Chandra FA, Kwun WH, Haas BT, Ahn SS. Changing pattern of surgical revascularization for critical limb ischemia over 12 years: Endovascular vs. open bypass surgery. *J Vasc Surg.* 2006;44:304–313.
7. Nasr MK, McCarthy RJ, Hardman J, Chalmers A, Horrocks M. The increasing role of percutaneous transluminal angioplasty in the primary management of critical limb ischemia. *Eur J Vasc Endovasc Surg.* 2002;23:398-403.
8. Dorros G, Jaff MR, Dorros AM, Mathiak LM, He T. Tibioperoneal (outflow lesion) angioplasty can be used as primary treatment in 235 patients with critical limb ischemia: Five-year follow-up. *Circulation.* 2001;104(17):2057–2062.
9. Kügler C, Rudofsky G. The challenges of treating peripheral arterial disease. *Vasc Med.* 2003;8(2):109–114.
10. Scheinert D, Peeters P, Bosiers M, O'Sullivan G, Sultan S, Gershony G. Results of the multicenter first-in-man study of a novel scoring balloon catheter for the treatment of infrapopliteal peripheral arterial disease. *Catheter Cardiovasc Interv.* 2007;70(7):1034–1039.
11. Bosiers, M, Deloose K, Cagiannos C, Verbist J, Peeters P. Use of the AngioSculpt scoring balloon for infrapopliteal lesions in patients with critical limb ischemia: 1-year outcome. *Vascular.* 2009;17(1):29–35.
12. Rabbi JF, Kiran RP, Gersten G, Dudrick SJ, Dardik A. Early results with infrainguinal cutting balloon angioplasty limits distal dissection. *Ann Vasc Surg.* 2004;18(6):640–643.
13. Kasirajan K, Schneider PA. Early outcome of "cutting" balloon angioplasty for infrainguinal vein graft stenosis. *J Vasc Surg.* 2004;39:702–708.
14. Miyamoto T, Araki T, Hiroe M, Marumo F, Niwa A, Yokoyama K. Stand-alone cutting balloon angioplasty for the treatment of stent-related restenosis: Acute results and 3- to 6-month angiographic recurrent restenosis rates. *Catheter Cardiovasc Intervent.* 2001;54:301–308.
15. Inoue T, Sakai Y, Hoshi K, Yaguchi I, Fujito T, Morooka S. Lower expression of neutrophil adhesion molecule indicates less vessel wall injury and might explain lower restenosis rate after cutting balloon angioplasty. *Circulation.* 1998;97:2511–2518.
16. Mauri L, Bonan R, Wiener BH, et al. Cutting balloon angioplasty for the prevention of restenosis: Results of the Cutting Balloon Global Randomized Trial. *Am J Cardiol.* 2002;90(10):1079–1083.

CHAPTER 21

Balloon-Assisted Thrombin Injection for Pseudoaneurysms with Wide or Short Neck Morphology

S. Lowell Kahn

Brief Description

Pseudoaneurysms after cardiac catheterizations are not uncommon, with a reported incidence of 0.1–1.1% following diagnostic catheterization and 3.5–5.5% following intervention.[1–4] Although most commonly they occur superficial to the common femoral artery, they are reported to occur at any location intentionally or unintentionally accessed, including the external iliac, profunda, and superficial femoral arteries. Risk factors for their development include age, female gender, high body mass index, low platelet count, high and low puncture sites, increased sheath size, urgent (vs. elective) procedures, inadvertent femoral artery and vein cannulation, and continued anticoagulation post procedure.[5]

Pseudoaneurysms present as a pulsatile mass near the site of catheterization. They are frequently associated with erythema, hematoma, and/or ecchymosis. A history of a slowly enlarging mass with associated tenderness is common. If auscultated, a bruit is may be appreciated. Although pseudoaneurysms are readily identifiable on computed tomography, the diagnosis is most commonly made on ultrasound (US), where a pulsatile mass is demonstrated with adjacent edema or hematoma. On duplex, a characteristic "yin and yang" pattern is observed with bidirectional flow toward and away from the neck of the pseudoaneurysm. US is a critical modality prior to treatment because it readily assesses the size, complexity (e.g., greater than one compartment), and neck of the pseudoaneurysms. An understanding of these features is essential prior to initiating therapy.

Historically, pseudoaneurysms were either managed conservatively (small) or repaired surgically. The advent of less invasive techniques has relegated surgery to a limited number of cases. Treatment options beyond surgery include ultrasound probe compression, placement of a covered stent across the neck of the pseudoaneurysm, coil embolization, or US-guided injection of various procoagulant agents to induce thrombosis.

Originally described by Cope and Zeit,[6] US-assisted thrombin injection has become the mainstay of therapy. Although variations exist regarding the optimal location, amount, and rate of thrombin injection, the superior outcomes, low complications, and low cost associated with this method render great appeal to its utilization.

Although rare (≤1%), the entrance of thrombin into the arterial vasculature can have disastrous consequences, including loss of limb. Most operators consider this risk to be greatest when treating small pseudoaneurysms or those with short and/or wide necks that more easily allow entrance of thrombin into the arterial vasculature. This chapter describes an adjunctive technique (as well as a simple modification) to prevent the entrance of thrombin to the vasculature using a balloon to isolate the pseudoaneurysm. Although typically not necessary, this technique is valuable in the treatment of high-risk pseudoaneurysms and is well described in the literature.[7–11]

Applications of the Technique

1. Management of central or peripheral pseudoaneurysms that meet criteria for treatment but have a hostile neck or small size for safe percutaneous treatment alone. Specifically, small pseudoaneurysms or those with short and/or wide necks that carry an elevated risk of thrombin escaping the pseudoaneurysm with consequent arterial thrombosis.

Challenges of the Procedure

1. With complex pseudoaneurysms, delineation of the neck can be challenging. For this reason, we advise that after the balloon is inflated and percutaneous access to the pseudoaneurysm is obtained, a small amount of contrast should be injected into the pseudoaneurysm to confirm isolation from the arterial system.

2. Occasionally, a pseudoaneurysm may be deep or located high from a poor access obtained above the inguinal ligament. Such scenarios, seen most commonly in obese patients, can limit visualization by ultrasound. We have managed this by obtaining femoral access and placing an occlusion balloon side by side with a microcatheter. The microcatheter is navigated directly into the pseudoaneurysm while the balloon is used to occlude the vessel and cover the neck. This method renders percutaneous needle access unnecessary and is described separately later.

Potential Pitfalls/Complications

1. As with all thrombin injections, extreme care must be taken to avoid injection of thrombin into the arterial vasculature. The consequent arterial thrombosis can lead to severe morbidity and possible loss of limb. If the neck is poorly delineated on digital subtraction arteriography (DSA) and US, it is possible that the interventionalist may inappropriately assume the pseudoaneurysm has been excluded from the arterial system with inflation of the balloon.

Steps of the Procedure

Standard Technique

1. Up-and-over catheterization of the contralateral superficial femoral artery is obtained with standard wire and catheter technique.
2. An appropriately sized 5 or 6 Fr up-and-over sheath is placed for added stability.
3. DSA is performed through the sheath with obliquity as necessary to profile the neck of the pseudoaneurysm. A steep ipsilateral oblique image typically profiles the femoral bifurcation and the neck of the pseudoaneurysm well.
4. A short balloon approximating the diameter of the vessel at the site of the pseudoaneurysm is chosen. This is typically between 5 and 8 mm in diameter and 2–4 cm in length.
5. The balloon is positioned over the neck of the pseudoaneurysm.
6. Under US guidance, a needle is inserted into the pseudoaneurysm at a location away from the neck. Duplex is performed, and the needle tip is positioned where the Doppler signal indicates flow is away from the neck. Our typical needle size ranges between 20 and 22 gauge, but use of larger and smaller needles is acceptable practice.
7. The balloon is inflated, and a test injection of contrast is performed. Isolation of the contrast from the arterial vasculature is confirmed.

8. The balloon is deflated to allow the contrast to escape and is then re-inflated.
9. Under US, thrombin is injected slowly into the pseudoaneurysm at a concentration of 1000 units/cc. Although variable, typically between 0.2 and 0.6 cc is required. The injection is slow at a rate of 0.1–0.3 cc per second.[1,12] Ultrasound with and without duplex verifies the formation of thrombus within the pseudoaneurysm.
10. The thrombin is allowed to dwell for no more than 5 minutes with the balloon inflated. The balloon is then deflated.
11. DSA and US are performed to verify complete thrombosis of the pseudoaneurysm with preserved blood flow in the native arterial vasculature.

Modified Technique for Deep Pseudoaneurysms with Poor Visualization Under Ultrasound

1. Up-and-over catheterization of the contralateral superficial femoral artery is obtained with standard wire and catheter technique.
2. An appropriately sized (typically 7 Fr) sheath is placed.
3. DSA is performed through the sheath with obliquity as necessary to profile the neck of the pseudoaneurysm.
4. A microcatheter is used to catheterize the pseudoaneurysm. The tip of the microcatheter is placed away from the neck and ideally in a position where blood flow is directed away from the neck.
5. Adjacent to the microcatheter, an appropriately sized short balloon is advanced side by side through the sheath and positioned at the neck of the pseudoaneurysm. As noted previously, typical occlusion balloon sizes range between 5 and 8 mm in diameter and are 2–4 cm in length.
6. The balloon is inflated over the neck of the pseudoaneurysm while a test injection of contrast is made through the microcatheter. Isolation of the contrast from the arterial vasculature is confirmed.
7. The balloon is deflated to allow the contrast to escape and is then re-inflated.
8. Thrombin is injected slowly through the microcatheter in a similar manner as described earlier.
9. The thrombin is allowed to dwell with the balloon inflated. The balloon is then deflated.
10. DSA is performed to verify complete thrombosis of the pseudoaneurysm with preserved blood flow in the native arterial vasculature.

Example
See Figure 21.1.

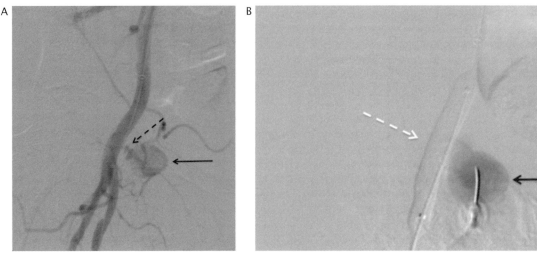

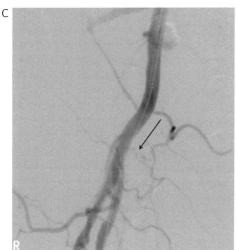

Figure 21.1 (A) DSA image of the right common femoral artery performed through the sheath prior to intervention. Note the short neck (dashed arrow) of the pseudoaneurysm (solid arrow) emanating from the common femoral artery. (B) A balloon (dashed arrow) has been advanced into the common femoral artery and positioned over the neck of the pseudoaneurysm (solid arrow). A needle was placed into the pseudoaneurysm under direct US guidance. Note an injection of contrast made into the pseudoaneurysm confirms isolation of the pseudoaneurysm from the arterial vasculature. Thrombin was subsequently injected into the pseudoaneurysm. (C) Final DSA image after thrombin injection and removal of the balloon. There is trace flow within the neck (arrow), but the pseudoaneurysm itself is otherwise completely thrombosed.

Source: From Popovic M, et al. Balloon occlusion assisted percutaneous femoral pseudoaneurysm treatment. Scientific paper, 2011. Courtesy the European Society of Radiology (ECR). DOI:10.1594/ecr2011/C-0604.

References and Suggested Readings

1. Saad WEA, Waldman DL. Management of postcatheterization pseudoaneurysms. In: Mauro MA, Murphy KPJ, Thomson KR, Venbrux AC, Zollikofer CL, eds. *Image-Guided Interventions*. Philadelphia: Elsevier; 2008:525–536.

2. Kronzon I. Diagnosis and treatment of iatrogenic femoral artery pseudoaneurysm: A review. *J Am Soc Echocardiogr.* 1997;10:236–245.

3. Altes M, Sahin S, Konuralp C, et al. Evaluation of risk factors associated with femoral pseudoaneurysms after cardiac catheterization. *J Vasc Surg.* 2006;43:520–524.

4. Ma M, Snook CP. Ruptured femoral pseudoaneurysm presenting as a lateral abdominal wall hematoma. *J Emerg Med.* 2005;29:147–150.

5. Stone PA, Campbell JE, AbuRahma AF. Femoral pseudoaneurysms after percutaneous access. *J Vasc Surg.* 2014;60(5):1359–1366.

6. Cope C, Zeit R. Coagulation of aneurysms by direct percutaneous thrombin injection. *AJR Am J Roentgenol.* 1986;147:383–387.

7. Lee TK, Jeon YS, Hong KC, Cho SG, Kim E. Balloon-assisted ultrasound-guided thrombin injection of a pseudoaneurysm in the posterior tibial artery: A case report. *J Korean Soc Radiol.* 2014;70(5):325–329.

8. Matson MB, Morgan RA, Belli AM. Percutaneous treatment of pseudoaneurysms using fibrin adhesive. *Br J Radiol.* 2001;74:690–694.

9. Loose HW, Haslam PJ. The management of peripheral arterial aneurysms using percutaneous injection of fibrin adhesive. *Br J Radiol.* 1998;71:1255–1259.

10. Owen RJ, Haslam PJ, Elliott ST, et al. Percutaneous ablation of peripheral pseudoaneurysms using thrombin: A simple and effective solution. *Cardiovasc Intervent Radiol.* 2000;23:441–446.

11. Samal AK, White CJ, Collins TJ, et al. Treatment of femoral artery pseudoaneurysm with percutaneous thrombin injection. *Cathet Cardiovasc Intervent.* 2001;53:259–263.

12. Vazquez V, Reus M, Pinero, A, et al. Human thrombin for treatment of pseudoaneurysms: Comparison of bovine and human thrombin sonogram-guided injection. *AJR Am J Roentgenol.* 2005;184:1665–1671.

CHAPTER 22

Distal Occlusion Thrombectomy Technique

S. Lowell Kahn

Brief Description

The distal occlusion balloon thrombectomy technique involves placement of an occlusion balloon immediately distal to the thrombus or embolus to be removed. The balloon overlaps the antegrade wire. With the balloon inflated, the thrombotic/embolic material is removed over the antegrade wire using the desired thrombectomy catheter or device. The inflated balloon prevents distal migration of the embolic material during removal. Intermittent digital subtraction angiography (DSA) is performed to assess for residual debris. When sufficiently extracted, the balloon is deflated and removed.

Most commonly, this is performed with the balloon inserted in a retrograde manner (e.g., 0.014- or 0.018-in. balloon via tibiopedal or popliteal access). However, if distal access is not feasible, the antegrade sheath can be upsized (typically 7 Fr or greater), and a 0.014-/0/018-in. balloon can be placed antegrade through the sheath over a buddy wire and positioned distal to the thrombus/embolus. Adjacent to the balloon, aspiration or pharmacomechanical thrombectomy can be performed.

Interestingly, the GuardWire Temporary Occlusion and Aspiration System (Medtronic Inc., Minneapolis, MN) is based upon a similar concept whereby a balloon is mounted on the tip of a guidewire that is inflated via use of a proprietary CO_2 injection system. The use of other embolic protection devices during thrombectomy is described in the literature, but these systems require intervention over a 0.014-in. platform and are limited with respect to the amount of embolic material successfully trapped from the distal circulation.[1,2]

Applications of the Technique

1. Most commonly, this technique is performed in the lower extremities during thrombus/embolus extraction, but it could be applied elsewhere as needed.
2. In select cases, the technique could be applied to embolus removal in the renal or visceral vasculature, but this would obviously require that the balloon be placed antegrade over a buddy wire.

Challenges of the Procedure

1. Advancing a retrograde balloon via the tibiopedal vessels requires that the vessels are suitable for access. Depending on the presence of disease and the size of the tibial vessels, the balloon may be advanced through a sheath or bareback with caution.
2. Advancing a balloon antegrade over a buddy wire requires sufficient size of the sheath so that there is minimal friction between the balloon and the thrombectomy catheter/device. Also, great care must be taken when advancing a balloon antegrade to prevent inadvertent dislodgment of the thrombus/embolus during distal balloon placement.

Potential Pitfalls/Complications

1. Although a relatively low risk, the tibial vessels can be traumatized with direct retrograde access, and this risk must be considered relative to the risk of further distal embolization.
2. Advancement of the occlusion balloon from the antegrade access carries a risk of dislodgment of the thrombus/embolus with potentially severe adverse sequelae.

Steps of the Procedure

1. From the antegrade sheath or a new retrograde access, the occlusion balloon is positioned immediately distal to the thrombus/embolus targeted for removal. If advanced from a retrograde access, the occlusion balloon will overlap the antegrade wire. If the balloon is to be advanced retrograde, the sheath must be adequately upsized (typically 7 Fr or greater) to accommodate the side-by-side advancement of the thrombectomy catheter/device adjacent to the occlusion balloon on a buddy wire. Regardless of the approach, we recommend use of a low-profile, short 0.014- or 0.018-in. balloon sized 1:1 with the vessel diameter.
2. DSA images are acquired to study the extent of the thrombus/embolus.

3. The balloon is inflated, and repeat imaging is performed to ensure occlusion.
4. With the balloon inflated, the thrombectomy catheter/device is utilized per the manufacturer's instructions for use to remove all thrombotic/embolic material.
5. Intermittent DSA images are acquired to verify complete removal and ensure there is no residual debris.

6. The occlusion balloon is deflated and removed from the antegrade or retrograde access. The procedure is then completed in standard fashion.

Example
See Figure 22.1.

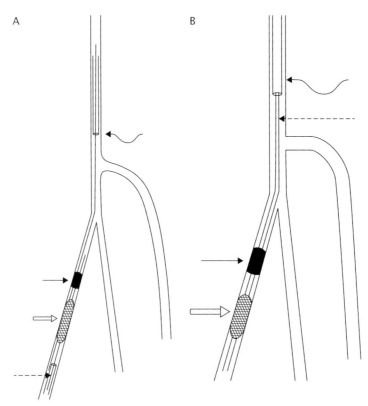

Figure 22.1 (A) Distal occlusion balloon thrombectomy technique. Schematic demonstrates acute embolus in the proximal posterior tibial artery of the left leg (solid arrow). An antegrade sheath (curved arrow) terminates in the distal popliteal artery. Antegrade wire access through the embolus has been obtained. Through a retrograde-placed sheath (dashed arrow) in the posterior tibial artery, an occlusion balloon (open arrow) has been inflated to protect the runoff. The balloon overlaps the antegrade wire. Thrombectomy is performed through the antegrade sheath. (B) Distal occlusion balloon thrombectomy technique. Schematic demonstrates acute embolus in the proximal posterior tibial artery of the left leg (solid arrow). Dual antegrade wire access (dashed arrow) through the embolus has been obtained from the antegrade sheath (curved arrow). An occlusion balloon (open arrow) is passed beyond the occlusion and inflated to provide distal protection during thrombectomy performed over the other guidewire.

References and Suggested Readings
1. Sedghi Y, Collins TJ, White CJ. Endovascular management of acute limb ischemia. *Vasc Med.* 2013;18(5):307–313.
2. Fujii K. Thrombus aspiration therapy and distal protection devices. *Nihon Rinsho.* 2011;69(Suppl 9):174–178.

CHAPTER 23

Techniques for Traversing Difficult Aortic Bifurcations and Aortobifemoral Grafts

S. Lowell Kahn

Brief Description

Although many lower extremity endovascular procedures are performed with an ipsilateral extremity access, contralateral extremity interventions remain a mainstay of endovascular therapy. Since its original description in 1979, the retrograde common femoral arterial access for contralateral infrainguinal interventions has remained one of the most common access sites.[1-4] The common femoral artery is desirable for access given its size, accessibility, and ease of compressibility against the femoral head for hemostasis post procedure.[2,5] Although an ipsilateral access confers the benefits of proximity for lesion traversal and intervention, there are various scenarios, including body habitus (obesity) and coexistent iliac disease, that may make a contralateral up-and-over approach desirable or necessary. Typically, traversing the aortic bifurcation for an up-and-over approach is readily accomplished with little difficulty, but sharp angulation, severe calcification, iliac occlusive disease, kissing common iliac stents, and surgical or endovascular (e.g., aortobifemoral or endovascular stent grafts) bifurcations can make this challenging or impossible.[2] Although other acceptable alternative accesses (radial, brachial, popliteal, and tibial) and techniques (catheter flipping) exist, these all have risks and limitations. Therefore, maximizing proficiency with the up-and-over approach remains imperative.

For reference in this chapter, *ipsilateral* refers to the point of access, and *contralateral* references the opposite extremity to which the intended intervention is performed. After obtaining retrograde ipsilateral access, a retrograde 4 or 5 Fr sheath is placed using the Seldinger technique. In comparison to the standard short 11-cm sheath, use of a longer 23- or 25-cm sheath straightens the ipsilateral iliac vasculature and provides added support for advancing a catheter over the aortic bifurcation.[1] If the groin is scarred, a stiff wire (e.g., Amplatz, Boston Scientific Inc., Marlborough, MA) and serial dilators may be necessary for sheath placement. Typically, passage of a Bentson (Cook Medical Inc., Bloomington, IN) or Glidewire (regular or stiff; Terumo Medical Corp., Somerset, NJ) over the bifurcation is readily accomplished with a RIM (Cook Medical Inc., Bloomington, IN), Omni Flush (AngioDynamics Inc., Latham, NY), or other reverse curve catheter (e.g., Sos and VCF, Cook Medical Inc., Bloomington, IN). In cases in which the bifurcation is more obtuse, a Cobra catheter (AngioDynamics Inc., Latham, NY) may be beneficial. Regardless of the catheter and wire combination selected, the wire should be advanced carefully (to avoid dissection) but as far as possible (common femoral or distally) for optimal support. In some instances, use of a stiff Glidewire is advantageous. If the initial catheter will not advance despite adequate sheath support, exchanging for a less angled catheter (e.g., straight or hockey stick configuration) with a hydrophilic coating (e.g., Slip-Cath [Cook Medical Inc.] and Glidecath [Terumo Medical Corp.]) is often helpful. Alternatively, a support catheter (e.g., CXI [Cook Medical Inc., Bloomington, IN] and Quick-Cross [Spectranetics Corp., Colorado Springs, CO]) may be used.

In rare cases in which the previously discussed equipment and techniques fail, compression on the contralateral groin (assuming the wire is at or beyond the common femoral artery) may provide traction on the wire and facilitate advancement of a catheter or sheath over the bifurcation.[1] Similarly, use of deflectable sheaths (Morph, BioCardia, San Carlos, CA) is occasionally required to provide the necessary catheter support for advancement.

Once catheter and wire access is obtained to the contralateral common femoral artery or beyond, the wire should be exchanged for a stiff wire providing optimal support for subsequent sheath or device advancement over the challenging bifurcation. If there is stenotic or occlusive ipsilateral or contralateral iliac disease, pretreatment with angioplasty and/or stenting may be required prior to sheath advancement. Finally, selecting the appropriate sheath is important, and we prefer use of braided (kink-resistant) and hydrophilic sheaths (e.g., Flexor, Cook Medical Inc.) for this purpose. Shaped sheaths (e.g., Balkin and Ansel 1, Cook Medical Inc.) may have an advantage over their straight (e.g., Raabe, Cook Medical Inc.) counterpart.

This chapter describes multiple techniques to optimize advancement of a sheath or device over the bifurcation, whether native or prosthetic. For those interested in additional reading, excellent review articles on this topic are provided by Herman[1] and Grenon et al.[2] The first technique, herein referred to as the *Wire Wiggle Technique*, was described by Grenon et al.[2] and involves rapidly advancing and withdrawing the support wire a short distance to remove tension and facilitate sheath advancement. As mentioned previously, a stiff wire splays the aortic bifurcation in and of itself and often allows passage of a sheath over the bifurcation. Generally, the stiffer the wire, the better (e.g., Amplatz and Meier [Boston Scientific Inc.] and Lunderquist [Cook Medical Inc.]), but interestingly, occasionally a semi-stiff wire (e.g., Rosen, Cook Medical Inc.,Bloomington, IN) performs better.

The second technique, referenced herein as the *Snared Wire Technique*, involves obtaining bilateral femoral sheath access. A snare is advanced from the contralateral sheath and used to grasp a wire advanced into the aorta. The wire is brought out the contralateral sheath, and with backtraction on both ends of the wire, the sheath is advanced over the bifurcation. Once the up-and-over sheath reaches the contralateral femoral artery, the wire is pulled back from the contralateral sheath and the case is continued as desired. This technique may be used alone or in conjunction with the *Buddy Wire Loop Technique*. The *Buddy Wire Loop Technique* involves placing a buddy wire deep into the lower extremity vasculature or obtaining a through-and-through stiff buddy wire access as described previously for the snared wire technique. Adjacent to this support wire, a catheter or device may be advanced and used over a second wire. This method was initially described by Viner and Kessel[6] in 2008 as a means to intervene on a transplant renal artery stenosis and to embolize an internal iliac artery with optimal sheath support. A variant of this technique was described by Etezadi and Powell[7] in 2010 whereby the stiff buddy wire was used to splay the aortic bifurcation and allow up-and-over passage of the Outback® LTD® Reentry Catheter (Cordis Corp, Milpitas, CA) over an adjacent 0.014-in. wire. Similarly, Zastro et al.[8] confirmed use of this technique in 2012 for embolization of an internal iliac artery.

The *Pay It Off The Dilator Technique* and the *Pay It Off The Balloon Technique* involve incremental advances of the sheath over the dilator or a deflating balloon, respectively. Both techniques carry a small risk of embolization, and some authors advocate periodic aspiration of the sheath while performing the pay it off the balloon technique.[1] Finally, the *Telescoping Sheaths Technique* involves placing the up-and-over sheath coaxially within a larger sheath that has been advanced within the ipsilateral common iliac artery to the level of the aortic bifurcation. Just as the longer 23- or 25-cm sheath supports passage of the initial catheter,

the larger outer sheath provides added support for passage of the up-and-over sheath.

The six techniques described herein are easily learned and readily accomplished with standard angiographic equipment available in most laboratories. Mastery of the techniques and approaching the bifurcation with an algorithm guarantee success in all but a very limited number of cases, including aortobifemoral and aortic endografts.

Applications of the Technique

Wire Wiggle Technique
1. Up-and-over sheath advancement with diseased, angled, or prosthetic (aortobifemoral/endografts) arterial anatomy at the bifurcation.
2. May be used for virtually any catheter or sheath advancement in tight or tortuous arterial or venous anatomy.
3. Has nonvascular applications as well, including advancement of biliary, urinary, or gastrointestinal tubes through tight or tortuous anatomy. Often useful for reducing an undesired redundant loop (i.e., fundal loop while advancing a gastrojejunostomy tube).

Snared Wire Technique
1. Up-and-over sheath advancement with diseased, angled, or prosthetic (aortobifemoral/endografts) arterial anatomy at the bifurcation.
2. May be used for a variety of arterial interventions when there is tight or tortuous vascular anatomy. The subintimal arterial flossing with antegrade–retrograde intervention (SAFARI) technique is essentially a variant of this technique. Similarly, the technique has potential application for subclavian and innominate artery interventions (femoral-to-brachial through-and-through wire access).
3. The technique could be employed for any of a variety of venous interventions in which there is tight or tortuous anatomy (e.g., brachiocephalic and superior vena cava) disease whereby femoral-to-upper extremity through-and-through venous wire access is obtained.
4. Biliary (rendezvous technique) and urinary (transrenal to transurethral wire access) for drain, scope, and device advancement as necessary.

Buddy Wire Loop Technique
1. The predominant use for this technique is for hypogastric embolization or device advancement, as has been described in the literature.[6–8]
2. We have not attempted to use the technique in this manner, but theoretically femoral to brachial wire

access could be employed for added system stability and support while performing innominate/subclavian or carotid interventions over a buddy wire.

3. The technique could also be employed for added support/stability during hypogastric venous interventions (e.g., pelvic congestion syndrome) by placing a buddy wire distally in the lower extremity veins or obtaining femoral-to-femoral through-and-through venous access.

Pay It Off The Dilator and Pay It Off the Balloon Techniques

1. Up-and-over sheath advancement with diseased, angled, or prosthetic (aortobifemoral/endografts) arterial anatomy at the bifurcation.
2. This technique is ubiquitous and can be used any time sheath advancement is necessary through tight or tortuous anatomy. We have used this extensively for sheath advancement within the visceral, renal, and peripheral arterial vasculature.
3. The technique is similarly useful for advancing a sheath within the venous vasculature.
4. As with the prior techniques, if sheath advancement is necessary for biliary or urinary procedures, it may be employed.

Telescoping Sheaths Technique

1. Up-and-over sheath advancement with diseased, angled, or prosthetic (aortobifemoral/endografts) arterial anatomy at the bifurcation.
2. The technique may be used for advancing a sheath into any arterial or venous territory. Obviously, the technique is performed at the expense of a larger sheath size at the point of access.

Challenges of the Procedure

Wire Wiggle Technique

1. No specific challenges have been encountered per se, but in the author's experience, this technique is applicable for short-distance sheath advancement only.

Snared Wire Technique

1. Requires a suitable site for secondary access.
2. Requires the ability to advance a snare or wire to a point accessible (e.g., aorta) for the opposite side.

Buddy Wire Loop Technique

1. *May require* a suitable site for secondary access if true through-and-through femoral access is desired for support. Can be performed with the buddy wire simply placed distally in the contralateral vasculature.
2. *May require* the ability to advance a snare or wire to a point accessible (e.g., aorta) for the opposite side.

3. The ipsilateral sheath must be upsized adequately to allow side-by-side advancement of the other catheter/device adjacent to the buddy wire.

Pay It Off The Dilator Technique

1. Advancement of the sheath over the dilator may cause the dilator to kick back with consequent little or no advancement of the overall system. Pulling the sheath back with a short quick motion with forward motion of the sheath sometimes overcomes this.

Pay It Off The Balloon Technique

1. The technique requires being able to successfully advance a balloon beyond the end of the sheath. We recommend use of a short balloon. At times, downsizing to a smaller balloon system (0.018 or 0.014 in.) may be necessary.

Telescoping Sheaths Technique

1. No specific challenges except that it requires being able to place a larger sheath at the point of access. Typically, a sheath will pass coaxially through another sheath that is two French sizes larger (e.g., a 6 Fr sheath will pass through an 8 Fr sheath).

Potential Pitfalls/Complications

Wire Wiggle Technique

1. Mindfulness of the wire position is mandatory with this technique. Specifically, it is possible to lose wire access with this method. We advise careful re-advancement of the wire as needed to ensure adequate purchase is maintained.
2. Wiggling of a stiff guidewire carries a small risk of vessel injury/dissection and should be performed cautiously.

Snared Wire Technique

1. There are no specific pitfalls or complications to this technique other than recognition of the fact that a second access is necessary and the vessel for this secondary access should be suitable for placement of a small sheath (although a sheath-less technique is possible, which is discussed later). There are inherent risks of vessel injury and bleeding associated with every additional vascular access.

Buddy Wire Loop Technique

1. As mentioned previously, the technique *may require* a suitable secondary access site (if true through-and-through femoral wire access is desired), and there are inherent risks of vessel injury and bleeding that exist with the addition of each access point. Also, as noted previously, if a second access is needed, it should

be able to accommodate a small sheath (although a sheath-less technique is possible).

2. Performance of this technique requires a larger ipsilateral sheath size to accommodate the additional buddy wire. A larger sheath is associated with a higher risk of access vessel injury/thrombosis and hemorrhage.

Pay It Off The Dilator Technique

1. The technique carries a small risk of lost access. In difficult cases, advancing the sheath over the dilator results in the dilator and therefore the system, including the wire, pulling back.

2. As the sheath is advanced over the stationary dilator, the normal taper between the dilator and sheath is lost. Consequently, there is a low associated risk of embolization because the free edge of the sheath could dislodge an unstable plaque during advancement.

Pay It Off The Balloon Technique

1. As with the former technique, advancing a sheath without its dilator in standard configuration carries an increased risk of embolization because the free edge of the sheath can dislodge an unstable plaque during advancement. Some authors advocate aspiration before and during balloon deflation/sheath advancement to mitigate this risk.

2. Inflation of a balloon always carries an associated risk of vessel trauma/dissection or rupture. The user must be mindful and prepared for this, given the potentially serious associated risks of this in the iliac vasculature.

Telescoping Sheaths Technique

1. As mentioned previously, performance of this technique requires a larger sheath size (typically two French sizes larger). A larger sheath is associated with a higher risk of access vessel injury/thrombosis and hemorrhage.

Steps of the Procedure

Wire Wiggle Technique

1. A stiff guidewire is advanced as far as possible to obtain optimal support and purchase.

2. If the sheath does not advance, the wire is wiggled in short bursts forward and backward while the sheath is advanced to lessen the tension/friction on the sheath. Alternatively, a fast, short-distance pullback of the wire can be performed while the sheath is advanced. As noted previously, it is important to be mindful of the wire position at all times during this maneuver.

Snared Wire Technique

1. After failed up-and-over sheath advancement to the contralateral femoral artery, retrograde catheterization of the contralateral femoral artery is obtained. Using the Seldinger technique, a 4 Fr sheath is placed. A stiff exchange length wire is advanced into the aorta from the contralateral access. *Note*: In multiple reports,[1,2,8] the snare is advanced from the contralateral side and used to grasp the wire from the ipsilateral side. We prefer to advance the snare on the ipsilateral side and the wire from the contralateral side so that the contralateral sheath remains small (e.g., 4 Fr). In theory, if a stiff exchange length wire can be advanced successfully to the aorta through the transitional dilator alone, a sheath may not be necessary, and simply the wire could be advanced to minimize the size of the access on the contralateral side. This may be beneficial later, particularly if the contralateral femoral artery is diseased and/or small in caliber.

2. A snare is advanced to the aorta from the ipsilateral access.

3. The wire advanced from the contralateral access is snared and brought out through the retrograde ipsilateral sheath.

4. With back tension applied to both ends of the wire, the sheath is carefully advanced to the contralateral external iliac or common femoral artery.

5. With the sheath having reached its desired position, the wire is removed and the case is continued with additional infrainguinal intervention as needed.

Buddy Wire Loop Technique

1. This technique is not intended for advancing the sheath over the bifurcation. Rather, it is designed to provide added sheath stability and support for internal iliac arterial interventions or to allow passage of a device (e.g., Outback® LTD® Re-entry Catheter) over a challenging bifurcation. For the technique to work, the ipsilateral sheath must be upsized accordingly to accommodate the added diameter necessary for the buddy wire. Obviously, the larger the buddy wire, the more upsizing of the sheath required (e.g., 0.035- vs. 0.014-in. buddy wire). Irrespective of the size chosen, the buddy wire should be stiff.

2. The stiff guidewire is advanced distally in the contralateral vasculature. The sheath is advanced to the desired position (proximal to the iliac bifurcation for internal iliac interventions).

3. *Optional*: Steps 1–3 of the *Snared Wire Technique* can be performed if desired for added sheath support obtained with through-and-through access. With back tension on both ends of the buddy wire, the sheath is advanced over the bifurcation to the desired

location (proximal to the iliac bifurcation for internal iliac interventions).

4. Adjacent to the buddy wire, the catheter or device to be used for the subsequent procedure (e.g., internal iliac embolization) is advanced with the firmly stabilized sheath position. As described by Etezadi and Powell,[7] this technique can be used to splay the bifurcation with a stiff buddy wire, thereby allowing passage of a device that is difficult over a sharp bifurcation (Outback® LTD® Re-entry catheter, atherectomy devices, etc.).

5. The procedure is completed as desired.

Pay It Off The Dilator Technique

1. The sheath and dilator are advanced over a stiff guidewire as far as possible.
2. When further advancement is not possible, the dilator is pinned and the sheath is carefully advanced and wiggled (spun) forward within the vessel.
3. The sheath position is maintained with forward pressure while the dilator is reinserted.
4. Steps 2 and 3 are repeated to advance the sheath as far as possible to its desired position.

Pay It Off The Balloon Technique

1. The sheath and dilator are advanced over a stiff guidewire as far as possible.
2. When further advancement is not possible, the dilator is removed.
3. A balloon is advanced through the sheath and placed just beyond the tip of the sheath. The chosen balloon should approximate or marginally exceed the diameter of the vessel it is in to allow for adequate apposition and traction (e.g., a 6- or 7-mm balloon for a 6-mm vessel). Typically, a short-length (20–40 mm) balloon is desirable for most interventions. The user should be mindful of the size of the balloon and coexistent plaque to ensure inadvertent vessel rupture/trauma/dissection does not occur.
4. The balloon is inflated at or below nominal pressure. The inflation should be just enough to allow apposition of the balloon to the vessel wall so that traction is obtained.
5. The balloon is then rapidly deflated. While the balloon is deflating, the sheath is advanced over it.
6. The balloon is re-advanced beyond the tip of the sheath, and steps 4 and 5 are repeated to obtain the desired sheath position.
7. *Optional*: As mentioned previously, some authors advocate aspiration of the sheath before and during balloon deflation to lessen the risk of embolization.

Telescoping Sheaths Technique

1. After failed up-and-over sheath advancement to the contralateral femoral artery, the sheath is removed over the stiff guidewire and exchanged for a 23- or 25-cm sheath that is two French sizes larger than the original sheath.
2. The large outer sheath is advanced just proximal to the aortic bifurcation, and its dilator is removed.
3. The original inner sheath is advanced with its dilator coaxially through the outer sheath. If successful, the outer sheath straightens the ipsilateral iliac vasculature and provides the necessary support to allow up-and-over sheath advancement as desired.

Example

See Figures 23.1–23.5.

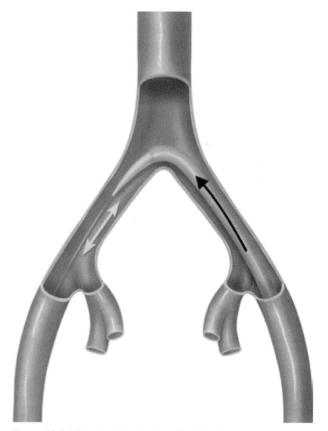

Figure 23.1 Wire wiggle technique. Rapid advancement and withdrawal of the wire (bidirectional white arrow) releases tension and allows forward advancement of the sheath (black arrow) over the aortic bifurcation. A variant of this technique involves a brisk, short pullback of the wire with simultaneous advancement of the sheath. Attention to wire position is critical with this method.

Source: From Grenon MS, et al. Technical endovascular highlights for crossing the difficult aortic bifurcation. *J Vasc Surg.* 2011;54:893–896. Courtesy Elsevier.

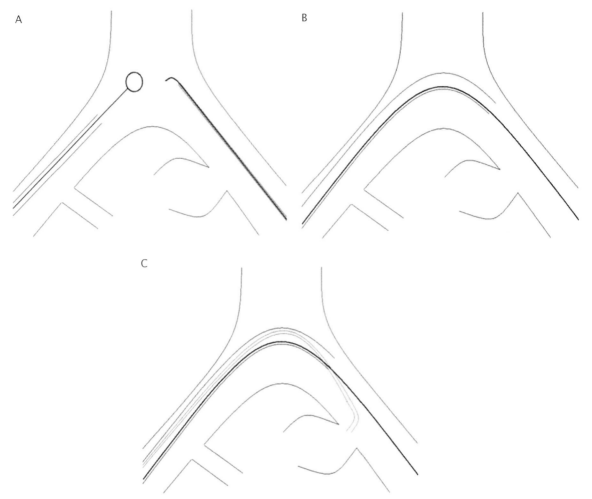

Figure 23.2 Snared wire technique and buddy wire loop technique. Bilateral femoral access has been obtained. (A) A snare is advanced to the aortic bifurcation through a sheath on the ipsilateral right side access. From the contralateral left side access, a catheter and wire are advanced to the bifurcation. (B) The wire is snared and brought out through the ipsilateral right side sheath. The ends of the wire exit the bilateral femoral sheaths, creating a wire loop. Tension applied to both ends of the wire allows easy advancement of the sheath over the bifurcation. (C) With the wire loop in place, a catheter is advanced adjacent to the wire loop through the ipsilateral sheath and used to catheterize the contralateral left internal iliac artery. The presence of the wire loop serves as a buddy wire and provides great stability during intervention on the contralateral left internal iliac artery.

Source: From Viner S, Kessel D. Wire-loop technique for stabilizing catheters over the aortic bifurcation for endovascular interventions. *Cardiovasc Intervent Radiol.* 2008;31(4):807–810. Courtesy Springer.

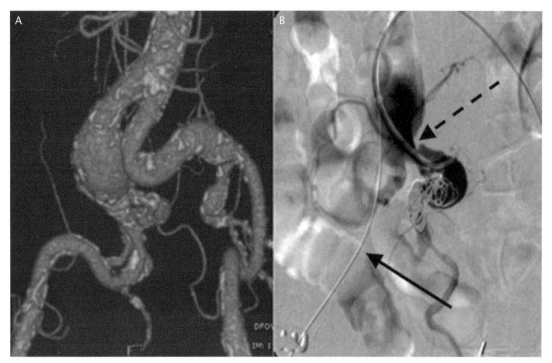

Figure 23.3 Buddy wire loop technique. (A) Three-dimensional computed tomography reconstruction shows profound tortuosity of the iliac vasculature with aneurysmal dilatation of the right common and right internal iliac arteries. (B) With bilateral femoral access and through-and-through wire access, a wire loop (solid arrow) has been made and is used as a stabilizing buddy wire. This provides excellent sheath stability and facilitates catheterization of the right internal iliac artery (dashed arrow) for embolization.

Source: From Zastrow C, et al. Femoral–femoral stabilizing buddy-wire for embolization of the internal iliac artery. *J Vasc Surg.* 2012;55:1526–1528. Courtesy Elsevier.

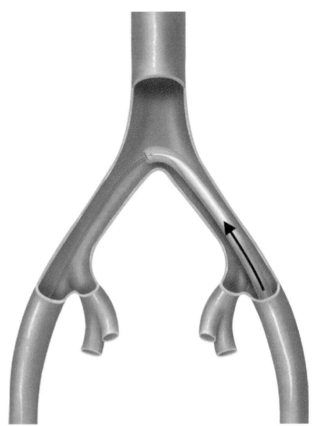

Figure 23.4 Pay it off the dilator technique. The sheath and dilator are advanced as far as possible as a unit. Once further advancement is not possible, the dilator is pinned, and the sheath is advanced forward over the pinned dilator (arrow). Forward pressure (to prevent kickback) is maintained on the sheath, and the dilator is again fully inserted. The dilator is again pinned and the sheath advanced. This is repeated, allowing incremental advancement of the sheath to its desired position.

Source: From Grenon MS, et al. Technical endovascular highlights for crossing the difficult aortic bifurcation. *J Vasc Surg.* 2011;54:893–896. Courtesy Elsevier.

References and Suggested Readings

1. Herman KC. Crossing the challenging aortic bifurcation. *Endovascular Today.* 2012 Jan;45–49.
2. Grenon MS, Reilly L, Ramaiah VG. Technical endovascular highlights for crossing the difficult aortic bifurcation. *J Vasc Surg.* 2011;54:893–896.
3. Bachman DM, Casarella WJ, Sos TA. Percutaneous iliofemoral angioplasty via the contralateral femoral artery. *Radiology.* 1979;130:617–621.
4. Narins CR. Access strategies for peripheral arterial intervention. *Cardiol J.* 2009;16:88–97.
5. Lyden SP. Techniques and outcomes for endovascular treatment in the tibial arteries. *J Vasc Surg.* 2009;50:1219–1223.

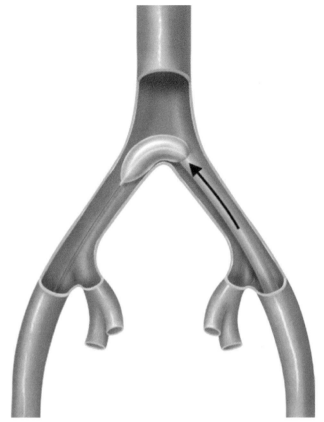

Figure 23.5 Pay it off the balloon technique. The sheath is advanced with the dilator as far as possible (not shown). The dilator is removed, and a balloon is advanced just beyond the end of the sheath. As the balloon is deflated, the sheath is advanced (arrow) over the deflating balloon. The maneuver is repeated until the desired sheath position is attained.

Source: From Grenon MS, et al. Technical endovascular highlights for crossing the difficult aortic bifurcation. *J Vasc Surg.* 2011;54:893–896. Courtesy Elsevier.

6. Viner S, Kessel D. Wire-loop technique for stabilizing catheters over the aortic bifurcation for endovascular interventions. *Cardiovasc Intervent Radiol.* 2008;31(4):807–810.
7. Etezadi V, Powell A. Widening the aortic bifurcation with super stiff wire to allow placement of an otherwise impossible-to-advance Outback catheter. *EJVES Extra.* 2011;21:e1–e3.
8. Zastrow C, Motaganahalli RL, Matsumura JS. Femoral–femoral stabilizing buddy-wire for embolization of the internal iliac artery. *J Vasc Surg.* 2012;55:1526–1528.

CHAPTER 24

Flip Techniques: Obtaining Antegrade and Retrograde Femoral Access Through a Single Access Site

S. Lowell Kahn

Brief Description

Despite the use of retrograde tibial access, brachial access, and radial access, the common femoral artery (CFA) remains the most ubiquitous point of access for lower extremity interventions.[1] Historically, retrograde catheterization of the vessel for ipsilateral iliac and up-and-over contralateral iliac-to-tibial interventions has been the mainstay of therapy. It is increasingly common, however, to employ ipsilateral antegrade access for infrainguinal occlusive disease. Proximity of the access site to the point of occlusion not only confers the benefits of a higher technical success rate, but may also provide an ergonomic benefit to the operator.

The value of converting an access is not new and has been described in the literature.[2–4] Variations of the technique using catheters and balloons are described.

This chapter provides three methods of conversion. The first technique, described by Hartnell,[3] involves using a reverse curve catheter in conjunction with a Glidewire (Terumo Medical Corp., Somerset, NJ) that is retracted to the point of femoral catheterization. With a small amount of wire extending beyond the tip of the catheter and into the superficial femoral artery (SFA), the catheter is retracted until it engages (hooks) on the point of insertion. The Glidewire is then threaded well into the SFA and preferably the popliteal artery. The catheter is advanced over the wire, and the wire is exchanged for a support wire over which sheath delivery and subsequent infrainguinal intervention can take place.

The second technique, by Ysa et al.,[4] describes a "rebound" method whereby a Fogarty catheter (Edwards Lifesciences Corp., Irvine, CA) is inflated just beyond the tip of a retrograde sheath to deflect a side-by-side Glidewire down the SFA and subsequently convert the retrograde sheath to antegrade.

Finally, we describe our own method of converting an antegrade sheath back to retrograde using a "buddy wire" technique.

The techniques described herein require no additional equipment beyond common catheters, balloons, and wires. With experience, all techniques are rapid, safe, and highly effective with multiple clinical applications, including the ability to treat both extremities from a single access.

Applications of the Techniques

Retrograde to Antegrade Methods 1 and 2

1. Utilization of a single access for treatment of bilateral lower extremity disease.
2. Ipsilateral treatment of inflow disease and outflow/runoff disease from a single access.
3. Unknown level of disease: Many patients arrive to the angiography suite without pre-procedural cross-sectional imaging. Often, the physical exam and noninvasive studies are inconclusive for the exact level(s) of disease. This technique allows a standard retrograde access to obtain a full aortic-to-tibial arteriogram. If disease is discovered below the inguinal ligament, the access is easily converted to antegrade, and the benefits of a standard antegrade access are conferred.
4. Obtaining antegrade access on patients in whom standard antegrade access would be difficult. Larger patients, particularly those with substantial pannus, are notoriously difficult for antegrade access. This technique affords the ease of obtaining retrograde access with the benefit of standard antegrade access.
5. In theory, conversion of an access could be beneficial in various fistula and venous interventions. If the caliber of the vessel is small (e.g., fistula), the second method as described by Ysa et al.[2] may be superior since it might prove difficult to form a reverse curve

catheter in a small vessel as required for the first method.

Antegrade to Retrograde

1. Utilization of a single access for treatment of bilateral lower extremity disease.
2. Ipsilateral treatment of inflow disease and outflow/runoff disease from a single access.
3. Use of a closure device requiring retrograde access after an antegrade intervention.

Challenges of the Procedure

Retrograde to Antegrade Method 1

1. Forming the reverse curve catheter: Ordinarily, this is a non-issue because the catheters most commonly employed in this technique are readily formed on the aortic bifurcation in most patients. Occasionally, forming the catheter in the thoracic aorta is necessary for patients with a particularly small abdominal aorta.
2. Retracting the formed reverse curve catheter from the aorta to the point of insertion in the femoral artery. Particularly with small or plaque-laden iliac arteries, this step can be difficult. Techniques for overcoming this are discussed later.
3. Advancing the wire a sufficient distance into the SFA to allow conversion without causing the reverse curve catheter to lose its curve and straighten into the iliac arteries.
4. Advancing the reverse curve catheter bareback without a sheath: Typically, this is easy, but in an obese patient and/or a patient with a scarred or plaque-laden vessel, this may be difficult. Under these scenarios, pre-dilatation and use of a stiffer wire may be required.
5. Converting a retrograde sheath (rather than a catheter) to antegrade is feasible but challenging with the method described by Hartnell.[3] Although we employ the Hartnell method more commonly, if a sheath has been placed first, we would advise using the method described by Ysa et al.[4] to convert the access.

Antegrade to Retrograde

1. The technique is detailed later, but converting from antegrade to retrograde is notoriously more difficult than the initial conversion from retrograde to antegrade and carries a risk of technical failure or loss of access.

Potential Pitfalls/Complications

Retrograde to Antegrade Method 1

1. Vessel dissection or embolization resulting from spinning and retracting the catheter in the iliac vasculature. The author has performed this procedure several hundred times and this has not occurred. Nonetheless, the catheter is spun aggressively to prevent the reverse curve catheter from losing its shape or engaging a plaque or side-branch vessel.
2. The catheter can be overspun while it is retracted, resulting in kinking. This is discussed further later, and tips are provided to avoid this.
3. Loss of access: This can occur with both retrograde-to-antegrade and antegrade-to-retrograde conversions.

Antegrade to Retrograde

1. Loss of access: As above, this is a risk with all types of access conversion.

Steps of the Procedure

Retrograde to Antegrade Method 1
See Hartnell.[3]

1. Retrograde catheterization of the femoral artery is performed with a steeper than usual angle of entry. We recommend that the vessel is catheterized with or without a micropuncture set at 60 degrees or greater. The more vertical the access, the easier the conversion of the access will be. A regular angled Glidewire is advanced to the upper abdominal aorta.
2. A reverse curve flush catheter is advanced to the abdominal aorta, and aortography is performed. The catheter can be retracted to the ipsilateral external iliac artery and lower extremity arteriography performed. At our institution, a Sos 2 catheter (Angiodynamics Inc., Latham, NY) is preferred, but Sos 1 or 3 (Angiodynamics Inc., Latham, NY), Simmons 1/Sidewinder (Angiodynamics Inc. Latham, NY), or a VCF flush catheter (Cook Medical Inc., Bloomington, IN) can be used. In small (diseased) iliac arteries, the tight loop of the VCF flush catheter may be desirable from the standpoint of retracting it with the curve intact through the iliacs, but this comes at the expense of less support for Glidewire advancement down the SFA and the potential for hematoma formation through the side holes if a wire is not maintained continuously within the catheter lumen.

3. The catheter is spun generously while it is slowly retracted. If the tip engages a branch vessel or plaque, the catheter is gently pushed forward and rotated the opposite direction. Optimal spinning is performed with two hands, one spinning the hub while the other spins the shaft. Often, spinning the catheter allows it to loop on itself, giving it a very low profile. However, care must be taken not to overspin the catheter because this can cause kinking and make advancing the wire in step 4 difficult. To prevent kinking, we often alternate the direction of spin as the catheter is retracted.

4. When the reverse curve catheter is located 1 or 2 cm above the entry site in the CFA, a Glidewire is spun and advanced approximately 5 cm down the SFA. It is important to obtain imaging demonstrating that the wire is in fact descending down the SFA and not the profunda. Use of a road map may be beneficial. It can be difficult to remedy the situation if the catheter inadvertently engages the profunda instead of the SFA. Care must be taken not to advance too much wire because this predisposes the catheter to buckling and straightening in the iliac artery, requiring returning to the aorta to form the catheter and repeating steps 1–4. Alternatively, extending too much wire could kick the catheter out of the femoral artery with consequent loss of access.

5. With the wire a short distance into the SFA, the catheter and wire are slowly retracted as a unit until the catheter engages itself at the entry site. This is where the apex of the reverse curve catheter is sitting at the entry site into the vessel and essentially hooks on it. In this position, the catheter is quite stable and unlikely to disengage.

6. With the catheter seated on the entry site, the system is now stable enough to advance the wire as far distally as possible into the SFA or popliteal artery. Sometimes it is beneficial to advance the reverse curve catheter over the wire distally and use it to exchange to a stiffer wire or obtain better below-knee angiographic images.

7. *Optional*: The Glidewire is obviously not an ideal support wire and may or may not be stiff enough to advance an antegrade sheath over. This obviously depends on patient factors (e.g., habitus and plaque). If exchanging the wire is necessary, we typically advance a 4 Fr Kumpe catheter (Cook Medical Inc., Bloomington, IN) over the wire and exchange for a stiffer wire.

8. Once adequate wire support has been obtained, an antegrade sheath of the desired size is placed in the standard fashion, and the procedure is completed.

9. *Note*: Although more difficult, the previous procedure can be performed with a sheath in place. This should not be attempted initially because it requires more practice since the sheath is nearly completely removed from the vessel when the catheter is retracted and engaged on the insertion site. This obviously carries the risk of loss of access and bleeding. If attempted, it is recommended that it be done with an assistant monitoring the sheath and under continuous fluoroscopic guidance. If interventions (which require a sheath) are to be performed above and below the common femoral insertion site, we typically advise either intervening on the infrainguinal segment first or employing the technique described by Ysa et al.[4] to flip a retrograde sheath. It is the author's experience that converting from antegrade to retrograde with a sheath is easier (safer) than converting from retrograde to antegrade with a sheath using the technique described by Hartnell.[3]

Retrograde to Antegrade Method 2
See Ysa et al.[4]

1. Retrograde catheterization of the femoral artery is performed with a steeper than usual angle of entry. We recommend that the vessel be catheterized with or without a micropuncture set at 60 degrees or greater. The more vertical the access, the easier the conversion of the access will be.

2. Using the Seldinger technique, an appropriately sized sheath (6 Fr or greater to allow adequate room for the balloon and wire) is placed, and the intervention for the ipsilateral iliac, contralateral lower extremity, or other location is performed and completed.

3. Through the sheath, a 4 Fr Fogarty catheter (Edwards Lifesciences Corp., Irvine, CA) is advanced just beyond the tip of the sheath and inflated with dilute contrast. The Fogarty catheter is withdrawn until it stops at the tip of the sheath.

4. The sheath and Fogarty are retracted as a unit until resistance is felt, indicating that the sheath is at the insertion site into the artery

5. The Fogarty catheter is then advanced 1 or 2 cm and then fully inflated to occlude the CFA.

6. Adjacent to the Fogarty catheter, a regular angled 0.035-in. Glidewire is advanced and deflected off the inflated balloon and steered well into the SFA.

7. The Fogarty catheter is deflated and removed.

8. The loop is reduced by pulling the wire and sheath back slightly.

9. The dilator is re-advanced over the Glidewire, and the sheath is now advanced in a antegrade fashion.

10. *Note*: Although it has not been attempted by the author, in theory, this method could be used to convert an antegrade sheath back to retrograde.

Antegrade to Retrograde

1. At completion of the antegrade procedure, the user ensures that a 5 Fr or greater size sheath is in place.
2. Through the sheath, a safety ("buddy") wire is left in place with the distal end in the popliteal artery. The ideal buddy wire is a stiff support wire (e.g., Amplatz, [Boston Scientific Inc., Marlborough, MA]). This is placed to ensure that access is not lost during the flipping process.
3. Adjacent to the buddy wire, an angled Glidewire is advanced to the tip of the sheath. At the operator's discretion, a torque is placed on the Glidewire for control.
4. The flat panel detector is rotated for oblique imaging. This can be performed with ipsi- or contralateral obliquity, depending on the operator's preference.
5. With the buddy wire maintained in position, the sheath and Glidewire are retracted carefully to the insertion site. Performing this procedure requires that the sheath is retracted to the anterior vessel wall and care is taken to bring it to this point but not beyond. The sheath should be essentially perpendicular to the vessel when it is in the appropriate location.
6. *Optional*: Contrast can be injected as the sheath approaches the insertion point to confirm location.
7. The Glidewire is retracted into the sheath and then advanced and spun beyond the tip. The Glidewire is maneuvered until it ascends the iliac vasculature and ideally into the aorta.
8. Once the Glidewire is advanced adequately to provide support, the buddy wire is removed from the sheath.
9. The sheath is advanced minimally over the Glidewire, and the dilator of the sheath is advanced over the Glidewire into the sheath.
10. The sheath is advanced to the desired position, and then the procedure or closure is conducted.

Example

See Figures 24.1–24.4.

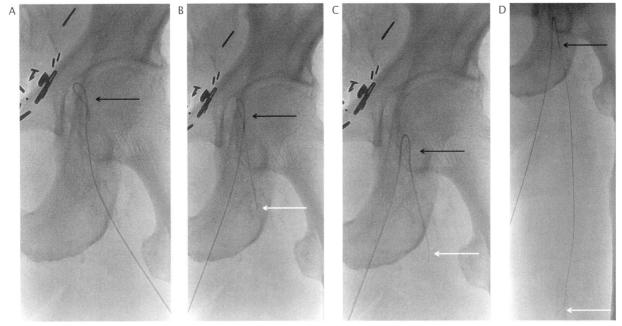

Figure 24.1 Retrograde-to-antegrade conversion using a Sos 2 catheter as described by Hartnell.[3] (A) After forming the catheter in the aorta, the Sos 2 catheter (arrow) has been retracted just above the insertion site in the common femoral artery (CFA). (B) The Sos 2 catheter (black arrow) is rotated so that the tip is directed toward the superficial femoral artery (SFA). A Glidewire (white arrow) has been advanced a short distance into the SFA. (C) As a unit, the Sos 2 catheter (black arrow) and Glidewire (white arrow) have been retracted until the catheter engages and the apex of the catheter is securely seated at the point of access in the CFA. (D) With the stable Sos 2 (black arrow), it is easy to advance the Glidewire (white arrow) well into the distal SFA or popliteal artery for added support. After obtaining adequate wire support (with or without exchange to a stiffer wire), the catheter is removed and an antegrade sheath is placed.

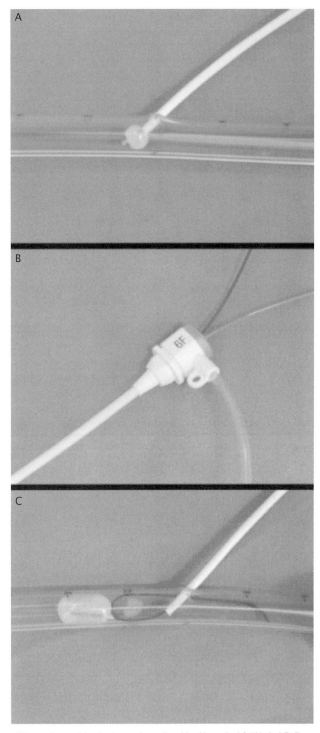

Figure 24.2 Model demonstration of the rebound technique described by Ysa et al.[4] (A) A 4-Fr Fogarty catheter is partly inflated with 0.2 cc of dilute contrast just past the tip of a 6-Fr sheath. The sheath and Fogarty are withdrawn until there is resistance, indicating the sheath is located at the anterior wall of the artery. (B) An angled Glidewire is inserted adjacent to the Fogarty catheter through the hub of the sheath. (C) The balloon on the Fogarty catheter is advanced 1 or 2 cm beyond the tip of the sheath and fully inflated to occlude the CFA more proximally. The Glidewire is then advanced and deflected off the inflated balloon. The Glidewire is advanced well into the SFA, after which the Fogarty catheter is deflated and removed. The sheath and wire are retracted slightly to remove the redundant loop, and the dilator is inserted back into the sheath to allow an antegrade advancement of the sheath.

Source: Images courtesy of the *Journal of Vascular Surgery*, Mosby/Elsevier.

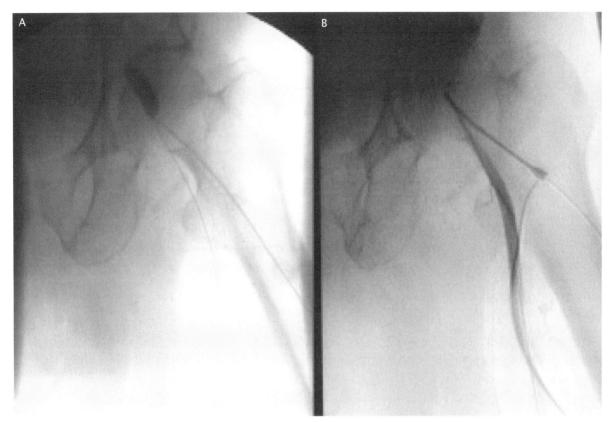

Figure 24.3 Fluoroscopic images of the rebound technique described by Ysa et al.[4] (A) With the Fogarty catheter inflated, a Glidewire is deflected off the balloon and advanced down the SFA. (B) The Fogarty catheter has been deflated and removed. The sheath can now be advanced antegrade down the SFA.

Source: Images courtesy of the *Journal of Vascular Surgery,* Mosby/Elsevier.

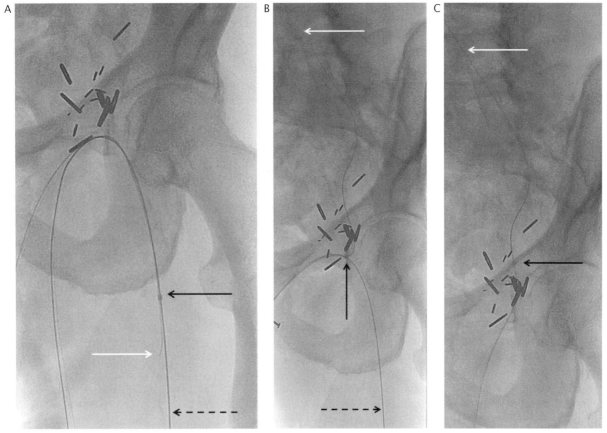

Figure 24.4 Antegrade-to-retrograde sheath conversion. (A) The tip of an antegrade 5-Fr sheath (black arrow) is at the level of the lesser trochanter with a safety ("buddy") wire (dashed arrow) advanced down to the popliteal artery. The tip of an angled Glidewire (white arrow) is located just beyond the tip of the sheath. (B) The sheath tip (black arrow) has been carefully retracted with the Glidewire to the point of insertion using the safety ("buddy") wire (dashed arrow) in the popliteal artery. Once the sheath was perpendicular to the vessel (without exiting the vessel), the Glidewire (white arrow) was advanced to the common iliac artery and subsequently the aorta. (C) With adequate support provided by the Glidewire (white arrow), the sheath tip (black arrow) has been flipped and advanced a short distance retrograde.

References and Suggested Readings

1. Lin PH, Poi MJ, Matos J, Kougias P, Bechara C, Chen C. Arterial disease. In: Brunicardi F, editor. *Schwartz's Principles of Surgery*. 10th ed. New York: McGraw Hill; 2015.
2. Giavroglou CE. "Retroantegrade" catheterization of the branches of the femoral artery: Technical note. *Cardiovasc Intervent Radiol*. 1989 Nov–1990 Dec;12(6):337–339.
3. Hartnell G. An improved reversal technique from retrograde to antegrade femoral artery cannulation. *Cardiovasc Intervent Radiol*. 1998;21(6):512–513.
4. Ysa A, Arruabarrena A, Bustabad M, Pena M. Easy technique for retro-antegrade superficial femoral artery catheterization. *J Vasc Surg*. 2008;48(4):1041–1043.

CHAPTER 25

Technical Pearls for Managing the Scarred Groin

S. Lowell Kahn

Introduction

Since its original description in 1979, the femoral artery has remained one of the most common access sites for endovascular interventions.[1] The common femoral artery is desirable because of its accessibility, size, and ease of compression over the femoral head post intervention.[1,2] Combined with the frequency with which the femoral artery is utilized in a variety of bypass and aortoiliac surgical interventions, scarred groins are frequently encountered. Further complicating femoral access are the rising rates of obesity that have doubled during the past 35 years, with more than two-thirds (68.6%) of American adults reported as overweight or obese as of 2012.[3,4] Despite its frequency, a scarred groin presents a unique challenge to the interventionalist, particularly in obese patients.

Patient Preparation

Assessing the patient for suitable alterative access points is imperative, particularly when known challenges exist at the groin. In many cases, the intervention can be safely performed from the contralateral femoral artery or a radial, brachial, popliteal, or tibiopedal access. Some authors advocate ultrasound-guided access of the superficial femoral artery in the presence of a hostile groin with limited common femoral access.[5] If the deep (pannus/obesity) or scarred femoral artery is to be used, an effort should be made to tape any excess pannus away from the access toward the contralateral shoulder. Minimizing the

percutaneous depth of the vessel facilitates easier access. In addition, ultrasound assessment of the femoral artery is helpful in the presence of scar tissue because the scar tissue produces acoustic shadowing. An area with less calcification and less shadowing may be identified and allows for a more suitable access. Also, approaching the vessel with a degree of obliquity (away from the standard 12 o'clock approach) may lessen traversal of scar tissue, but this may make compression post intervention more challenging.

Access and Needle Considerations

In the setting of a scarred groin, making an initial 5- to 10-mm incision with a number 11 blade followed by generous blunt dissection with curved hemostats is beneficial. Although some operators prefer to access the vessel first and then make an incision along the shaft of the needle, we consistently make our incision first to minimize the chance of a skin/tissue tag between the needle shaft and the incision. An effort should be made to extend the dissection to the level of the vessel. These strategies are particularly important when scar tissue is present.

Many practices have abandoned access with a conventional 18 gauge Seldinger or hollow needle (Figure 25.1) in favor of the smaller 21 gauge micropuncture sets (Cook Medical Inc., Bloomington, IN) because of the theoretically less traumatic nature of these needles. Interestingly, the safety benefit of the smaller micropuncture sets is not proven. Of note, a study published in 2012 examined 3243

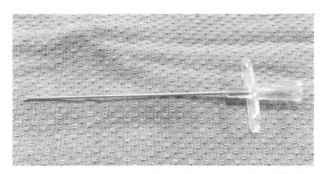

Figure 25.1 Standard 19 gauge hollow beveled needle (Argon Medical Devices Inc., Plano TX). Use of a 19 gauge needle in a scarred groin allows introduction of a stiff 0.035-in. wire without the need for a transitional dilator.

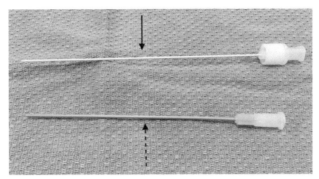

Figure 25.2 Micropuncture access set with stiffened cannula. The stiff inner dilator (solid arrow) is introduced coaxially into the outer cannula (dashed arrow) and facilitates transition to a 0.035-in. wire in a scarred groin.

consecutive patients who had 18 and 21 gauge accesses and found no significant safety benefit in those accessed with the micropuncture set; in fact, it found a higher rate of retroperitoneal hematomas in the micropuncture group.[6] Despite a lack of proven benefit, many operators still prefer use of the micropuncture set. In the setting of a scarred groin, selection of a micropuncture set may be disadvantageous because the ultimate goal is to transition to a stiff 0.035-in. wire over which further dilatation and sheath placement are performed.

If a micropuncture set is selected, a set with a stiffened cannula (Figure 25.2) should be employed because it passes more readily over the 0.018-in. wire into the artery. Of note, the outer cannula of the transitional dilator is identical in both regular and stiffened micropuncture sets. In a severely scarred groin, a high level of friction can make it difficult to remove the outer cannula after threading the 0.035-in. wire. In this scenario, the cannula is prone to stretching and breaking that, if not recognized, could result in a retained foreign body (Figure 25.3). It is therefore important that the operator remove the outer cannula carefully, grasping it close to the skin and inspecting it to ensure that it has been completely removed. It may be helpful to maximally advance the microwire and then retract the wire and transitional dilator as a unit, being careful not to lose wire access.

In our practice, we advocate use of an 18 or 19 gauge needle (see Figure 25.1) for scarred groins because it allows immediate advancement of a 0.035-in. wire without necessitating use of a transitional dilator. If available, a Seldinger 18 gauge needle may be beneficial because the tip lacks a bevel once the inner stylet is removed. Absence of the sharp bevel allows direct advancement of a stiff Glidewire (Terumo Medical Corp., Somerset, NJ) or Glidewire Advantage (Terumo Medical Corp., Somerset, NJ), both of which are beneficial in this scenario with their combined support and navigation properties. The selection of the optimal wire is discussed next.

Wire Selection

Whether using an 18/19 gauge needle or a 21 gauge micropuncture platform, the objective is to advance a stiff guidewire well into the abdominal aorta to facilitate dilator and sheath placement. Stiff guidewires, such as the Rosen (Cook Medical Inc., Bloomington, IN), Amplatz and Extra/Ultra Stiff Amplatz (Cook Medical Inc., Bloomington, IN), Meier (Boston Scientific Inc., Marlborough, MA), and Lunderquist (Cook Medical Inc., Bloomington, IN), provide the necessary support. Unfortunately, these wires track poorly in tortuous and/or plaque-laden iliac arteries. If these wires fail to advance through the 18/19 gauge needle

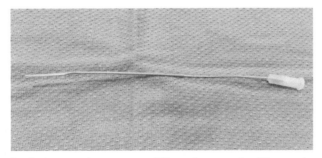

Figure 25.3 Stretched outer cannula of micropuncture access set. The outer cannula of the regular and stiffened micropuncture access set is identical and is composed of a soft plastic. In a scarred groin with a high friction coefficient, the cannula is prone to stretching/elongation. This compromises its structural integrity and can result in disruption of the cannula. If not recognized, the retained fragment could be pushed intravascularly with subsequent catheter/dilator/sheath advancement over the wire. The outer cannula should always be grasped near the skin during removal. If stretching occurs, the wire and outer cannula should be retracted as a unit while ensuring wire access is not sacrificed (intermittent re-advancement of the wire).

or transitional dilator, using a stiff hydrophilic guidewire (stiff Glidewire and Glidewire Advantage) to obtain initial access to the aorta may be beneficial. A 4 Fr dilator or hockey stick catheter can then be used to exchange for one of the aforementioned stiff guidewires if the dilators or a sheath will not pass over the Glidewire.

Dilatation and Sheath Placement

Judicious stepwise use of dilators is advantageous in the management of the scarred groin. We typically start with a 4 or 5 Fr dilator and serially dilate (at increments of one or two French sizes) until the desired degree of dilatation is obtained. Lubrication of the dilators with mineral oil or Surgilube (Savage Laboratories Inc., Melville, NY) reduces the friction coefficient and facilitates advancement. Also, manual rotation of the dilator during insertion allows easier insertion. Dilatation should be continued to a French size that is two sizes larger than the desired sheath size to match the outer diameter of the sheath (e.g., 8 Fr dilator for a 6 Fr sheath). On occasion, dilatation one French size larger than the device to be inserted is helpful, but must be done with cautious subsequent monitoring of the groin for bleeding around the device. As with the dilators, lubrication and spinning of sheath aid advancement.

The selection of a sheath is equally important. Choosing a sheath with a braided core and hydrophilic exterior (e.g., Flexor, Cook Medical Inc., Bloomington, IN) is helpful. Alternatively, the Super Arrow-Flex Sheath (Medline Industries Inc., Mundelein, IL) is preferred by some because it offers a kink-resistant metallic platform with enhanced longitudinal strength.

Bailout Strategies for Inadequate Wire Support

If the operator underestimates the degree of scar tissue present, a 0.035-in. wire with inadequate support may be advanced to the aorta. A wire with inadequate stiffness may not allow passage of the dilators or a sheath. Ideally, the wire is exchanged for a stiffer guidewire, but in a severely scarred groin, this may prove difficult. We typically attempt placement of the outer cannula of a transitional dilator first because it is smaller than a 4 Fr dilator. In most cases, this will advance over the wire and allow wire exchange. On rare occasions, we have found that advancing the outer cannula of a coaxial 18 or 19 gauge needle (without the stylet) over the wire allows for a successful exchange (Figure 25.4). To do this, a gentle curve is made on the outer cannula to follow the curve of the wire as it enters the femoral artery. The cannula is advanced over the wire and subsequently used to exchange it for a stiffer wire. Once a stiff guidewire is in place, dilatation and sheath placement are performed as described previously.

Closure

Obtaining hemostasis in the scarred groin is typically performed with manual pressure alone because the use of closure devices is relatively contraindicated. If a closure device is deemed necessary, those devices that are suture (Perclose ProGlide Suture-Mediated Closure System, Abbott Vascular Inc., Santa Clara, CA) or clip (StarClose SE Vascular Closure System, Abbott Vascular Inc.) based should be avoided because they are more prone to failure in this scenario. Although relatively contraindicated, a collagen plug-based system (Angio-Seal [St. Jude Medical Inc., St. Paul, MN] and MYNXGRIP [Cordis Corp., Milpitas, CA]) can be used successfully, but they should be performed only after ensuring adequate tract dilatation to facilitate delivery and with fluoroscopic guidance (e.g., balloon of MYNXGRIP) when possible.

The presence of scar tissue paradoxically limits hematoma formation and typically allows for excellent hemostasis with manual pressure alone.

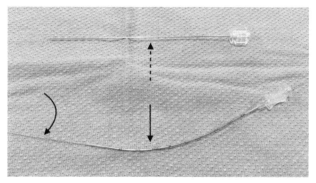

Figure 25.4 A 19 Gauge Co-Axial Introducer Needle (Argon Medical Devices Inc.) with Cope wire (Cook Medical Inc.). The outer cannula of the coaxial needle (solid arrow) can be used as a bailout when the initial wire lacks adequate support for catheter, dilator, or sheath advancement. The stylet (dashed arrow) is removed, and a gentle curve is made in the blunt tip outer cannula to match the angle of entry to the femoral artery. The curved outer cannula can then be passed over a 0.018-in. wire (Cope wire as shown by the curved arrow) if a micropuncture transitional dilator will not pass over a 0.035-in. wire to allow exchange for a stiffer 0.035-in. support wire. This should be done cautiously and under fluoroscopic guidance to avoid vessel injury.

Approaching the scarred groin with a treatment algorithm and knowledge of alternative techniques is important for success. The methods described in this chapter are easily applied and require no additional inventory beyond standard lab equipment.

References and Suggested Readings

1. Bachman DM, Casarella WJ, Sos TA. Percutaneous iliofemoral angioplasty via the contralateral femoral artery. *Radiology*. 1979;130:617–621.
2. Narins CR. Access strategies for peripheral arterial intervention. *Cardiol J*. 2009;16:88–97.
3. Ogden CL, Carroll MD, Kit BK, Flegal KM. Prevalence of childhood and adult obesity in the United States, 2011–2012. *JAMA*. 2014;311(8):806–814.
4. Fryar DC, Carroll MD, Ogden CL. Prevalence of overweight, obesity, and extreme obesity among adults: United States, 1960–1962 through 2011–2012. National Center for Health Statistics Health E-Stat. 2014. http://www.cdc.gov/nchs/data/hestat/obesity_adult_11_12/obesity_adult_11_12.htm. Accessed May 2015.
5. Marcus AJ, Lotzof K, Howard A. Access to the superficial femoral artery in the presence of a "hostile groin": A prospective study. *Cardiovasc Intervent Radiol*. 2007;30(3):351–354.
6. Ben-Dor I, Maluenda G, Mahmoudi M, et al. A novel, minimally invasive access technique versus standard 18-gauge needle set for femoral access. *Catheter Cardiovasc Interv*. 2012;79(7):1180–1185.

Visceral and Pelvic Vascular Interventions

Use of a Fogarty Occlusion Balloon During Splenic Artery Embolization to Prevent Distal Coil Migration

S. Lowell Kahn

Brief Description

Splenic embolization has become a mainstay of therapy in the setting of splenic trauma for patients not requiring urgent surgery.[1] Compared to surgery, splenic embolization offers a lower morbidity and mortality as well as preservation of splenic function.[2] Unlike the distal embolization performed for hypersplenism and pancytopenia, embolization for the trauma patient is typically performed proximally, except in scenarios in which definitive extrasplenic hemorrhage is identified, in which case distal or combined proximal and distal embolization may be employed.[3] Proximal embolization is typically sufficient to decrease the perfusion pressure to the spleen and hence control hemorrhage. Proximal embolization decreases the risk of splenic infarction given the rich collateral blood supply to the spleen.[3]

Although proximal embolization is generally obtained with standard technique, distal migration of deployed coils is a well-known phenomenon and carries an increased risk of splenic infarction.[4] This is secondary to a variety of factors, including the high flow nature of the vessel, inadequate compaction of the deployed coils, and undersizing of the coils resulting in inadequate radial force of the coils to provide traction. Undersizing is common in the setting of hemodynamic shock because vasospasm can significantly reduce the perceived diameter of the splenic artery.

A variety of devices exist on the market to lower the risk of distal migration, including detachable balloons, plugs, and coils, as well as specialty coils such as hydrocoils. These devices are typically effective, but they may be prohibitively expensive or unavailable to the operator.

This chapter describes a simple balloon occlusion technique to facilitate proximal embolization of the target splenic artery. Although the example presented is for a splenic artery, the technique may be extrapolated for other embolization procedures as described later. Briefly, an occlusion balloon is delivered and supported proximally in the splenic artery, ideally distal to the dorsal pancreatic artery. After inflation of the occlusion balloon, the guidewire is removed and embolization is performed with standard 0.035-in. coils. This method allows for a dense packing of the coils and the use of fewer coils to obtain vascular stasis.

Applications of the Technique

1. Traumatic embolization of the spleen.
2. Embolization of the spleen prior to planned splenectomy.
3. General trauma embolization procedures (e.g., pelvic trauma). Can be used with combined distal and proximal vessel occlusion.
4. Other solid organ embolization procedures (e.g., proximal renal artery embolization prior to nephrectomy).

Challenges of the Procedure

1. In the author's experience, the single challenge encountered involves obtaining adequate stability of the platform. Specifically, advancing a 6 Fr sheath into the celiac or splenic artery can be difficult, particularly in a sharply angled celiac artery or when atherosclerotic disease/vasospasm results in a narrow caliber of the vessel. If placement of a sheath is not possible within the celiac or splenic artery, a curved sheath or 8 Fr guide catheter may provide adequate support to deliver the Fogarty balloon over a stiff guidewire into the proximal splenic artery.

Potential Pitfalls/Complications

1. As with all embolization procedures, nontarget embolization is a risk.
2. Trauma (dissection) of the splenic artery with placement of the 6 Fr sheath or over-inflation of the occlusion balloon.

3. Distal migration of the coils after deflation of the balloon secondary to inadequate oversizing of the coils, poor packing of the coils, or use of too few coils.

Steps of the Procedure

1. After catheterization of the femoral artery, a 6 Fr sheath is advanced to the upper abdomen. A variety of sheaths can be used, but we typically select either an Ansel 1 or Ansel 2 45-cm sheath (Cook Medical Inc., Bloomington, IN).

2. The celiac artery is selectively catheterized. A variety of catheters are well suited for this indication. Our most commonly used catheter is the SOS Omni 2 (AngioDynamics Inc., Latham, NY). However, multiple other catheters work well, including the Cobra (AngioDynamics Inc., Latham, NY), Sidewinder (AngioDynamics Inc., Latham, NY), and RC (AngioDynamics Inc., Latham, NY) shapes. Use of a specific catheter is based on anatomy and operator preference. For celiac arteries with sharp angulation or proximal narrowing, the Sidewinder (Simmons) catheters offer greater support and may be beneficial.

3. Selective digital subtraction angiography imaging in the splenic artery is performed. For this technique and most traumatic splenic artery embolizations, the proximal splenic artery will be embolized.

4. After the catheter and wire are used to select the celiac and subsequently the splenic artery, the sheath is carefully advanced, ideally into the celiac artery. Often, the catheter is exchanged for a standard hockey stick catheter (e.g., Kumpe, Cook Medical Inc., Bloomington, IN), which can be used to obtain more distal splenic artery catheterization. In some cases, advancing the sheath into the celiac and splenic artery can be difficult. In these scenarios, placement of a stiff guidewire distally in the splenic artery is helpful, and replacement of the inner dilator may be required. Alternatively, the sheath can be advanced over a balloon as it is deflated in the celiac and proximal splenic artery. If the sheath cannot be advanced into the celiac or splenic artery, the 6 Fr sheath or an 8 Fr guide catheter should be placed as close as possible to the celiac ostium for maximal support over a stiff guidewire.

5. A 5.5 Fr 80-cm over-the-wire Fogarty embolectomy catheter (Edwards Lifesciences Corp., Irvine, CA) is advanced to the proximal splenic artery, ideally distal to the dorsal pancreatic artery.

6. The balloon on the Fogarty catheter is inflated to the diameter required (maximum 11 mm). For most splenic arteries, a standard Fogarty balloon is appropriate. Other occlusion balloons can be used as needed (e.g., Python Balloon (range, 5–14 mm), Applied Medical, Rancho Santa Margarita, CA).

7. Embolization is performed through the 0.035-in. lumen of the Fogarty catheter. The selected coil is operator dependent because the coil should not migrate distally with the balloon inflated. At our institution, we employ Nester embolization coils (Cook Medical Inc., Bloomington, IN) given their length and relative expense. Regardless of coil chosen, we advise oversizing by at least 20% because many splenic arteries are in spasm in the trauma setting and the true vessel size is larger than appreciated by angiography. The first one or two coils are placed by push wire. Subsequent coils can be injected with a 1- or 3-cc syringe. The coils should be tightly packed. With this method, typically no more than three to five coils are required to obtain stasis.

8. The occlusion balloon is slowly deflated under live fluoroscopy. If the coils begin to move during deflation, the balloon is reinflated and additional coils are deployed. The process is repeated until stability of the coils is demonstrated with near or complete vascular stasis.

9. Final angiography is performed through the sheath (after deflation of the occlusion balloon) to confirm vascular stasis.

Example
See Figure 26.1.

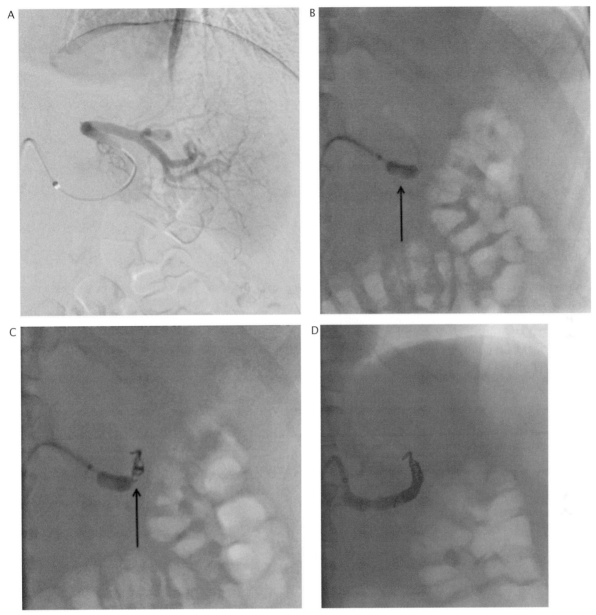

Figure 26.1 A 49-year-old female with a grade IV splenic laceration on computed tomography angiography and hemodynamic instability. (A) A splenic arteriogram did not show active extravasation, although there were clear areas of an absent parenchymal stain, particularly at the upper pole. (B) Through a 6-Fr sheath positioned in the proximal splenic artery, a Fogarty balloon (arrow) has been inflated and is fully occlusive of the vessel. (C) Through the wire lumen of the Fogarty balloon, coil embolization (arrow) is performed. (D) Final arteriogram in the proximal splenic artery demonstrates the coil plug, which is fully occlusive.

References and Suggested Readings

1. Ahuja C, Farsad K, Chadha M. An overview of splenic embolization. *AJR Am J Roentgenol.* 2015;205(4):720–725.
2. Dehli T, Bagenholm, A, Trasti NC, Monsen SA, Bartnes K. The treatment of spleen injuries: A retrospective study. *Scand J Trauma Resusc Emerg Med.* 2015;23(1):85.
3. Raikhlin A, Baerlocher MO, Asch MR, et al. Imaging and transcatheter arterial embolization for traumatic splenic injuries: Review of the literature. *Can J Surg.* 2008;51(6):464–472.
4. Ekeh AP, Khalaf S, Ilyas S, Kauffman S, Walusimbi M, McCarthy MC. Complications arising from splenic artery embolization: A review of an 11-year experience. *Am J Surg.* 2013;205(3):250–254.

CHAPTER 27

Combined Endovascular and Surgical Retrograde Superior Mesenteric Artery Recanalization

Syed M. Peeran

Brief Description

Acute mesenteric ischemia is a highly morbid condition that can result from plaque disruption or rupture in the setting of long-standing mesenteric atherosclerotic stenosis. It may also manifest with acute superior mesenteric artery (SMA) occlusion because of embolic events. Without timely restoration of perfusion, bowel ischemia, septic shock, and patient demise can be expected. Thus, it is imperative that these patients be promptly diagnosed and treated. This disease process is a life-threatening vascular emergency associated with a very high mortality rate. Prior to the endovascular era, the standard of care for acute mesenteric artery thrombosis was mesenteric arterial bypass grafting; however, the perioperative mortality has been reported to be as high as 45%.[1] This is largely attributable to the operation time required and the need for aortic or iliac cross-clamping in these critically ill patients.

Retrograde SMA recanalization via an open approach is a relatively new technique first described in the literature by Milner et al.[2] in 2004 and subsequently verified by others.[2-7] It is recognized as a vital means of restoring perfusion when patients present with acute-on-chronic mesenteric ischemia in the setting of SMA occlusion.

The procedure is performed in a hybrid operating room in which an exploratory laparotomy is performed for evaluation of compromised or necrotic bowel. After necrotic bowel has been resected during the laparotomy, the peritoneum is opened transversely at the root of the mesentery, and the SMA is readily identified by palpation due to arterial calcification. The superior mesenteric vein is identified first. The SMA is then exposed and dissected circumferentially and its terminal branches are controlled with vessel loops. Doppler ultrasound is used to assess flow. A retrograde puncture is performed distal to the lesion in the SMA with a micropuncture set allowing subsequent wire exchange and placement of a sheath. Using a braided hydrophilic-tipped catheter or crossing catheter in conjunction with a straight or angled Glidewire (Terumo Medical Corp., Somerset, NJ), the lesion is traversed in a retrograde fashion. After pre-dilatation, a balloon-expandable iCast (Atrium Medical Corp., Hudson, NH) stent is positioned at the origin of the SMA, dilated to the appropriate diameter, and flared within the aorta. Occasionally, an over-the-wire Fogarty catheter is needed to remove thrombus or soft atheromatous debris from the diseased artery. Prior to recanalization, a completion retrograde angiogram is performed to verify patency. After copious flushing and fore-bleeding, the puncture site is closed with a vein patch or primarily, depending on the size of the vessel and the size of the puncture site. The bowel mesentery is evaluated clinically and with Doppler signals to verify adequate bowel perfusion.

Applications of the Technique

1. Acute thrombotic or embolic SMA occlusion with co-existent bowel necrosis necessitating open laparotomy. In a hybrid operating room equipped with live fluoroscopy, retrograde SMA recanalization can be performed at the time of surgery.
2. Failed percutaneous antegrade treatment via femoral, radial, or brachial access. Antegrade revascularization can be challenging in the setting of advanced calcification, absence of a vessel stump from the aorta, and when there is sharp angulation and/or tortuosity relative to the access. In these scenarios, direct retrograde traversal may be more favorable. In the rare case where retrograde traversal fails, a traditional bypass may be required.

Challenges of the Procedure

1. Exposure of the mesenteric root requires the assistance of a vascular surgeon or an experienced general surgeon.
2. As with all arterial occlusions, traversal can be difficult and may require sheath support immediately adjacent to the occlusion, crossing catheters, and specialized chronic total occlusion (CTO) wires. Occasionally, more aggressive techniques (e.g., back end of the a Glidewire) may be required. Ultimately,

one should be prepared for failure to cross the lesion, and a vascular surgeon should be on hand to perform a bypass in such cases.

3. A multidisciplinary approach is ideal for these cases. Depending on local resources, a team consisting of a general surgeon, vascular surgeon, interventional radiologist, anesthesiologist, radiology technician, and critical care physician should be assembled. These patients commonly require intensive care unit admission as well as multiple trips to the operating room for bowel assessments.

4. The patient who presents with frank bowel necrosis and abdominal contamination requires expeditious source control with bowel resection, abdominal washout, and appropriate IV antibiotic coverage.

Potential Pitfalls/Complications

1. Distal embolic phenomenon may occur in the process of traversing and treating an SMA ostial lesion. This can be avoided with adequate control of the SMA distal to the access site with atraumatic clamping as well as control of branch vessels.

2. SMA dissection may occur if access to the vessel is performed in a diseased segment or if the access is performed too distal on a smaller segment of the artery.

3. SMA rupture may occur with aggressive balloon dilatation of the SMA ostial lesion. It is important to realize that stents may not expand to profile in the heavily calcified SMA ostium. Caution should be taken when treating a circumferentially calcified artery.

4. Inadequate heparinization: When access to the SMA is performed, the patient should be adequately heparinized. Thus, meticulous hemostasis should be achieved when dissecting and exposing the SMA.

5. Polytetrafluoroethylene-covered stents should not be employed in a grossly contaminated abdomen. Stent graft infections are very challenging with regard to vascular reconstruction.

Steps of the Procedure

1. Exposure of the SMA via a midline laparotomy: The root of the mesentery is identified, and palpation often reveals a calcified SMA. First, the superior mesenteric vein should be identified. Often, a vessel loop may be used for gentle retraction. Care must be taken not to injure the vein, and hemostasis is key because the patient will need to be heparinized. The SMA may not have a palpable pulse, so a Doppler probe may be used to help identify the vessel. Proximal and distal control, as well as identification and preservation of SMA braches, should be achieved prior to access.

2. Heparin should be administered systemically with a target activated clotting time of greater than 250 seconds.

3. A retrograde puncture is performed distal to the lesion in the distal SMA with a micropuncture needle. A 0.014- or 0.018-in. wire is directed under fluoroscopic imaging through the SMA more proximally, and the 4 Fr transitional dilator is passed over the access wire. A retrograde angiogram may be performed to visualize the proximal lesion and to ensure luminal access. A 6 or 7 Fr 23 or 45 cm sheath is introduced over a Bentson wire (Cook Medical Inc., Bloomington, IN). A longer sheath is used so that the operator may remove his or her hands from the radiation field.

4. A 0.035 angled or straight Glidewire will traverse the majority of these short occlusions with proper sheath and catheter support. On occasion, a stiff Glidewire or dedicated 0.014 CTO wire may be required. In rare cases, the back end of a Glidewire can be employed over a short distance, but this technique should be employed cautiously because of the risk of vessel dissection or perforation.

5. Once the SMA ostial lesion is crossed, the wire is exchanged for a stiff support wire (e.g., Amplatz, Cook Medical Inc., Bloomington, IN).

6. If there is thrombus or "soft" atheromatous debris, as suggested by computed tomography imaging, then over-the-wire Fogarty balloon embolectomy may be performed.

7. Predilation of the SMA ostial lesion is performed with a 4-mm low-profile angioplasty balloon.

8. Stent is delivered and deployed:

   a. In the case of a "clean" abdomen without bowel compromise or resection, a covered Atrium iCast 5- or 6-mm balloon-expandable stent reduces the risk of bleeding and allows for a more aggressive inflation.

   b. In the case of a "contaminated" abdomen (bowel necrosis or bowel content spillage), an uncovered balloon-expandable stent should be used.

9. Completion angiography should be performed to assess patency of the stent and treatment of the ostial lesion.

10. The sheath should be removed with the distal vessel clamped to prevent distal embolization. The arteriotomy should be adequately fore-bled and irrigated with heparinized saline. Patch closure of the arteriotomy is most favorable to ensure that the lumen of the vessel at the access site is not narrowed.

11. Doppler evaluation of the bowel, the SMA, and its branches should be performed to ensure that revascularization of the bowel has been achieved.

12. Depending on the clinical scenario, the abdomen may be left open for re-evaluation in 24–36 hours.

Example
See Figures 27.1–27.4.

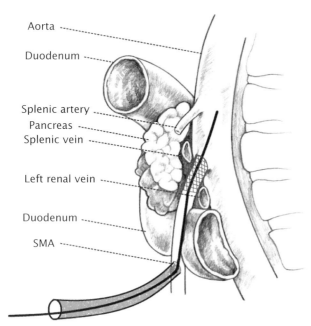

Aorta
Duodenum
Splenic artery
Pancreas
Splenic vein
Left renal vein
Duodenum
SMA

Figure 27.1 Coronal schematic of retrograde SMA stenting via open access.

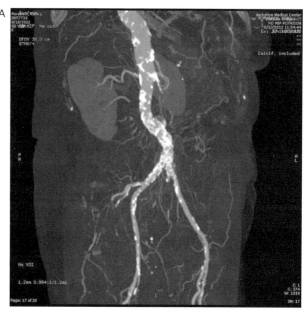

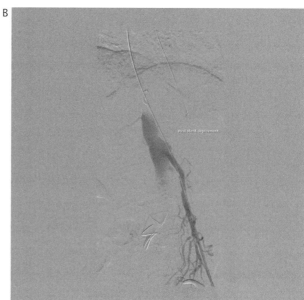

Figure 27.2 Example case of acute-on-chronic mesenteric ischemia. A Three-dimensional computed tomography angiogram of a 90-year-old male who presented with an acute abdomen. The patient was taken to the operating room, and an exploratory laparotomy revealed dusky but viable small bowel.

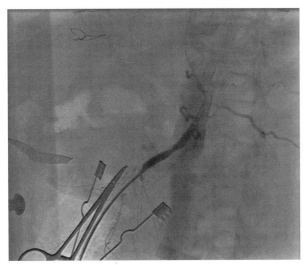

Figure 27.3 Retrograde SMA stenting of an occluded SMA ostial lesion. Retrograde access of the distal SMA with successful deployment of a balloon-expandable Atrium iCAST stent. Distal SMA flow is verified via retrograde angiogram.

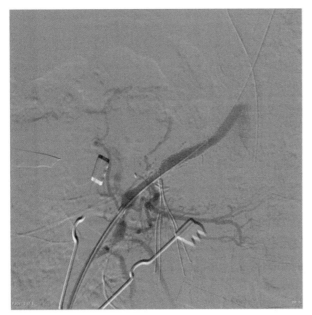

Figure 27.4 (A) Retrograde SMA angiogram access. A 74-year-old male with an acute abdomen was explored by general surgery and found to have necrotic bowel. SMA was not palpable. Retrograde canalization was performed. (B) Retrograde SMA stent deployment. After bowel resection, retrograde stenting was performed to re-establish perfusion to the remaining bowel with a balloon-expandable stent. The patient required re-evaluation and critical care support, but no further bowel resection was needed after the stenting at initial operation. The patient survived hospitalization and was discharged tolerating a regular diet.

Disclosure

The views and clinical opinions presented in this chapter do not reflect a consensus opinion of the Mayo Clinic, nor its faculty.

References and Suggested Readings

1. Schermerhorn ML, Giles KA, Hamdan AD, Wyers MC, Pomposellie FB. Mesenteric revascularization: management and outcomes in the United States, 1988–2006. *J Vasc Surg.* 2009;50(2):341–348.

2. Milner R, Woo EY, Carpenter JP. Superior mesenteric artery angioplasty and stenting via a retrograde approach in a patient with bowel ischemia. *Vasc Endovasc Surg.* 2004;38(1):89–91.

3. Pisimisis GT, Oderich GS. Technique of hybrid retrograde superior mesenteric artery stent placement for acute-on-chronic mesenteric ischemia. *Ann Vasc Surg.* 2011;25:132

4. Do N, Tayyarah M, et al. Retrograde superior mesenteric artery stenting for acute mesenteric arterial occlusion. *Vasc Endovasc Surg.* 2010:44(6):468–471.

5. Wyers MC, Powell RJ, Nolan BW, Cronenwett JL. Retrogreade mesenteric stenting during laparotomy for acute occlusive mesenteric ischemia. *J Vasc Surg.* 2007;45(2):269–275.

6. Tallarita T, Oderich GS, Macedo TA, et al. Reinterventions for stent restenosis in patients treated for atherosclerotic mesenteric artery disease. *J Vasc Surg.* 2011;54:1422–1429.

7. Sonesson B, Hinchliffe RJ, Dias NV, Resch TA, Malina M, Ivancev K. Hybrid recanalization of superior mesenteric artery occlusion in acute mesenteric ischemia. *J Endovasc Ther* 2008;15:129–132.

8. Park WM, Cherry KJ, Chua HK, et al. Current results of open revascularization for chronic mesenteric ischemia: A standard for comparison. *J Vasc Surg.* 2002;35(5):853–859.

9. Cho JS, Carr JA, Jacobsen G, Shepard AD, Nypaver TJ, Reddy DJ. Long-term outcome after mesenteric artery reconstruction: A 37-year experience. *J Vasc Surg.* 2002;35(3):453–460.

10. Davenport DL, Shivazad A, Endean ED. Short-term outcomes for open revascularization of chronic mesenteric ischemia. *Ann Vasc Surg* 2012;26:447–453.

CHAPTER 28

Techniques for Treating Visceral Aneurysms and High-Flow Arteriovenous Malformations of the Renal and Visceral Vasculature

Nikhil Mehta and Bulent Arslan

Brief Description

Aneurysm Treatments

Techniques for treating visceral aneurysms are based on location and anatomic region. Visceral artery aneurysms typically require treatment if they are greater than 2 cm. Aneurysms that are favorable for endovascular therapy include saccular aneurysms, preferably with a narrow neck, and/or aneurysms that have good collateral blood flow to the target organ.[1] The technique chosen depends on the location of the aneurysm and whether the aneurysm is a true aneurysm or pseudoaneurysm.

For aneurysms involving large arteries, treatment options include trapping the aneurysm between coils—that is, coiling distal to proximal, effectively trapping the aneurysm between the coil packs. This allows elimination of both antegrade and potential retrograde flow. This works for saccular or fusiform aneurysms.

For visceral aneurysms that arise from a large parent artery (>6 mm), the aneurysm can potentially be excluded using covered stents. Because of the rigidity of the delivery systems, the tortuosity of the vessel must be considered.

For narrow-necked saccular aneurysms, direct coiling within the aneurysm is possible to allow for occlusion of the aneurysm and preserve flow to the parent artery.

For broad-necked aneurysms in which the parent artery cannot be sacrificed, a stent coil technique can be utilized. A stent is placed to cover the neck of the aneurysm. A microcatheter is then placed through the struts of the stent. Coils are deployed into the aneurysm sac, and the stent acts as a scaffold to prevent the coils from herniating into the parent vessel.

For pseudoaneurysms, a covered stent or direct puncture and injection of thrombin can be considered for treatment. If good collateral flow is identified, a trapping technique may also be performed.

Arteriovenous Malformation Treatments

Endovascular techniques for treating arteriovenous malformations (AVMs) are multifaceted and require appropriate identification of AVMs using multiple imaging modalities in addition to angiography. AVMs can be defined as slow flow, intermediate flow, and high flow. The location of the AVM will also dictate treatment. The goal of AVM treatment is obliteration of the nidus. If the nidus is not adequately treated, then the AVM will recur and may grow beyond its original size if inappropriately managed.[2]

Slow-flow AVMs can be treated with direct puncture using a small butterfly needle. Once blood is able to be aspirated, contrast is injected to confirm intranidal location and to identify draining outflow veins. The outflow veins can be compressed with either manual compression or a tourniquet. Next, a mixture of 25 mg/ml of contrast/doxycycline is administered to allow for obliteration of the nidus. This must be administered slowly to prevent toxicity to the outflow veins. This is allowed to dwell for 5 minutes, and then the needles are removed. Typically, these can be treated in one session, depending on the size.[2]

For intermediate-flow AVMs, treatment can be performed with sclerotherapy, as described previously. In order to slow the flow, simultaneous arterial balloon occlusion or coil embolization can be performed to allow for a longer sclerosant dwell time. In addition, a tourniquet can be applied to slow venous outflow. The key is to reduce flow long enough to allow the sclerosant to work.[2]

For high-flow AVMs or diffuse lesions, a multidisciplinary approach is necessary. These are the riskiest AVMs to treat and they require a combination approach typically involving reduction of flow followed by injection of a sclerosing agent including alcohol, ethiodol, or sotradecol. Alternative agents include Onyx (ev3 Endovascular Inc., Plymouth, MN) and n-BCA (Trufill, Codman & Shurtleff Inc., Raynham, MA). The choice of agent is dependent on the location of the lesion and the ability to reduce flow to the lesion.[2]

Applications of the Technique

1. Aneurysms of the visceral vasculature that are greater than 2 cm.
2. Visceral pseudoaneurysms secondary to a variety of etiologies, including pancreatitis, biliary procedures, liver transplants, and trauma.
3. Sclerosis of slow, intermediate, and high-flow AVMs.

Challenges of the Procedure

Aneurysm Treatments

1. Choosing the appropriate technique in the appropriate setting.
2. Recognizing the collateral supply and predicting infarction.
3. Navigating through tortuous vascular anatomy and around the aneurysm, including getting distal to the aneurysm.
4. End-organ infarction.
5. Persistent endotension on the aneurysm wall despite adequate treatment.

AVM Treatments

1. Nontarget embolization.
2. Recruitment of new vessels.
3. End-organ infarction, which is particularly important in treating subcutaneous/cutaneous malformations.
4. Choice of embolic agent.
5. Staging therapy.

Potential Pitfalls/Complications

AVM and Aneurysm Treatments

1. For renal artery aneurysms that require compromise of the renal parenchyma, incomplete embolization may result in hypertension due to chronic renal ischemia without infarction.
2. Potential for intraprocedural aneurysm rupture.
3. Nontarget embolization: Ensure that the anatomy is well known prior to embolization.

Steps of the Procedure

Renal Bifurcation Aneurysms

1. Determine the anatomy. High frame-rate digital subtraction angiography in multiple projections allows appropriate delineation of anatomy.

2. Determine if a part of the kidney needs to be sacrificed, then particle embolization is recommended to prevent ischemic but perfused parenchyma resulting in hypertension.
3. Subsequently, wire access across the aneurysm is needed along with an appropriately sized covered stent. The authors use a Viabahn (W.L. Gore & Associates Inc., Flagstaff, AZ) or iCast stent (Atrium Medical Corp., Hudson, NH) to exclude the aneurysm.
4. Repeat DSA angiography to ensure no endoleak is present.
5. COnsider angioplasty if endoleak is present and if that fails extending the seal zones with an additional stent.

Peripheral AVM

A. For high-flow AVMs, the treatment is staged. Always approach high flow AVMs with a plan. For large multimeric AVM assume to treat in multiple stages. The plan should consist of proper evaluation of a diagnostic angiogram. Plan which arterial pedicles are to be treated. Identify important collateral vessels that cannot be compromised. Consider embolic agent, is it safe for a liquid embolic? Is the lesion too superficial, will Onyx result in skin discoloration? Would NBCA or alcohol be better?

B. In the distal branches of multimeric AVMs, embolization is performed as close to the nidus as possible—ideally with a liquid embolic to facilitate nidus obliteration.

C. Nidus obliteration is the ultimate goal. If there are no arterial pedicles that are easily accessible, a retrograde transvenous approach should be considered. Using a dual microcatheter/coil trapping technique or balloon occlusion microcatheter, a liquid embolic could be pushed into the nidus in retrograde fashion. This approach should be considered after exhaustion of arterial approaches.

D. The final result after multiple rounds should be complete angiographic nidus obliteration and clinical success.

Example

See Figures 28.1–28.2.

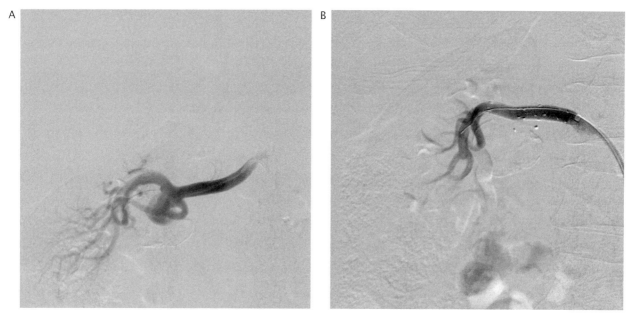

Figure 28.1 (A) An aneurysm of the right renal artery is demonstrated at the bifurcation. The neck is wide, limiting treatment options. (B) Initially, a 2.5 covered Viabahn stent was utilized to cover the neck of the aneurysm and direct all blood flow to the upper pole branch. Unfortunately, this was complicated with an endoleak, and a second Viabahn was placed and telescoped into the first Viabahn. There was a persistent endoleak arising from the overlap that responded to angioplasty, allowing for a good seal. A one-month follow-up computed tomography angiography study demonstrated complete exclusion of the aneurysm.

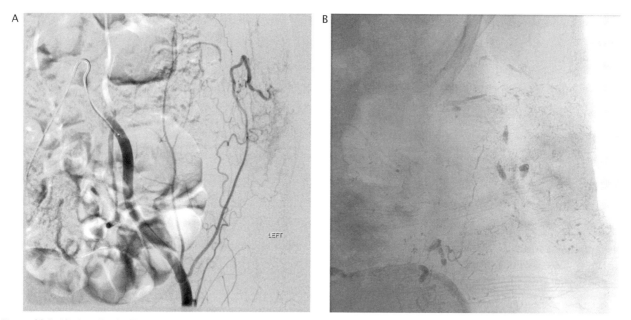

Figure 28.2 (A) A patient with a large left flank pulsatile mass. On angiography, the AVM was supplied from multiple branches, including the left iliac circumflex, the left T12 intercostal, and L2 and L3 lumbar arteries. This was staged with the patient returning for a total of four treatments. (B) Post-treatment appearance of the AVM, with the nidus obliterated with a combination of ethiodol and alcohol.

References and Suggested Readings

1. Hemp J, Sabri S. Techniques in vascular and interventional radiology. *Technical Interv Radiol.* 2015;18(1):14–23.
2. Hyodoh H, Hori M, Akiba H, Tamakawa M, Hyodoh K, Hareyama M. Peripheral vascular malformations: Imaging, treatment, approaches, and therapeutic issues. *Radiographics.* 2005;25:S159–S171.

CHAPTER 29

Proximal Arterial Occlusion During Treatment of Pelvic High-Flow Arteriovenous Malformations

Roshni A. Parikh and David M. Williams

Brief Description

Pelvic arteriovenous malformations (AVMs) are a cause of significant morbidity, with symptoms ranging from discomfort and pressure to considerable vaginal/rectal bleeding and high-output heart failure. Surgical management of AVMs is precarious and poses a risk of massive intraoperative hemorrhage, surrounding organ injury, and incomplete removal of the nidus with a consequent high recurrence rate.[1] Therefore, endovascular management is the preferred modality for treatment of pelvic AVMs. However, the high-flow nature of these and other AVMs poses a challenge to endovascular management. During endovascular treatment of pelvic AVMs, it is important to provide adequate proximal arterial occlusion before injecting the therapeutic agent. Failure to do so can result in ineffective sclerosis of the AVM itself and the potential for systemic distribution of the sclerosant, an event which could have catastrophic or fatal sequelae.

Effective sclerosis of a malformation depends on adequate contact time between the injected sclerosant and the vessel wall and prevention of inadvertent retrograde passage of the agent into normal vessels. In long-standing, high-volume, rapid-transit AVMs, ectatic and tortuous feeder vessels can prevent effective placement of occlusion balloons in distal feeder arteries. The technique described below presents a mechanism to create temporary stasis in an enlarged distal vessel to extend contact time between an injected sclerosant and the recipient vessel wall.

Two coaxial catheters are advanced adjacent to one another into the same distal feeder artery, one stopping 5–10 mm short of the other. Through the more proximal (or "occlusion") catheter, a retrievable coil or plug is deployed, creating temporary stasis in the vessel, while through the more distal (or "injectable") catheter, alcohol or other sclerosant is injected. After the desired contact time has elapsed, the coil or plug is retracted into the occlusion catheter, and flow is reassessed through the injectable catheter. If flow remains vigorous, the plug or coil is redeployed, and more sclerosant is injected. Bilateral or tandem single common femoral arterial access may be used. Once treatment is complete, the detachable coil or plug is retracted and removed.

Applications of the Technique

1. Treatment of a high-flow pelvic AVM with a sclerosing agent, when inflow vessels are too large or too tortuous to accommodate a balloon occlusion catheter.

Challenges of the Procedure

1. Dual selection of the pelvic AVM can be a technical challenge; however, careful wire and catheter manipulation will guide both catheters into the same arterial feeder of the pelvic AVM.

Potential Pitfalls/Complications

1. Dual common femoral arterial access is potentially required, which increases the risk for groin complications (i.e., hematoma, pseudoaneurysm, or arteriovenous fistula). Careful attention to both access points is needed to prevent these complications.
2. Premature retraction of the coil: Coil occlusion needs to be maintained in place until the treatment sets within the AVM. If the coil is retracted before thrombosis of the AVM, the sclerosant may travel retrograde and result in nontarget treatment.
3. Premature detachment of the coil: The goal of this technique is to retract the coil after treatment so that residual flow volume can be estimated and, if necessary, additional sclerosing agent can be injected. Although reliable, retractable microcoils and microplugs carry a risk of spontaneous deployment while the operator attempts to retract them. If this occurs, standard foreign body retrieval methods should be used to retrieve the device. Because the goal of this procedure is to sclerose a branch artery, inadvertent loss of an occlusive device may not be critical or organ threatening; however, the operator should consider the ramifications of inadvertent, more proximal occlusion, which may complicate additional sclerosis procedures.

Steps of the Procedure

1. Obtain dual common femoral arterial access with placement of two 5 French sheaths (or larger). Dual

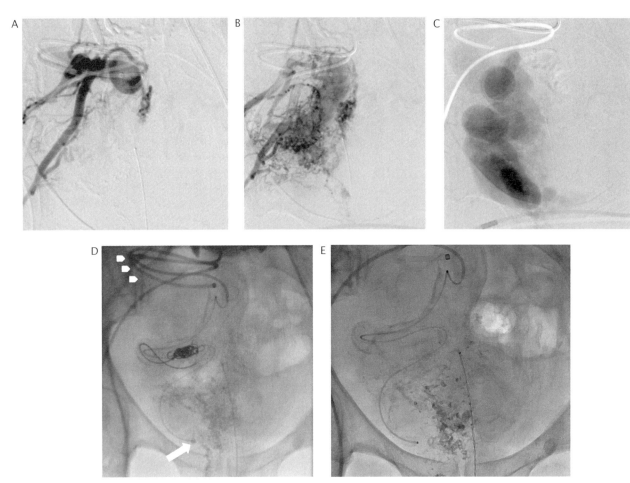

Figure 29.1 (A-C) Pelvic angiogram (arterial-to-venous phase) showing the extensive arteriovenous malformation. Bilateral access to the proximal AVM has been obtained. (D) Deployment of a detachable coil (not detached) from the occlusion microcatheter located more proximally in the arteriovenous malformation. Note redundant curves in internal iliac artery (arrowheads). Sclerosant is being delivered from the injection microcatheter (arrow) located distally in the arteriovenous malformation. (E) The coil has been retracted from the proximal occlusion microcatheter. The distal injection microcatheter is still in place. Sclerosant is seen staining the pelvic arteriovenous malformation.

selection of the proximal arterial feeder (i.e., internal iliac artery) of the pelvic AVM using a 4 or 5 French catheter with distal advancement into a feeder branch.
   a. Stabilization of the access within the proximal arterial feeder may require a longer reinforced sheath.
2. Dual microcatheter advancement deeper into an arterial feeder of the pelvic AVM.
   a. Placement of one microcatheter proximal in the arterial end of the AVM (occlusion microcatheter) and the other microcatheter slightly more distal in the arterial end of the AVM (injectable microcatheter).
3. Selection of an appropriately sized detachable coil (or microplug) that is subsequently advanced through the occlusion microcatheter upstream in the target feeder artery. (Do not detach the coil.)
4. Contrast injection through the injectable microcatheter more distal in the feeder artery to confirm stasis. This confirms that the coil is occlusive or nearly so.
5. Delivery of treatment (i.e., sclerosant) via the access with the injectable microcatheter in the feeder vessel.

6. Allow the treatment to set with the coil still in place (i.e., approximately 5–10 minutes).
7. Slow retraction of the coil back within the occlusion microcatheter.
8. Treatment can be repeated in the same or new arterial feeders as required.
9. Final arteriogram through one of the two 4 or 5 French proximal access catheters outlining the AVM to confirm effective treatment.
10. Removal of all catheters, wires, sheaths. Achieve hemostasis at both access sites.

Example

See Figure 29.1.

Reference and Suggested Reading

1. Christenson BM, Gipson MG, Smith MT. Pelvic vascular malformations. *Semin Intervent Radiol.* 2013;30:364–371.

Venous and Pulmonary Arterial Interventions

Reverse Deployment of the Gore Excluder Contralateral Iliac Limbs for Central Venous Occlusive Disease

S. Lowell Kahn

Brief Description

Central venous occlusive disease is a common entity, occurring in as much as 40% of the dialysis population.[1] The incidence of central venous occlusions is increasing, largely because of the expanded use of central venous catheters and pacer wires[2-4] and the growing dialysis population. The pathophysiology is thought to be multifactorial, with etiologies including direct trauma from a catheter or wire, turbulent flow from an arteriovenous (AV) fistula, and inflammatory processes. The clinical sequelae of central venous occlusions are highly variable and depend on the site of occlusion, the presence of collaterals, and the presence of an AV fistula on the affected side.[5] Many patients have occult disease, but often the disease presents with failure of the AV access and swelling of the involved extremity, breast, neck, and face. Rarely, a pleural effusion may be present.[5] Occlusions involving the superior vena cava (SVC) can present with the aforementioned symptoms, but the swelling can be bilateral and severe. Other symptoms may develop, including dyspnea, chest pain, dysphagia, orthopnea, headache, nausea, stridor, nasal stuffiness, and cough.[6]

Secondary to the associated risks of surgery, endovascular management of central venous occlusion has become the mainstay of therapy despite the efficacy of surgery.[7] Although angioplasty and treatment with bare-metal stents produce excellent short-term results, both methods are hindered by the need for repeat interventions to maintain patency. In addition, it is not clear that bare-metal stenting provides any benefit over angioplasty alone.[8] There are early data suggesting the superiority of covered stents versus bare-metal stents in managing central venous occlusions, and although the results are promising, further randomized studies are necessary to confirm benefit.[9-11]

At our institution, we routinely treat central venous occlusions with covered stent grafts. Unfortunately, options for covered stent grafts can be limited when treating large central venous occlusions. The largest Viabahn (W. L. Gore & Associates, Flagstaff, AZ) and Fluency (C.R. Bard Inc., Tempe, AZ) are 13 and 13.5 mm, respectively. These stent grafts are appropriate for many stenoses, but they may be undersized when treating stenoses of the subclavian and brachiocephalic veins as well as the SVC.

The desirable stent graft for treating central venous occlusions has an increasing diameter as the veins become larger centrally. In theory, a conventional aorto-uni-iliac device could be used, but this would require an unacceptably large access for a peripheral upper extremity vein (18–22 Fr) and would be prohibitively expensive. At our institution, we have made use of Gore Excluder iliac limbs for some large central venous occlusions.

The Gore Excluder contralateral limb is a flexible self-expanding stent graft available in lengths ranging from 9.5 to 14 cm. The proximal diameter of all grafts is 16 mm, and the distal diameter ranges between 12 and 27 mm. Depending on the size selected, these grafts require a femoral access between 12 and 15 Fr, but 12 Fr is adequate for virtually all grafts selected for central venous occlusion. Occasionally, these grafts deployed with conventional technique may be suitable for central venous occlusions, but this necessitates that the more central end of the stent will always be 16 mm and the peripheral end can have a variety of sizes. If one reverses the Gore Excluder limb, the 16-mm end will be in the subclavian vein, and a variety of larger sizes are available for the more central end of the stent graft. Given that the normal adult subclavian vein varies in size between 10 and 20 mm, a 16-mm graft is appropriate for many patients.

This chapter describes a simple and safe method for reversing deployment of the Gore Excluder contralateral limb. Reversal of the limb allows a larger central diameter of 18–27 mm (for the innominate, brachiocephalic, or SVC end) with a fixed subclavian diameter of 16 mm. Two important considerations must be made prior to utilization of this technique. First, the short shaft length of the Gore Excluder limbs necessitates that the device be deployed from an upper extremity vein or fistula. The 12 Fr sheath may be unacceptably large for this access. Second, if treating right-sided disease, the distance between the subclavian/cephalic vein confluence and the confluence of the left and right brachiocephalic veins may be unacceptable. The shortest contralateral limb is 9.5 cm, and deployment of this limb may result in covering of the cephalic vein or the left brachiocephalic vein.

Applications of the Technique

1. Central venous stenoses/occlusions, particularly in the setting of failing dialysis access, upper extremity, face, or neck swelling, and SVC syndrome.
2. Aortoiliac interventions for occlusive or aneurysmal disease.[12]
3. Bailout technique for type I or type III endoleaks during conventional endovascular aneurysm repair.

Challenges of the Procedure

1. Removing the graft from its delivery system can be challenging, and it is advisable to have an assistant as described during the steps of the procedure (discussed later).
2. As described later, the sheath must be modified in that the sheath dilator is cut to a blunt end to create the push rod necessary for deployment of the graft. The wire lumen is often compromised during this process, preventing the dilator from being loaded on the wire. We remedy this situation by passing the back end of an Amplatz Super Stiff Guidewire (Boston Scientific Inc., Marlborough, MA) through the hub end of the dilator and forcing it through the compromised lumen on the other end.
3. After the graft is removed from its manufactured delivery system, it is reversed and then placed in a 12 Fr sheath, where it is deployed. After deployment in the sheath, the actual graft deployment is a simple pin-pull system with unsheathing of the graft. With practice, this is highly accurate, but it is advised that the operator attempt this technique outside of the patient prior to first clinical use.
4. The 12 Fr access for this technique may be unacceptably large for an upper extremity peripheral vein or AV fistula access.

Potential Pitfalls/Complications

1. Several steps are required to remove the graft from its delivery system. These must be adhered to carefully for the technique to work. Most important, the string of the Gore Excluder delivery system must be cut very close to the knob with care taken not to pull the string to prevent inadvertent deployment of the graft.
2. It is advised that the ends of the Gore Excluder be marked with a sterile marker to ensure that the graft is deployed in the desired orientation within the patient. Once the graft is removed from its delivery system, the ends of the undeployed graft look identical even though their diameters are different.
3. There is a risk of graft dislodgement, particularly if the stent is undersized relative to the diameter of the vein undergoing treatment. The consequences can be catastrophic if the graft migrates into the cardiac circulation. Several techniques can be employed to prevent this.
   a. A long wire can be employed that is advanced well beyond the treatment site. For example, an innominate vein stenosis treated from the right arm should have the wire advanced distally in the inferior vena cava or into the iliac vasculature. Some authors even advise snaring it and externalizing it through a femoral vein access. Nonetheless, a long wire provides options if the graft maldeploys to prevent loss of the graft within the heart.
   b. Oversizing the graft (10–20%) in diameter and using a stent that is longer than needed increases the radial force of the graft relative to the vessel wall and increases the points of contact of the stent. Both measures decrease the risk of stent migration.
   c. We routinely angioplasty the stent 1 or 2 mm below the rated diameter of the graft. For example, a 14-mm stent would be angioplastied to 12 mm. This ensures that the graft exerts constant radial force against a smaller diameter vein.
4. The shortest contralateral Gore limb is 9.5 cm in length. It is important to consider this when planning treatment. For example, if treating occlusive disease of the right subclavian and/or innominate vein, the distance between the right cephalic vein confluence and the confluence of the brachiocephalic and innominate vein may be less than 9.5 cm. Covering the cephalic and/or brachiocephalic veins may have untoward consequences, and this needs to be considered in treatment planning.
5. The large sheath required for this technique could damage the peripheral vein or AV fistula used for access. Also, prolonged pressure is required for hemostasis with the large sheath required.

Steps of the Procedure

For deployment steps, see Figures 9.1–9.3 in Chapter 9.

1. Over a guidewire, advance a 12 or 15 Fr sheath (depending on the size of the bell-bottom Gore

Excluder limb selected) beyond the intended location for the graft deployment. Remove the dilator.

2. With heavy scissors, cut the tip of the dilator off near the transition point between the taper and the shaft of the dilator. It is common for the wire lumen to become compromised where the dilator is cut. This is easily repaired by passing the back end of an Amplatz guidewire through the hub end of the dilator and pushing it though forcefully. It is imperative that the lumen be intact because the cut dilator is necessary for graft deployment.

3. Carefully unscrew the deployment knob of the Gore Excluder. With caution, the knob should be barely pulled to expose the white string to which it is attached. Once exposed, cut it with a thin blade. It is imperative that the string is not pulled any further than is necessary to visualize the back of the knob where the string is attached. Pulling it further than required will result in inadvertent deployment of the graft.

4. The graft is now ready to be removed from its delivery shaft. For this step, it is useful to have an assistant. The assistant should place one hand on the graft and should pull on the tip (olive) with the other hand. When this is performed properly, the metal stylet is exposed. With heavy-duty (e.g., sternal) wire cutters, the stylet is cut. Be careful not to damage the graft during this process.

5. The graft should now slide easily off the distal end of the delivery system. At this point, the graft should be in its constrained configuration with the white string attached. Mark the end(s) of the graft with a sterile marker so that the proximal and distal ends are not confused.

6. With the distal end of the graft loaded first, the undeployed graft should be advanced into the sheath over the guidewire. The blunt back end of the dilator should be used to push the graft a few inches into the sheath. The string of the graft will be hanging out of the back end of the sheath.

7. With forward pressure on the blunt dilator (acting as a push rod at this point), the string should be pulled to deploy the graft within the sheath. The blunt dilator ensures that the graft does not come back out of the sheath during deployment. The string is discarded.

8. Push the graft to its desired place of deployment under fluoroscopic guidance.

9. With a pin (blunt dilator)-pull (sheath) method, deploy the graft at its intended location. When the graft first begins to deploy, slight adjustments in the proximal or distal position can be made. We have found that the deployment of this technique is remarkably accurate, arguably more so than when the graft is deployed per the instructions for use with pulling of the string.

10. Complete the procedure by removing the blunt dilator and ballooning the graft as necessary.

Example
See Figures 30.1 and 30.2.

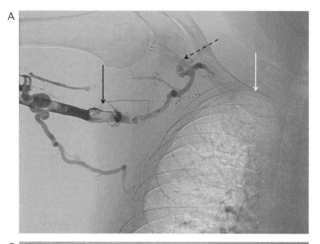

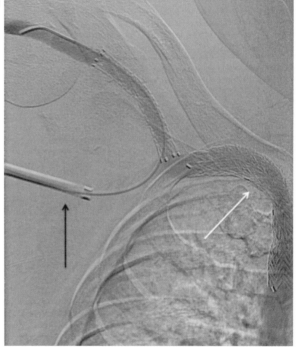

Figure 30.1 Patient with a right upper extremity brachial-to-cephalic AV fistula presents with arm swelling and elevated venous pressures. (A) The basilic vein is catheterized, and venography demonstrates thrombus (solid black arrow) occluding the axillary and subclavian veins. A Luminexx stent (C.R. Bard Inc., Murray Hill, NJ) is present in the cephalic vein (dashed black arrow) and is also occluded. By duplex (not shown), the fistula remains patent as it drains through collateral veins. There is an occluded Viabahn stent centrally (white arrow) within the subclavian vein. (B) A 12-Fr sheath has been placed in the basilic vein (black arrow). After thrombectomy and balloon angioplasty, a reversed Gore Excluder limb (white arrow) has been placed just distal to the cephalic vein and proximal to the confluence of the left brachiocephalic vein. Venography performed through a hockey stick catheter in the venous outflow of the fistula demonstrates patency of the fistula and central veins.

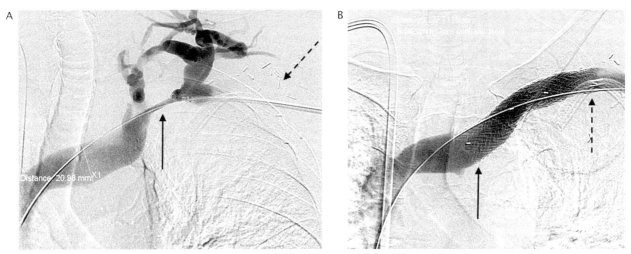

Figure 30.2 Patient with severe left upper extremity swelling after creation of a left upper arm AV fistula. Venous duplex revealed incidental occlusion of the left subclavian vein secondary to thoracic outlet syndrome. The patient underwent thrombectomy and venous angioplasty immediately prior to decompressive surgery with resection of the first rib. Unfortunately, the patient developed immediate recurrent swelling of the left upper extremity after the surgery. (A) He returned for venography, which revealed an occlusion (solid arrow) at the prior site of occlusion, indicating severe chronic injury to the vein. Contrast is seen passing through the occlusion in this image because the sheath had already been advanced through this segment prior to obtaining this image. Note the surgical clips (dashed arrow) and JP drain in the surgical bed. (B) The subclavian vein proximal to the occlusion (not shown) measured approximately 14 mm, and the brachiocephalic vein distal to the occlusion measured 20 mm. The left jugular vein was occluded by ultrasound. A flipped bell-bottom Gore Excluder contralateral limb was employed. The 20-mm end was placed in the brachiocephalic vein (solid arrow), and the 16 mm end was placed in the subclavian vein (dashed arrow).

References and Suggested Readings

1. Glanz S, Gordon DH, Lipkowitz GS, Butt KMH, Hong J, Sclafani SJA. Axillary and subclavian vein stenosis: Percutaneous angioplasty. *Radiology.* 1988;168:371–373.

2. Agarwal AK, Patel BM, Farhan NJ. Central venous stenosis in hemodialysis patients is a common complication of ipsilateral central vein catheterization. *J Am Soc Nephrol.* 2004;15:368A–369A.

3. Vanherweghem JL, Yasine T, Goldman M, et al. Subclavian vein thrombosis: A frequent complication of subclavian cannulation for hemodialysis. *Clin Nephrol.* 1986;26:235–238.

4. Trerotola SO, Kuhn-Fulton J, Johnson MS, Shah H, Ambrosius WT, Kneebone PH. Tunneled infusion catheters: Increased incidence of symptomatic venous thrombosis in subclavian versus internal jugular venous access. *Radiology.* 2000;217:89–93.

5. Kundu S. Central venous obstruction management. *Semin Intervent Radiol.* 2009;26(2):115–121.

6. Rice TW, Rodriguez RM, Light RW. The superior vena cava syndrome: Clinical characteristics and evolving etiology. *Medicine (Baltimore).* 2006;85(1):37–42.

7. Mansour M, Kamper L, Altenberg A, Haage P. Radiological central vein treatment in vascular access. *J Vasc Access.* 2008;9:85–101.

8. Bakken AM, Protack CD, Saad WE, Lee DE, Waldman DL, Davies MG. Long-term outcomes of primary angioplasty and primary stenting of central venous stenosis in hemodialysis patients. *J Vasc Surg.* 2007;45:776–783.

9. Anaya-Ayala JE, Smolock CJ, Colvard BD, et al. Efficacy of covered stent placement for central venous occlusive disease in hemodialysis patients. *J Vasc Surg.* 2011;54(3):754–759.

10. Verstandig AG, Berelowitz D, Zaghal I, et al. Stent grafts for central venous occlusive disease in patients with ipsilateral hemodialysis access. *J Vasc Interv Radiol.* 2013;24(9):1280–1287.

11. Jones RG, Willis AP, Jones C, et al. Long-term results of stent-graft placement to treat central venous stenosis and occlusion in hemodialysis patients with arteriovenous fistulas. *J Vasc Interv Radiol.* 2011;22:1240–1245.

12. van der Steenhoven TJ, Heyligers JM, Tielliu IF, Zeebregts CJ. The upside down Gore Excluder contralateral leg without extracorporeal predeployment for aortic or iliac aneurysm exclusion. *J Vasc Surg.* 2011;53(6):1738–1741.

CHAPTER 31

Branched Stent Graft Placement in the Vena Cava Using the Endologix AFX

S. Lowell Kahn

Brief Description

Originally described in 1757, superior vena cava syndrome (SVCS) comprises a constellation of symptoms resulting from stenosis, occlusion, or thrombosis of the SVC of benign and malignant etiologies.[1] Historically, SVCS resulted most commonly from infections such as tuberculosis or syphilis.[2-4] Currently, the diagnosis is most commonly seen with thoracic malignancies, with primary lung cancer accounting for up to 70% of cases.[5-7] Up to 4% of lung cancer patients present with SVCS at the time of diagnosis, and many more develop it at a later time.[8] In younger patients with SVCS, lymphoma is commonly responsible.[9] Recently, there has been a rise in benign SVCS secondary to the increased use of central venous catheters and pacemakers. In some series, device-related SVCS may be responsible for up to 40% of cases.[3,10,11] As of 2006, there were roughly 15,000 new cases of SVCS in the United States annually, and the incidence is rising.[12]

Occlusion or stenosis of the SVC results in decreased cardiac preload and impaired venous drainage of the head, neck, and upper extremities. The presentation of SVCS is variable, but facial and neck swelling is most common, occurring in 82% of patients.[3] Unilateral or bilateral upper extremity swelling, dyspnea, cough, and dilated neck and chest wall veins are common.[3] Orthopnea, dysphagia, stridor, and neurologic symptoms occur in severe cases.[13-15] SVCS most commonly presents late in the sixth decade, but it can be seen in children and young adults as well.[3,9] The presentation is frequently subacute occurring over days to weeks, but acute and more insidious presentations occur as well.[9,16] The diagnosis is predominantly clinical, but contrast-enhanced computed tomography (CT) is essential to delineate the etiology of the obstruction and evaluate the extent of the disease for treatment planning.[17] Secondary findings of obstruction, such as dilated chest wall collaterals, are commonly appreciated as well.

Interestingly, SVC stenosis or occlusion has implications beyond SVCS in the dialysis population. Specifically, occlusion of the central veins can cause malfunction of dialysis catheters and shunts, and it may reduce the number of peripheral veins available for catheterization.[18,19] The importance of central vein patency in this population is reflected in the current National Kidney Foundation Guidelines, which advocate for stent placement for patients with immediate elastic recoil or greater than 30% residual stenosis post angioplasty and those with recurrent stenosis within 3 months.[20]

Benign and malignant SVCS have considerably different prognoses, and this may have implications for treatment decisions. The median life expectancy for malignant SVCS is a 6 months,[16,21,22] but there is wide variability, with one recent study yielding a median survival of only 1.6 months.[9] In contrast, patients with malignant SVCS secondary to lymphoma fare considerably better with a median survival of 80.1 months according to a recent study.[9] Although multiple factors influence prognosis, malignant etiology, advanced age (>50 years), history of smoking, and use of steroids are associated with a poor outcome.[9]

Patients presenting with benign and malignant SVCS should be promptly provided with supplemental oxygen, head elevation, diuretics, and a course of steroids.[23] Although such measures are beneficial, more definitive treatment is required. Historically, definitive management of malignant SVCS consisted of radiotherapy and chemotherapy, but the efficacy of this approach is controversial, and the response to therapy is delayed.[24,25] Similarly, surgery to relieve SVCS is of high risk and is only rarely performed.[26]

Endovascular stenting of the SVC for SVCS has been described for more than 25 years and is now the first-line treatment of choice for benign and malignant SVCS.[27-30] Stent placement relieves symptoms in 81–100% of patients, which is superior to the efficacy of chemotherapy and radiation.[31-33] Moreover, most patients will experience relief within 24–72 hours after the intervention, and the placement of stents does not interfere with the adjunctive use of chemotherapy and radiation.[31,34] Stenting of the SVC is generally regarded as safe, with a peri- and post-procedural complication and mortality rate of 6% and 3%, respectively.[13,26,27] Complications include venous rupture, stent migration, pulmonary embolism, and cardiac tamponade. Migration to the heart or pulmonary arteries is a particularly dreaded outcome and may be more likely to occur with covered stents given the lesser endothelialization of the stents. Migration incidence has been reported as high as 3%, but with proper oversizing and placement technique, this percentage should be lower.[33,35]

Although stenting of the SVC is broadly accepted, the optimal technique has yet to be elucidated, and considerable variation exists in the literature. Traditionally, bare-metal stents are most commonly used, and it has been established that nitinol stents have lower rates of SVCS recurrence compared to stainless-steel stents.[28] The ideal bare-metal stent for the SVC should have a large diameter, long length, flexibility, and high radial force.[36] There are limited options for self-expanding stents with these properties. In the United States, most self-expanding stents have a maximum diameter of 14 mm, except for the Wallstent (Boston Scientific, Marlborough, MA), but this stent is limited by poor radial strength and elongation, making accurate deployment more challenging. Recently, Andersen et al.[36] reported a 92% rate of SVCS resolution in patients treated with the Zilver Vena stent (Cook Medical Inc., Bloomington, IN) for malignant SVCS. This stent is designed for iliac stenting, but it has these desired properties for the SVC. Unfortunately, the stent is currently unavailable in the United States.

One limitation of bare-metal stents is that they are prone to restenosis, particularly in the setting of malignancy. Recurrence is reported in up to 41% of cases of malignant SVCS secondary to tumor ingrowth and thrombosis.[8,13,30,33,37] However, patients with malignant SVCS have a short life expectancy, and in the majority of cases, adequate patency is maintained until death, particularly with secondary reintervention.[8,14,31] The consequences of restenosis are more likely significant for those patients with longer life expectancies and for those patients with benign SVCS with ongoing needs for dialysis access.

When a stent is placed, most commonly it descends from one of the two brachiocephalic veins into the SVC. Particularly if a covered stent is used, this effectively jails the contralateral brachiocephalic vein. Although likely of consequence to the dialysis patient with respect to the availability of the contralateral side for future access, the clinical significance of this is otherwise controversial. It has not been proven that unilateral stenting adversely impacts venous drainage in the patient. In fact, it has been argued that unilateral stenting is a cost-effective, equally efficacious solution with a low complication and recurrence rate.[29,30,34,38] Despite this, investigators have attempted bilateral venous stenting to preserve physiologic bilateral drainage. Methods include the creation of a "Y stent" via deployment of a second stent through the interstices of the primary stent or by deploying kissing stents into both brachiocephalic veins. Interestingly, it has

been shown that although bilateral stents confer equal initial technical and clinical success, bilateral stenting has a shorter patency and higher complication rate than unilateral stenting.[38]

There is now increased interest in the use of covered stents, particularly for patients with malignant SVCS. Until recently, the use of covered stents was limited to emergent repair (e.g., trauma) or after failed bare-metal stenting.[39–42] In theory, covered stents may offer superior patency relative to bare metal by preventing tumor ingrowth and limiting endothelialization. In 2012, Gwon et al.[43] reported outcomes of two patients with malignant SVCS treated with stent grafts. Both patients achieved palliation of their symptoms, and the stents remained patent until their deaths without the need for reintervention. Similarly, in 2014, Cho et al.[31] reported the outcomes of 40 patients with malignant SVCS treated with unilateral stent grafts. The technical success rate was 100%, and 92% of patients had full resolution of their symptoms within 8 days of implantation. Cumulative stent patency at 1, 3, 6, and 12 months was 95%, 92%, 86%, and 86%, respectively. A single prospective study compared bare-metal and covered stents and found a higher patency rate with covered stents. Patency at 1, 3, 6, and 12 months for covered stents was 97%, 94%, 94%, and 94% versus 97%, 79%, 67%, and 48% for bare-metal stents, but survival did not differ between the two groups.[44]

Selection of a stent graft for SVCS has similar limitations to those discussed with respect to bare-metal stents because the options are limited. The maximal diameter of the Viabahn (W. L. Gore & Associates, Flagstaff, AZ) is 13 mm, and this is available in 2.5-, 5-, and 10-cm lengths. Successful use of the Viatorr (W. L. Gore & Associates, Flagstaff, AZ) has also been described for SVC stenting because it confers the potential benefit of preserving jugular flow by landing the uncovered portion of the stent over the jugular–subclavian confluence.[18] The Viatorr has a maximal diameter of 12 mm, so use of this stent in the SVC and brachiocephalic veins may be limited. In our practice, we have commonly used Gore Excluder AAA Endoprosthesis iliac limbs (W. L. Gore & Associates, Flagstaff, AZ) deployed in either standard configuration or reversed (allows bell-bottom deployment at the atriocaval junction) with a 100% success rate. Nonetheless, an ideal covered stent for the SVC that offers preservation of bilateral brachiocephalic flow, high radial strength, large diameter, accurate deployment, and optimal fixation to prevent migration does not currently exist.

This chapter describes use of the Endologix AFX AAA System (Endologix, Irvine, CA) for the treatment of SVCS. Although not appropriate for all cases, the AFX is a covered, branched unibody aortic stent graft delivered by a 17 Fr primary access and an 8 or 9 Fr secondary contralateral access. Placement of the graft in the SVC and bilateral brachiocephalic veins is technically feasible and confers the benefits of a large-diameter covered graft with preservation of both brachiocephalic veins. The benefits of this technique are most likely to be realized in the dialysis population with central venous stenosis/occlusion and those patients with malignant SVCS with a longer life expectancy. In addition, we demonstrate use of the AFX stent graft in the treatment of a patient with chronic lower extremity pain, swelling, and venous stasis ulceration secondary to a remote surgical ligation of the inferior vena cava (IVC). Although obsolete because of the advent of filters and the high rate of complications, ligation of the IVC was formerly performed for the prevention of pulmonary embolism in the setting of deep venous thrombosis (DVT).[45] Indications for the use of the AFX in the IVC will be infrequent relative to the SVC given the satisfactory results of bilateral iliac stenting for chronic DVT and unilateral stenting for May–Thurner syndrome.[46,47] Nonetheless, the AFX offers the most physiologic repair of both the SVC and the IVC, and use of the device may be warranted under various circumstances.

Applications of the Technique

1. Revascularization of benign and malignant stenoses or occlusions involving the superior vena cava with involvement of one or both brachiocephalic veins. This technique provides an optimal physiologic revascularization with preservation of bilateral upper extremity venous drainage.

2. Revascularization of stenoses or occlusions involving the IVC with involvement of one or both common iliac veins. Again, use of the AFX preserves the iliac vein confluence, providing the most physiologic endovascular repair.

Challenges of the Procedure

1. The main body of the Endologix AFX requires insertion of a 17 Fr sheath. In theory, this sheath can be introduced from either internal jugular or subclavian vein, providing four potential access sites where the main body can be introduced. Placement of the 17 Fr sheath via a brachial or basilic vein might be possible, but it would not be advisable because this might result in bleeding or irreversible injury to the vein.

2. There are size constraints of the Endologix AFX device that may make use of this technique undesirable. First, except for a single 22-mm-diameter configuration with a length of 40 mm, the shortest main body measures 60 mm in length and the SVC must be long enough to accommodate the graft. The short 40- and 60-mm-length devices both have a minimum of 40-mm-length limbs, whereas the longer 70-, 90-, and 110-mm-length devices offer shorter 30-mm limbs. Therefore, the brachiocephalic veins should measure greater than 30 or 40 mm in length (depending on the graft chosen) to avoid exclusion of the subclavian or internal jugular vein. Further information on the sizes available is provided later.

3. The Endologix AFX main bodies range in diameter between 22 and 18 mm, and the limbs range between 13 and 20 mm in diameter. Fortunately, the device tolerates oversizing well because the fabric lies on the outside of the metallic endoskeleton. Nonetheless, oversizing should ideally be in the range of 10–20%. Further information on sizes available is provided later.

4. SVC and brachiocephalic stenoses may be quite refractory to dilatation, which poses two important implications: First, the stenoses should be predilated to allow delivery of the device. A high degree of recoil should be viewed with caution because this could make sheath delivery or removal of the delivery system post deployment difficult. In our experience, a minimum of 10-mm diameter should be attained with pre-dilatation angioplasty to safely perform this technique. Second, the main body of the Endologix AFX lacks high radial strength, and reinforcement of the graft with a large balloon-expandable bare-metal stent (e.g., Palmaz, Cordis, Hialeah, FL) after deployment may be necessary to achieve the desired luminal gain.

5. The Endologix AFX requires snaring of the contralateral limb for deployment. In the aortic aneurysm setting, this is achieved with little difficulty. However, in the presence of severe caval stenosis, snaring in the SVC may be difficult. In these situations, the wire can be safely snared in the right atrium or in the retrohepatic IVC.

Potential Pitfalls/Complications

1. The 17 Fr sheath required for insertion of the Endologix AFX carries a risk of bleeding or vessel trauma/shearing with consequent thrombosis. Careful review of the vessels with pre-procedural CT and intraoperative ultrasound and venography is imperative for case planning. Because of the potential difficulty in maintaining hemostasis with a subclavian access, it is recommended that a secondary ipsilateral extremity venous access be obtained as a safety measure because this would allow bailout balloon tamponade or covered stent placement in the setting of an uncontrolled subclavian venous bleed.

2. The operator should monitor carefully for recoil of the brachiocephalic vein or SVC stenosis/occlusion. As stated previously, obtaining a suitable (e.g., ≥10 mm) lumen with pre-dilatation is imperative prior to device delivery. With severe recoil, delivery of the sheath may be impossible. Alternatively, recoil could prevent retrieval of the delivery system as the

nose cone is retracted through the newly deployed graft. This is a potentially serious complication.

3. The operator should monitor the sheaths carefully for the development of thrombus or air, both of which could embolize to the pulmonary circulation with adverse sequelae. It is advised that the sheaths be maintained to a continuous heparinized saline flush.

4. Introduction of the stiff wires and large sheath could result in traumatic injury to the heart, pericardium, mediastinum, and lungs. Potentially serious arrhythmias could result as well. Advancement of the wires and devices should therefore be performed with continuous hemodynamic monitoring and under live fluoroscopy at all times.

5. Although highly unlikely given the oversizing of the Endologix AFX and the multiple points of contact of the graft with the brachiocephalic veins and SVC, migration of the stent graft into the heart or IVC is possible.

Steps of the Procedure

Endologix AFX Deployment in the SVC

1. Pre-procedural contrast-enhanced Computed Tomography Venography (CTV) or Magnetic Resonance Venography (MRV) should be obtained for planning. Specific attention should be paid to the degree of stenosis or obstruction and the underlying etiology. Delineation of the extent of vascular involvement should be made (SVC, one or both brachiocephalic veins, etc.). Diameters of the uninvolved SVC (just above the right atrium) and of the brachiocephalic veins should be determined. In addition, the length from the right atrium to the brachiocephalic vein and the lengths of each brachiocephalic vein (prior to the confluence of the subclavian and jugular veins) should be measured and compared with the sizing chart to ensure that an appropriate graft meets the size criteria. The Endologix AFX tolerates oversizing well because the fabric is external to the metallic endoskeleton, and the graft diameters should be oversized at least 10–20% relative to the uninvolved SVC and brachiocephalic measurements. Also, when choosing a length, the graft typically foreshortens modestly, and this should be taken into account (e.g., a 70-mm graft will typically measure approximately 65 mm in actual length). Finally, an assessment of the potential access vessels (subclavian and jugular) should be made to ensure delivery of the 17 French sheath is possible.

2. Prior to commencing the procedure, ultrasound of the jugular and subclavian veins should be performed to verify the CT findings and confirm vessel selection for the primary access.

3. A subclavian or jugular vein should be chosen for the primary access (anticipated 17 Fr sheath delivery). Both veins are typically more than adequate to accommodate the sheath, and technically, any of the four veins could be used. The jugular vein is easier to compress post procedure, but the subclavian vein may be more optimally located. Specifically, the jugular veins (particularly the right side) lie close to the intended graft landing zones in the brachiocephalic veins. Therefore, the sheath will barely lie within the jugular vein during graft deployment, and dislodgement of the sheath from the vein altogether is possible. Consideration of this should be made as well as the ergonomics of the case and room configuration (a long table should be placed adjacent to the planned access to accommodate the device). In the case demonstrated in this chapter, we chose the left subclavian vein. *Note*: If the subclavian vein is chosen as the primary access, a secondary (safety) access in the ipsilateral arm should be obtained with wire access across the subclavian insertion point. This secondary access could be used to control unanticipated bleeding with either balloon tamponade or covered stent placement after removal of the 17 French sheath. After the primary access is chosen, the vessel is accessed and an 8 Fr sheath is placed initially.

4. Obtain contralateral upper extremity venous access, and advance an 8 or 9 Fr × 45-cm sheath to the central veins.

5. Central venography through the bilateral sheaths should be performed to study the SVC and brachiocephalic occlusion.

6. Wire access to the common iliac veins should be obtained from both accesses. A stiff wire such as a Lunderquist (Cook Medical) is ideal. If a third safety access is obtained for a subclavian primary access, the wire from this access need simply be placed across the subclavian access point.

7. Primary angioplasty should be performed as necessary to attain a suitable lumen for device delivery and deployment. Generally, a diameter of 10 mm or more is ideal to ensure safe sheath delivery and device deployment.

8. The Endologix AFX is then deployed per the manufacturer's instructions for use (IFU). This requires snaring of a wire from the contralateral access to deploy the limb in the contralateral brachiocephalic vein. Snaring can be performed in the SVC, but in the setting of stenosis, it may be easier to snare the wire in the right atrium or IVC.

9. After deployment, the graft is angioplastied and follow-up venography performed. If there is residual stenosis, reinforcement with a balloon-expandable stent is performed.

10. The accesses are removed, and hemostasis is obtained with manual pressure. If a subclavian access is used for the 17 Fr sheath, prolonged manual pressure (e.g., 15–20 minutes) is applied and follow-up venography is performed through the safety sheath in the ipsilateral extremity. If bleeding is present, additional pressure or treatment with balloon tamponade or covered stent placement is performed as required.

Endologix AFX Deployment in the IVC

1. A pre-procedural CTV or MRV is ideal but not mandatory. Adequate information for planning can be obtained via bilateral iliac venography/cavography. Regardless of the imaging modality, attention should be paid to the degree of stenosis or obstruction and the underlying etiology. Delineation of the extent of vascular involvement should be made (IVC, one or both common iliac veins, etc.). Diameters of the uninvolved IVC (above the stenosis or occlusion) and of the common iliac veins should be determined. In addition, the length of the infrarenal IVC and the lengths of each common iliac vein should be measured and compared with the sizing chart to ensure that an appropriate graft meets the size criteria. As stated previously, the Endologix AFX tolerates oversizing well, and the graft diameters should be oversized at least 10–20% relative to the uninvolved IVC and common iliac veins. Remember that the length of the graft will foreshorten slightly, and this should be considered. Finally, an assessment of the common femoral veins should be made to ensure delivery of the 17 Fr sheath is possible on at least one of the sides.

2. Ultrasound of both common femoral veins is performed to select the appropriate ipsilateral (17 Fr) and contralateral (8 or 9 Fr) sides, and access is obtained.

3. Bilateral iliac venography and cavography is performed through both sheaths to study the stenosis/occlusion and verify measurements for case planning.

4. Bilateral wire access, ideally to the SVC, is obtained with use of stiff wires.

5. Pre-dilatation is performed through the stenosis/occlusion with the goal of obtaining an adequate lumen (ideally ≥10 mm) to ensure sheath delivery and device deployment.

6. After placement of the 17 Fr sheath into the IVC and advancement of a snare from the contralateral access, the Endologix AFX is deployed per the manufacturer's IFU.

7. The graft is angioplastied, and follow-up venography is performed.

8. If there is significant residual stenosis, reinforcement with a balloon-expandable stent should be considered.

9. The procedure is terminated with removal of both accesses, and manual pressure is applied for hemostasis.

Example

See Figures 31.1–31.3.

Main Body Options									
Body Diameter	Limb Diameter	Body Length	Limb Length	Model #	Body Diameter	Limb Diameter	Body Length	Limb Length	Model #
☐22 mm	13 mm	40 mm	40 mm	BA22-40/I13-40	☐22 mm	16 mm	90 mm	30 mm	BA22-90/I16-30
☐22 mm	13 mm	60 mm	40 mm	BA22-60/I13-40	☐22 mm	20 mm	70 mm	30 mm	BA22-70/I20-30
☐22 mm	16 mm	60 mm	40 mm	BA22-60/I16-40	☐22 mm	20 mm	80 mm	40 mm	BA22-80/I20-40
☐22 mm	16 mm	70 mm	30 mm	BA22-70/I16-30	☐22 mm	20 mm	90 mm	30 mm	BA22-90/I20-30
☐22 mm	16 mm	80 mm	40 mm	BA22-80/I16-40					
☐25 mm	13 mm	80 mm	40 mm	BA25-80/I13-40	☐25 mm	16 mm	120 mm	40 mm	BA25-120/I16-40
☐25 mm	16 mm	60 mm	40 mm	BA25-60/I16-40	☐25 mm	20 mm	70 mm	30 mm	BA25-70/I20-30
☐25 mm	16 mm	70 mm	30 mm	BA25-70/I16-30	☐25 mm	20 mm	80 mm	40 mm	BA25-80/I20-40
☐25 mm	16 mm	80 mm	40 mm	BA25-80/I16-40	☐25 mm	20 mm	90 mm	30 mm	BA25-90/I20-30
☐25 mm	16 mm	80 mm	55 mm	BA25-80/I16-55	☐25 mm	20 mm	100 mm	40 mm	BA25-100/I20-40
☐25 mm	16 mm	90 mm	30 mm	BA25-90/I16-30	☐25 mm	20 mm	110 mm	30 mm	BA25-110/I20-30
☐25 mm	16 mm	100 mm	40 mm	BA25-100/I16-40	☐25 mm	20 mm	120 mm	40 mm	BA25-120/I20-40
☐25 mm	16 mm	110 mm	30 mm	BA25-110/I16-30					
☐28 mm	16 mm	60 mm	40 mm	BA28-60/I16-40	☐28 mm	20 mm	70 mm	30 mm	BA28-70/I20-30
☐28 mm	16 mm	70 mm	30 mm	BA28-70/I16-30	☐28 mm	20 mm	80 mm	40 mm	BA28-80/I20-40
☐28 mm	16 mm	80 mm	40 mm	BA28-80/I16-40	☐28 mm	20 mm	90 mm	30 mm	BA28-90/I20-30
☐28 mm	16 mm	90 mm	30 mm	BA28-90/I16-30	☐28 mm	20 mm	100 mm	40 mm	BA28-100/I20-40
☐28 mm	16 mm	100 mm	40 mm	BA28-100/I16-40	☐28 mm	20 mm	110 mm	30 mm	BA28-110/I20-30
☐28 mm	16 mm	110 mm	30 mm	BA28-110/I16-30	☐28 mm	20 mm	120 mm	40 mm	BA28-120/I20-40
☐28 mm	16 mm	120 mm	40 mm	BA28-120/I16-40					

Figure 31.1 Sizing sheet for the Endologix AFX main body.

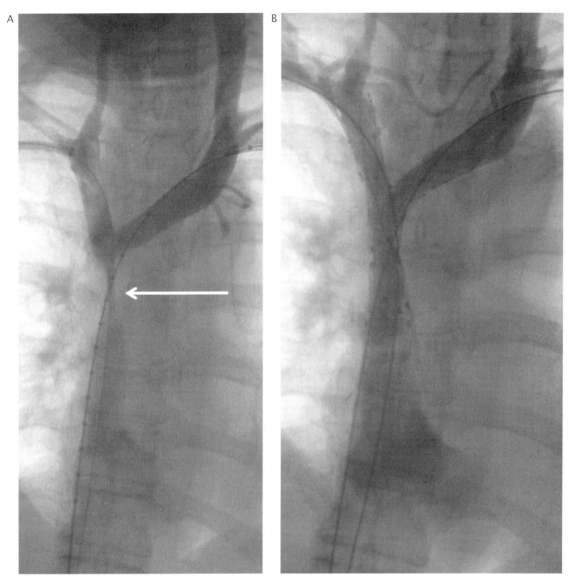

Figure 31.2 Endologix AFX deployment in the SVC for symptomatic malignant SVCS secondary to primary lung cancer. (A) A critical stenosis is present within the SVC (arrow). Three accesses have been obtained. The primary access for the 17-Fr sheath is the left subclavian vein. A secondary (safety) access with wire placement across the left subclavian access was obtained in the left basilic vein. Finally, the contralateral access required for deployment of the AFX was obtained in the right basilic vein. (B) After deployment of the graft, venography was performed through the bilateral accesses and showed unimpeded blood flow through the bilateral brachiocephalic veins and the SVC.

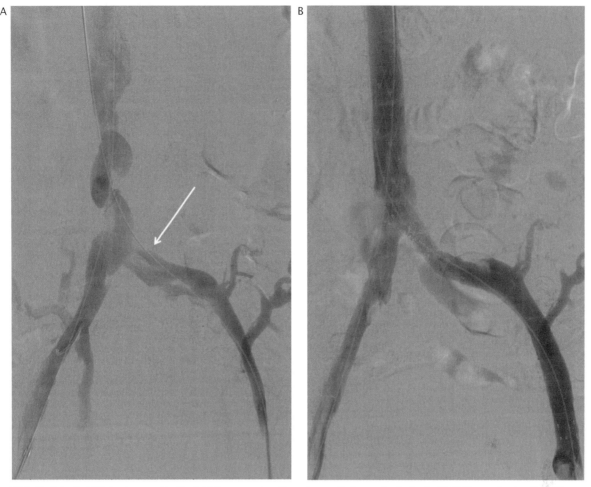

Figure 31.3 Endologix AFX deployment in the IVC for reconstruction of a partially surgically ligated IVC. The patient suffered from severe bilateral lower extremity edema, venous claudication, and venous stasis ulcers. (A) Preliminary venography shows marked narrowing of the left common iliac vein (arrow) and profound irregularity and narrowing of the IVC. (B) After deployment of the graft, venography was performed through the bilateral femoral accesses and showed unimpeded blood flow through the bilateral iliac veins and IVC.

References and Suggested Readings

1. Hunter W. History of aneurysm of the aorta with some remarks on aneurysm in general. *Med Obser Inq.* 1757;1:323–357.
2. Nunnelee JD. Superior vena cava syndrome. *J Vasc Nurs.* 2007;25:2–5.
3. Rice TW, Rodriguez RM, Light RW. The superior vena cava syndrome: Clinical characteristics and evolving etiology. *Medicine.* 2006;85:37–42.
4. Zisis C, Skevis K, Kefaloyannis E, Avgoustou K, Bellenis I. Mediastinal tuberculous lymphadenitis presenting as superior vena cava syndrome. *J Thorac Cardiovasc Surg.* 2006;131:e11–e12.
5. Flounders J. Superior vena cava syndrome. *Oncol Nurs Forum.* 2003;30(4):E84–E88.
6. Ahmann FR. A reassessment of the clinical implications of the superior vena caval syndrome. *J Clin Oncol.* 1984;2(8):961–969.
7. Hassikou H, Bono W, Bahiri R, Abir S, Benomar M, Hassouini NH. Vascular involvement in Behçet's disease: Two case reports. *Joint Bone Spine.* 2002;69(4):416–418.
8. Rowell NP, Gleeson FV. Steroids, radiotherapy, chemotherapy and stents for superior vena caval obstruction in carcinoma of the bronchus: A systematic review. *Clin Oncol (R Coll Radiol).* 2002;14:338–351.
9. Chiu-Lung Chan R, Chan YC, Wing-Keung Cheng S. Mid- and long-term follow-up experience in patients with malignant superior vena cava obstruction. *Interact Cardiovasc Thorac Surg.* 2013;16:455–458.
10. Schifferdecker B, Shaw JA, Piemonte TC, Eisenhauer AC. Nonmalignant superior vena cava syndrome: Pathophysiology and management. *Catheter Cardiovasc Interv* 2005;65:416–423.
11. Rizvi AZ, Kalra M, Bjarnason H, Bower TC, Schleck C, Gloviczki P. Benign superior vena cava syndrome: Stenting is now the first line of treatment. *J Vasc Surg.* 2008;47:372–380.
12. Higdon ML, Higdon JA. Treatment of oncologic emergencies. *Am Fam Physician.* 2006;74:1873–1880.
13. Uberoi R. Quality assurance guidelines for superior vena cava stenting in malignant disease. *Cardiovasc Intervent Radiol.* 2006;29(3):319–322.
14. Kee ST, Kinoshita L, Razavi MK, Nyman UR, Semba CP, Dake MD. Superior vena cava syndrome: Treatment with catheter-directed thrombolysis and endovascular stent placement. *Radiology.* 1998;206(1):187–193.

15. Wan JF, Bezjak A. Superior vena cava syndrome. *Hematol Oncol Clin North Am.* 2010;24(3):501–513.

16. Schraufnagel DE, Hill R, Leech JA, Pare JA. Superior vena caval obstruction: Is it a medical emergency? *Am J Med.* 1981;70:1169–1174.

17. Qanadli SD, El Hajjam M, Bruckert F, et al. Helical CT phlebography of the superior vena cava: Diagnosis and evaluation of venous obstruction. *AJR Am J Roentgenol.* 1999;172:1327–1333.

18. Quaretti P, Galli F, Paolo Moramarco LP, et al. Dialysis catheter-related superior vena cava syndrome with patent vena cava: Long term efficacy of unilateral Viatorr stent-graft avoiding catheter manipulation. *Korean J Radiol.* 2014;15(3):364–369.

19. Agarwal AK. Central vein stenosis. *Am J Kidney Dis.* 2013;61:1001–1015.

20. National Kidney Foundation/KDOQI. *2006 Updates: Clinical Practice Guidelines for Hemodialysis Adequacy.* New York: National Kidney Foundation; 2006.

21. Yellin A, Rosen A, Reichert N, Lieberman Y. Superior vena cava syndrome: The myth–The facts. *Am Rev Respir Dis.* 1990;141(5 Pt 1):1114–1118.

22. Marcy PY, Magne N, Bentolila F, Drouillard J, Bruneton JN, Descamps B. Superior vena cava obstruction: Is stenting necessary? *Support Care Cancer.* 2001;9:103–107.

23. Cheng S. Superior vena cava syndrome: A contemporary review of a historic disease. *Cardiol Rev.* 2009;17:16–23.

24. Dyet JF, Nicholson AA, Cook AM. The use of the Wallstent endovascular prosthesis in the treatment of malignant obstruction of the superior vena cava. *Clin Radiol.* 1993;48: 381–385.

25. Urban T, Lebeau B, Chastang C, Leclerc P, Botto MJ, Sauvaget J. Superior vena cava syndrome in small-cell lung cancer. *Arch Intern Med.* 1993;153:384–387.

26. Picquet J, Blin V, Dussaussoy C, Jousset Y, Papon X, Enon B. Surgical reconstruction of the superior vena cava system: Indications and results. *Surgery.* 2009;145:93–99.

27. Andersen PE, Duvnjak S. Palliative treatment of superior vena cava syndrome with nitinol stents. *Int J Angiol.* 2014;23(4):255–262.

28. Fagedet D, Thony F, Timsit JF, et al. Endovascular treatment of malignant superior vena cava syndrome: Results and predictive factors of clinical efficacy. *Cardiovasc Intervent Radiol.* 2013;36(1):140–149.

29. Urruticoechea A, Mesía R, Domínguez J, et al. Treatment of malignant superior vena cava syndrome by endovascular stent insertion: Experience on 52 patients with lung cancer. *Lung Cancer.* 2004;43(2):209–214.

30. Lanciego C, Pangua C, Chacón JI, et al. Endovascular stenting as the first step in the overall management of malignant superior vena cava syndrome. *AJR Am J Roentgenol.* 2009;193(2):549–558.

31. Cho Y, Gwon DI, Ko GY, et al. Covered stent placement for the treatment of malignant superior vena cava syndrome: Is unilateral covered stenting safe and effective? *Korean J Radiol.* 2014;15(1): 87–94.

32. Watkinson AF, Yeow TN, Fraser C. Endovascular stenting to treat obstruction of the superior vena cava. *BMJ.* 2008;336:1434–1437.

33. Nguyen NP, Borok TL, Welsh J, Vinh-Hung V. Safety and effectiveness of vascular endoprosthesis for malignant superior vena cava syndrome. *Thorax.* 2009;64:174–178.

34. Nicholson AA, Ettles DF, Arnold A, Greenstone M, Dyet JF. Treatment of malignant superior vena cava obstruction: Metal stents or radiation therapy. *J Vasc Interv Radiol.* 1997;8:781–788.

35. Wilson LD, Detterbeck FC, Yahalom J. Superior vena cava syndrome with malignant causes. *N Engl J Med.* 2007;356:1862–1869.

36. Andersen PE, Midtgaard A, Brenoe AS, Elle B, Duvnjak S. A new nitinol stent for use in superior vena cava syndrome: Initial clinical experience. *J Cardiovasc Surg (Torino).* 2015;56(6):877–881.

37. Ganeshan A, Hon LQ, Warakaulle DR, Morgan R, Uberoi R. Superior vena caval stenting for SVC obstruction: Current status. *Eur J Radiol.* 2009;71:343–349.

38. Dinkel HP, Mettke B, Schmid F, Baumgartner I, Triller J, Do DD. Endovascular treatment of malignant superior vena cava syndrome: Is bilateral Wallstent placement superior to unilateral placement? *J Endovasc Ther.* 2003;10:788–797.

39. Chin DH, Petersen BD, Timmermans H, Rosch J. Stent-graft in the management of superior vena cava syndrome. *Cardiovasc Intervent Radiol.* 1996;19:302–304.

40. Gill K, Ettles DF, Nicholson AA. Recurrent superior vena caval obstruction due to invasion by malignant thymoma: Treatment using a stent-graft. *Br J Radiol.* 2000;73:1015–1017.

41. Azizzadeh A, Pham MT, Estrera AL, Coogan SM, Sa HJ. Endovascular repair of an iatrogenic superior vena caval injury: A case report. *J Vasc Surg.* 2007;46:569–571.

42. Mansour M, Altenburg A, Haage P. Successful emergency stent implantation for superior vena cava perforation during malignant stenosis venoplasty. *Cardiovasc Intervent Radiol.* 2009;32:1312–1316.

43. Gwon DI, Paik SH. Successful treatment of malignant superior vena cava syndrome using a stent-graft. *Korean J Radiol.* 2012;13(2):227–231.

44. Gwon DI, Ko GY, Kim JH, Shin JH, Yoon HK, Sung KB. Malignant superior vena cava syndrome: A comparative cohort study of treatment with covered stents versus uncovered stents. *Radiology.* 2013;266(3):979–987.

45. Donaldson MC, Wirthlin LS, Donaldson GA. Thirty-year experience with surgical interruption of the inferior vena cava for prevention of pulmonary embolism. *Ann Surg.* 1980;191(3):367–372.

46. Hartung O, Loundou AD, Barthelemy P, Arnoux D, Boufi M, Alimi YS. Endovascular management of chronic disabling iliocaval obstructive lesions: Long-term results. *Eur J Vasc Endovasc Surg.* 2009;38(1):118–124.

47. Ahmed O, Ng J, Patel M, et al. Endovascular stent placement for May–Thurner syndrome in the absence of acute deep vein thrombosis. *J Vasc Interv Radiol.* 2016;27(2): 167–173.

Needle Recanalization of Chronic Venous Total Occlusions

Adam N. Plotnik and Stephen Kee

Brief Description

The needle recanalization of chronic venous total occlusions (NRCVTO) technique may be employed for difficult chronic venous occlusions where standard initial techniques have failed. Initial efforts to cross the occlusion should always begin with an angled or straight 0.035-in. Glidewire (Terumo Medical Corp., Somerset, NJ) together with a 4 Fr diagnostic catheter (e.g., angled Glide Cath [Terumo Medical Corp., Somerset, NJ] or Quick-Cross catheter [Spectranetics Corp., Colorado Springs, CO]). If these efforts fail, consider using the stiff-end/back-end of a 0.035-in. Glidewire or even a 0.035-in. Amplatz wire (Cook Medical Inc., Bloomington, IN); however, this can create a large hole with no ability to "steer" the wire. Ferral et al.[1] first described sharp recanalization of occluded central veins in 1996 with subsequent further variations reported in the literature.[2–6] Our variant NRCVTO technique employs the use of a trans-septal needle (e.g., Mullins trans-septal needle [Medtronic Inc., Minneapolis, MN] or BRK trans-septal needle [St. Jude Medical Inc., St. Paul, MN]) together with a 0.014-in. guidewire (e.g., Balance Middleweight, Abbott Vascular Inc., Santa Clara, CA). The trans-septal needle can pass through a 5 or 6 Fr guide catheter; however, a 7 Fr introducer sheath (e.g., Destination [Terumo Medical Corp., Somerset, NJ] or Brite Tip [Cordis Corp., Milpitas, CA]) is usually employed because it gives more stability. The trans-septal needle, which has a curve, can be "steered" and is then gently advanced across the occlusion. Alternatively, the NRCVTO technique can be performed using a 22 gauge Chiba needle (Cook Medical Inc., Bloomington, IN), usually 20–25 cm long, with a gentle curve placed to aid "steering." A target is then provided in the vessel distal to the occlusion in the form of a 4 Fr 10-mm snare, which is usually placed via a transfemoral or, less commonly, transhepatic approach. Following this, the 0.014-in. guidewire is passed across the occlusion into the patent distal vessel. At this stage, the wire can be snared, and with "through-and-through" access achieved, the occlusion can be crossed with the necessary peel-away sheath, balloon dilatation, and/or stenting as per standard technique.

Applications of the Technique

1. Chronic venous occlusions whereby standard methods to cross the occlusion have failed, including using an angled or straight 0.035-in. Glidewire together with a 4 Fr catheter (e.g., angled Glide Cath or Quick-Cross catheter) or even attempting to cross with the back end of a 0.035-in. Glidewire.

2. Common scenarios of chronic venous occlusion include the following: hemodialysis patients with chronic central venous occlusions needing placement of a tunneled dialysis catheter; patients with short gut syndrome and long-standing total parenteral nutrition (TPN) dependency with central venous occlusion now requiring placement of central venous access for TPN; patients with symptomatic superior vena cava (SVC) syndrome secondary to benign chronic venous occlusion of the SVC and/or brachiocephalic veins; patients with malfunctioning arteriovenous (AV) grafts or fistulas secondary to chronic central venous occlusions.

Challenges of the Procedure

1. Staying intraluminal: During sharp recanalization, contrast medium should be injected intermittently to assess for extra-anatomic passage or the need to adjust the trajectory. In addition, fluoroscopy in both the true anterior–posterior (AP) and lateral to the target occlusion is essential to help guide the needle trajectory. For more difficult cases, we prefer to perform the procedure in a biplane angiography suite for ease of switching between the AP and lateral plane.

2. Patient comfort: Sharp recanalization can be a lengthy procedure and at times uncomfortable for the patient. As a result, we often perform these procedures under general anesthesia.

3. Puncture from a lower pressure system: Some authors[3,5] stress the importance of puncturing from a lower pressure territory central to the occlusion to reduce the risk of bleeding in case of a false passage. In many cases, however, this may be difficult to

achieve secondary to the location and length of the occlusion.

4. Radiation exposure can often be increased to the patient and operator. Passage of the needle under fluoroscopic guidance can expose the operator's hands to excess radiation. It is important to be cognizant during the case and use fluoroscopy sparingly.

Potential Pitfalls/Complications

1. Increased risk of pericardial tamponade: When performing sharp recanalization, particularly in the region of the SVC, it is important to be aware of the pericardial recesses that extend cranially to cover the pulmonary trunk, SVC, and ascending aorta. This risk increases as the recanalization extends inferiorly, with little risk above the clavicle, moderate risk between the clavicle and azygos arch, and high-risk recanalizing below the azygos arch. A covered stent (e.g., Viabahn, W. L. Gore & Associates Inc., Flagstaff, AZ) should always be ready in the room in case of rupture into the pericardium. In high-risk cases, a pericardial drain should be available in case of pericardial tamponade, with backup cardiothoracic surgery services on hand in the event of an urgent thoracotomy or sternotomy.

2. Increased risk of venous rupture: Once sharp recanalization has been performed, there is an increased risk of venous rupture during balloon dilatation. Again, a covered stent (e.g., Viabahn) should be ready in the room in case of such an event.

3. Luminal gain: Once across the occlusion, only balloon dilate up to the size necessary to perform the endpoint of the case. For example, if the endpoint is to place a hemodialysis catheter, then the interventionalist does not need to restore venous patency, which is known to be of a limited durability, but simply gain sufficient track diameter to permit passage of the catheter.[2] In addition, this technique will ensure the catheter will completely occupy the recanalized venous segment, thereby safeguarding from any extravasation from the tract.

4. Stent occlusion: When a venous stent is placed across a chronic venous occlusion, there is a high risk of stent reocclusion.[7] Therefore, at least 3 months of anticoagulation should be considered.

5. Snare position within the uppermost aspect of the SVC/right atrium inferior to the venous occlusion: A common pitfall is to advance the snare as "high" as possible on the AP projection; however, this may result in the targeting device being displaced posterior in the azygos arch, which is not optimal for recanalization. Careful monitoring in two orthogonal projections should prevent this.

Steps of the Procedure

1. Pre-procedural imaging: A key step in successfully executing a sharp recanalization is pre-procedural imaging. This will help the interventionalist identify a suitable recanalization route, ideally with a straight-line trajectory that does not violate important mediastinal structures such as aorta, carotid vessels, lung, and pericardium.

2. Access the vein proximal to the occlusion: This is usually performed under ultrasound guidance using a micropuncture kit. Often, the access is within an upper extremity or the internal jugular vein given that most chronic venous occlusions occur in the central or upper extremity veins. Right-sided neck or internal jugular vein access is preferred when dealing with chronic SVC occlusions, due to the resultant straight-line trajectory. The initial venogram is generally performed through a 4 Fr diagnostic catheter to help define the length of the occlusion.

3. Simultaneous access within the vein distal/central to the occlusion: This is usually performed via the right femoral vein with a 6 Fr sheath (e.g., Destination) advanced through the heart to the level of the occlusion. A snare (e.g., 10-mm Amplatz GooseNeck [ev3 Endovascular Inc., Plymouth, MN] or EN Snare [Merit Medical Systems Inc., South Jordan, UT]) is then placed to provide a target in anticipation of snaring the wire when the chronic venous occlusion has been traversed.

4. Sharp recanalization: Via the upper extremity access, a 7 Fr sheath is placed proximal to the occlusion, and through this a trans-septal needle (e.g., Mullins or BRK trans-septal needle) is then placed. The 18 gauge trans-septal needle has a curve so it can be "steered" and is then gently advanced across the chronic venous occlusion. Contrast medium should be injected intermittently to assess for extra-anatomic passage or the need to correct the needle trajectory. In addition, fluoroscopy in both the true AP and lateral projections to the target occlusion will help guide the needle trajectory.

5. Alternatively, a 22 gauge Chiba needle, usually 20 or 25 cm long with a gentle curve placed on it to aid "steering," can be used to advance through the chronic venous occlusion instead of using the transseptal needle. We often use the 22 gauge Chiba needle when recanalizing the SVC via a right transjugular approach in a straight-line trajectory. This is usually advanced through a 5 Fr Kumpe catheter (Cook Medical Inc., Bloomington, IN), which is positioned at the superior end of the central venous occlusion. The 5 Fr Kumpe catheter will need to be cut short to allow passage of the Chiba needle. It is important to gently spin the 22 gauge Chiba needle as it is advanced through the 5 Fr Kumpe catheter to prevent

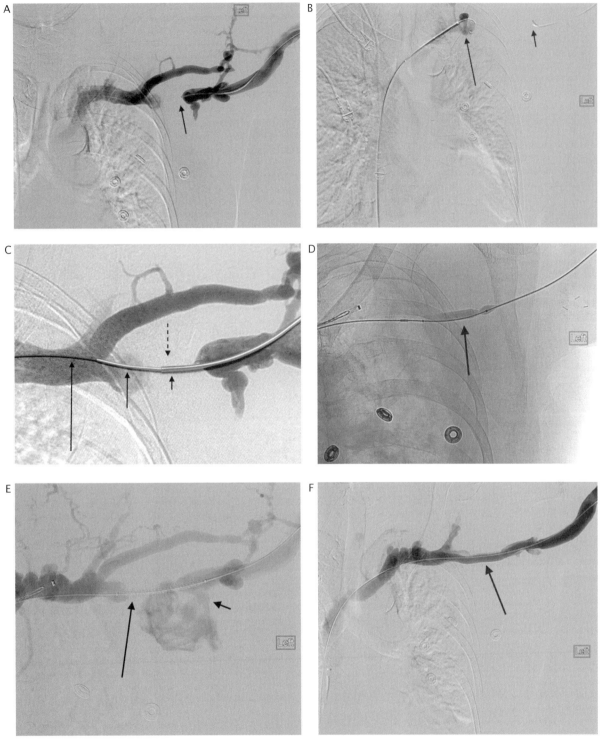

Figure 32.1 (A) Left brachial venogram demonstrates complete occlusion of the axillary vein (arrow), with evidence of bridging collaterals draining into the brachiocephalic vein. This is the etiology for the poorly functioning AV graft. (B) Venogram is then performed through a 6-Fr sheath in the left brachiocephalic vein (long arrow), central to the occlusion, which has been placed via the right common femoral vein. A 4-Fr catheter is noted at the point of occlusion in the axillary vein (short arrow). (C) Sharp recanalization schematic. Recanalization is shown with the needle (medium arrow) and sheath (short arrow) of the trans-septal needle (BRK) traversing the occluded axillary vein (dashed arrow), with an 0.014-in. wire (long arrow) passed into the patent left brachiocephalic vein. (D) With through-and-through access achieved into the patent central vein, the 0.014-in. wire is exchanged for a 0.035-in. wire, and venoplasty using a 6 mm × 4-cm balloon (arrow) has been performed. (E) Post balloon dilatation. Extravasation of contrast (short arrow) is present at the site of venoplasty secondary to a venous rupture. Therefore, a self-expanding covered stent (large arrow) has been inserted in preparation for deployment. (F) Post deployment of covered stent (arrow) venogram. Excellent venous flow is now demonstrated without residual stenosis or extravasation.

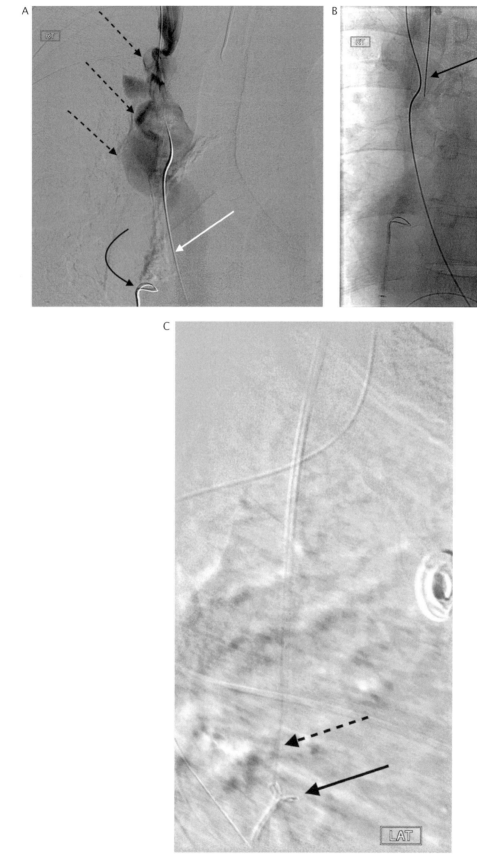

Figure 32.2 (A) Alternative approach using a 22 gauge Chiba needle. Venogram via a right transjugular approach demonstrates a large collateral vessel draining into the azygos vein (dashed arrows). A wire remains in the azygos vein after removal of a previously malpositioned dialysis catheter (white arrow). A "target" snare (curved arrow) is seen in the lower SVC. (B) Sharp recanalization. A curved 22 gauge Chiba needle begins to traverse the long-segment occlusion (arrow). (C) Lateral projection. The snare remains anterior (solid arrow), thereby aiding the straight-line trajectory of the 22 gauge Chiba needle (dashed arrow).

the needle from puncturing through the side of the catheter. With the 22 gauge Chiba needle at the superior end of the occlusion, sharp recanalization is then performed as described in step 4.

6. Snare "target" placement: When recanalizing an occluded SVC, it is important to place the "target" snare in the uppermost aspect of the SVC, inferior to the occlusion, to assist with directing the 22 gauge needle along the appropriate trajectory.

7. Through-and-through access: Once the trans-septal needle (or the 22 gauge Chiba needle) has punctured into the patent distal/central venous lumen, and this has been confirmed with contrast injection, an exchange length 0.014-in. wire (e.g., Balance Middleweight) is passed through the lumen of the trans-septal needle and snared by the previously placed snare. Consequently, through-and-through access is achieved from the upper and lower extremity access sites. The snare itself can be used as the target with the snare tightened on the tip of the needle. The wire can then be advanced several cm beyond the needle tip and the needle can be carefully released and removed leaving the snare grasping the wire tip again providing through-and-through access.

8. Balloon dilation: With through-and-through access achieved, the tract is dilated to the size needed for the clinical situation. As discussed previously, balloon dilatation should be kept to a minimum required size to achieve the endpoint of the case. With venous access, for example, all that is needed is passage of the peel-away sheath.

9. Stent placement: This should be considered depending on the end goal of the case. In the setting of recanalization for the placement of dialysis catheters, there is no need to expand the lumen greater than the size of the catheter and, as such, no need for stent placement. When recanalizing a chronic occluded vein in the setting of a malfunctioning AV graft, a bare-metal stent is usually placed as per standard protocol to ensure adequate luminal size for dialysis.

In the setting of a venous rupture, a covered stent is often employed.

10. Catheter placement: Following balloon dilatation appropriately sized to the catheter placed, the dialysis or central venous line is advanced over a stiff 0.035-in. wire.

Examples

Example 1: A 65-year-old male with a poorly functioning left-side AV graft secondary to chronic axillary venous occlusion (Figure 32.1).

Example 2: **A** 34-year-old male requiring a dialysis catheter with chronic right brachiocephalic/SVC occlusion (extending below the azygos confluence; i.e., high risk) (Figure 32.2).

References and Suggested Readings

1. Ferral H, Bjarnason H, Wholey M, Lopera J, Maynar M, Castaneda-Zuniga WR. Recanalization of occluded veins to provide access for central catheter placement. *J Vasc Interv Radiol.* 1996;7(5):681–685.

2. Athreya S, Scott P, Annamalai G, Edwards R, Moss J, Robertson I. Sharp recanalization of central venous occlusions: A useful technique for haemodialysis line insertion. *Br J Radiol.* 2009;82(974):105–108.

3. Farrell T, Lang EV, Barnhart W. Sharp recanalization of central venous occlusions. *J Vasc Interv Radiol.* 1999;10(2 Pt 1):149–154.

4. Gupta H, Murphy TP, Soares GM. Use of a puncture needle for recanalization of an occluded right subclavian vein. *Cardiovasc Intervent Radiol.* 1998;21(6):508–511.

5. Lang EV, Reyes J, Faintuch S, Smith A, Abu-Elmagd K. Central venous recanalization in patients with short gut syndrome: Restoration of candidacy for intestinal and multivisceral transplantation. *J Vasc Intervent Radiol.* 2005;16(9):1203–1213.

6. Murphy TP, Webb MS. Percutaneous venous bypass for refractory dialysis-related subclavian vein occlusion. *J Vasc Intervent Radiol.* 1998;9(6):935–939.

7. Rizvi AZ, Kalra M, Bjarnason H, Bower TC, Schleck C, Gloviczki P. Benign superior vena cava syndrome: Stenting is now the first line of treatment. *J Vasc Surg.* 2008;47(2):372–380.

Recanalization of Chronic Central Venous Occlusions: Techniques to Cross Difficult Venous Occlusions

Sreekumar Madassery and Bulent Arslan

Brief Description

With approximately 400,000 patients on hemodialysis in the United States alone,[1] there are increasingly more patients who eventually develop central venous occlusions, mostly because of numerous central venous catheterizations, and the placement of arteriovenous fistulas and grafts. With improving technical abilities to obtain central venous access for catheters and maintain fistula/graft patency, increasingly more patients present with signs of central venous stenosis/occlusion. For many, the underlying occlusion is chronic, with well-formed collateral vessels that have developed over time, thus allowing for continued dialysis or asymptomatic function. However, for many patients there is a gradual progression of symptoms, including upper extremity/neck swelling, pain, increased bleeding during dialysis, poor dialysis flow rates, and dyspnea. Other conditions associated with central venous occlusions include extrinsic tumor compression, the presence of pacemaker wires, and hypercoagulable states.

Chronic occlusions present particular difficulty to the interventionalist due to the likelihood that the native occluded vessel will become obliterated once well-formed collaterals develop. Acute occlusions and severely stenotic lesions are far less problematic because recanalization/traversal is typically achieved quickly. With chronic occlusions, imaging usually demonstrates a beak-like stump or "nubbin," beyond which the chronic occlusion continues. There tends to be a hard, possibly calcified cap at this location that needs to be traversed first.

Some lesions can be treated with antegrade access using a combination of an angled catheter with hydrophilic guidewire and sheath, with the access being the outflow vein/graft of the dialysis access or the brachial/basilic/cephalic vein if the patient does not have a surgical access. If there is difficulty, the back end of the hydrophilic wire can be used for sharper recanalization. More difficult cases require a retrograde access to perform the flossing technique, in which femoral venous access is obtained and a combination of sheath and catheters are used to snare a needle and/or wire from the upper extremity access once the lesion is crossed. Once through-and-through access is obtained, serial balloon dilation is performed with intermittent contrast injection to ensure no rupture is encountered. Balloon dilation alone usually provides temporary patency, whereas most choose to place stents, preferable self-expanding covered stents if possible, to improve the duration of patency. If hydrophilic guidewire recanalization is unsuccessful, other methods have provided success at our institution, including use of a chronic total occlusion (CTO) device (TruePath, Chronic Total Occlusion Device Boston Scientific Inc., Marlborough, MA) through the hard cap of the occlusion, as well as through a long-standing port-a-catheter. Use of a radiofrequency guidewire (PowerWire Radiofrequency Guidewire, Baylis Medical Company Inc., Montreal, QC, Canada) in treating chronic occlusions has gained some traction.[2] Although limited available reports show strong success rates, the potential deleterious consequences include arterial injury, and even tracheal injury has been reported by Sivananthan et al.[3] One reason for the high risk of extravascular complications is that the radiofrequency wire does not have the tactile feedback that conventional guidewires provide. Also, due to the energy used, a tract can be made in any tissue, unlike with conventional hydrophilic guidewires, in which there is far less likelihood of entering/injuring mediastinal structures such as the pleura, pericardium, arteries, and airways.[3]

Once patency has been achieved, many patients require repeat, sometimes frequent, interventions because there is a high likelihood of in-stent thrombosis/stenosis and re-occlusion, particularly when covered stents cannot be used due to attempts to preserve native veins such as the internal jugulars and innominate vein/superior vena cava (SVC) confluence.

Applications of the Technique

1. Chronic central venous occlusions in symptomatic patients.
2. Chronic central venous occlusions in dialysis patients with access issues.
3. Can be utilized in chronic arterial occlusions.

Challenges of the Procedure

1. Some lesions cannot be recanalized into an intraluminal segment despite all possible techniques. These patients may need to be referred for surgical bypass.
2. False passage along an extraluminal tract is common, particularly if using radiofrequency wire.
3. Some chronic occlusions have very long occluded segments, decreasing the likelihood of successful recanalization.

Potential Pitfalls/Complications

1. Potential for venous rupture during balloon dilation of the tract.
2. Injury to the mediastinal structures, including the pleura, pericardium, arteries, and central airways with use of a radiofrequency wire.
3. Obtaining optimal stent positioning due to the location of central vessels that should be preserved (i.e., internal jugular veins and contralateral confluence of the SVC and innominate vein).
4. Recurrent in-stent restenosis/occlusion is common and should be expected.

Steps of the Procedure

1. After access into the peripheral vein on the affected side, or through the outflow vein of the arteriovenous fistula/graft, perform a venogram to determine the length of occlusion, target site, and beaking of the occlusion. Beaking refers to the tapering seen at the point of an occlusion and is the best location to attempt traversal. Successful venogram requires prolonged delay of digital subtraction angiography to show the actual distal/central target.
2. Advance a sheath (typically 6 or 7 Fr) for support. Then, advanced an angled 4 or 5 Fr catheter with hydrophilic guidewire to the location of the point of beaking at the occlusion. Attempts should be made to "drill" the guidewire across the occlusion, with the support of the angled catheter and the sheath. If unsuccessful, the stiff back end

of the guidewire can be used to perform sharp recanalization. When using the back end of the wire care should be taken to only pass the wire a relatively short distance to avoid extravasation or injury to adjacent structures.
3. If antegrade recanalization is initially unsuccessful, retrograde access can be gained through the common femoral vein with a sheath, angled catheter, and hydrophilic guidewire. Attempt the previously mentioned technique in reverse by attempting to traverse the occlusion from the distal end.
4. If both antegrade and retrograde attempts are unsuccessful, a snare can be advanced into the retrograde access. Then, through the antegrade access, sharp needle recanalization as described in the previous chapter can be attempted. Alternatively, recanalization using a CTO device (e.g., TruePath device or Crosser system [C.R. Murray Hill, NJ]) or weighted-tip crossing wires can be attempted through a microsupport catheter. The crossing device/wire can be advanced toward the snare and then, once successfully captured, brought out the retrograde access, thus providing through-and-through access ("flossing").
5. If these methods are still unsuccessful, radiofrequency guidewire placement can be attempted, after discussion of the increased risks with the patient.
6. Once the recanalization has been performed, the tract needs to be dilated. Over a stiffer support guidewire, serial angioplasty can be performed starting with a 4-mm balloon and eventually noncompliant 10-/12-mm balloons. Intermittent venograms are recommended to monitor for rupture, which if seen should be treated with prolonged angioplasty or covered stenting. If not under general anesthesia, concerning signs such as onset of chest pain should be monitored and evaluated.
7. After achieving satisfactory tract dilation, typically self-expanding covered/uncovered stenting is deployed. Care should be taken to preserve any nearby central vessels such as the ipsilateral internal jugular vein or the contralateral SVC/innominate vein junction.
8. SVC/inferior vena cava stenting can be performed with covered stents/endografts.
9. It is important to maintain anticoagulation during the procedure (i.e., maintain activated clotting time >200 seconds).

Example

See Figures 33.1 and 33.2.

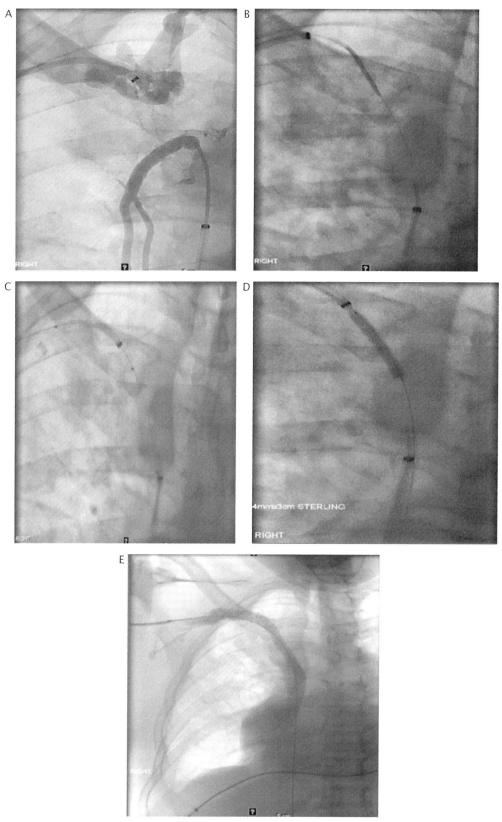

Figure 33.1 Patient with hemodialysis fistula and chronic central venous occlusion. (A) Venogram with simultaneous injection from antegrade upper extremity sheath and retrograde femoral sheath showing chronic-appearing central occlusion with collaterals extending across the neck as well as opacification of the azygous vein. (B) Eventual successful crossing of the occlusion using the back end of a hydrophilic guidewire. (C) Support catheter and guidewire positioned within the right atrium, extending into the IVC, which was then snared from the retrograde access, thus providing through-and-through access. (D) Pre-dilation of the recanalized tract. (E) Completion image post covered stenting.

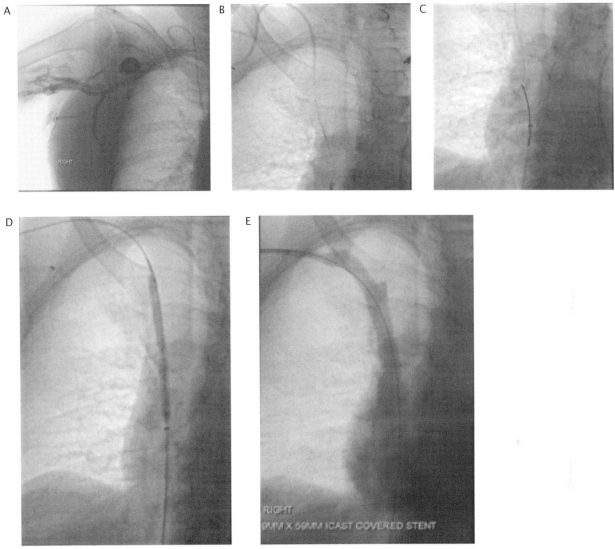

Figure 33.2 Chronic central occlusion successfully recanalized using the existing portacatheter and TruePath device. (A) Initial venogram shows chronic central occlusion with collateral vessels. Old portacatheter noted. (B) After failed antegrade and retrograde recanalization attempts, the nonfunctional port chamber was dissected out, and through its catheter, the TruePath wire was advanced and used to successfully drill through the occlusion. (C) Snaring of the wire from the groin retrograde access. Subsequently, retrograde access into the right subclavian vein was achieved after snaring retrograde wire through upper extremity sheath, providing "flossing" access. (D) Pre-dilation of the tract was performed. (E) Completion image showing post covered stenting patent antegrade flow with venogram performed through the upper extremity sheath.

References and Suggested Readings

1. United States Renal Data System. https://www.usrds.org/2012/view/v2_01.aspx.
2. Iafrati M, Maloney S, Halin N. Radiofrequency thermal wire is a useful adjunct to treat chronic central venous occlusions. *J Vasc Surg.* 2012;55(2):603-606.
3. Sivananthan G, MacArthur DH, Daly K, Allen DW, Hakkan S, Halin NJ. Safety and efficacy of radiofrequency wire recanalization of chronic central venous occlusions. *J Vasc Access.* 2015;16(4):309–314.

CHAPTER 34

Managing Chronic Iliac Venous Occlusions That Extend Below the Inguinal Ligament

Roshni A. Parikh and David M. Williams

Brief Description

Inferior vena cava and iliac vein thrombosis is a cause of significant morbidity. Re-establishment of the flow in the iliocaval lumen(s) ensures venous outflow from the lower extremities. Recanalization of chronic occlusion(s) with venoplasty and stenting is currently the treatment of choice. This treatment, combined with adequate anticoagulation, can significantly improve patients' quality of life. Stent patency, however, is highly dependent on venous inflow.

Preoperative imaging with ultrasound, computed tomography, or magnetic resonance imaging can fail to define the extent of venous inflow disease, resulting in an underestimation or overestimation. Contrast enhancement or flow signal characterize veins with flowing blood rather than anatomically competent (i.e., recruitable) veins, in which blood is static due to diversion of inflow into collaterals bypassing an outflow obstruction. Poor timing of contrast may fail to opacify inflow channels, simulating obstruction. In addition, ultrasound has difficulty characterizing the deep femoral vein.

The failure mode of stents is thrombosis, and poor flow trumps anticoagulation. Therefore, the success of treating iliocaval venous obstruction with recanalization, venoplasty, and stenting depends on connecting good inflow to good outflow. Without good inflow, the outflow stents will inexorably fail (i.e., thrombose).[1]

This chapter describes the management of venous occlusion that extends below the level of the inguinal ligament. The first step involves exploring the saphenofemoral junction, femoral vein confluence, and/or the saphenous vein directly, followed by recanalization of the occluded segment(s). Ultimately, extending the stents into the femoral vein, deep femoral vein, or, rarely, the greater saphenous vein will improve the venous inflow and the sustainability of the venous outflow.

Sometimes, however, extending the stents into the femoral vein alone does not provide enough venous inflow to maintain venous outflow patency. In these situations, endophlebectomy or a femoral arteriovenous fistula may be necessary for adequate venous inflow.

Applications of the Technique

1. Iliocaval deep vein thrombosis with unilateral or bilateral femoral vein (or deep femoral vein) extension.
2. May–Thurner syndrome with femoral vein extension.

Challenges of the Procedure

1. Inability to recanalize the chronically occluded segments via the traditional vertebral tip catheter and Glidewire (Terumo Medical Corp., Somerset, NJ). If this occurs, sharp recanalization techniques may be necessary (e.g., loop snare and a BRK-1 needle (St. Jude Medical Inc., St. Paul, MN) or re-entry needle/catheter) using popliteal and internal jugular approaches.
2. Inadequate venous inflow despite extending the stents to the femoral and/or deep femoral veins. In this situation, a femoral arteriovenous fistula or surgical endophlebectomy may be necessary to improve the venous inflow.

Potential Pitfalls/Complications

1. Vessel perforation/rupture: Extravascular passage can occur during routine (and sharp) recanalization. Short segments, however, are usually not a problem because small venous perforations will thrombose quickly. A major venous tear may require a stent graft.

Steps of the Procedure

1. Right internal jugular and unilateral (or bilateral) greater saphenous vein (may also use common femoral vein) access with placement of 6 Fr or larger sheaths.
2. Venous outflow recanalization:
   a. Using a vertebral tip catheter and a straight stiff Glidewire, begin to recanalize from the saphenofemoral vein to the inferior vena cava.

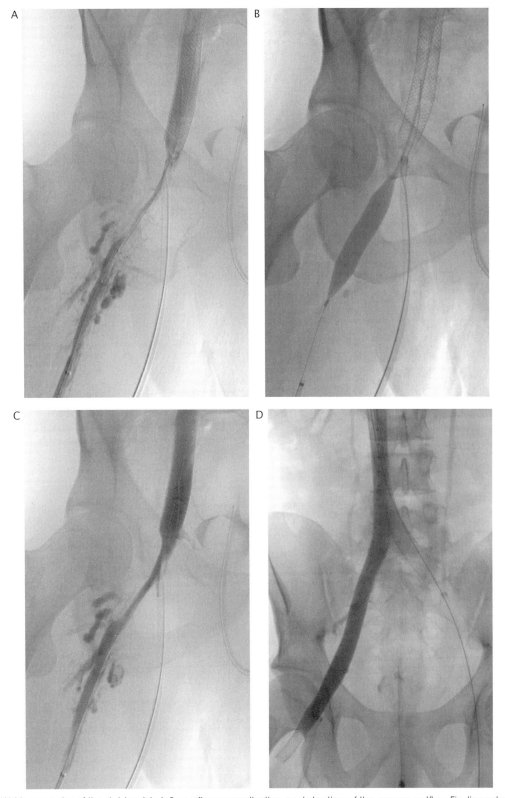

Figure 34.1 (A) Venography of the right pelvic inflow, after recanalization and stenting of the venous outflow. Findings show poor right pelvic inflow disease with surrounding collaterals. (B) Venoplasty of the right pelvic inflow. (C) Post-venoplasty venography of the right pelvic inflow shows some improvement, but significant residual obstruction remains. (D) Final venography of the right pelvic venous system after the stents were extended beyond the inguinal ligament. Venography shows a widely patent pelvic inflow and outflow.

b. Occasional contrast injections will guide the catheter and wire and verify an intravenous path. Redirect the path as needed.

c. Continue work from both the internal jugular vein access and the greater saphenous vein access until a complete through-and-through channel is present.

d. Occasionally, advanced sharp recanalization techniques may be necessary.

3. Confirmation of the venous outflow channel: contrast/CO_2 injection or intravascular ultrasound (IVUS) are employed.

4. Venoplasty of the venous outflow tract: The venous outflow channel is sequentially dilated followed by contrast injections to verify integrity of the venous wall.

a. Maximum dilation: Inferior vena cava (18 mm), common iliac veins (16 mm), and external iliac and common femoral veins (14 mm).

5. Stenting of the venous outflow tract: Stent across the area of the newly recanalized segment (approximately 18–20 mm in the inferior vena cava).

6. Evaluation of the venous inflow:

a. Once the venous outflow is achieved, advance a flush catheter from the transjugular vein access into each thigh for lower extremity venography.

    i. Flow through numerous collaterals indicates venous obstruction.

b. IVUS evaluation of the pelvic and proximal lower extremity venous channels that are not already stented.

    i. IVUS will detect the areas of stenosis requiring venoplasty and stenting.

    ii. IVUS will show confluences of venous collateral pathways, which we prefer not to jail.

7. Establishment of the venous inflow: Perform venoplasty with subsequent stenting from the caudal venous outflow stents to the saphenofemoral junction. Stents may need to be extended into the femoral vein, deep femoral vein, or, rarely, the greater saphenous vein.

a. Only venoplasty below the saphenofemoral junction is performed, unless a critical stenosis, unresponsive to angioplasty, jeopardizes inflow from the femoral or deep femoral vein.

8. Once the venous inflow and outflow recanalization is complete, immediate therapeutic anticoagulation must be initiated without delay to prevent stent thrombosis. We give patients a dose of Lovenox before they leave the angiography suite.

Example
See Figure 34.1.

Reference and Suggested Reading

1. Williams DM. Iliocaval reconstruction in chronic deep vein thrombosis. *Tech Vasc Interv Radiol.* 2014;17(2):109–113.

CHAPTER 35

Management of Acute Iliocaval Thrombosis

Jordan C. Tasse and Bulent Arslan

Brief Description

Acute deep vein thrombosis (DVT) occurs in approximately 300,000 people per year in the United States. Iliocaval thrombosis is most commonly related to the progression of lower extremity DVT. Inferior vena cava (IVC) thrombosis occurs in approximately 4–15% of patients with acute DVT.[1] Vena cava thrombosis is frequently associated with neoplastic disease. Foreign body placement such as IVC filter or a venous catheter is a frequently reported cause of iliocaval thrombosis. External compression due to right common iliac artery mass effect (May–Thurner syndrome), tumor, lymphadenopathy, or aortic aneurysm are also commonly seen. Anticoagulation has been the mainstay of therapy for acute DVT and iliocaval thrombosis for many years. However, anticoagulation typically does not work to clear the burden of thrombosis within the iliac veins and IVC, and therefore associated complications often occur. These complications may include limb pain and swelling, potential limb or life-threatening complications, organ dysfunction such as renal or liver failure, and pulmonary embolism. In recent years, catheter-directed therapies have been instituted to help prevent the complications of acute iliocaval thrombosis.

Applications of the Technique

1. Patients with acute iliocaval thrombosis to treat or prevent secondary complications such as lower extremity edema or pain, limb-threatening occlusion, organ dysfunction, or life-threatening pulmonary embolism.

Challenges of the Procedure

1. Patients will often need to be prone for popliteal vein access if there is thrombus extending below the femoral vein.
2. Bilateral venous access is frequently necessary for bilateral disease.

3. Patients with a contraindication to thrombolytics present a challenging subset of patients.

Potential Pitfalls/Complications

1. Bleeding: Access site, retroperitoneal or cerebral hemorrhage. Contraindications to catheter-directed thrombolytic therapy must be screened prior to procedure start.
2. Pulmonary embolism (PE): We do not place an IVC filter for PE protection in most our iliocaval occlusion cases because thrombus migration is rare. We consider protective IVC filter placement if a patient is hemodynamically unstable, already has pulmonary emboli, or if the clot burden from the iliocaval thrombosis is so large that migration of the thrombus to the lungs would be catastrophic. Most patients undergo overnight catheter-directed thrombolysis in the acute setting and this, in itself, would treat any embolism in the rare event that it did occur.

Steps of the Procedure

1. Determine site of access—femoral, popliteal, tibial, peroneal, or small saphenous vein: Use ultrasound to determine the most peripheral site of thrombus, and access the patent vein just below. Alternatively, the internal jugular vein can be used. Most commonly, access will be in the popliteal vein with the patient in the prone position. Bilateral access is frequently needed. Ultrasound-guided puncture is recommended to help minimize bleeding during potential thrombolysis.
2. Diagnostic venography: Contrast injection should be obtained to determine the extent of occlusion.
3. Traverse occlusion with guidewire: In the acute setting, thrombus is generally soft, and crossing the occlusion should not be difficult. We start with a 5 Fr Berenstein

shape catheter and a 0.035-in. Glidewire (Terumo Medical Corp., Somerset, NJ). After gaining access into the IVC, contrast should be injected to confirm patency of the IVC centrally and to assess the extent of the iliocaval thrombus.

4. Determine course of action:

a. Rheolytic or suction thrombectomy with or without thrombolysis is our preferred treatment course. We bolus the patients with 5000 U of heparin. After traversing the occlusion, we perform rheolytic thrombectomy throughout the occluded segment. In patients who are candidates, we perform overnight thrombolysis for 12–18 hours with 0.5–1 mg/hour of Alteplase while simultaneously infusing subtherapeutic heparin (300–500 U/hour) through the vascular sheath, keeping the partial thromboplastin time less than 60 seconds. Concomitant systemic anticoagulation is not recommended during catheter-directed thrombolysis because this has been shown to increase bleeding risk without

improving outcomes.[2] The infusion catheter should be embedded within the occluded segment with an infusion catheter side hole length that matches the length of thrombus. The patient is then brought back the following day for follow-up venography. In acute occlusion, the clot is frequently completely resolved. If there is near-complete resolution, further rheolytic or suction thrombectomy can be performed.

b. Recently, we have begun performing large-bore thrombectomy with the Angiovac thrombectomy device (Angiodynamics Inc., Latham, NY) in patients unable to receive or resistant to thrombolysis. This requires extracorporeal circulatory support. The preferred route for treatment is via right internal jugular vein access with a 26 Fr sheath. A second access, usually 16 or 18 Fr, is also necessary for reperfusion. The large-bore catheter is inserted into the iliocaval thrombus, and suction is initiated.

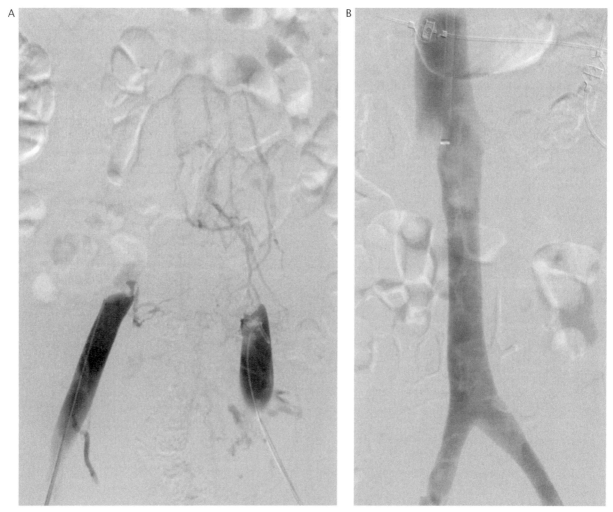

Figure 35.1 (A) A 60-year-old male developed acute onset of severe bilateral lower extremity swelling after being immobile for 7 days following orthopedic surgery. Initial venogram shows complete occlusion of both iliac veins and the IVC. (B) Inferior vena cavagram demonstrates complete resolution of thrombus following rheolytic thrombectomy and catheter-directed thrombolysis.

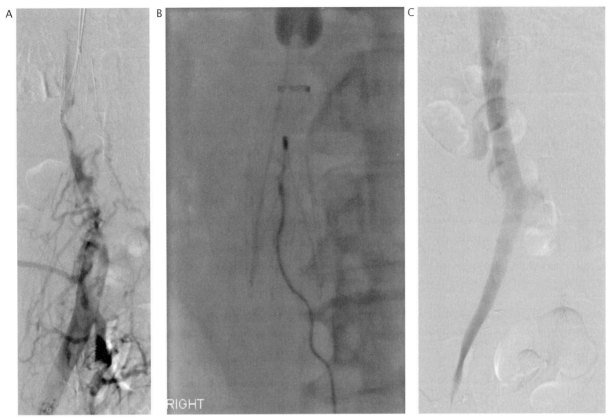

Figure 35.2 (A) A 65-year-old male with metastatic bladder cancer was transferred from an outside hospital to the Interventional Radiology department for treatment of an indwelling vena cava filter and iliocaval thrombus extending up to the filter. (B) Large-bore suction thrombectomy device via internal jugular vein access with mechanical thrombectomy device for clot maceration via femoral access. (C) Widely patent right iliac vein and IVC following suction and mechanical thrombectomy.

Tip: We combine this technique with uni- or bilateral femoral vein access. Through 7 Fr sheaths, the Cleaner mechanical thrombectomy device (Argon Medical Devices Inc., Plano, TX) can be used to macerate thrombus. This has greatly decreased our procedural time in these cases.

5. Fix mechanical culprit, if any: If there is an underlying stenosis, such as the left iliac vein due to external compression, angioplasty with stent placement can be performed.

Example
See Figures 35.1–35.2.

References and Suggested Readings

1. Anderson FA Jr, Wheeler HB, Goldberg RJ, et al. A population-based perspective of the hospital incidence and case-fatality rates of deep vein thrombosis and pulmonary embolism: The Worcester DVT Study. *Arch Intern Med*. 1991;151:933–938.
2. Stein PD, Matta F, Yaekoub AY. Incidence of vena cava thrombosis in the United States. *Am J Cardiol*. 2008;102:927–929.

CHAPTER 36

Management of Chronic Iliocaval Thrombosis

Osmanuddin Ahmed

Brief Description

Chronic deep venous thrombosis (DVT) is defined by thrombus persisting beyond 28 days of initial onset and represents a condition that leads to long-standing venous hypertension, valvular incompetence, and ultimately chronic venous insufficiency and occlusion.[1] As chronic thrombus organizes, it contracts and becomes adherent to the vein wall, causing scarring and consequent atresia of the lumen. The sequelae of such disease are manifested by limb edema, pain, discoloration, exercise intolerance, and ulceration—all encompassed within a clinical spectrum known as post-thrombotic syndrome.[2]

Prior literature has indicated that proximal (defined as iliocaval or iliofemoral) DVT compared to distal DVT poses a greater absolute risk in the overall incidence and severity of post-thrombotic syndrome.[3] For this reason, attempts at recanalization with venoplasty and stenting of chronic inferior vena cava (IVC) and iliac occlusions are performed to restore the main venous outflow of the extremities to reverse or arrest the morbidity associated with this disease.

Applications of the Technique

Endovascular reconstruction of the iliac veins and IVC can be attempted for patients suffering from the lifestyle-limiting morbidity of chronic venous obstruction, which can present clinically as severe post-thrombotic syndrome and/or venous claudication. No duration of chronic iliocaval occlusion should be considered a contraindication for an attempt at revascularization. However, the risks and benefits of intervention should be carefully considered and discussed with asymptomatic patients who experience no significant morbidity from their chronic iliocaval occlusion due to the compensation provided by well-developed collateral veins returning blood to the heart.

Challenges of the Procedure

1. The main challenge in any recanalization attempt for chronic iliocaval thrombosis is crossing the chronically occluded segment.

2. Multiple or bilateral access points are often required to revascularize the IVC and iliac veins.

3. Chronic IVC occlusions may be secondary to pre-existing IVC filters. Retrieval of the filter is often necessary to successfully recanalize the IVC and maintain patency.

4. Initiating appropriate anticoagulation is necessary to ensure long-term patency of stents after revascularization.

Potential Pitfalls/Complications

1. Maintaining an intravascular position during recanalization can be a challenge, particularly with advanced "sharp recanalization" techniques. Advancement of guidewires or catheters into the extravascular space should be promptly recognized and/or confirmed with gentle contrast injection. The probability of technical success is increased when the operator can quickly recognize that the course of his or her instruments no longer follows the path of the occluded vessel.

2. Caution should be given to attempts using sharp recanalization techniques near the left iliac vein confluence due to the presence of the overlying right iliac artery. For similar anatomical reasons, the risk for arterial complication is also increased near the level of the renal vein.

3. Frequent contrast injections in different obliquities may be necessary to fully comprehend the venous anatomy and identify the points of occlusion.

4. Hemorrhagic complications can occur after aggressive venoplasty or extravascular perforations. Typically, balloon tamponade is sufficient to arrest bleeding, but occasionally stents or covered stent grafts may be necessary for treatment.

5. Venoplasty for chronic iliac and IVC occlusion is frequently inadequate to achieve long-term patency. Stenting of the chronically occluded iliac or IVC segments provides the best chance at restoring flow through the vessel and preventing rethrombosis.

6. When stenting the IVC, the inflow of the renal vessels should be clearly identified to avoid coverage of the renal veins.

7. Achieving adequate inflow from the extremities is critical to maintaining patency of the recanalized and stented iliocaval segments. For this reason, stenting into the femoral segments may be necessary to achieve the required inflow to the central veins.

Steps of the Procedure

1. The level of sedation chosen can vary and is often left to individual operator preference. Some experienced individuals choose to utilize moderate sedation because patients often can verbally relay a sensation of pain when the wire or catheter are extravascular. This has the disadvantage of patient discomfort in longer cases. Alternatively, general anesthesia can be used for these procedures because it provides the benefit of patient immobility.

2. The initial step for any iliocaval recanalization procedure is choosing appropriate access sites. The right internal jugular vein access is often utilized for purposes of attempting recanalization from a cephalad approach or, alternatively, to obtain through-and-through access after recanalization from below is achieved. Access from below is typically obtained in the common femoral or proximal femoral vein depending on the extent of venous occlusion. In the instance of bilateral iliac vein occlusion, bilateral femoral vein access is needed. If possible, obtaining a preoperative computed tomography venogram (CTV) is very helpful for decision making in access site planning.

3. Once access is obtained, venography is performed to identify the points of occlusion both distally and proximally. Although many venous collaterals opacify with contrast injection, the object of interest is the main occluded vessel, which often forms a thread-like or nipple appearance. Initial attempts at recanalization of this target can be performed using a 5 Fr end-hole catheter (KMP, Berenstein, VERT, etc.) and angled or straight Glidewire (Terumo Medical Corp., Somerset, NJ). A sheath is necessary to provide support for the guidewire and catheter and to prevent buckling.

4. If the occlusion cannot be crossed with a hydrophilic guidewire and catheter combination, more advanced techniques can be attempted at the discretion and comfort level of the operator. Such techniques may include using the back end of the wire, weighted wires such as the Astato 30 (Asahi Intecc USA Inc., Santa Ana, CA) or Approach (Cook Medical Inc., Bloomington, IN), or a sharp recanalization approach by placing a 21 or 22 gauge Chiba needle through a metal or stiff sheath. Additional techniques include the use of crossing devices such as the TruePath (Boston Scientific Inc., Marlborough, MA) and Ocelot (Avinger Inc., Redwood City, CA) systems, as well as the radiofrequency wire.

5. Once the occlusion is crossed, the wire can be snared and pulled through from an access on the opposite end to obtain through-and-through access. Over the wire, the occlusion can be serially venoplastied to allow upsizing of the system to a 0.035-in. wire. Intermittent venograms should be performed to confirm that the recanalization was intraluminal and to assess vessel patency and size. After venoplasty of the IVC and iliac veins up to 14 mm, we routinely perform stenting of the veins that demonstrate residual stenosis or scarring. The IVC is sized fluoroscopically by assessing the diameter of a nondiseased segment and often stented using either Wallstents (Boston Scientific Inc., Marlborough, MA) up to 24 mm in size or alternatively a stent graft. For iliac segments, we routinely prefer to place 14-mm self-expanding nitinol stents for the common iliac vein and extend to the level of the diseased segments in the external iliac and common femoral veins with 12- or 10-mm self-expanding nitinol stents. Occasionally, 16-mm Wallstents can also be used for the common iliac vein in patients with larger caliber vessels. Although not performed commonly at our institution, intravascular ultrasound has also been proposed as a mechanism for sizing stents and choosing the segments that require coverage. Upon completion, a final venogram is performed from the bilateral femoral veins to ensure brisk inflow and appropriate stent sizing.

6. In situations of chronic iliocaval occlusions secondary to an implanted IVC filter, filter retrieval is routinely attempted to prevent the filter serving as a nidus for recurrent thrombosis. In situations in which filter retrieval is not feasible, the filter can be crushed against the IVC wall with a stent graft.

7. Anticoagulation is initiated periprocedurally once the occlusion is crossed using unfractionated heparin at 50 U/kg. The patient is maintained at an activated clotting time >200 seconds with transition to 1 mg/kg BID low-molecular-weight heparin dosing at the conclusion of the procedure. Long-term anticoagulation should be initiated in coordination with a hematologist and based on the extent of venous segments that required stenting and any underlying thrombophilia. In general, completely stented iliocaval segments should be managed with life-long anticoagulation with or without an antiplatelet agent; however, withdrawal of anticoagulation can be made after close coordination with the patient's hematologist after at least 2 years.

Example

Figure 36.1 are from a 40-year-old female patient with antiphospholipid syndrome who presented with chronic limb swelling and pain.

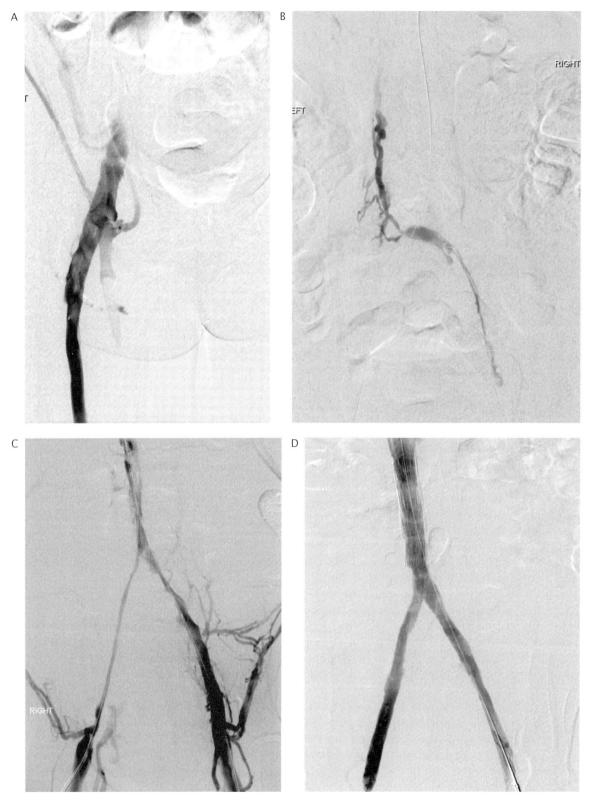

Figure 36.1 (A) Initial venogram from the left femoral vein demonstrates tapering and chronic occlusion at the level of the left external iliac vein. Collateral veins peripheral to the level of the tapered occlusion are seen opacifying with contrast. (B) Venogram from the right common iliac vein demonstrates the chronic occlusion involving the right common and external iliac segments. No contrast is seen opacifying the IVC with drainage via an ascending lumbar vein. The occlusion on the left has already been crossed with a guidewire. (C) Repeat venogram from the bilateral femoral access sites after venoplasty with an 8-mm high-pressure balloon demonstrates chronic narrowing and near-complete occlusion of the IVC and right greater than left iliac veins. (D) Post IVC 26-mm stent graft placement in the IVC with bilateral 12-mm common iliac vein self-expanding nitinol stents placed in a "kissing" fashion. The right external iliac vein was also stented with a 12-mm self-expanding nitinol stent.

References and Suggested Readings

1. Franzeck UK, Schalch I, Jäger KA, et al. Prospective 12-year follow-up study of clinical and hemodynamic sequelae of deep venous thromboses in patients with low risk (Zurich study). *Wien Med Wochenschr*. 1999;149(2-4):78–84.

2. Labropoulos N, Jen J, Jen H, et al. Recurrent deep vein thrombosis: Long-term incidence and natural history. *Ann Surg*. 2010;251(4):749–753.

3. Kahn SR, Shrier I, Julian JA, et al. Determinants and time course of the postthrombotic syndrome after acute deep venous thrombosis. *Ann Intern Med*. 2008;149(10):698–707.

CHAPTER 37

Directional AngioJet Thrombectomy with Guide Catheter Helical Spin Technique

S. Lowell Kahn

Brief Description

The presence of thrombus in the central veins (iliac and inferior vena cava [IVC]) is associated with a substantially higher risk of development post-thrombotic syndrome (PTS).[1] The morbidity of PTS is considerable; therefore, removal of acute deep venous thrombus (DVT) in this segment is recommended by current guidelines.[2]

The AngioJet (Boston Scientific Inc., Marlborough, MA) Solent Proxi (90 cm) and Omni (120 cm) catheters are commonly used peripheral thrombectomy devices indicated for acute arterial and venous thrombus removal. Both catheters are 6 Fr sheath/8 Fr guide catheter compatible, and both offer the Power Pulse feature, allowing the direct infusion of tissue plasminogen activator into the thrombus. The catheters are indicated for use in vessels greater than 3 mm, with an optimal vessel range between 6 and 20 mm.[3] Their use in the removal of iliac vein and IVC thrombus is frequent.

Although the system is purported to provide effective thrombectomy capabilities in larger vessels; incomplete thrombus removal is common with larger vessels.[4] Incomplete thrombus removal is not surprising given that the average adult IVC measures 20 mm with a range of 13 to 30 mm.[5] The common iliac vein is similarly variable in size, with an average diameter of 11.5 mm.[6] The presence of residual thrombus after use of the AngioJet system likely reflects inadequate contact between the thrombus and the catheter.

Newer devices, such as the AngioVac (Angiodynamics Inc., Latham, NY), are designed to remove thrombus from large-diameter vessels, including the pulmonary arterial vasculature. However, the device is costly, requires a 22 Fr sheath, and requires extracorporeal bypass. Similarly, the new Zelante catheter (Boston Scientific Inc., Marlborough, MA) is the largest AngioJet catheter and designed for large vessel DVT extraction, but it requires a larger access and it is expensive, limiting its availability.

This chapter proposes a simple modification in the standard use of the AngioJet Solent Proxi and Omni catheters. Briefly, the catheters are placed within an 8 Fr guide catheter with the tip of the Proxi or Omni catheter extending 1 or 2 cm beyond the tip of the guide catheter. The guide catheter and thrombectomy catheter are advanced beyond the thrombus. The wire is retracted to allow deflection of the guide catheter. The guide catheter and thrombectomy catheter are then slowly retracted with a "spinning" motion through the entirety of the thrombus. This method allows thrombectomy in a helical (rather than straight) pattern, thereby significantly enhancing the contact between the catheter and the thrombus. The employment of this technique has been described by others,[7] and its use substantially decreases the required time for AngioJet thrombectomy.

Applications of the Technique

1. Thrombectomy of peripheral and central veins. At our institution, this method is used only in larger (>10 mm) central veins because the standard over-the-wire technique is typically effective for smaller veins.
2. Arteriovenous fistula and graft thrombectomy, particularly at sites of aneurysmal dilatation.
3. Pulmonary thrombectomy: Note that use of the AngioJet in the setting of pulmonary embolism is associated with major complications, including death. Use in this territory should be executed within the operator's scope of practice and with extreme caution.

Challenges of the Procedure

1. The guide catheter is trimmed and the hub removed so that the Proxi or Omni catheter is slightly longer (i.e., 1 or 2 cm) than the guide catheter. It is desirable to secure the guide catheter to the thrombectomy catheter to ensure that the thrombectomy catheter consistently extends just beyond the guide catheter.

This is typically done with Steri-Strips (3M Co., St. Paul, MN) and/or a thin layer of Dermabond (Ethicon Inc., Somerville, NJ). Frequently, despite these measures, fluid runs between the thrombectomy catheter and guide catheter, which loosens the Steri-Strips. Therefore, we routinely hold and spin both catheters in one hand to retain their relationship and spin the guide catheter shaft with the other hand as they are withdrawn. The assistant maintains the sheath position.

2. Although we attempt to perform complete thrombectomy in a single setting, the amount of thrombus in iliocaval cases is considerable, and limitations on the amount of AngioJet use must be respected to prevent serious complications, including renal failure.[7] Separating the case with overnight catheter-directed thrombolysis may be prudent.

3. Wire access must be given up for this procedure to work well. In our experience, even with a floppy (e.g., Bentson) guidewire, there is inadequate deflection of the guide catheter if the wire is kept in place. Therefore, after traversing the thrombus, the guidewire is withdrawn to the midportion of the guide catheter. In our experience, traversing acute thrombus is typically not difficult and therefore sacrificing wire access is acceptable practice. However, if traversal is difficult, we would not advise this technique or would advise placing a soft 0.014-in. wire to spin the catheters over. After thrombectomy, the soft wire could be exchanged for a stronger 0.035-in. support wire.

Potential Pitfalls/Complications

1. Securing the AngioJet catheter to the guide catheter is more difficult than expected. The AngioJet catheter can easily slip inside of the guide catheter, obviously preventing effective thrombectomy.

2. Loss of wire access is intentional and is an acceptable risk in most cases. However, this technique should not be considered if obtaining wire access across the thrombus was difficult. As mentioned previously, a compromise (not as effective as fully pulling the wire back) is to use this technique while spinning the guide catheter/thrombectomy catheter combination over a soft 0.014-in. wire.

3. Standard risks of thrombolysis (e.g., hemorrhage) and mechanical thrombectomy (bradycardia/arrhythmia, hemoglobinuria, renal failure, etc.) exist for this technique.

Steps of the Procedure

1. Ultrasound-guided catheterization of the venous system is obtained proximal to the thrombus,

commonly within the posterior tibial, popliteal, or common femoral vein.

2. Using the Seldinger technique, an 8 Fr sheath is placed.

3. Through the sheath, the occluded segment is traversed with standard catheter and wire technique.

4. An Amplatz guidewire (Boston Scientific Inc., Marlborough, MA) is placed distal to the occlusion.

5. An 8 Fr guide catheter is selected. At the author's institution, the Launcher series of guide catheters (Medtronic Inc., Minneapolis, MN) is typically employed. These catheters are 90 cm in length. We trim the catheter so that it is slightly (e.g., 1 or 2 cm) shorter than the chosen AngioJet thrombectomy catheter. The AngioJet catheters are quite rigid and therefore will straighten the guide catheter considerably. Considering this, we choose a guide catheter with sharp angulation (e.g., the JL family of catheters) to maximize deflection of the AngioJet catheter.

6. The selected guide catheter is advanced over the AngioJet catheter with the distal 1 or 2 cm of the AngioJet catheter extending beyond the end of the guide catheter.

7. The AngioJet catheter is secured to the guide catheter using Steri-Strips and/or Dermabond.

8. The thrombectomy catheter and guide catheter are advanced as a unit through the sheath and beyond the distal end of the thrombus.

9. The wire is retracted to the midportion of the guide catheter.

10. The thrombectomy mode (or Power Pulse mode if desired first) is activated. While active, the guide catheter and thrombectomy catheter are slowly withdrawn and spun as a unit. This is optimally performed with two hands—one hand securing the hub of the AngioJet catheter and guide catheter and the other grasping the midportion of the guide catheter shaft. The assistant should ensure that the sheath does not move.

11. Venography is performed after completely withdrawing the catheters through the thrombotic occlusion. If significant thrombus remains, steps 3–10 are repeated within the time parameters outlined in the AngioJet instructions for use.

12. When thrombectomy is complete, the involved segment is again traversed with standard catheter and wire technique.

13. Additional maneuvers, including balloon maceration/sweeping, angioplasty, and stenting, are performed at the operator's discretion.

Example
See Figures 37.1 and 37.2.

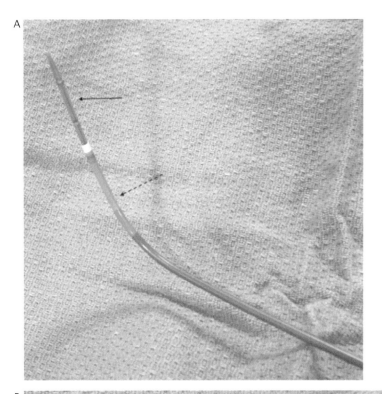

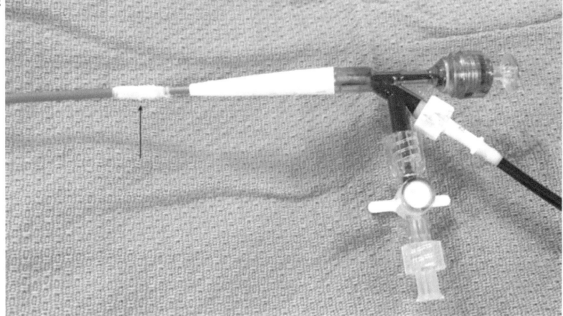

Figure 37.1 Configuration of the guide catheter and AngioJet catheter. (A) An image of the tip reveals the AngioJet Solent catheter (solid arrow) extending minimally beyond the tip of the 8-Fr guide catheter (dashed arrow). (B) Image taken of the proximal end shows that the 8-Fr guide catheter has been cut. It is secured to the AngioJet Solent catheter with Steri-Strips (arrow).

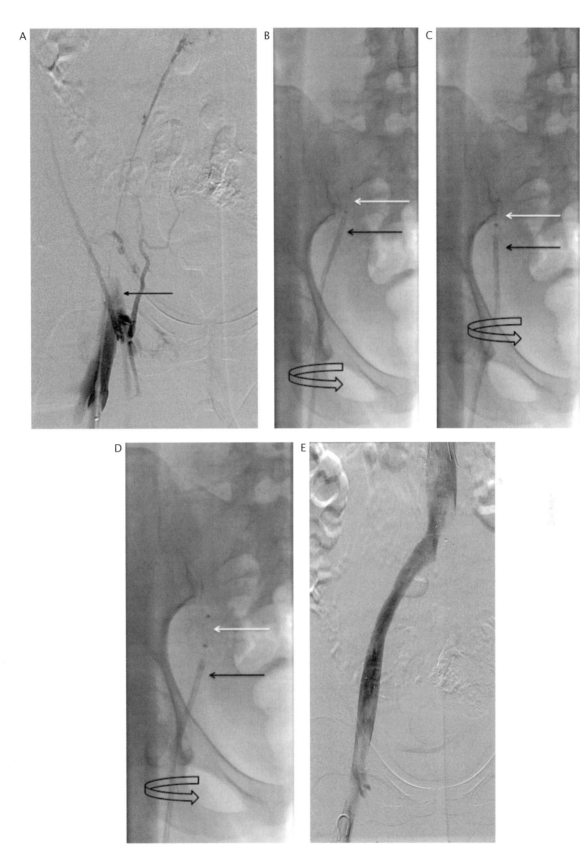

Figure 37.2 A 27-year-old female with left leg pain and swelling. Acute DVT was demonstrated by ultrasound (not shown). (A) Left leg venography with the patient in the prone position reveals abrupt occlusion of the common femoral (arrow) and iliac veins with filling of collateral pelvic veins. Wire access across the occlusion and into the IVC is obtained (not shown). (B–D) Over the wire, an AngioJet Solent Omni catheter (white arrow) was advanced within an MB2 guide catheter (black arrow) into the IVC. The guide catheter and AngioJet are spun and withdrawn slowly as a unit during thrombectomy, providing optimal contact with the thrombus circumferentially. Wire access to the IVC was then regained. (E) Final venography after additional angioplasty and stenting with a 14-mm Luminexx stent (C.R. Bard Inc., Murray Hill, NJ) shows wide patency of the previously occluded veins.

References and Suggested Readings

1. Tick LW, Kramer MH, Rosendaal FR, Faber WR, Doggen CJ. Risk factors for post-thrombotic syndrome in patients with a first deep venous thrombosis. *J Thromb Haemost.* 2008;6:2075–2081.

2. Meissner MH1, Gloviczki P, Comerota AJ, et al.; Society for Vascular Surgery. American venous forum. *J Vasc Surg.* 2012;55(5):1449–1462.

3. http://www.bostonscientific.com/en-US/products/thrombectomy-systems/angiojet-thrombectomy-system.html

4. Sildiroglu O, Ozer H, Turba UC. Management of the thrombosed filter-bearing inferior vena cava. *Semin Intervent Radiol.* 2012; 29(1):57–63.

5. Prince MR, Novelline RA, Athanasoulis CA, Simon M. The diameter of the inferior vena cava and its implications for the use of vena caval filters. *Radiology.* 1883;149(3):687–689.

6. Amin VB, Siegelbaum RH, Fischman AM, Lookstein, RA. Interventional management of DVT: Top 10 technical tips. Approaches, techniques, and preprocedure considerations for successful interventional management of DVT. *Endovascular Today* July 2013, pp. 48–55.

7. Arslan BA, Turba UC, Matsumoto AH. Acute renal failure associated with percutaneous mechanical thrombectomy for iliocaval venous thrombosis. *Semin Intervent Radiol.* 2007; 24(3):288–295.

CHAPTER 38

Dual and Balloon-Assisted AngioJet Thrombectomy for Iliofemoral Deep Venous Thrombosis

Zubin Irani and Sara Zhao

Brief Description

Lower extremity deep venous thrombosis (DVT) may be complicated by pulmonary embolism, post-thrombotic syndrome, and phlegmasia cerulea dolens. Due to these complications, the American Venous Forum now recommends thrombus removal for large or symptomatic thrombus burden.[1] The AngioJet Solent Proxy and Omni thrombectomy sets (Boston Scientific Inc., Marlborough, MA) are indicated for use in iliofemoral and lower extremity veins with a diameter ≥3 mm.[2] The device has quickly become a preferred device among the available mechanical thrombectomy options.

The AngioJet system has been demonstrated as both efficacious and safe as a method of thrombectomy in lower extremity DVT.[3-7] Complete removal of thrombus has been reported in 65–75% of patients and partial removal in another 25–35% of patients.[4,6] Immediate (defined as <24 hours) improvement in symptoms has been demonstrated in 72–81% of patients.[4,6] In addition, the use of the AngioJet pharmacomechanical thrombectomy device has been shown to decrease the time of overall treatment, which includes both time in the interventional suite and time in the intensive care unit (ICU) and overall hospital stay.[3-6] Lin et al.[6] reported a reduction of time in the ICU and in overall hospital stay by at least 50% in patients who underwent thrombectomy using the AngioJet compared to catheter-directed thrombolysis (0.6 vs. 4.6 days in the ICU and 2.4 vs. 8.4 days in the hospital, respectively). Finally, Garcia et al.[5] found excellent long-term patency rates of 94%, 87%, and 83% at 3, 6, and 12 months, respectively.

Although it may reduce health care costs and the potential complications of prolonged hospital stay, mechanical thrombectomy has the potential to lengthen both patient and operator radiation exposure, particularly in larger caliber veins, in which several passes may be required for the catheter to clear the entire width of the thrombus. This chapter presents two techniques for wider coverage of thrombus in the iliofemoral veins and more rapid clearance of thrombus. One technique utilizes two AngioJet devices used in parallel. This technique is achieved by gaining access in both popliteal veins and running one device from the contralateral lower extremity up and over the bifurcation into the thrombus burden. The second technique uses an inflated angioplasty balloon to guide thrombus toward the AngioJet device.

Applications of the Technique

1. Iliofemoral venous thrombectomy in the attempt to avoid post-thrombotic syndrome: The balloon-assisted technique has been successfully utilized in patients with occlusive thrombus as extensive as the involvement of the venous system from an infrarenal inferior vena cava (IVC) filter to both popliteal veins.
2. Iliofemoral venous thrombectomy in patients at increased risk for hemorrhage with the use of tissue plasminogen activator (tPA), such as in the immediate postsurgical period.

Challenges of the Procedure

1. Use of two AngioJet devices requires the use of two Ultra Thrombectomy System consoles. This may require coordination with other clinicians or, occasionally, the company to ensure that two consoles are available for use. A balloon-assisted technique can be employed when two consoles are not available.
2. Access up and over the bifurcation with a wire: The wire from the contralateral access must be snared to be guided into the ipsilateral limb. This is best accomplished in a segment of vein that is thrombus free and may occasionally need to be done in the suprarenal IVC.
3. Navigation through the ipsilateral thrombosed vein from the popliteal vein: A prerequisite for this technique, particularly in gaining up-and-over access from the contralateral limb.
4. Sheath selection must be proper: 6 Fr for the contralateral limb, to accommodate the AngioJet catheter,

and 8 Fr for the ipsilateral limb (to also accommodate the contralateral wire guide).

5. Mechanical thrombectomy carries a risk of macerated clot embolization to the lungs. Therefore, an IVC filter should be considered prior to carrying out thrombectomy. In at least one case, an embolus was successfully removed using the balloon-assisted AngioJet thrombectomy technique in the region of the IVC filter. This technique utilized bilateral popliteal access, with an inflated angioplasty balloon to guide clot toward the AngioJet tip. This procedure was performed in a patient with recent intracranial surgery; thrombectomy was performed due to concern for bleeding with the use of excessive tPA.

Potential Pitfalls/Complications

1. Standard risks related to the use of AngioJet apply to this technique (proximal embolization including cerebrovascular accident [in the setting of a patent foramen ovale], bleeding, hemolysis, and vessel wall or valve damage).

2. The second, contralateral puncture always introduces risks of bleeding, vessel damage, and thrombosis related to puncture site.

3. As with AngioJet systems in general, there is a risk of acute renal failure. This can be mitigated by being mindful of the duration of use.

4. The balloon-assisted technique typically requires a percutaneous transluminal angioplasty balloon 6–8 mm in diameter and upwards of 10 cm in length. This size may not be available. A shorter length balloon can be utilized, although it may require frequent repositioning.

Steps of the Procedure

Dual AngioJet Thrombectomy

1. Ultrasound is utilized to access the right internal jugular vein.

2. A 5 Fr pigtail catheter is advanced to the distal IVC and venogram performed.

3. The catheter is exchanged for an IVC filter sheath, and an IVC filter is placed for prevention of a large pulmonary embolism during mechanical thrombectomy.

4. A short 10 Fr sheath is left in place in the right jugular access site.

5. The patient is then moved to the prone position.

6. The popliteal fossae are prepped, and the popliteal vein ipsilateral to known DVT is accessed.

7. A 4 Fr catheter is advanced to a level distal/inferior to the known DVT, and venogram is performed.

8. An 8 Fr, 10-cm-long sheath is placed into the ipsilateral vein, and 10 mg tPA is administered.

9. The contralateral popliteal vein is then accessed, and via a 6 Fr sheath, a guidewire is advanced to the IVC.

10. A snare is advanced through the venous system ipsilateral to the DVT and is used to pull the guidewire from the IVC out through the sheath in the popliteal vein ipsilateral to the DVT, such that the guidewire is now through-and-through from one popliteal vein to the other.

11. One AngioJet device is advanced over the wire from the popliteal fossa contralateral to the DVT to the level of the DVT.

12. A second guidewire is introduced into the popliteal vein sheath ipsilateral to the DVT and advanced to the IVC.

13. A second AngioJet device is advanced over this wire until it is parallel to the first AngioJet device. With the help of an assistant, both are used in tandem for wider coverage of venous caliber.

Balloon-Assisted AngioJet Thrombectomy

1. Ultrasound is utilized to access the right internal jugular vein.

2. A 5 Fr pigtail catheter is advanced to the IVC and venogram performed.

3. The catheter is exchanged for an IVC filter sheath, and an IVC filter is placed for prevention of a large pulmonary embolism during mechanical thrombectomy.

4. A short 10 Fr sheath is left in place in the right jugular access site.

5. The patient is then moved to the prone position.

6. The popliteal fossae are prepped, and the popliteal vein ipsilateral to known DVT is accessed.

7. A diagnostic catheter is advanced to a level distal/inferior to the known DVT, and venogram is performed.

8. An 8 Fr, 10-cm-long sheath is placed into the ipsilateral vein and 10 mg tPA administered.

9. The contralateral popliteal vein is then accessed, and via a 6 Fr sheath, a guidewire is advanced to the IVC, over the bifurcation and beyond the level of thrombosis.

10. An AngioJet device is advanced to the level of thrombosis over the wire from the popliteal fossa ipsilateral to the DVT.

11. A 10-mm angioplasty balloon is advanced from the contralateral popliteal fossa to the level of thrombosis and inflated.

12. The AngioJet device is used adjacent to the inflated balloon for mechanical thrombectomy.

Examples

For an example of dual AngioJet thrombectomy, see Figure 38.1.

For an example of balloon-assisted AngioJet thrombectomy, see Figure 38.2.

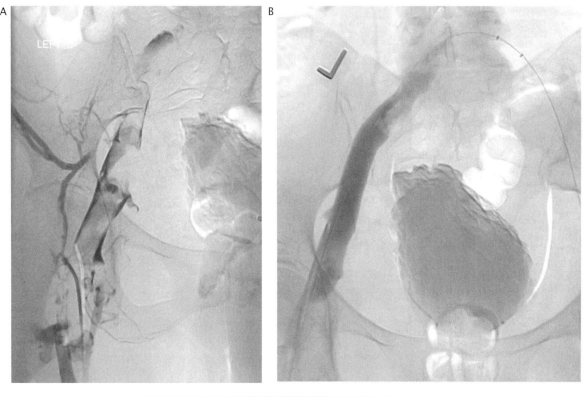

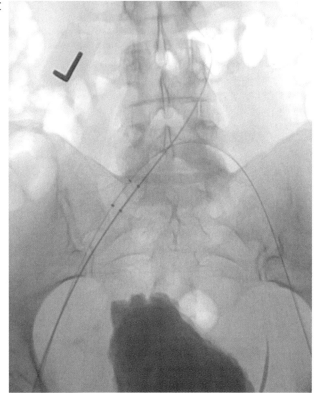

Figure 38.1 (A) A 60-year-old female with a history of acute DVT extending to the level of the left common femoral vein with severe pain and cramping, which limit the patient's mobility. After placement of an IVC filter and access obtained via both popliteal veins, the patient was turned to the prone position and venogram performed in the left lower extremity. This image demonstrates a lengthy region of non-occlusive thrombus in the left common femoral and external iliac veins. (B) One AngioJet device was advanced from the contralateral popliteal vein up and over the IVC bifurcation. (C) Dual AngioJet technique. This image demonstrates the two AngioJet devices in parallel. Underlying severe stenosis of the left common iliac vein was treated with stent placement. Follow-up venogram obtained during IVC filter removal 2 months later demonstrated no new thrombosis in the left lower extremity.

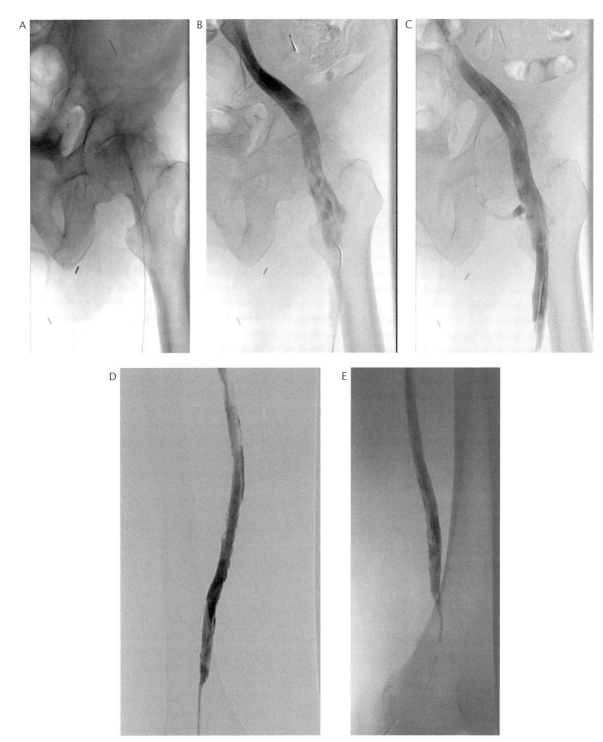

Figure 38.2 (A) A 62-year-old male with a history of malignancy presented with right lower extremity pain and swelling. Ultrasound was positive for DVT. After overnight tPA infusion, residual thrombus was demonstrated throughout the right femoral vein. This figure shows the balloon-assisted technique, in which an inflated angioplasty balloon is placed in parallel with the AngioJet device via access from the contralateral popliteal vein. (B) Upper femoral vein; before and (C) after balloon-assisted thrombectomy using the AngioJet device. (D) Lower femoral vein; before and (E) after balloon-assisted thrombectomy using the AngioJet device.

References and Suggested Readings

1. Gloviczki P. *Handbook of Venous Disorders: Guidelines of the American Venous Forum.* 3rd ed. London: Arnold; 2009.

2. http://www.bostonscientific.com/en-US/products/thrombectomy-systems/angiojet-thrombectomy-system.html

3. Arko FR, Davis CM 3rd, Murphy EH, et al. Aggressive percutaneous mechanical thrombectomy of deep venous thrombosis: Early clinical results. *Arch Surg.* 2007;142(6):513–518.

4. Bush RL, Lin PH, Bates JT, Mureebe L, Zhou W, Lumsden AB. Pharmacomechanical thrombectomy for treatment of symptomatic lower extremity deep venous thrombosis: Safety and feasibility study. *J Vasc Surg.* 2004;40(5):965–970.

5. Garcia MJ, Lookstein R, Malhotra R, et al. Endovascular management of deep vein thrombosis with rheolytic thrombectomy: Final report of the prospective multicenter PEARL (Peripheral Use of AngioJet Rheolytic Thrombectomy with a Variety of Catheter Lengths) registry. *J Vasc Interv Radiol.* 2015;26(6):777–785.

6. Lin PH, Zhou W, Dardik A, et al. Catheter-direct thrombolysis versus pharmacomechanical thrombectomy for treatment of lower extremity deep venous thrombosis. *Am J Surg.* 2006;192(6):782–788.

7. Rao S, Konig G, Leers SA, et al. Pharmacomechanical thrombectomy for iliofemoral deep vein thrombosis: An alternative to contraindications to thrombolysis. *J Vasc Surg.* 2009;50(5):1092–1098.

CHAPTER 39

Tips and Tricks of the AngioVac Device

David C. Stevens and Sabah Butty

Brief Description

The AngioVac system (AngioDynamics Inc., Latham, NY), which consists of a 22 Fr suction cannula, bypass circuit, bubble trap/filter, and an 18 Fr reinfusion cannula, allows for the percutaneous removal of unwanted vascular debris, such as venous thrombus and cardiac vegetations. The suction cannula has two novel features that contribute to its efficacy: (1) the coil-reinforced construction that endows the cannula with sufficient structural rigidity to transmit significant external suction without collapsing and (2) the balloon actuated tip that expands to 48 Fr when inflated. When external suction is applied via a centrifugal bypass pump, debris is funneled into the cannula and trapped in the bubble trap/filter. The blood is then returned through an 18 Fr venous reinfusion cannula. The AngioVac system is a versatile tool for removing thrombus and other unwanted debris from the central venous system and the right heart.

Applications of the Technique

1. Proximal venous thrombus: We have found the AngioVac to be a safe and extremely effective device for removing proximal thrombus in the inferior vena cava (IVC) and iliac veins.[1]
2. Right heart debris: Unwanted material in the right heart can include mobile thrombus (which carries a very high mortality rate), fibrin sheaths, and septic vegetations.[1] All have been successfully removed using the AngioVac device.[2-6] Possible complications specific to the right heart include valvular damage, arrhythmia, perforation, and/or cardiac tamponade. Due to the complex anatomy of the right heart and the potentially life-threatening nature of complications, we recommend monitoring all right heart thrombectomies with a transesophageal echocardiogram. In addition, it is wise to communicate with cardiothoracic surgery prior to initiating the procedure, in case emergent surgical intervention is required. Despite these risks, we find that the AngioVac device is well suited for removal of right heart debris.
3. Pulmonary artery thrombus: Although successful pulmonary artery thrombectomies have been reported using the AngioVac device, its rigid nature and limited maneuverability make it difficult to direct into the pulmonary artery.[7,8] For this reason, in addition to the fact that there are reasonable alternatives, such as catheter-directed thrombolysis, our use of the device in this area is limited.

Challenges of the Procedure

1. Maintaining flow through the cannula: Hemofiltration and clot removal depend on flow through the system. If the distal end of the suction cannula is completely occluded, adequate suction cannot be generated, and the system will not function. Thus, the pump should be initiated in a location free of thrombus. The target material is then drawn toward the cannula, or the cannula is advanced slowly to the material. Large thrombi are approached with a "to and fro" motion, allowing for small pieces to be removed while maintaining adequate flow through the circuit. Occasionally, the circuit may become occluded. Quickly altering the circuit's flow by clamping and unclamping the bypass tubing (not the suction cannula) often dislodges the offending clot. To augment insufficient flow, blood or saline can be infused through a catheter placed distal to the suction cannula.
2. Large and resistant thrombus: In suitable patients, the pre-application of recombinant tissue plasminogen activator and use of the AngioJet device (Boston Scientific Inc., Marlborough, MA) in power pulse mode can significantly reduce procedural time and improve results. Alternative adjunctive therapies, such as balloon maceration, balloon mobilization, and percutaneous thrombectomy using the Trerotola device (Teleflex Medical Europe Ltd., Westmeath, Ireland), can be considered.
3. Indwelling IVC filters: Proximal venous thrombus can occur in conjunction with IVC filters, and the approach varies depending on clot location and filter dwell time. When possible, the filter is removed via standard technique to avoid inadvertent displacement or removal of the filter with the suction cannula. When the filter cannot be removed and is sufficiently established in the vein, the cannula can

usually be advanced through the filter. Smith and colleagues[9] reported a technique called "pulling the cannula" to help maneuver through obstacles such as vena cava filters. This technique involves cannulating the suction catheter with an angioplasty balloon, inflating the balloon, and using it to pull the suction catheter through the offending obstacle. This technique requires opposing access sites, such as an internal jugular vein and femoral vein.

Potential Pitfalls/Complications

1. Usage on Iliocaval Thrombus:
   a. Pulmonary emboli
   b. Venous perforation
   c. Displacement of IVC filters
   d. Inability to establish adequate flow
2. Usage on Pulmonary Artery and Right Heart Thrombus:
   a. Valvular damage
   b. Arrhythmia
   c. Venous perforation, hemopericardium, and cardiac tamponade

Steps of the Procedure

1. Obtain venous access via surgical cut down or percutaneously using a modified Seldinger technique. We regularly obtain three percutaneous venous access sites: one each for a suction cannula, reinfusion cannula, and a diagnostic catheter. Femoral and internal jugular veins are the most common access sites, but specific site selection depends on the location of the target material and the patient's anatomy. To facilitate hemostasis after removal, a purse-string suture is placed around the suction and reinfusion cannulas.
2. Dilate the selected vein and place a 26-Fr Gore DrySeal sheath (W.L. Gore & Associates Inc., Flagstaff, AZ).
3. Advance the suction cannula and internal stiffener through the 26-Fr sheath over a stiff wire.
4. Prime and de-air the veno-venous bypass system, ideally with the assistance of a trained perfusionist.
5. Anticoagulate the patient with intravenous heparin or bivalirudin to an activated clotting time >300 seconds.
6. Inflate the tip of the suction cannula and initiate bypass.
7. Advance the cannula through the thrombus or toward the vegetation. When removing cardiac vegetations, continuous monitoring with a transesophageal echocardiogram aids in safety and efficacy.

Example

See Figures 39.1–39.4.

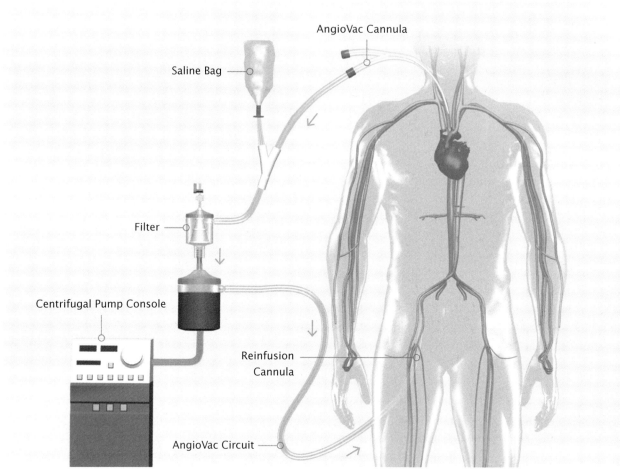

Figure 39.1 Schematic of the AngioVac system.

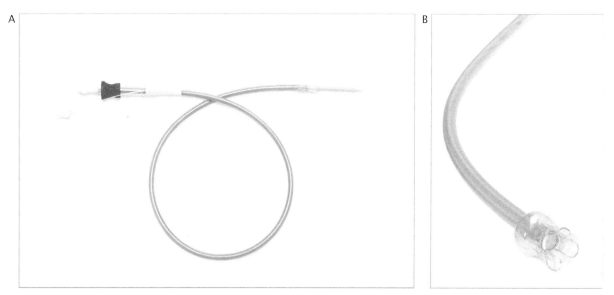

Figure 39.2 Photographs of the AngioVac suction cannula with deflated (A) and inflated (B) tip.

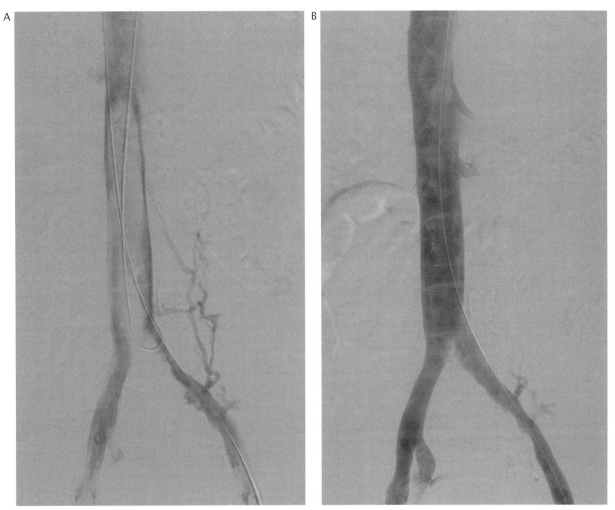

Figure 39.3 Angiographic images of the IVC. (A) Large filling defect of the inferior vena cava consistent with large-volume thrombus. (B) Post AngioVac thrombectomy demonstrates complete thrombus removal.

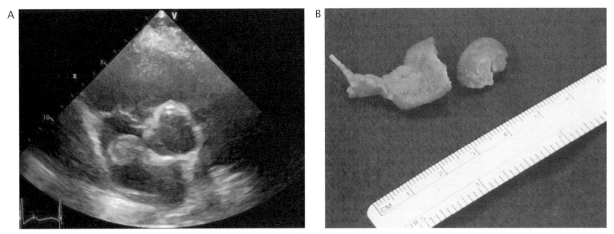

Figure 39.4 (A) Transthoracic echocardiogram demonstrating a lesion tethered to the tricuspid valve. (B) Photograph of tricuspid vegetation extracted using the AngioVac device.

References and Suggested Readings

1. Stevens DC, Garbett D, Casciani T, Butty S. Percutaneous thrombectomy with the AngioVac aspiration device: A single center-experience. *J Vasc Intervent Radiol.* 2015;26(1):150.

2. Al-Hakim R, Patel K, Moriarty JM. AngioVac aspiration for paradoxical emboli protection through a fenestrated Fontan during central venous thrombus manipulation. *Cardiovasc Intervent Radiol.* 2015;38(3):752–754.

3. Divekar AA, Scholz T, Fernandez JD. Novel percutaneous transcatheter intervention for refractory active endocarditis as a bridge to surgery—AngioVac aspiration system. *Catheter Cardiovasc Interv.* 2013;81(6):1008–1012.

4. Dudiy Y, Kronzon I, Cohen HA, Ruiz CE. Vacuum thrombectomy of large right atrial thrombus. *Catheter Cardiovasc Interv.* 2012;79(2):344–347.

5. Patel N, Azemi T, Zaeem F, et al. Vacuum assisted vegetation extraction for the management of large lead vegetations. *J Cardiac Surg.* 2013;28(3):321–324.

6. Todoran TM, Sobieszczyk PS, Levy MS, et al. Percutaneous extraction of right atrial mass using the AngioVac aspiration system. *J Vasc Interv Radiol.* 2011;22(9):1345–1347.

7. Donaldson CW, Baker JN, Narayan RL, et al. Thrombectomy using suction filtration and veno-venous bypass: Single center experience with a novel device. *Catheter Cardiovasc Interv.* 2015;86(2):E81–E87.

8. Pasha AK, Elder MD, Khurram D, Snyder BA, Movahed MR. Successful management of acute massive pulmonary embolism using AngioVac suction catheter technique in a hemodynamically unstable patient. *Cardiovasc Revasc Med.* 2014;15(4):240–243.

9. Smith SJ, Behrens G, Sewall LE, Sichlau MJ. Vacuum-assisted thrombectomy device (AngioVac) in the management of symptomatic iliocaval thrombosis. *J Vasc Interv. Radiol.* 2014;25(3):425–430.

CHAPTER 40

Optimal Technique for Catheterizing the Pulmonary Arteries Without Dedicated Pulmonary Catheters

George Carberry and Michael Brunner

Brief Description

With the emergence of high-resolution computed tomography pulmonary angiography (CTPA), the number of transcatheter pulmonary arteriograms being performed has steeply declined. For this reason, many interventional departments no longer stock dedicated pulmonary artery (PA) catheters such as the pre-shaped 7 Fr Grollman catheter (Cook Medical Inc., Bloomington, IN) for a femoral vein approach.[1] Interventionalists are therefore required to improvise with catheters that are available on hand. The following technique describes the use of the 5 Fr Omniflush catheter (AngioDynamics Inc., Latham, NY), a common diagnostic catheter found in most interventional departments, to gain access to the pulmonary arteries from either a superior or an inferior vena cava approach.[2,3]

Applications of the Technique

1. Diagnostic and therapeutic pulmonary arteriography when there is limited availability of dedicated PA catheters. Common indications for intervention include embolotherapy for arteriovenous malformations and catheter-directed thrombolysis for PA embolism.

Challenges of the Procedure

1. In patients with a dilated right atrium and/or ventricle, the guidewire may not take the proper angle to access the main PA. Varying wire stiffness (0.035 vs. 0.038 in.) and the amount of wire advanced beyond the end of the catheter will provide control over the angle needed to access the ventricular outflow tract.[4]
2. Despite modifying the catheter shape/angle, obtaining wire access to the main PA can remain difficult. If the wire is still unable to access the main PA, threading the wire a short distance through the tricuspid valve into the proximal right ventricle, and orienting the catheter so the curve faces the pulmonary valve may help. Gentle manipulation of the catheter will usually guide it into the main PA.

3. Depending on operator preference and patient anatomy, an alternative off-the-shelf PA catheter is a pigtail flush catheter (Angiodynamics Inc., Latham, NY), which can be manipulated with a tip deflecting wire to access either the right or the left PA from the right ventricular outflow tract.

Potential Pitfalls / Complications

1. Right heart catheterization in patients with a left bundle branch block (BBB) may result in the development of complete heart block. Before pulmonary angiography, always evaluate a recent electrocardiogram. If a left BBB is present, the patient may need temporary transvenous pacemaker placement prior to pulmonary arteriography.
2. Chronic heart disease is associated with increased arrhythmogenicity of the heart. Short runs of atrial and ventricular tachycardia usually respond to altering the position of the catheter and/or retracting the guidewire. If there is sustained or recurrent ventricular tachycardia, administer 150 mg amiodarone intravenously over 10 minutes.

Steps of the Procedure

1. Gain access to the common femoral, internal jugular, or brachial vein in standard fashion, and place a 5 Fr vascular sheath.
2. Use a soft-tipped guidewire to position the 5 Fr Omniflush catheter in the right atrium with the curve facing the tricuspid valve. We prefer the 0.038-in. Bentson guidewire (Cook Medical Inc., Bloomington, IN), but a 0.035- or 0.038-in., 3-mm, J-tipped guidewire can also be used. Long tapered hydrophilic wires such as a Glidewire (Terumo Medical Corp., Somerset, NY), which mimic the properties of a Bentson guidewire but are more lubricious, are an alternative option and may facilitate moving from the left to the right PA.

3. Slowly advance the wire through the end of the catheter. This will open the curve of the catheter approximately 90 degrees, which, in most cases, will be the angle needed to advance the guidewire into the main PA.

4. Pin the wire and advance the catheter to the proximal PA. Retraction of the wire will re-form the curve. Diagnostic arteriography can then be performed.

5. The catheter preferentially guides into the left PA from a right femoral vein approach. If access to the right PA is required, the curve should face the right PA to direct the soft-tipped wire into the right PA. In addition, decreasing the amount of wire in the distal catheter (e.g., retracting the guidewire back from the distal 15 cm of the catheter) can improve flexibility of the catheter when trying to access the right PA from the right ventricular outflow tract.

Example

See Figures 40.1–40.3.

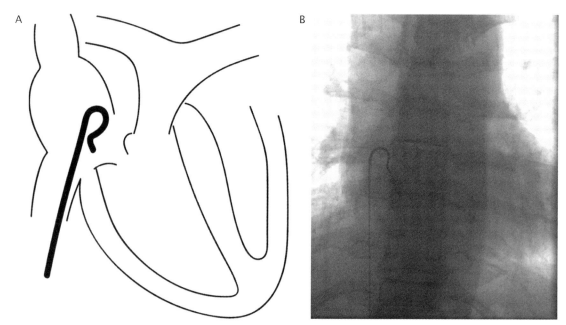

Figure 40.1 (A) Illustration and (B) corresponding fluoroscopic image demonstrating the orientation of the 5-Fr Omniflush catheter in the right atrium.

Source: Images courtesy of Jason Pinchot, MD.

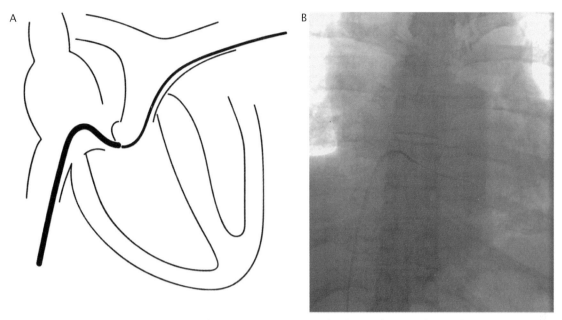

Figure 40.2 (A) Illustration and (B) corresponding fluoroscopic image revealing how advancing the guidewire through the Omniflush catheter results in a 90-degree curve on the guidewire, which is usually the correct angle for the wire to enter the right ventricular outflow tract.

Source: Images courtesy of Jason Pinchot, MD.

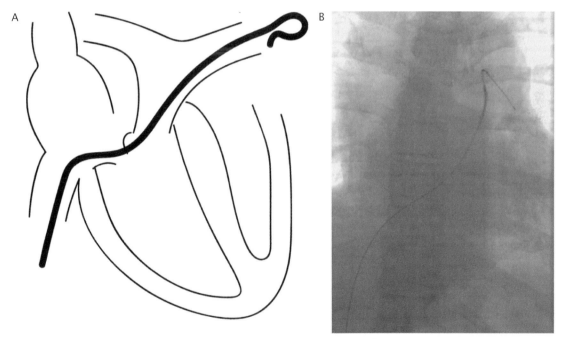

Figure 40.3 (A) Illustration and (B) corresponding fluoroscopic image showing the appearance of the reformed catheter in the left pulmonary artery.

Source: Images courtesy of Jason Pinchot, MD.

References and Suggested Readings

1. Grollman JH, Renner JW. Transfemoral pulmonary angiography: Update on technique. *AJR Am J Roentgenol.* 1981;136(3):624–626.
2. Valji K. Pulmonary and branch arteries. In: *Vascular and Interventional Radiology.* 2nd ed. Philadelphia: Saunders; 2006:347–373.
3. Velling, T, Brennan F, Hall L. Pulmonary angiography with use of the 5-F Omniflush catheter: A safe and efficient procedure with a common catheter. *J Vasc Interv Radiol.* 2000;11(8):1005–1008.
4. Waltman AC, Walker TG. A technique for pulmonary artery catheterization in patients with right ventricular enlargement. *AJR Am J Roentgenol.* 1989;152(2):391–392.

Venous Access and Dialysis Interventions

CHAPTER 41

Minimally Invasive Repair of Azygos Catheter Migration

Mikin V. Patel and Steven Zangan

Brief Description

Central venous catheter (CVC) placement is a common procedure to facilitate the care of patients requiring access for hemodialysis, long-term intravenous drug administration, or parenteral nutrition. The desired location of the catheter tip varies on societal guidelines and purpose of the catheter; the cavoatrial junction is a commonly accepted landmark signifying appropriate positioning. CVCs are not static once placed, and with changes in patient position, the catheter tip can shift by up to a few centimeters. Although initial placement may be optimal, numerous reports have described migration of the catheter tip out of the superior vena cava (SVC) into various locations, often the azygos arch.[1-3] Of note, left-sided CVC placement has been reported as a risk factor for tip migration into the azygos vein, probably due to the orientation of the left brachiocephalic vein toward the azygos opening. This abnormal catheter position can lead to an increased number of complications, including catheter malfunction, thrombosis, or even rupture of the azygos vein requiring surgical intervention.[3] Recognition of CVC tip malposition is important, and several factors are considered before deciding to intervene and reposition the catheter. Although invasive repositioning of the catheter is always an option, minimally invasive options can be attempted to repair azygos catheter malposition. This technique involves caudally retracting the port hub on the skin to move the catheter tip cranially. The patient is then instructed to take a deep inspiration to redirect the catheter. The position of the catheter can then be verified fluoroscopically.

Applications of the Technique

1. Abnormal position of a CVC tip in the azygos vein.
2. Patients with azygos catheter tip position with relatively minor symptoms, such as inability to flush or aspirate.

Challenges of the Procedure

1. Repositioning of the catheter tip may be more difficult if a significant length of catheter is in the azygos vein.

2. Endothelialization of the catheter tip into the azygos wall may also increase the difficulty of this technique.
3. Added radiation exposure to the patient and operator is expected because this manipulation should be done under fluoroscopic guidance. Use of leaded undergloves can be considered.

Potential Pitfalls/Complications

1. After correction, there is risk of the catheter tip again migrating into the azygos arch.
2. Failure of this conservative technique may require invasive intervention to reposition the catheter.
3. Patients with perforation of the azygos vein may ultimately require more aggressive endovascular or surgical intervention.

Steps of the Procedure

1. Retraction of the port hub caudally: As the catheter tip is tethered in soft tissues superiorly, this moves the catheter tip cranially out of the azygos opening. This step can be performed under fluoroscopy to verify movement of the CVC tip.
2. Patient takes a deep inspiration: The expansion of the thorax during inspiration expands the venous structures relative to the fixed length of the CVC and increases venous blood flow through the SVC. These effects help redirect the catheter toward the cavoatrial junction.
3. Release of the port hub and verification of CVC tip position: Once the CVC is directed appropriately, the port hub can be released, and proper tip position in the SVC can be documented fluoroscopically.

Example

See Figure 41.1.

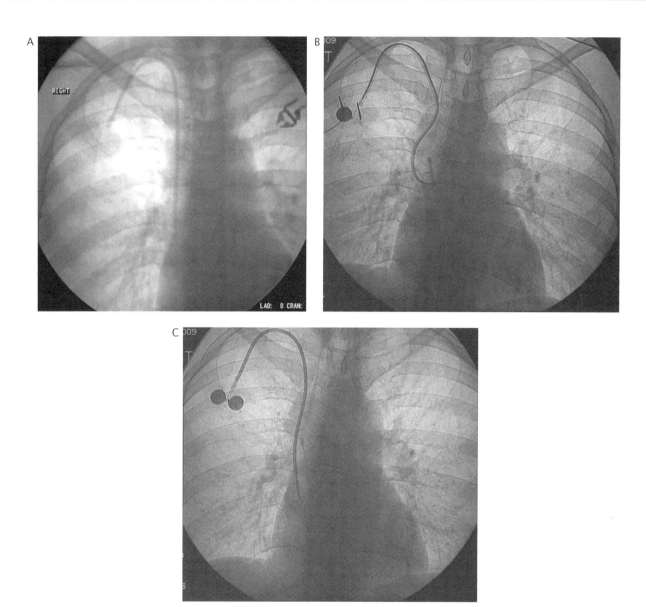

Figure 41.1 (A) Fluoroscopic image of dual-lumen port at time of initial placement. Note the appropriate position of the port catheter tip just above the cavoatrial junction. (B) Fluoroscopic image of malfunctioning dual-lumen port. Patient was active with yoga and had a history of a port catheter that did not flush or aspirate two months after placement. Note port tip in the azygos vein, likely apposed to the wall. (C) Fluoroscopic image of dual-lumen port after repositioning. After retraction of the port and deep patient inspiration under fluoroscopy, the catheter tip is now seen in an appropriate position near the cavoatrial junction.

References and Suggested Readings

1. Haygood TM, Malhotra K, Ng C, et al. Migration of central lines from the superior vena cava to the azygos vein. *Clin Radiol.* 2012;67:49–54.
2. DiGiacomo JC, Tarlian HS. Spontaneous migration of long-term indwelling venous catheters. *J Parenter Enteral Nutr.* 1991;15(5):574–577.
3. Bankier AA, Mallek R, Wiesmayr MN, et al. Azygous arch cannulation by central venous catheters: Radiographic detection of malposition and subsequent complications. *J Thor Imag.* 1997;12:64–69.

CHAPTER 42

Endovascular Snaring Technique for Shortening of Central Venous Port Catheters in Children

Mahmoud Zahra and Ganesh Krishnamurthy

Brief Description

Implantation of venous ports in children is increasingly performed by pediatric interventional radiologists and surgeons due to increasing need for long-term central venous access. The most common indication for venous port placement is chemotherapy. Additional indications include total parenteral nutrition (TPN), antibiotic therapy, administration of blood products, fluid administration, and apheresis.[1,2]

Venous ports have a lower infection rate, are more socially acceptable, and are less restrictive to children than other central catheters.[1]

Venous ports are usually inserted via the subclavian or internal jugular vein. Internal jugular vein access is preferred because of fewer complications compared to subclavian access.[3,4]

The ideal port catheter tip is either in the cavoatrial junction or right atrium. The cavoatrial junction has been defined as two vertebral bodies below the carina.[2] Short catheters with the tip located in the upper superior vena cava (SVC) or brachiocephalic vein have an increased risk of fibrin sheath formation and thrombosis,[5] whereas long catheters with the tip deep in the right atrium and right ventricle have an increased risk of cardiac dysrhythmias, cardiac perforation,[6] tamponade, and thrombosis. Because children have a shorter SVC and smaller right atrium, proper location of the catheter tip is more important to maintain the port function and decrease the risk of complications in children compared to adults.

The catheter tip in children is more variable than in adults based on inspiration/expiration, body habitus, and position (supine vs. upright). The endovascular snaring technique is used for the revision of long catheters. Compared to conventional open surgical revision[6], the technique confers multiple benefits and has been proven to be effective, feasible, and safe.[7] First, it obviates the need for opening the port pocket and therefore results in fewer procedure related complications, including bleeding and infection. Second, it is a considerably shorter procedure with reduced anesthesia and radiation time. Lastly, the lack of a surgical incision allows for less patient discomfort.[5]

Applications of the Technique

The decision to revise a long catheter is based on the length of the catheter, the function of the port, and the presence or absence of palpitations. Revision of the catheter is indicated if the catheter tip is in the right ventricle with or without symptoms. This may be detected with echocardiography or plain film. An upright chest radiograph should be obtained before the revision to confirm the location of the catheter tip. The other indication for catheter revision is the presence of a dysrhythmia or catheter dysfunction secondary to the tip location deep in the right atrium.

Challenges of the Procedure

1. Access: The right internal jugular vein is the preferred access since anatomically it provides the most direct access to the catheter tip for snaring. However, this access may not be available either secondary to the presence of another device/catheter or because of occlusion. The right subclavian vein is a potentially suitable site for access, but the angle relative to the catheter position is suboptimal. Similarly, both the left internal jugular and subclavian veins may potentially be used, but the catheter tip must be long enough to allow externalization from these sites. If there is no safe cephalad access secondary to occlusion, trauma, burn, or infection, the procedure cannot be performed.

2. Snaring of the Tip: This is usually accomplished with little difficulty, but a catheter tip that is within the right ventricle or abutting the atrial wall can be more difficult to grasp. Care should be made to monitor the patient's ECG for dysrhythmia during this step.

Potential Pitfalls/Complications

Complications for this procedure are very rare, but include the following[2]:

1. Hemorrhage: Patients with coagulopathy or those taking anticoagulant medications should be treated first until the international normalized ration is <1.5. Patients with thrombocytopenia should be treated first until their platelet count is ideally >50,000.
2. Procedure Related Sepsis: Patients with active infection or bacteremia should be treated until the infection has resolved.
3. Pneumothorax or Hemothorax
4. Air Embolism

Steps of the Procedure

1. Required Equipment:
   a. Vascular sheath of choice
   b. Ultrasound with hockey stick probe
   c. Fluoroscopy machine
   d. 21-Gauge micropuncture needle
   e. Micropuncture set
   f. Serial dilator(s) based on vascular sheath of choice
   g. Scissors
   h. Amplatz GooseNeck Snare (ev3 Endovascular Inc., Plymouth, MN) or other snare as available
2. Pre-Procedural Preparation:
   i. Review the imaging studies and port placement report if available.
   j. The choice of sedation is based on the patient's age and anticipated cooperation. General anesthesia is required for younger ages while conscious sedation is appropriate for older children.
   k. The choice of the sheath size is based on the port catheter diameter. The sheath should be at least 1.5 times larger than the port catheter.
   l. Prophylactic antibiotics are not routinely given.
3. Initial clinical and ultrasound assessment of the neck, including the internal jugular vein of choice is required before starting sedation or anesthesia.
4. Mild extension of the neck during the procedure is preferred.
5. The neck is prepped and draped in the usual sterile fashion.
6. Local anesthesia is infiltrated into the subcutaneous tissues.
7. Ultrasound-guided access of the internal jugular vein: High access at the 12 o'clock position of the internal jugular vein in the mid neck is preferred. Care is taken to avoid placing the carotid artery in the path of the needle trajectory. Puncture of the vein should be done with a quick stick during expiration. Avoid puncture of the posterior wall to decrease the risk of bleeding.
8. A 0.018-in. micropuncture wire is advanced into the jugular vein under fluoroscopic guidance.
9. A small neck incision is performed along the needle using a number 11 scalpel. Some operators prefer to make the incision prior to needle insertion.
10. The needle is exchanged for a 4 or 5 Fr micropuncture set.
11. The inner dilator of the micropuncture set as well as the micropuncture wire are exchanged for a 0.035-in. Glidewire (Terumo Medical Corp., Somerset,

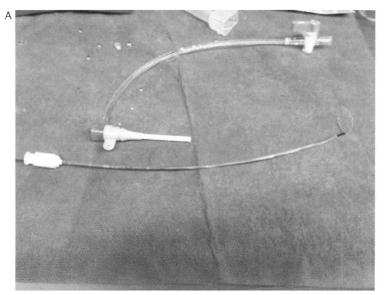
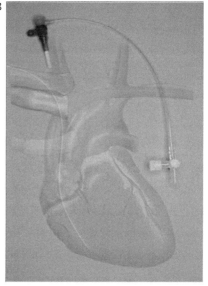

Figure 42.1 (A) Picture demonstrating a shortened sheath and an accompanying Amplatz GooseNeck Snare (ev3 Endovascular Inc., Plymouth, MN). (B) The shortened sheath is optimally placed in the internal jugular vein (IJV) ipsilateral to the catheter to be trimmed. The sheath is just long enough to allow access to the IJV.

NJ) or regular 3-mm J-wire (Cook Medical Inc., Bloomington, IN), which is advanced under fluoroscopic guidance into the IVC.

12. The shortest sheath length available should be utilized. A short sheath allows externalization of the port catheter. The hemostatic valve can be removed if necessary. In this situation, care should be taken to decrease the risk of an air embolism with cross clamping if needed.[5]

13. The Amplatz GooseNeck snare is advanced through the sheath into the right atrium, and the catheter tip is snared.

14. The port catheter tip is pulled through the sheath and externalized outside the patient.

15. The line is easily shortened by cutting it with a sterile scissors. Grasping the line with the snare close to the hub of the sheath during cutting prevents slippage of the line back into the sheath.

16. Reinsertion of the catheter into the right atrium/SVC junction is performed by advancing the shortened catheter with the aid of the snare back into a satisfactory position.

17. The snare is then removed.

18. The sheath is removed, and hemostasis is achieved with gentle manual compression. The sterile dressing is left in place for at least 24 hours.

Example

See Figures 42.1–42.6.

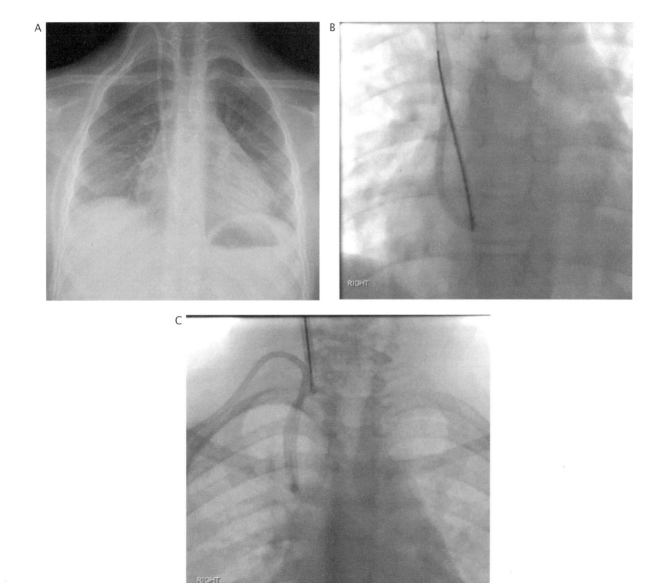

Figure 42.2 (A–C) Snaring the device line in the right atrium (RA). A GooseNeck snare is advanced through the IJV sheath into the RA and the catheter tip is snared and subsequently externalized through the sheath.

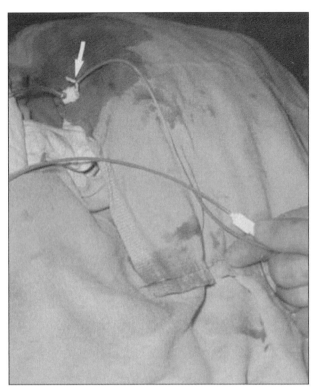

Figure 42.3 Externalization of the device line. The port catheter tip is snared and pulled through the IJV sheath (arrow) and externalized outside the patient.

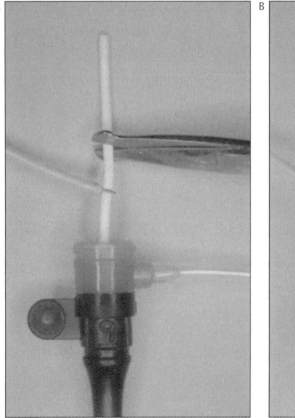

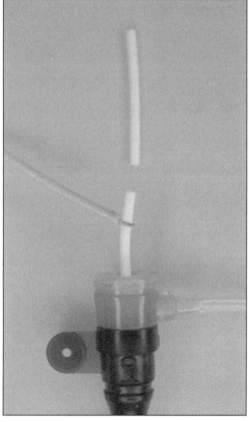

Figure 42.4 Shortening the device line. (A) The line is easily shortened by cutting with a sterile scissors. (B) Grasping the line with the snare close to the hub of the sheath during cutting prevents slippage of the line back into the sheath.

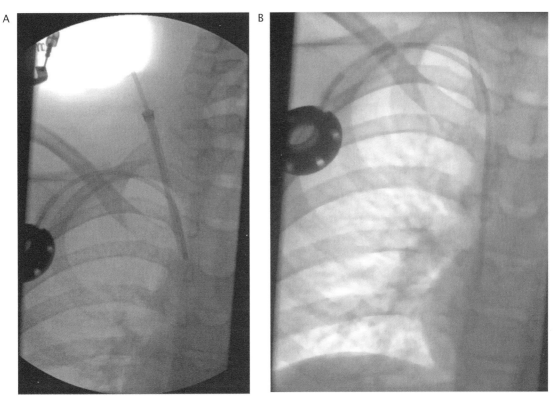

Figure 42.5 Reinsertion of the catheter into the RA/SVC junction. (A) This is performed by advancing the shortened line with the aid of the snare back into a satisfactory position at the SVC/RA junction. (B) The snare is then removed via the sheath.

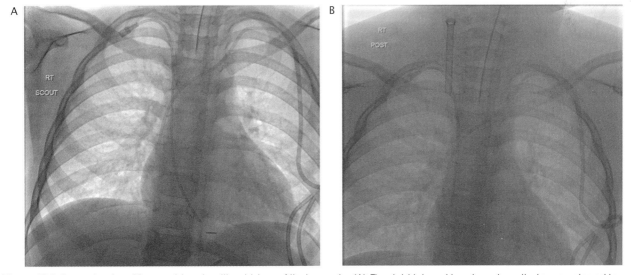

Figure 42.6 Example of an 11-year-old male with a history of thalassemia. (A) The right internal jugular vein catheter was placed in an outpatient setting with the catheter tip in right ventricle. (B) After revision, the catheter tip sits at the atriocaval junction.

References and Suggested Readings

1. Barnacle A, Arthurs OJ, Roebuck D, Hiorns MP. Malfunctioning central venous catheters in children: A diagnostic approach. *Pediatr Radiol*. 2008;38(4):363–378.

2. Dariushnia SR, Wallace MJ, Siddiqi NH, et al.; Society of Interventional Radiology Standards of Practice Committee. Quality improvement guidelines for central venous access. *J Vasc Interv Radiol*. 2003;14(9 Pt 2):S231–S235.

3. Gebauer B, Teichgraber UK, Podrabsky P, Werk M, Hanninen EL, Felix R. Radiologic intervention for correction of central venous port catheter migrations. *Cardiovasc Intervent Radiol* 2007;30(4):668–674.

4. Funaki B. Central venous access: A primer for the diagnostic radiologist. *AJR Am J Roentgenol*. 2002;179(2):309–318.

5. Murthy R, Arbabzadeh M, Richard H 3rd, Levitin A, Lund G, Stainken B. Endovascular technique for revision of excess catheter length in subcutaneous implanted venous access devices. *Cardiovasc Intervent Radiol*. 2004;27(3):259–261.

6. Kaufman JA, Fan CM, Geller SC, Rieumont MJ, Waltman AC. Percutaneous revision of excess length from an implanted long-term central venous access device. *AJR Am J Roentgenol*. 1997;169(6):1732–1734.

7. Bessoud B, de Baere T, Kuoch V, et al. Experience at a single institution with endovascular treatment of mechanical complications caused by implanted central venous access devices in pediatric and adult patients. *AJR Am J Roentgenol*. 2003;180(2):527–532.

CHAPTER 43

Placing a Jugular Port Without Direct Percutaneous Jugular Vein Access

Michael Rush, Cynthia Toot Ferguson, and S. Lowell Kahn

Brief Description

Although subcutaneous ports consisting of a port reservoir attached to a single or dual lumen central venous catheter have traditionally been placed by surgeons, an increasing number are placed in the interventional suite.[1] Subcutaneous ports are now routinely implanted by interventionalists utilizing ultrasound and fluoroscopic guidance. Interventional radiologists have demonstrated proficiency in inserting subcutaneous ports with high success and low complication rates.[2–5]

The internal jugular vein has been shown to be the vessel of choice for placement of the subcutaneous chest port catheter.[6–8] Proficiency with image guidance eliminates the need for a surgical cutdown for direct visualization of the vessel targeted for central venous cannulation. Interventionalists most often pierce the jugular vein by performing a direct percutaneous puncture under ultrasound guidance with a stab wound in the neck. A port pocket is subsequently created at an infraclavicular location, and the port catheter is tunneled from the pocket to the jugular access site in the neck.

This chapter describes an alternative single-incision technique for port placement. Specifically, with ultrasound guidance, the central venous catheter of a port can easily be placed from the port pocket, thereby negating the need for a second percutaneous access site to the jugular vein. This approach allows for the placement of the subcutaneous port reservoir and the catheter via a single site because the only interruption in the skin is the incision where the pocket is created for the port reservoir. Single-incision techniques for successful implantation of a subcutaneous chest port for central venous access have been reported by others in the literature.[9–12] In our practice, we have used this technique successfully in hundreds of patients with a low complication rate.

There are several advantages to placing a port without direct percutaneous jugular vein access. First, the procedure has been received very positively by patients who may be concerned about the cosmetic appearance of a stab wound in the neck for vascular access. Second, the risk of a surgical site infection is minimized because the skin is interrupted with only a single incision. Finally, an experienced operator can perform the procedure (skin-to-skin) in an expeditious manner.

Applications of the Technique

1. Placement of left- or right-sided chest ports.
2. Modification of this technique can be employed for placement of other tunneled catheters whereby a needle is inserted from the catheter exit site to the jugular vein, through which a wire is threaded ultimately to the inferior vena cava (IVC). Dilatation and subsequent placement of the tunneled catheter can be performed over this wire, thus obviating the need for a separate neck access.

Challenges of the Procedure

1. As described later, a needle is advanced from the port pocket to the internal jugular vein, through which a wire is subsequently advanced. Inevitably because of the angle of entry, the wire will tend to ascend within the jugular vein rather than turning inferiorly toward the IVC. Strategies to remedy this are discussed later.
2. Advancement of the peel-away sheath over the wire is sometimes difficult. We routinely curve the peel-away sheath to facilitate passage. At times, advancement of the dilator first is helpful.
3. Placement of the port in the pocket causes the catheter to "knuckle" with focal kinking where the catheter attaches to the port. Retraction of the incision in a caudal direction while placing the port in the pocket and careful readvancement of the catheter into the tunnel with small hemostats resolves this issue in most cases.

Potential Pitfalls/Complications

1. Performance of this technique requires continuous monitoring of the needle tip under ultrasound guidance. This is more challenging because a single transverse or longitudinal plane does not work as is typically employed with a standard jugular puncture.

It is therefore theoretically easier to inadvertently puncture the carotid artery.

2. Attention should be paid to the wire tip under fluoroscopy given the tendency for the wire to ascend within the jugular vein. This could result in bleeding if the wire tip were to enter and penetrate the cavernous sinus.

Steps of the Procedure

1. Preliminary ultrasound is performed to identify a suitable access vessel (preferably the internal jugular vein) prior to prepping the site for placement of the port. This noninvasive assessment allows the radiologist to assess the proximity of the internal jugular vein relative to the carotid artery; approximate vessel size; and determine patency of the jugular vein, which is compressible and relatively phasic with respiration. Phasic changes with respiration may be dampened if the internal jugular vein is patent at the point of intended access but becomes occluded in the chest. It is acceptable to access either the right or the left internal jugular vein for placement of the port's catheter. Rarely, access to the central venous structures cannot be accomplished via an internal jugular vein. In such cases, the external jugular vein or subclavian vein may be catheterized for central venous access.

2. The patient's neck and chest are subsequently prepped and draped in the usual fashion for port placement. The ultrasound transducer is placed in a sterile sleeve for use on the field. Lidocaine 2% with epinephrine is injected for local anesthesia, and a skin incision large enough to accommodate insertion of the selected port reservoir is made approximately 2 cm below the inferior margin of the clavicle and approximately 2 cm lateral to the lateral margin of the internal jugular vein. Gentle blunt dissection is used to create a pocket for the port reservoir so that it will reside inferior to the incision.

3. Imaging of the jugular vein is performed just above the superior margin of the clavicle over the site where the operator expects to introduce the catheter into the vessel. Vascular access is achieved by passing an introducer needle through the skin incision while directing the needle toward the internal jugular vein. The needle is introduced near the midpoint of the incision and advanced in a cephalad direction to a point just above the clavicle. The needle is then torqued and directed medially and slightly inferior as it is advanced to the target vessel while being observed with ultrasound. Real-time ultrasound imaging using an in-plane technique allows the operator to detect needle movement to the target vessel, ensuring that the tip of the needle reaches the intended location. The introducer needle can be curved or straight depending on operator preference. A curved needle confers the advantage of directing subsequent wire passage inferiorly, but following the tip of a curved needle under ultrasound is more challenging. An 18 or 21 gauge needle can be used for this step, and there are advantages to both. The 18 gauge needle torques better and is more visible by ultrasound, but the 21 gauge needle is less traumatic if there is inadvertent carotid puncture. With practice, both needles work well.

4. Advancement of the guidewire must be observed under fluoroscopic imaging because the wire may tend to ascend within the jugular vein. Once it is observed that the guidewire moves inferiorly toward the right atrium, the introducer needle is removed. If a 21 gauge needle is used, a Micropuncture Access Set (Cook Medical Inc., Bloomington, IN) will be necessary to transition to the 0.035-in. wire. Curving the needle and placing a gentle curve in the wire will help steer the wire inferiorly. If the guidewire ascends the jugular vein in a cephalad direction, it may need to be manipulated and repositioned. This can be accomplished by introducing a shepherd hook catheter over the guidewire. Given the short distance required, the catheter should be cut 15 cm from the distal end. This allows for insertion of the catheter while maintaining access via the guidewire. Under fluoroscopy, the catheter is advanced into the cervical jugular vein, where standard techniques for reforming the catheter are employed. Once reformed, the catheter and guidewire are pulled down slightly so that the tip engages the innominate vein. The guidewire can then be advanced to its intended position in the atriocaval junction or, more preferably, into the IVC for added support.

5. Gentle curvature is made to the peel-away sheath to facilitate advancement inferiorly. The peel-away sheath is then inserted over the wire.

6. The radiopaque port catheter (cut to approximately 30 cm) is advanced thru the peel-away sheath, and correct placement is confirmed under fluoroscopy. The peel-away sheath is removed, the catheter is trimmed to its final length, and the proximal end of the catheter is attached to the port reservoir. With the reservoir tucked into the pocket, the incision is closed with vertical interrupted absorbable sutures with the knots buried deep in the incision. A dermal adhesive is applied to the surface. Finally, Steri-Strips (3M Co., St. Paul, MN) and a protective sterile dressing are applied to the site.

Example

See Figures 43.1–43.5.

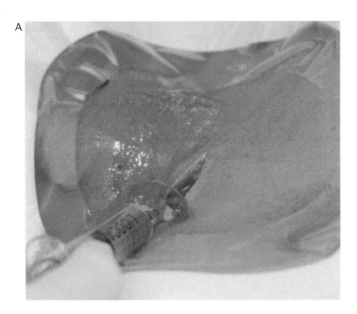

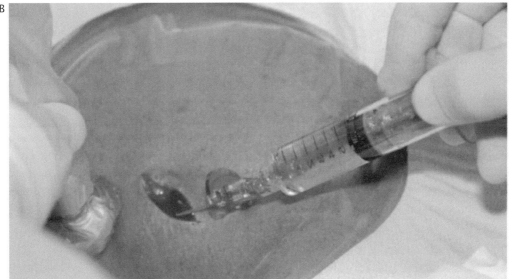

Figure 43.1 (A) A 19 gauge needle is directed from the port pocket incision toward the jugular vein with gentle aspiration applied to the connected syringe. (B) The ultrasound is placed just above the clavicle, and the needle tip is inserted into the internal jugular vein under real-time guidance. The needle typically enters the vein obliquely. Torque is applied to the needle whereby the hub is rotated cranially and the tip is deflected inferiorly to favor wire passage toward the atriocaval junction.

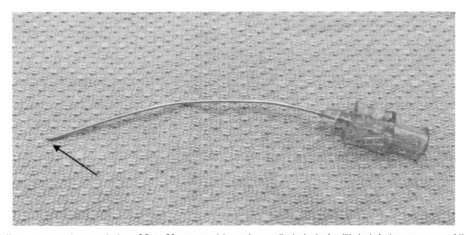

Figure 43.2 A gentle curve can be made in a 19 or 21 gauge (shown) needle to help facilitate inferior passage of the wire (see Figure 43.3). Note that the bevel (arrow) directs the wire inferiorly.

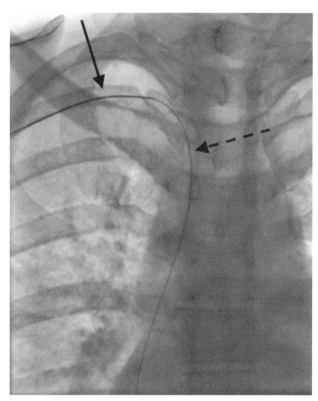

Figure 43.3 A right internal jugular port is placed with the single incision technique. Note the curved 21 gauge needle (solid arrow) is torqued and directs the microwire (dashed arrow) inferiorly toward the atriocaval junction. The needle was subsequently removed and the wire transitioned for a 0.035-in. Rosen wire (Cook Medical Inc., Bloomington, IN) over which the peel-away sheath was advanced.

A

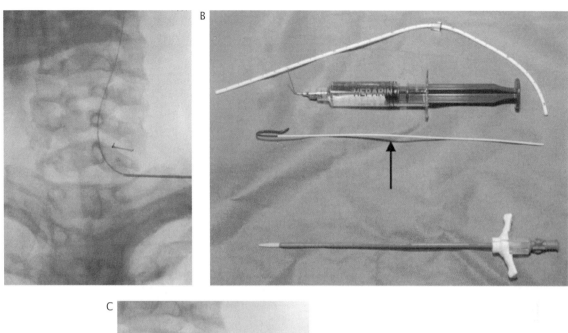

C

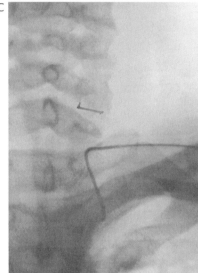

Figure 43.4 (A) On occasion, the wire will pass cranially into the cervical jugular vein with this technique. This is usually remedied by retracting and redirecting the wire with added torque on the needle hub. Backing the needle tip away from the medial wall of the vein is also helpful. (B) When these techniques fail, a reverse curve catheter can be cut (arrow) to facilitate redirection of the wire. (C) The catheter is inserted over the wire and formed in the cervical jugular vein. It is then retracted until the apex of the curve engages the point of entry into the vein and allows redirection of the wire inferiorly.

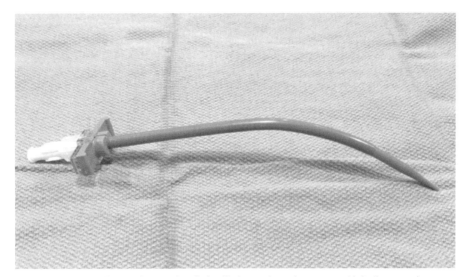

Figure 43.5 Making a gentle curve on the peel-away sheath facilitates easier advancement into the superior vena cava over the wire.

References and Suggested Readings

1. Reeves AR, Seshadri R, Trerotola SO. Recent trends in central venous catheter placement: A comparison of interventional radiology with other specialties. *J Vasc Interv Radiol.* 2001;12:1211–1214.

2. Morris SL, Jaques PF, Mauro MA. Radiology-assisted placement of implantable subcutaneous infusion ports for long-term venous access. *Radiology.* 1992;184(1):149–151.

3. De Gregorio MA, Miguelena JM, Fernandez JA, De Gregorio C, Tres A, Alfonso ER. Subcutaneous ports in the radiology suite: An effective and safe procedure for care in cancer patients. *Eur Radiol.* 1996;6:748–752.

4. Lorch H, Zwaan M, Kagel C, Weiss HD. Central venous access ports placed by interventional radiologists: Experience with 125 consecutive patients. *Cardiovasc Intervent Radiol.* 2001;24:180–184.

5. Shetty PC, Mody MK, Kastan DJ, et al. Outcome of 350 implanted chest ports placed by interventional radiologists. *J Vasc Interv Radiol.* 1997;8:991–995.

6. Funaki B, Szymski GX, Hackworth CA, et al. Radiologic placement of subcutaneous infusion chest ports for long-term central venous access. *Am J Roentgenol.* 1997;169(5):1431–1434.

7. Yip D, Funaki B. Subcutaneous chest ports via the internal jugular vein: A retrospective study of 117 oncology patients. *Acta Radiol.* 2002;43(4):371–375.

8. Charvát J, Linke Z, Horáèková M, Prausová J. Implantation of central venous ports with catheter insertion via the right internal jugular vein in oncology patients—Single center experience. *Supportive Care Cancer.* 2006;14(11):1162–1165.

9. Glenn BJ. Single-incision method for the placement of an implantable chest port or a tunneled catheter. *J Vasc Interv Radiol.* 2007;18(1):137–140.

10. Hearns CW, Miguel T, Kovacs S, Gohari A, Arampulikan J, McCann JW. Chest port placement with use of the single-incision insertion technique. *J Vasc Interv Radiol.* 2009; 20(11):1464–1469.

11. Marino AG, Larjani H, Perosi NA, Gonzalez-Beicos A. A "how-to" demonstration highlighting the single-incision insertion technique of chest port placement. *J Vasc Interv Radiol.* 2013;24(4):S173.

12. Romero Jaramillo A, Perez Lafuente M, Salmeron Alemany N, Gelabert Barragan A, Diez Miranda I, Segarra Medrano A. One year using the modified single-incision technique (MSIT) for subcutaneous chest port placement: One center experience. Presented at the Proceedings of the European Society of Radiology, 2012, Vienna, Austria.

CHAPTER 44

Transhepatic Snare Placement for Translumbar Inferior Vena Cava Access

Mikin V. Patel and Steven Zangan

Brief Description

In patients requiring long-term chemotherapy, antibiotics, hemodialysis, or parenteral nutrition, central venous access is typically inserted using a jugular, subclavian, or femoral approach. As these routes become complicated by thrombosis, stenosis, infection, or surgical intervention, the options for central venous catheter (CVC) placement become limited. Alternative sites to consider for patients who have few remaining options for central venous access include the hepatic veins and the inferior vena cava (IVC).[1-5] Translumbar catheterization of the IVC has been shown to be safe and effective, but direct access using anatomic landmarks can be challenging.[1] To aid in appropriate placement of an IVC catheter, the hepatic veins can first be accessed using sonographic guidance.[1] After performing a hepatic venogram to confirm appropriate access, an Amplatz GooseNeck snare (ev3 Endovascular Inc., Plymouth, MN) snare can be advanced into the IVC at the level of the renal veins. Under fluoroscopic guidance, a 21 gauge needle can be advanced toward the snare from a translumbar approach. A 0.018-in. wire is then passed through the snare, and the wire is grasped and pulled into the IVC. A central venous catheter is then placed in the routine fashion using a 5 Fr dilator, stiff 0.035-in. wire, and peel-away sheath. The catheter is also tunneled in the usual fashion with a subcutaneous Dacron cuff to help secure the catheter in place and prevent infection.

Applications of the Technique

1. End-stage renal disease patients in whom other central venous access options have been exhausted.
2. Patients with IVC filter thrombosis that cannot be recanalized.
3. Select patients who prefer translumbar access for aesthetic reasons.

Challenges of the Procedure

1. The CVC must course through the subcutaneous and muscular tissues before entering the IVC, so there is potential for it to become kinked. The needle should

be advanced in a caudo-cranial oblique direction to reduce the angle between the IVC and the needle.

Potential Pitfalls/Complications

1. Hepatic hemorrhage or injury is possible with the transhepatic access.[5] Judicious use of ultrasound to obtain access to the hepatic veins peripherally rather than centrally will decrease this risk. Additionally, embolization of the tract with gelfoam/coils during removal of the transhepatic access should be considered.
2. Retroperitoneal bleeding is a risk of the translumbar puncture as the needle passes through the musculature near lumbar arterial branches and near the renal vasculature.
3. Ureteral injury is also a potential complication of the procedure, either due to injury during initial catheter placement or due to erosion from prolonged contact of the catheter with the ureter.
4. Over time, the patient's voluntary and respiratory movement may dislodge the catheter or even cause the catheter to fracture.
5. The translumbar IVC catheter can migrate and enter the renal or phrenic veins. If needed, the catheter can be repositioned under fluoroscopy with a guidewire.
6. Catheter malfunction due to fibrin sheath or thrombus formation is a possible complication of all catheters, regardless of insertion site, and can be treated similarly to catheters placed via jugular, subclavian, or femoral approaches.
7. Catheter-related sepsis is a complication of central venous access that also applies to the translumbar IVC approach and may ultimately require removal. The infection rate of IVC catheters is slightly higher than that reported for all central venous catheters; however, this may be related to the relatively higher number of comorbidities in these patients.

Steps of the Procedure

1. The right hepatic vein is accessed with a 21 gauge needle under sonographic guidance. A small amount

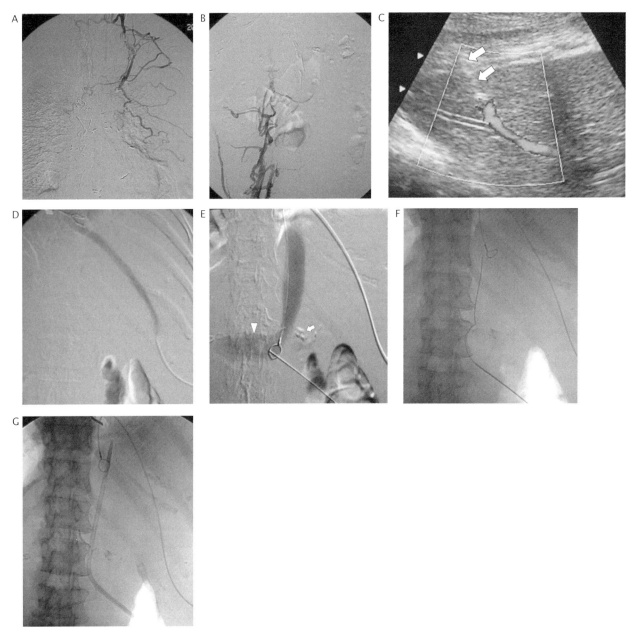

Figure 44.1 Digital subtraction angiography images of the left internal jugular and right femoral veins. Patient with need for hemodialysis with exhausted jugular, subclavian, femoral, and infrarenal IVC access. Venograms obtained from the left internal jugular vein (A) and the right femoral veins (B) show both supradiaphragmatic and subdiaphragmatic central venous stenosis and occlusion. Also note the numerous collateral vessels, indicating chronic obstruction. (C) Sonographic image in the right lobe of the liver. Right hepatic vein was accessed using a 21 gauge AccuStick needle (arrows). (D) Right hepatic venogram with the patient prone. Injected contrast outlines the right hepatic vein. (E) Amplatz GooseNeck snare (ev3 Endovascular Inc., Plymouth, MN) advanced into the IVC at the level of the left renal vein (arrowhead). Note the calcifications in the right renal artery (arrow). A 21 gauge needle was advanced from a translumbar approach into the opened snare using a single puncture. (F) A 0.018-in. wire is advanced through the translumbar needle, snared, and pulled into the IVC. This allows access for introduction of a 5 Fr sheath and placement of CVC using conventional methods. (G) Fluoroscopic image of the IVC showing successful translumbar placement of a CVC using a snare from the right hepatic vein to guide initial access.

of contrast is then injected under fluoroscopy to verify needle location in the right hepatic vein.

2. A sheath is placed, and a 4 Fr 10-mm Amplatz GooseNeck snare is advanced into the IVC to the level of the renal veins and opened. A larger snare can be used if desired, but this must be weighed against the increased risk of bleeding with a larger transhepatic access. Also, a larger snare may be more difficult to advance caudally within the IVC.

3. Under fluoroscopy, a 21 gauge needle is advanced toward the open snare using a translumbar approach. A caudo-cranial oblique approach targeting the IVC more proximally will reduce the kinking of the subsequently introduced sheath.

4. A 0.018-in. wire is introduced, snared, and pulled into the proximal IVC.

5. A 5 Fr sheath is introduced over the 0.018-in. wire, which is then replaced with a 0.035-in. stiff wire.

6. The central venous catheter is then tunneled subcutaneously to the translumbar venotomy site. The catheter is then cut to appropriate length such that the tip ends in the proximal IVC.

7. A peel-away sheath is advanced into the IVC over the 0.035-in. wire, and the catheter is placed into the IVC.

8. The hepatic venous access is removed, and the IVC catheter is secured in place.

Example
See Figure 44.1.

References and Suggested Readings

1. Lorenz JM, Regalado S, Navuluri R, et al. Transhepatic guidance of translumbar hemodialysis catheter placement in the setting of chronic infrarenal IVC occlusion. *Cardiovasc Intervent Radiol.* 2010;33(3):635–638.

2. Bennett JD, Papadouris D, Rankin RN, et al. Percutaneous inferior vena caval approach for long-term central venous access. *J Vasc Interv Radiol.* 1997;8:851–855.

3. Kade G, Les J, Buczkowska M, et al. Percutaneous translumbar catheterization of the inferior vena cava as an emergency access for hemodialysis: 5 years of experience. *J Vasc Access.* 2014;15:306–310.

4. Elduayen B, Martinez-Cuesta A, Vivas I, et al. Central venous catheter placement in the inferior vena cava via the direct translumbar approach. *Eur Radiol.* 2000;10:450–454.

5. Qureshi AM, Prieto LR, Bradley-Skelton S, et al. Complications related to transhepatic venous access in the catheterization laboratory: A single center 12-year experience of 124 procedures. *Cathet Cardiovasc Interv* 2014;84:94–100.

CHAPTER 45

Fibrin Sheath Removal Techniques

S. Lowell Kahn

Brief Description

Although autogenous arteriovenous fistula creation is the gold-standard dialysis access, catheters represent between 40% and 60% of dialysis access in the United States.[1] Catheters are placed for a variety of reasons, commonly as temporary access for acute renal failure or as a bridge to a more permanent access in patients with end-stage renal disease. Irrespective of their indications, maintenance of these catheters is imperative because complications arising from their use result in an annual national expenditure of greater than $1 billion in healthcare costs.[1–4]

Fibrin sheaths represent a heterogeneous matrix of cells and debris that form around catheters and are a known common cause of catheter failure and central venous stenosis.[1] Their formation is ubiquitous in the dialysis population, occurring in 80–100% of catheters within 1 week of inplantation.[1] A fibrin sheath is intimately related with the biofilm, and its presence is known to be associated with bacterial colonization, vessel stenosis, and thrombosis.[5] If the fibrin sheath extends around the tip of the catheter, the catheter will typically fail either completely or have significantly reduced flow rates and efficiency. In addition to the risks of catheter failure and infection, fibrin sheaths also carry a risk of catheter retention, making removal risky with potentially serious consequences.[6–9] Finally, although not common, a fibrin sheath can result in an air embolism after catheter removal because the fibrin sheath itself serves as a portal for vascular entry.[10–12] Incidents of serious complications are reported in the literature.[12]

There has been substantial industry investment with respect to catheter design and coatings to reduce the development and impacts of fibrin sheaths.[5,13] Nonetheless, fibrin sheaths remain a common problem encountered by the interventionalist. A variety of techniques exist for the treatment of fibrin sheaths, most commonly pharmacologic with tissue plasminogen activator infusion or with a simple catheter exchange. Unfortunately, these methods, although readily performed, are commonly inadequate.

This chapter presents several techniques for the management of the fibrin sheath. The first method described, the traditional catheter stripping technique, is a commonly employed method[14–17] for fibrin sheath removal. With this technique, a snare is advanced to the catheter tip via a femoral or upper extremity approach and is used to grab and strip the fibrin sheath from the end of the catheter. This method confers the benefit of intervention away from the catheter, thereby obviating the need for an exchange and minimizing the risks of infection or bleeding at the catheter site. However, if the catheter is adherent to the wall (e.g., superior vena cava or right atrium), it may be difficult to advance the snare around the tip of the catheter. Moreover, there are reports in the literature of the stripped fibrin sheath embolizing to the lungs.[17]

A modified catheter stripping technique involving a snare, the internal catheter stripping technique, is described by Reddy et al.[18] and involves looping a 0.035-in. guidewire and passing the loop (as a snare) through the proximal (red) and distal (blue) lumens of a dialysis catheter. The rigidity of the loop snare exerts force on the catheter lumen, thereby disrupting the fibrin sheath. The sheath is stripped from the catheter as the loop (snare) exits the catheter tip. In addition, after the snare exits the proximal (red lumen), it can be brought around the tip of the catheter (blue lumen) and used to strip the fibrin sheath from the posterior aspect of the catheter. In a small series, Reddy et al.[18] reported 100% technical and clinical success at 2, 4, and 6 weeks of follow-up. This method is simple and similarly obviates the need for a catheter exchange and the associated complications.

A final method presented here is the fibrin sheath angioplasty technique. Although variations exist, this method is also well described in the literature with excellent results.[1,15,19,20] This method is easily performed during a routine catheter exchange. After the existing catheter is removed over a wire, a balloon is passed over the wire and used to angioplasty and disrupt the fibrin sheath. The balloon is removed, and a new catheter is subsequently placed. This method may provide the most definitive removal of the fibrin sheath, but there is conflicting evidence as to whether inflation of the balloon predisposes the patient to central venous stenosis or occlusion through endothelial trauma and hyperplasia. For example, a study by Ni et al.[21] showed that patients whose fibrin sheath underwent angioplasty had a 14.2% incidence of subsequent central venous stenosis compared to a 7% incidence for patients who underwent catheter exchange alone. Conversely, a study by Hacker et al.[1] utilized angioplasty during catheter removal or exchange to prevent subsequent central venous stenosis. Although limited by a small sample size ($N = 43$), 91% of the treated patients remained patent and did not require subsequent intervention. A separate study by Shanaah et al.[19] compared patients whose fibrin sheaths were angioplastied to patients who had catheter exchanges without the presence of a fibrin sheath and found equivalent outcomes with respect to infection and catheter dysfunction, suggesting that treated fibrin sheaths carry no significant increased risk.

Among the described techniques, no technique is proven superior to another. A study by Janne d'Othée et al.[16] compared catheter exchange, catheter stripping, and balloon dilatation of the fibrin sheath. Technical success and patency rates were not significantly different among the three groups. All the techniques described herein are technically easy, readily performed with standard angiography equipment, and associated with relatively low risk.

Applications of the Technique

All Techniques
1. Fibrin sheath removal in the setting of a failing central venous catheter.

Fibrin Sheath Angioplasty Technique
1. Prevention of delayed central venous stenosis.

Challenges of the Procedure

Traditional Catheter Stripping Technique
1. This procedure is most commonly performed by obtaining a femoral vein access. Many end-stage renal disease patients have had numerous prior central lines and, consequently, venous occlusion is possible. Compromised femoral vein patency may limit the ability to perform this technique.
2. A catheter that is adherent to the vessel/atrial wall secondary to a chronic fibrin sheath may limit the ability to advance a snare around the catheter and therefore preclude successful performance of this technique.

Internal Catheter Stripping Technique[18]
1. Advancing a looped 0.035-in. Glidewire (Terumo Medical Corp., Somerset, NJ) through the lumen of a dialysis catheter may be challenging, and the operator may encounter a high level of friction, preventing advancement.
2. Although traditionally considered "kink resistant," the looped Glidewire may exceed the wire's elastic tolerance, resulting in a kink.
3. Attempting this technique on a smaller catheter (e.g., port) may require use of a smaller 0.018-in. nitinol wire.

Fibrin Sheath Angioplasty Technique
1. Advancing a balloon "bareback" through the subcutaneous tract can be difficult, but it is typically accomplished with little difficulty. At our institution, a stiff Glidewire (Terumo Medical Corp., Somerset, NJ) is optimal in terms of its low friction coefficient and adequate level of support.

Potential Pitfalls/Complications

Traditional Catheter Stripping Technique
1. The catheter could be stretched or otherwise damaged with this maneuver if it is pulled too aggressively.
2. Embolization of the fibrin sheath to the lungs has been reported as clinically significant with this method.[17]

Internal Catheter Stripping Technique[18]
1. It is theoretically possible that an excessive bend in the Glidewire could exceed the wire's elastic tolerance and result in a kink in the wire. If the kinked wire were to exit the catheter and pass over the catheter tip, removal could be difficult, and complete removal of the catheter and wire might be required.
2. Although we have not encountered this problem, it is possible for the structural integrity of the catheter to be compromised by the passing of the looped Glidewire.

Fibrin Sheath Angioplasty Technique
1. Injury to the superior vena cava, jugular vein, or subclavian vein is possible with overaggressive dilatation and could result in severe bleeding complications (e.g., hemothorax and hemopericardium).
2. There are reports of long-term central venous stenosis with this method.[21]
3. Removal of the catheter from the subcutaneous tunnel carries a very small risk of an air embolism during the exchanges for placement of the balloon and the subsequent new catheter placement.[10-12] It is therefore advisable to maintain gentle pressure on the tract during catheter/balloon exchanges.

Steps of the Procedure

Traditional Catheter Stripping Technique
1. *Optional*: Contrast can be injected into the catheter to study the extent and confirm the presence of the fibrin sheath.
2. Femoral vein access is obtained, and using the Seldinger technique, an appropriately sized sheath (adequate to accommodate selected snare) is advanced into the inferior vena cava.

3. A snare is advanced to the distal end of the catheter. A variety of snares work adequately. At our institution, we have obtained good results using a 20-mm Amplatz GooseNeck Snare (ev3 Endovascular Inc., Plymouth, MN).

4. The snare is opened and advanced carefully over the catheter tip as far as possible in a cranial direction.

5. The snare is tightened (not overly to prevent movement or stretching of the catheter tip).

6. The tightened snare is withdrawn over the length of the catheter.

7. The central venous catheter is intermittently tested for flushing and aspiration.

8. Steps 3–6 are repeated until the central venous catheter functions appropriately.

Internal Catheter Stripping Technique[18]

1. *Optional*: Contrast can be injected into the catheter to study the extent and confirm the presence of the fibrin sheath.

2. For a standard dialysis catheter, a 0.035-in. Glidewire is looped. For smaller catheters (e.g., port), a 0.018-in. nitinol wire may be used.

3. The apex of the Glidewire is advanced through the proximal (red) lumen of the catheter.

4. The passage of the loop through the catheter lumen naturally stretches and fractures the fibrin sheath surrounding the catheter. A to-and-fro motion is applied within the catheter for optimal effect.

5. As the loop exits the catheter, it is similarly rotated and passed in a to-and-fro motion to break up the fibrin sheath. The loop is also passed over the distal (blue) catheter lumen to clear the fibrin sheath from the posterior aspect of the catheter.

6. Steps 2–4 are repeated for the distal (blue) lumen of the catheter.

7. *Optional*: If difficulty is encountered passing the loop of the Glidewire though the catheter, a small bend can be placed at the loop of the wire with a Kelly clamp prior to placing it into the lumen of the catheter. The single end of the wire exiting the catheter is then pulled in a similar manner after the apex of the loop exits the catheter tip, again activating the snare.

Fibrin Sheath Angioplasty Technique

1. *Optional*: Contrast can be injected into the catheter to study the extent and confirm the presence of the fibrin sheath.

2. The existing catheter is removed over a wire. At our institution, this is typically performed over a stiff Glidewire. Gentle pressure is maintained at the catheter exit site during each exchange to minimize the risk of introducing an air embolism into the pulmonary vasculature.

3. Over the Glidewire, a balloon (commonly 8–12 mm) is passed directly (through the subcutaneous tunnel if it is a tunneled catheter) into the central venous vasculature.

4. *Optional*: Some authors advocate placing a sheath first either directly into the vein or through the subcutaneous tract if tunneled. In our experience, the sheath is not typically necessary.

5. The balloon is then inflated along the course of the catheter to rupture and remove the fibrin sheath. This can be performed with multiple sequential balloon inflations and deflations, or the balloon can be inflated once proximally and pushed over the wire distally.

6. A new catheter is then placed over the stiff Glidewire. In our experience, a single stiff Glidewire is adequate for placement of a new dialysis catheter (not split tip). The wire is passed through the distal (blue) lumen of the catheter, and the catheter is spun as it is advanced into the subcutaneous tunnel. Use of a second wire or peel-away sheath is typically not necessary.

Example
See Figures 45.1–45.3.

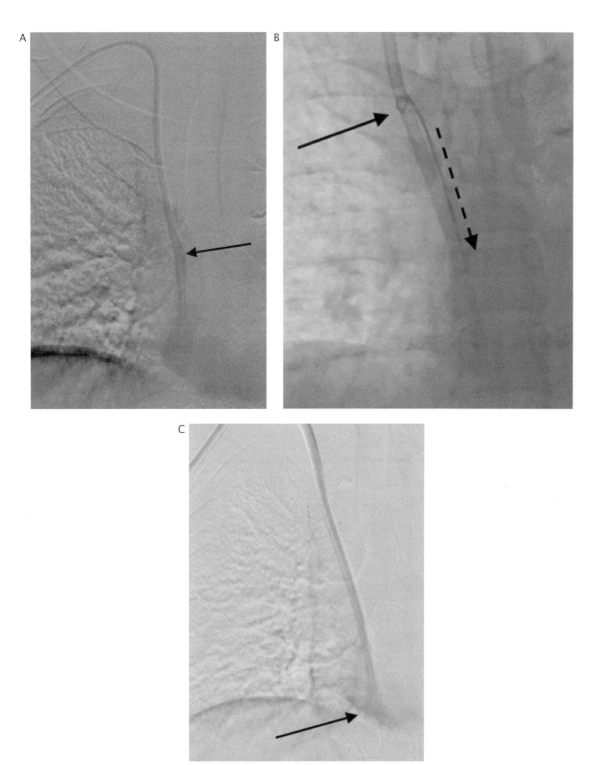

Figure 45.1 Traditional catheter stripping technique. (A) A venogram performed through a tunneled right internal jugular catheter shows contrast ascending along the shaft of the catheter (arrow) consistent with a fibrin sheath. (B) A snare is advanced from a right femoral vein access and ascends around the catheter (solid arrow). The snare is tightened and withdrawn (dashed arrow) along the shaft of the catheter. The maneuver is repeated as necessary to remove the entirety of the fibrin sheath. (C) Repeat venogram after removing the fibrin sheath shows contrast only at the tip of the catheter (arrow), indicating successful removal of the fibrin sheath.

Source: From Mohamad Ali AF, et al. Dialysis catheter fibrin sheath stripping: A useful technique after failed catheter exchange. *Biomed Imaging Interv J.* 2012;8(1):e8. Courtesy of the Department of Biomedical Imaging, University of Malaysia.

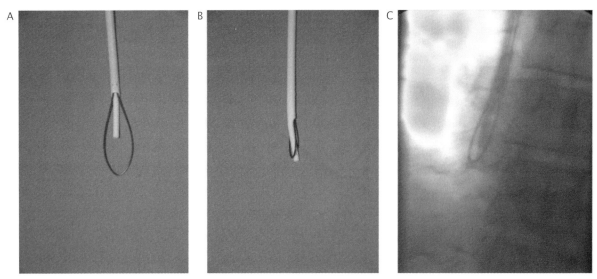

Figure 45.2 Internal catheter stripping technique. (A) A looped Glidewire is advanced through the proximal port of a dialysis catheter. As the loop passes through the catheter, force is distributed to the fibrin sheath causing disruption. A to-and-fro motion can be employed as the wire exits the catheter tip. (B and C) After the loop exits the tip, the loop is passed over the distal end of the catheter tip to disrupt the fibrin sheath from the posterior aspect of the catheter. The maneuver is repeated with passage of the looped Glidewire through the distal port of the catheter.

Source: From Reddy AS, et al. Fibrin sheath removal from central venous catheters: An internal snare manoeuvre. *Nephrol Dial Transplant* 2007;22:1762–1765. Courtesy Oxford University Press.

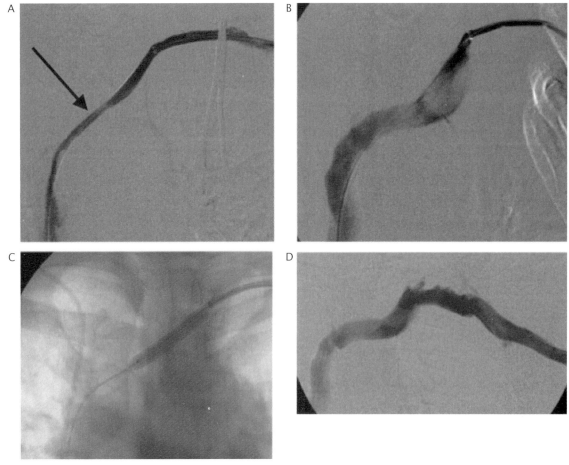

Figure 45.3 Fibrin sheath angioplasty technique. Venogram obtained after the catheter is removed showing the narrow fibrin sheath (solid black arrow) before (A) and after (B) angioplasty. (C) A balloon may be advanced either bare or through a sheath to angioplasty and disrupt the fibrin sheath. (D) Venogram obtained 1 year after angioplasty reveals wide patency of the left axillary, subclavian, and brachiocephalic veins.

Source: Hacker RI, et al. Fibrin sheath angioplasty: A technique to prevent superior vena cava stenosis secondary to dialysis catheters. *Int J Angiol.* 2012;21:129–134. Courtesy Thieme Medical Publishers, Inc.

References and Suggested Readings

1. Hacker RI, Garcia LD, Chawla A, Panetta TF. Fibrin sheath angioplasty: A technique to prevent superior vena cava stenosis secondary to dialysis catheters. *Int J Angiol.* 2012;21:129–134.

2. Dwyer A. Surface-treated catheters—A review. *Semin Dial.* 2008;21(6):542–546.

3. Oliver MJ, Mendelssohn DC, Quinn RR, et al. Catheter patency and function after catheter sheath disruption: A pilot study. *Clin J Am Soc Nephrol.* 2007;2(6):1201–1206.

4. Centers for Medicare and Medicaid Services. Office of Clinical Standards and Quality: 2004 Annual Report: The ESRD Clinical Performance Measures Project. Baltimore: US Department of Health and Human Services; 2004.

5. Ibeas-Lopez J. New technology: Heparin and antimicrobial-coated catheter. *J Vasc Access.* 2015;16(Suppl 9):S48–S53.

6. Garcarek J, Gołębiowski T, Letachowicz K, et al. Balloon dilatation for removal of an irretrievable permanent hemodialysis catheter: The safest approach. *Artif Organs.* 2016;40(5):E84–E88.

7. Jafferbhoy SF, Asquith JR, Jeeji R, Levine A, Menon M, Pherwani AD. A stuck haemodialysis central venous catheter: Not quite open and shut! *J Surg Case Rep.* 2015;2015(4):rjv032.

8. Arnáiz-García ME, Gutiérrez-Diez F, Arnáiz-García AM, et al. Successful retrieval of an irretrievable jugular Tesio catheter using a Fogarty arterial embolectomy catheter. *Vasc Endovascular Surg.* 2014;48(4):349–351.

9. Teeple EA, Shiels WE, Nwomeh BC, Rocourt DV, Caniano DA. Difficult central venous access removal: Case reports of the use of endovascular snare shearing of endothelialized tetherings. *J Pediatr Surg.* 2011;46(5):e13–e15.

10. Marco M, Roman-Pognuz E, Anna B, Allesio S. Air embolism after central venous catheter removal: Fibrin sheath as the portal of persistent air entry. *Case Rep Crit Care.* 2013;2013:403243.

11. Bellasi A, Brancaccio D, Maggioni M, Chiarelli G, Gallieni M. Salvage insertion of tunneled central venous catheters in the internal jugular vein after accidental catheter removal. *J Vasc Access.* 2004;5(2):49–56.

12. Roberts S, Johnson M, Davies S. Near-fatal air embolism: Fibrin sheath as the portal of air entry. *South Med J.* 2003;96(10):1036–1038.

13. Bridges C. New heparin coating reduces thrombosis and fibrin sheath formation in HD catheters. *Nephrol News Issues.* 2007;21(3):32, 34.

14. Mohamad Ali AF, Uhwut E, Liew S. Dialysis catheter fibrin sheath stripping: A useful technique after failed catheter exchange. *Biomed Imaging Interv J.* 2012;8(1):e8.

15. Faintuch S, Salazar GM. Malfunction of dialysis catheters: Management of fibrin sheath and related problems. *Tech Vasc Interv Radiol.* 2008;11(3):195–200.

16. Janne d'Othée B, Tham JC, Sheiman RG. Restoration of patency in failing tunneled hemodialysis catheters: A comparison of catheter exchange, exchange and balloon disruption of the fibrin sheath, and femoral stripping. *J Vasc Interv Radiol.* 2006;17(6):1011–1015.

17. Winn MP, McDermott VG, Schwab SJ, Conlon PJ. Dialysis catheter "fibrin-sheath stripping": A cautionary tale! *Nephrol Dial Transplant.* 1997;12(5):1048–1050.

18. Reddy AS, Lang EV, Cutts J, Loh S, Rosen MP. Fibrin sheath removal from central venous catheters: An internal snare manoeuvre. *Nephrol Dial Transplant.* 2007;22:1762–1765.

19. Shanaah A, Brier M, Dwyer A. Fibrin sheath and its relation to subsequent events after tunneled dialysis catheter exchange. *Semin Dial.* 2013;26(6):733–737.

20. Watorek E, Golebiowski T, Letachowicz K, et al. Balloon angioplasty for disruption of tunneled dialysis catheter fibrin sheath. *J Vasc Access.* 2012;13(1):111–114.

21. Ni N, Mojibian H, Pollak J, Tal M. Association between disruption of fibrin sheaths using percutaneous transluminal angioplasty balloons and late onset of central venous stenosis. *Cardiovasc Intervent Radiol.* 2011;34(1):114–119.

CHAPTER 46

Obtaining Hemostasis at Puncture Sites

Sreekumar Madassery

Brief Description

This chapter pertains to femoral artery access. Deciding whether to perform arterial access closure using the gold standard of manual compression versus a vascular closure device (VCD) requires the operator to evaluate many characteristics of the patient. The location of the arteriotomy, vessel size, degree of calcification, use of anticoagulants, and sheath size during the procedure are the primary factors that need to be considered. The 2014 ISAR-CLOSURE study by Schulze-Stephanie et al.[1] reported that use of VCDs was not inferior to manual compression.

The most important aspect of the arterial closure is in fact the initial access. Attaining an "ideal" access is essential for maximizing the chances of maintaining effective hemostasis. Attaining an ideal access entails using the standard landmarks under fluoroscopy to enter the midportion of the common femoral artery (CFA) so that the arteriotomy will be superior to the bifurcation of the CFA into the superficial and profunda femoral arteries and inferior to the hypogastric artery. In approximately 10% of patients, there may be a high bifurcation, which can result in access into the superficial femoral artery (SFA) or profunda femoral arteries, thus increasing the risk of pseudoaneurysm or arteriovenous fistula.[2] For this reason, many employ ultrasound in all cases to obviate the risk of catheterization below the bifurcation. For manual pressure, 10–15 minutes of gradually decreasing pressure is generally sufficient to maintain hemostasis.

However, in obese patients, those with a high risk of bleeding (activated clotting time (ACT) >180 seconds), those who cannot tolerate prolonged bed rest, and those who are immobile, a VCD may be beneficial. During the past two decades, the number of different closure devices on the market has increased. Some VCDs are intravascular using collagen (Angio-Seal, Terumo Medical Corp., Somerset, NJ) or sutures (Perclose ProGlide Suture-Mediated Closure System, Abbott Vascular Inc., Santa Clara, CA), whereas others are extravascular and use bioabsorbable components (e.g., MYNXGRIP, Cordis Corp., Milpitas, CA), Vascade (Cardiva Medical Inc., Santa Clara, CA) or clips (StarClose SE, Abbott Vascular Inc., Santa Clara, CA). Compared to manual pressure, VCDs carry an increased risk of infection due to the presence of a foreign body and due to potential hematoma formation with device failure.[3] Evaluating for heavy atherosclerotic burden near the arteriotomy site on angiogram is vital because experience has shown that plaque can cause premature deployment of some of the VCDs. The luminal diameter, determined on angiography, needs to be considered as well, for which manufacturer recommendations may dictate each device's safe use (e.g., ≥ 4 mm for Angio-Seal, ≥ 6 mm for Vascade and ≥ 5 mm for MYNXGRIP). Some diagnostic cases, and most interventional cases, involve anticoagulation. Depending on how much estimated anticoagulant is still in the patient's system at the completion of the case (typically assessed by ACT level), manual compression may have a high risk for bleeding. Some operators choose to give protamine to reverse the heparin prior to sheath removal; however, this needs to be used with caution, especially in diabetics. Therefore, due to the risk of bleeding, a VCD may be a good option. Overall, the decision to deploy a VCD or to hold manual pressure is operator dependent, with many factors that need to be considered.

Applications of the Technique
1. Diagnostic and therapeutic arteriograms

Challenges of the Procedure
1. The patient may have extensive atherosclerotic disease.
2. The patient may have had multiple prior arterial interventions, thus limiting the use of VCDs.
3. Some vasculopathic patients may have had prior surgical interventions of the groin, such as bypass grafts, stenting, endarterectomies, which similarly limit the use of VCDs.
4. A large body habitus may make manual pressure difficult.

Potential Pitfalls/Complications
1. Use of VCDs can result in ischemia due to embolism (e.g., a footplate) from the device.
2. Circulating anticoagulants may cause excessive bleeding times and increase the risk of hematoma formation with manual pressure.
3. There is a potential for infection when using a VCD.

4. Use of a VCD in a plaque laden vessel or a vessel smaller than specified by the device instructions for use (IFU) can result in occlusion of the access vessel.

Steps of the Procedure

1. Prior to deciding whether to use manual pressure or a closure device, perform an arteriogram of the ipsilateral iliofemoral vessels through the existing sheath, with medial deviation of the sheath and in the ipsilateral oblique (~30°–45°) projection. This can be performed with non-ionic contrast or CO_2.

2. If the access is deemed appropriate for use of a closure device, a sterile re-preparation of the sheath and groin should be performed and new sterile gloves should be donned by the interventionalist. Some physicians choose to administer an IV antibiotic (e.g., Ancef) prior to using the closure device. The device can then be deployed according to the manufacturer IFU.

3. After deployment, typically light manual pressure and observation are performed for approximately 5 minutes. If there is visible bleeding or hematoma, immediate manual pressure should be held for at least 10 additional minutes.

4. If, after the sheath arteriogram, manual pressure is deemed the best option, the physician performs this with strong pressure held approximately 1 or 2 cm above the skin entry site immediately after removal of the sheath. This position accounts for the fact that the arteriotomy is located above the skin incision because of the traditional 45-degree angle at which the needle enters the vessel.

5. After the first 5 minutes of deep pressure, the force is gradually decreased. Usually, an average of 15 minutes is sufficient to obtain hemostasis. Assuming an ACT < 180, the following time guidelines are typically reliable for the duration of manual compression (note the time increase of 5 minutes for every Fr increase in sheath size):
   a. 4 Fr Sheath: 10 minutes
   b. 5 Fr Sheath: 15 minutes
   c. 6 Fr Sheath: 20 minutes
   d. 7 Fr Sheath: 25 minutes

6. After cessation of manual pressure, the site should be observed for approximately 5 minutes. If there is persistent bleeding from the skin site or a developing hematoma, immediate manual pressure should again be applied for at least 10 minutes.

7. Regardless of manual pressure versus VCD use, the lower extremity pulses should be checked by palpation and/or with Doppler and compared to pre-procedure findings.

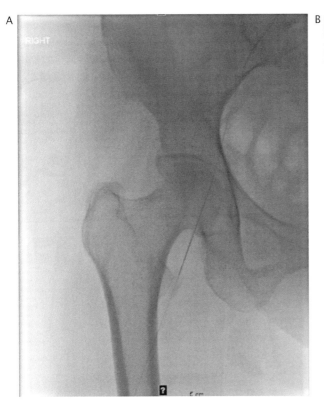 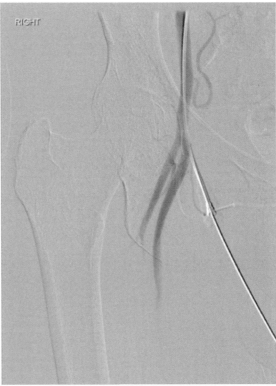

Figure 46.1 High common femoral artery bifurcation. A high femoral artery was identified on ultrasound utilized to obtain access (not shown). (A) Fluoroscopic image obtained after femoral artery catheterization shows needle entry just above the mid femoral head. (B) Digital subtraction angiography performed through the sheath at completion of the case confirms the high femoral bifurcation. Note that the acquisition is obtained with RAO obliquity and with the sheath pulled medially. This combination allows excellent visualization of the bifurcation and shows the sheath entering the common femoral artery just above the bifurcation.

References and Suggested Readings

1. Schulze-Schupke S, Helde S, Gewalt S, et al. Comparison of vascular closure devices vs manual compression after femoral artery puncture: The ISAR-CLOSURE randomized clinical trial. *JAMA*. 2014;312(19):1981–1987.

2. Kaufman JA, Lee MJ. *Vascular and Interventional Radiology: The Requisites*. St. Louis, MO: Saunders; 2004.

3. Johanning JM, Franklin DP, Elmore JR, Han DC. Femoral artery infections associated with percutaneous arterial closure devices. *J Vasc Surg*. 2001;34(6):983–985.

CHAPTER 47

Elimination of Post-Procedural Bleeding After Placement of Tunneled Dialysis Catheters

Almas Syed, Robert Evans Heithaus, and Chet R. Rees

Brief Description

Tunneled intravenous chest catheters, particularly dialysis catheters, sometimes result in oozing or bleeding from the neck or chest incisions during the first 24 hours after placement.[1] The problem is exacerbated by the large diameter of tunneled catheters, their stiffness, and the frequently abnormal hemostasis profiles of patients who require them.[1] Many patients have altered international normalized ratios (INR), thrombocytopenia, or abnormal platelet function due to uremia. Bleeding can lead to morbidity and results in discomfort due to soaked bandages and clothes, increased nursing requirements, repeated physician visits, and the application of pressure dressings that frequently do not work. It also increases the risks of exposure to those around the patient and increases the cost of care.

Attempts to inject flowable hemostatic agents into the tract were initially met with limited success at our institution. However, our improved method described in this chapter is simple and has eliminated postoperative bleeding in these patients at our institution.

The salient features of the technique are as follows: A 0.018 in. wire is advanced along with the tunneler and remains in the tunneled tract after the tunneler is disconnected from the catheter. A 3 Fr dilator is then passed over the wire, and the wire is removed. Next, a hemostatic slurry is injected into the tunnel while the dilator is retracted. All potential bleeding sites throughout the operative site and tract are well coated and permeated by the hemostatic agent with this technique. This provides superior coating compared to simply pushing the catheter into the incision and injecting the material.

Applications of the Technique

1. Tunneled chest catheter placement, particularly in patients with abnormal hemostasis profiles.

Challenges of the Procedure

1. The wire can dislodge from the tunneler during aggressive tunneling.

2. Advancing the 3 Fr dilator over the wire can be difficult.

Potential Pitfalls/Complications

1. Retracting the dilator too quickly may not allow for adequate injection of hemostatic material.
2. If enough hemostatic material is not injected it may compromise the success of the technique.
3. Failure to apply pressure at the neck incision during injection can result in the hemostatic material oozing out of the tract or potentially even passing into the vein.

Steps of the Procedure

1. A standard 0.018-in. wire, leftover from the micropuncture kit used to access the jugular vein, is sandwiched inside the tunneler and tunneler cap assembly together with the catheter.
2. Tunneling is performed as usual, dragging the wire through the tract along with the tunneler.
3. The wire is detached from the tunneler and left in place through-and-through the tract.
4. The 3 Fr dilator from the micropuncture kit is passed over the wire until its distal tip is revealed from the neck incision.
5. The wire is removed from the 3 Fr dilator.
6. Focal pressure is applied to the neck site.
7. Injectable thrombin hemostatic (D-Stat Flowable Hemostat, Vascular Solutions Inc., Minneapolis, MN) is injected into the dilator and into the peri-tract/peri-vein tissues while the dilator is withdrawn.
8. The full tract is massaged to allow complete permeation of the tract and exposure to tissues while expressing excess material.

Example

See Figure 47.1.

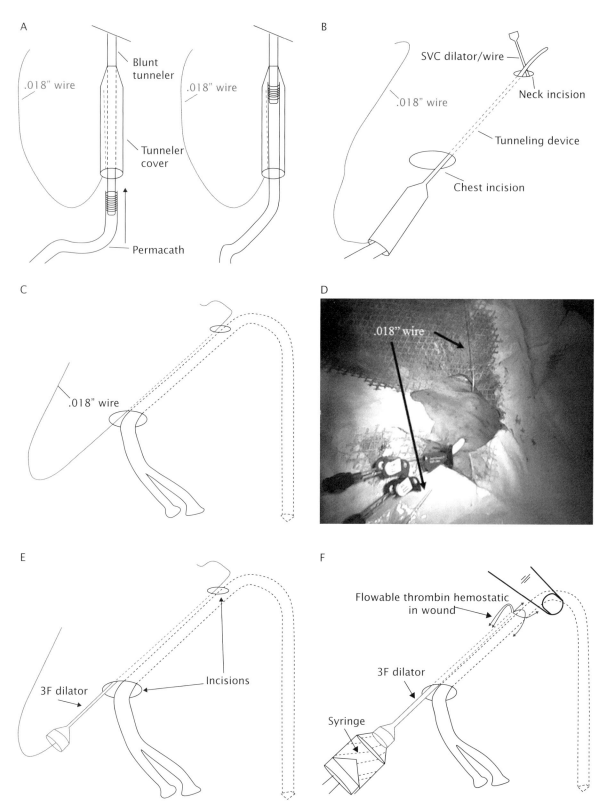

Figure 47.1 (A) The standard 0.018-in. wire, leftover from the micropuncture kit used to access the jugular vein, is sandwiched inside the tunneler and tunneler cap assembly as shown. Bending or kinking of the wire may occur but will have no adverse effects. (B) Tunneling is performed as usual, thereby dragging the wire through the tract along with the tunneler.   (C) After tunneling, the wire is detached from the tunneler (D) and left in place through-and-through the tract. (E) A 3 Fr dilator from the micropuncture kit is passed over the wire until its distal tip is revealed from the neck incision. (F) The wire is removed and flowable thrombin hemostatic (D-Stat Flowable Hemostat, Vascular Solutions, Inc., Minneapolis MN) is injected into the dilator and into the peri-tract/peri-vein tissues. Focal pressure is applied to the neck site from which it would otherwise ooze. The dilator is withdrawn as material is injected, permeating the entire tract. The full tract must be massaged to allow complete permeation of the tract and exposure to tissues while expressing excess material. The material does not pass into the vein because of the catheter and the manual pressure applied to the neck.

Reference and Suggested Reading

1. Kerr A, Pathalapati R, Qiuhu S, Baumstein D. Purse-string suture to prevent bleeding after tunneled dialysis catheter insertion. J Vasc Interv Radiol. 2008 Aug;19(8):1176-9.

CHAPTER 48

Balloon-Assisted Removal of the Trapped Catheter

S. Lowell Kahn

Brief Description

Although uncommon, a trapped central venous catheter (CVC) can present a significant problem for the interventionalist and pose considerable risk to the patient. The use of chronic long-term CVCs is on the rise, with an average catheter dwell time of 10 months.[1] This is likely attributable to an aging population, exhaustion of sites for vascular access, urgent hemodialysis needs, and the failure or non-maturation of an arteriovenous fistula.[2,3] Although all CVCs are prone to complications, including vessel thrombosis or injury, infection, and catheter dysfunction, chronic catheters exhibit a higher rate of such complications, namely sepsis.[4-7] In addition, chronic catheters are at risk of becoming trapped, whereby they cannot be removed by standard technique.[8] Because of this rare but serious hazard, some advocate prophylactic catheter exchanges every 16–18 months, but this is not recommended by the National Kidney Foundation/Kidney Disease Outcomes Quality Initiative (NKF KDOQI).[9,10]

A trapped catheter typically occurs secondary to the development of a fibrin sheath, but iatrogenic causes are reported, including suture entrapment during cardiothoracic surgery and fissuring or penetration of the catheter with consequent adhesion.[6,11,12] Fibrin sheaths begin to form within 24 hours of catheter placement,[13] and their incidence is high, occurring in 13–57% of placements.[14] Although this commonly causes catheter dysfunction, it is rarely complicated by entrapment. A fibrin sheath results from damage to the endothelium from catheter contact resulting in thrombosis, smooth muscle proliferation, and venous stenosis.[2,12] Although many catheters encased in a fibrin can be safely removed with added or slow gentle traction, excessive traction can result in a fracture of the catheter with retained fragments or a potentially fatal vascular injury.[2,4,6,15] Retained fragments pose a risk of pulmonary embolization, vessel thrombosis, or may serve as a nidus for infection.[9,16] The incidence of trapped catheters is not known, but reports estimate it to range from 0.92% to 22%.[8,17] Factors that may favor entrapment include prolonged dwell time, female gender (smaller vessels), and left-sided catheter placement, secondary to increased surface contact between the vein and catheter.[2]

The management of the trapped catheter varies considerably in the literature. Due to the risks of an aggressive surgical removal, some groups advocate for conservative management, either leaving the entire catheter in situ or burying the remaining catheter subcutaneously after failed retrieval.[4,15,18,19] Unfortunately, conservative management bears its own risks due to the aforementioned risks of sepsis or vascular occlusion.

Subtle variations in retrieval technique for trapped catheters are described in the literature. Gladman et al.[20] describe successful retrieval of a catheter by applying slow, gentle traction over a prolonged period. An alternative technique whereby the stuck catheter is advanced into the patient over a guidewire to free it from the fibrin sheath before retracting it from the patient has been described as well.[21] More aggressive surgical and hybrid endovascular/surgical removal is well described in the literature, but an open thoracotomy with or without cardiopulmonary bypass is highly invasive and is not appropriate for most patients.[9,22,23]

In lieu of surgery, minimally invasive endovascular methods for retrieval of a trapped catheter have gained favor. Use of a snare to free the catheter from one or more accesses has been described on a limited basis.[2,24,25] Similarly, advancement of a sheath over a trapped catheter is also reported both with and without use of a laser.[26,27] Unfortunately, delivery of a coaxial sheath may prove quite difficult along a subcutaneous or tortuous tract, and the laser has inherent risks and expense associated with its use.[2]

In 2011, Hong[28] described a simple, elegant technique to remove a trapped CVC via inserting an angioplasty balloon into the lumen of a stuck catheter. The elastic nature of most catheters accommodates this dilatation without fragmentation of the catheter. Balloon dilatation expands the fibrin sheath (and hence the vein) and releases the adhesion between the catheter and the fibrin sheath. After dilatation, the catheter is readily removed. This technique has been confirmed by others.[17,29] Quaretti et al.[2] modified the technique with inclusion of a hemostatic sheath and a stiff guidewire inserted into the cut catheter to ensure hemostasis, prevent air embolism or endoluminal thrombosis, and avoid injury to the central veins and heart. Quaretti's group also endorses use of the balloon at a lower pressure to grip the catheter after dilatation and facilitate removal.

In our practice, we have embraced the methods described by both Hong and Quaretti et al. with great success. Although there is limited experience with this new technique, it appears to be a highly efficacious, safe, and cost-effective alternative. We have also found that this method works well on encrusted urinary catheters even though the pathophysiology of the encrustation varies greatly from the fibrin sheath of a trapped CVC.[30] Examples of both applications are provided later in this chapter.

Applications of the Technique

1. Removal of a trapped central venous catheter secondary to a fibrin sheath.
2. Removal of an encrusted urinary drainage catheter (e.g., nephrostomy, nephroureteral stent, and suprapubic tube).
3. Removal of other encrusted, chronic drainage catheters (e.g., biliary and abscess).

Challenges of the Procedure

1. If the catheter or drainage tube is occluded, a balloon may not pass, with or without a wire. We perform the technique with initial passage of a wire, but occasionally we have had difficulty passing the wire. Initial flushing of the catheter with subsequent passage of a stiff hydrophilic wire (e.g., stiff Glidewire, Terumo Medical Corp., Somerset, NJ) may be beneficial.
2. There is no size formula for the balloon because there are numerous different catheter, drainage tube, and balloon sizes. The technique can be performed with 0.014-, 0.018-, and 0.035-in. balloons. The chosen balloon should be low profile with good trackability, and it should readily pass through the lumen of the trapped catheter or drainage tube. We typically choose an initial balloon diameter that is approximately 30–50% larger than the diameter of the catheter or tube being removed. Larger balloons are then used as needed.
3. With tunneled catheters, some authors advocate dissection and removal of the tunneled portion with a cutdown to expose the catheter near the venotomy site. This provides a more direct access for advancement of the balloon and removal of the catheter. Depending on the catheter location and the patient's body habitus, this exposure can be challenging in some patients. Obviously, the cuff of any catheter must be freed prior to removal, but we have used this technique via a cutdown near the venotomy with transection of the catheter as well as through the hub of the intact catheter.

Potential Pitfalls/Complications

1. Reports in the literature indicate that this procedure is safe, and this is consistent with our own experience. However, the reports are limited to small series. In theory, there is a risk of catheter or tube fragmentation with consequent retained or embolized fragments. As noted previously, the elastic nature of most catheters and drainage tubes allows dilatation, but we nonetheless advocate starting with a small balloon and increasing size only as needed.
2. There is a small risk of hemorrhage with balloon dilatation, with a hemopericardium/tamponade being the most feared consequence. The balloon sizes needed for this technique are small and unlikely to result in this complication.
3. Similarly, when the technique is used in the urinary tract, there exists a small risk of bleeding or injury to the surrounding urothelial tissues (e.g., ureter).

Steps of the Procedure

1. The catheter or tube should be flushed with normal saline at the beginning of the procedure. If a heparin lock exists within the catheter, this should be aspirated first. Flushing the catheter or tube facilitates guidewire advancement in step 3.
2. If removing a tunneled catheter, the cuff of the catheter is freed from the subcutaneous tract. Occasionally, this is more difficult than usual because the trapped catheter does not retract to allow better exposure of the cuff. Therefore, in some cases, it may be beneficial to make an incision near the venotomy site to expose the catheter. The catheter is then cut, which allows removal of the tunneled segment and cuff and provides a more direct access to the stuck catheter.
3. Either through the cut catheter or through the hub of the intact catheter, a stiff hydrophilic guidewire is advanced beyond the tip. In the venous system, the wire is ideally advanced into the inferior vena cava for added stability. In the urinary tract, the wire can be advanced into the ureter or bladder. *Optional*: If a venous catheter is cut, an appropriately sized hemostatic sheath can be inserted into the cut end. This technique, described by Quaretti et al.,[2] has several advantages. The sheath prevents an air embolism or thrombosis because the catheter can be flushed. It also facilitates easier guidewire and balloon advancement.
4. A balloon is advanced into the trapped catheter or drainage tube. As stated previously, a 0.014-, 0.018-, or 0.035-in. wire can be chosen, depending on the size and make of the catheter or drainage tube being removed. We commonly select a 0.018-in. platform using a V-18 wire (Boston Scientific Inc.,

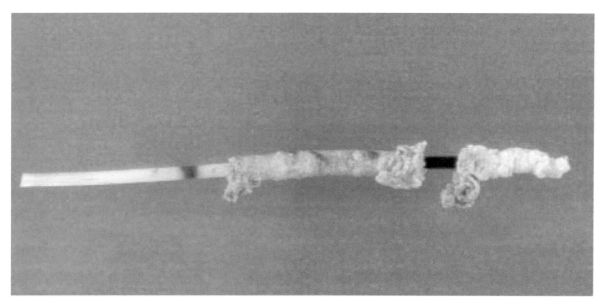

Figure 48.1 Central venous catheter tip with a surrounding fibrin sheath.
Source: From Filan PM, et al. Stuck long line syndrome. *Arch Dis Child.* 2005;90(6):558. Courtesy BMJ Publishing, Inc.

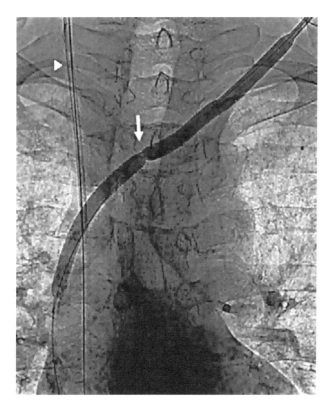

Figure 48.2 Balloon dilation of a Tesio catheter (Medical Components Inc., Harleysville, PA) during removal from a left internal jugular vein access. The right internal jugular Tesio catheter was removed over a wire (arrowhead) without incident. Note the waist (arrow) at the point of attachment during balloon dilation of the left internal jugular catheter.

Source: From Quaretti P, et al. A refinement of Hong's technique for the removal of stuck dialysis catheters: An easy solution to a complex problem. *J Vasc Access.* 2014;15(3):183–188. Courtesy Wichtig International Limited, Cheshire, UK.

Marlborough, MA), given its stiffness and hydrophilic tip that advances well through most catheters or drainage tubes. A low-profile balloon (e.g., Sterling, Boston Scientific Inc., Marlborough, MA) is then advanced over the wire. There is no specific formula for selecting the balloon. The balloon should pass easily into the trapped catheter/tube. We recommend an initial balloon diameter that is approximately 30–50% larger than the diameter of the catheter/tube being removed.

5. The balloon is inflated at the anticipated location of the fibrin sheath or encrustation. Commonly, a waist is seen at the point of attachment.

6. After dilatation, an attempt is made to remove the catheter or tube over a wire. Some authors suggest that the balloon be left partially inflated to provide greater traction (grip) during removal.[2]

7. If removal is unsuccessful, the balloon can be upsized, and steps 4–6 are repeated until successful removal is attained.

Example
See Figures 48.1–48.3.

References and Suggested Readings

1. Cetinkaya R, Odabas A, Unlu Y, Selcuk Y, Ates A, Ceviz M. Using cuffed and tunneled central venous catheters as permanent vascular access for hemodialysis: A prospective study. *Ren Fail.* 2003;25:431–438.

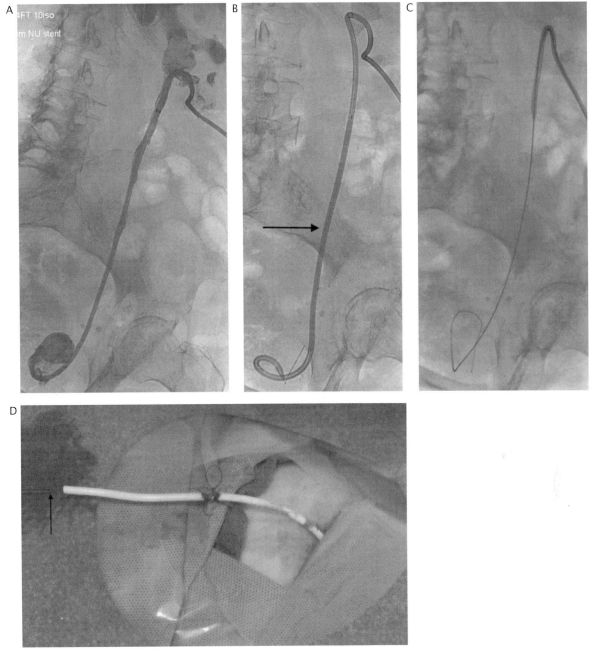

Figure 48.3 Removal of an encrusted 8.5 Fr nephroureteral stent. (A) Contrast injection through an existing nephroureteral stent outlines extensive debris and stones within the collecting system. The catheter would not remove over a wire. (B and C) A 3-mm × 150 mm Sterling balloon (arrow) was inserted and inflated at multiple locations within the encrusted nephroureteral stent over a V-18 wire that was advanced past the tip of the nephroureteral stent. (D) After dilatation, the nephroureteral stent was easily removed and exchanged for a new catheter.

2. Quaretti P, Galli F, Fiorina I, et al. A refinement of Hong's technique for the removal of stuck dialysis catheters: An easy solution to a complex problem. *J Vasc Access.* 2014;15(3):183–188.

3. Ethier J, Mendelssohn DC, Elder SJ, et al. Vascular access use and outcomes: An international perspective from the Dialysis Outcomes and Practice Patterns Study. *Nephrol Dial Transplant.* 2008;23(10):3219–3226.

4. Field M, Pugh J, Asquith J, Davies S, Pherwani AD. A stuck hemodialysis central venous catheter. *J Vasc Access.* 2008;9: 301–303.

5. Kanada DJ, Jung, RC, Ishihara S. Superior vena cava syndrome due to a retained central venous pressure catheter. *Chest.* 1979;76(6):734–735.

6. Schon D, Whittman D. Managing the complications of long-term tunneled dialysis catheters. *Semin Dial.* 2003;16(4): 314–322.

7. Sequeira A, Sachdeva B, Abreo K. Uncommon complications of long-term hemodialysis catheters: Adhesion, migration, and perforation by the catheter tip. *Semin Dial.* 2010;23(1):100–104.

8. Vellanki VS, Watson D, Rajan DK, Bhola CB, Lok CE. The stuck catheter: A hazardous twist to the meaning of permanent catheters. *J Vasc Access.* 2015;16(4):289–293.

9. Jafferbhoy SF, Asquith JR, Jeeji R, Levine A, Menon M, Pherwani AD. A stuck haemodialysis central venous catheter: Not quite open and shut! *J Surg Case Rep.* 2015;2015(4):rjv032.

10. Liu T, Hanna N, Summers D. Retained central venous hemodialysis catheters. *Nephrol Dial Transplant.* 2007;22:960–961.

11. Kong H, Chen S, Wen X. Suture of the right internal jugular vein catheter in a mitral valve replacement: A case report. *J Med Case Rep.* 2014;8:129.

12. Forauer AR, Theoharis C. Histologic changes in the human vein wall adjacent to indwelling central venous catheters. *J Vasc Interv Radiol.* 2003;14(9 Pt 1):1163–1168.

13. Filan PM, Woodward M, Ekert PG. Stuck long line syndrome. *Arch Dis Child.* 2005;90(6):558.

14. Suhocki PV, Conlon PJ, Knelson MH, Harland R, Schwab SJ. Silastic cuffed catheters for hemodialysis vascular access: Thrombolytic and mechanical correction of malfunction. *Am J Kidney Dis.* 1996;28:379–386.

15. Ndzengue A, Kessaris N, Dosani T, Mustafa N, Papalois V, Hakim NS. Mechanical complications of long-term Tesio catheters. *J Vasc Access.* 2009;10(1):50–54.

16. Thein H, Ratanjee SK. Tethered hemodialysis catheter with retained portions in central vein and right atrium on attempted removal. *Am J Kidney Dis.* 2005;46(3):e35–e39.

17. Ryan SE, Hadziomerovic A, Aquino J, Cunningham I, O'Kelly K, Rasuli P. Endoluminal dilatation technique to remove "stuck" tunneled hemodialysis catheters. *J Vasc Interv Radiol.* 2012;23(8):1089–1093.

18. Mira-Marceli NA, Gallego Mellado N, Mira Navarro J, et al. Conservative management of retained central venous catheters. *Cir Pediatr.* 2012;25(2):61–65.

19. Hassan A, Khalifa M, Al-Akraa M, Lord R, Davenport A. Six cases of retained central venous hemodialysis access catheters. *Nephrol Dial Transplant.* 2006;21:2005–2008.

20. Gladman G, Sinha S, Sims DG, Chiswick ML. Staphylococcus epidermidis and retention of neonatal percutaneous venous catheters. *Arch Dis Child.* 1990;65:234–235.

21. Huang SC, Tsai MS, Lai HS. A new technique to remove a "stuck" totally implantable venous access catheter. *J Pediatr Surg.* 2009;44(7):1465–1467.

22. Akgun S, Ak K, Tugrular S, Civelek A, Isbir C, Arsan S. Median sternotomy for an unexpected complication of permanent hemodialysis catheters: "Stuck catheter." *VASA.* 2008;37(3):293–296.

23. Wacker F, Cholewa D, Waldschmidt J, Wolf KJ. Percutaneous removal of a brachiocephalic vein anchored venous catheter with wire loop and mini-laparoscopy scissors. *RöFo.* 1999;170(2):225–227.

24. McIntyre CW, Taal MW, Fluck RJ, Hinwood D. Adherence of tunneled haemodialysis catheter to superior vena caval stent: Successful percutaneous removal. *Nephrol Dial Transplant.* 2003;18(2):432-433.

25. Foley PT, Carter RM, Uberoi R. Endovascular removal of long-term hemodialysis catheters. *Cardiovasc Intervent Radiol.* 2007;30(5):1079–1081.

26. Carrillo RG, Garisto JD, Salman L, Merrill D, Asif A. A novel technique for tethered dialysis catheter removal using the laser sheath. *Semin Dial.* 2009;22(6):688–691.

27. Bastian D, Fessele K, Bednarski P, Bodenschatz K, Pauschinger M, Göhl K. Laser extraction of a trapped infected port catheter in a child using existing experience from pacemaker and ICD lead removal. *Pacing Clin Electrophysiol.* 2011;34(1):e9–e10.

28. Hong JH. A breakthrough technique for the removal of a hemodialysis catheter stuck in the central vein: Endoluminal balloon dilatation of the stuck catheter. *J Vasc Access.* 2011;12(4):381–384.

29. Farooq A, Jones V, Agarwal S. Balloon dilatation: A helpful technique for removal of a stuck dialysis line. *Cardiovasc Interv Radiol.* 2012;35(6):1528–1530.

30. Stickler DJ, Feneley RC. The encrustation and blockage of long-term indwelling bladder catheters: A way forward in prevention and control. *Spinal Cord.* 2010;48(11):784–790.

CHAPTER 49

The Rapid Fistula Declot

Dean C. Preddie and Gregg A. Miller

Brief Description

The rapid fistula declot is an endovascular approach to efficiently salvage the acutely thrombosed dialysis arteriovenous fistula (AVF). Thrombectomy of the AVF has historically been performed in the inpatient setting, but the advent of the outpatient vascular access center has vastly improved the efficiency and cost-effectiveness of dialysis access management.[1] Fistula surveillance has generally been accepted to improve the life span of the AVF;[2] however, due to the contribution of multiple factors, including uremia-induced vascular dysfunction,[3] acute access thrombosis remains an issue. Fistula declot techniques have improved in safety, effectiveness, and durability over time.[4,5] As such, our rapid fistula declot technique combines best practices gleaned from several accepted methods[6] to achieve safe, effective, and rapid turnaround with maximal durability.[7]

Critical to our procedure is assessing the volume of thrombus burden and determining the hemodynamically significant stenoses that contributed to access thrombosis. The approach to removing thrombus is entirely dependent on the volume of thrombus. For example, a small forearm AVF may contain as little as 5 cc of thrombus and require nothing more than balloon maceration of the clot. Conversely, a large upper arm fistula may contain 60 cc of clot and require a combination of thrombolysis with tissue plasminogen activator (tPA), rotational thrombectomy devices, manual thromboaspiration, or even direct incision techniques with manual debulking of clot depending on the size of the aneurysms. In short, the greater the thrombus burden, the more tools may be required to ensure thorough clot removal.

Furthermore, it is useful to preoperatively determine if the critical lesion is in the outflow, inflow, or conduit. A detailed physical exam combined with ultrasound evaluation helps to stage the procedure and identifies the appropriate site for vascular sheath placement. Prior fluoroscopic images provide historical precedent, helping to finalize the plan for the procedure.

The rapid fistula declot is encapsulated in a simple algorithm of (1) clot removal, (2) repair of culprit stenoses, and (3) flow restoration. The preferred approach to each step is discretionary as long as near-complete evacuation of the fistula and venous outflow pathways of thrombus precedes flow restoration.

Clearing fresh thrombus as well as mural fibrin can be achieved through manual catheter-directed thromboaspiration techniques, with or without antecedent thrombolytic agents or rotational thrombectomy devices. Repair of culprit AVF and venous outflow stenoses completes the establishment of a clean AVF cannulation zone and venous outflow pathway. Now, removal of the arterial plug restores unobstructed AVF blood flow that need only to be enhanced by potential repair of hemodynamically significant arterial inflow stenoses. Final fluoroscopic confirmation is then performed.

Applications of the Technique

1. Acutely or subacutely thrombosed mature AVF or arteriovenous graft (AVG).
2. Thrombosed AVF (or AVG) with extensive thrombus burden.
3. Thrombosed AVF (or AVG) with convincing evidence of a venous outflow stenosis or obstruction, where clot removal is necessary for both immediate and long-term success.

Challenges of the Procedure

1. Complete evacuation of adherent thrombus may prove impossible, thus leaving laminar remnants that are refractory to thrombolytic agents or remain after restoration of blood flow.
2. Chronic mural fibrin deposition may become unroofed and impossible to aspirate, necessitating conversion to an open thrombectomy procedure for removal.
3. Subacute thrombus burden may at best be partially liquefied with thrombolytic agents prior to thromboaspiration techniques, especially in the significantly enlarged or aneurysmal AVF.
4. The immature clotted AVF tends to be more fragile, and venous perforation can complicate any attempt to declot the fistula. Of note, all balloons and mechanical devices can seriously damage the fistula pathway. In nearly all cases, tPA should be used with a small amount of contrast to help determine the true access pathway.

Potential Pitfalls/Complications

1. Risk of pulmonary embolism: The angled suction catheter can inadvertently dislodge adherent thrombus, embolizing fragments to the central venous circulation and ultimately the lungs. In addition, mechanical maceration techniques using rotational thrombectomy devices can sequentially encourage embolization of mounting thrombus burden into the pulmonary vasculature. Clearly, paradoxical embolization can prove catastrophic in the setting of a patent foramen ovale. Preemptive thrombolysis may reduce this risk significantly.

2. Risk of downstream arterial embolism: Intentional care must be taken to avoid inadvertently embolizing the arterial plug by attempting to aspirate thrombus via the retrograde vascular sheath. Again, the angled catheter can dislodge the arterial plug during placement.

3. Risk of venous rupture: The relatively thin-walled conduit and venous outflow pathways, especially in the setting of the uremic milieu, can easily rupture in response to percutaneous transluminal angioplasty (PTA) or during use of any of the mechanical rotational devices.

Steps of the Procedure

1. Gain bidirectional AVF access: Initial antegrade (outflow) access is necessary to prioritize the clearance of the fistula and venous outflow pathways of thrombus. The retrograde (inflow) sheath is used to determine the anatomy of the arterial anastomosis. Ultrasound should be used to identify the anatomy prior to the use of fluoroscopy.

2. Confirm central venous patency: After gaining access in the antegrade direction, central venous patency is confirmed using a guidewire-directed diagnostic catheter. This step ensures a patent venous outflow pathway for optimal access function as well as excludes potentially life-threatening central venous thrombus burden. If a large amount of thrombus is present in the central veins, then one must be prepared to stent the thrombus in place or abandon the procedure. Alternatively, a patient can be admitted to the intensive care unit for an overnight tPA infusion.

3. Pullback venogram: A pullback venogram defines the venous anatomy, critical venous outflow stenoses, and extent of thrombus burden. Furthermore, commingled contrast and tPA help to "loosen" the thrombus, rendering it easier to aspirate.

4. Mechanical thromboaspiration: We use a firm "hockey stick" angled 7 Fr catheter with a wide lumen and atraumatic tip to make direct contact with the most proximal limit of the thrombus. Manual thromboaspiration is performed using a 60-cc (Luer-Lock) syringe while the catheter is slowly dragged back with rapid seesaw movements, which help to further detach laminar thrombus for aspiration. Manual compression of the access during aspiration generates improved wall contact, especially in enlarged or aneurysmal fistulas. Each time the catheter is removed from the access, it is flushed through gauze to demonstrate the quantity of aspirated thrombus. This step is repeated until the entire thrombus burden is largely cleared. The completion of this step cannot be overstated because the restoration of fresh blood flow into an insufficiently cleared fistula is a recipe for rethrombosis.

5. Mechanical rotational devices: Multiple devices have been shown to be very effective in lysing and removing thrombus from the AVF, but we have narrowed our scope to three such devices. First, the Arrow Trerotola Percutaneous Thrombectomy Device (Teleflex Medical Europe Ltd., Westmeath, Ireland) is either an over-the-wire or a self-guided rotational device that is directed into the thrombus and rotates at 3000 rpm to recanalize the efferent venous pathway.[8] It is equipped with a side port into which tPA can be instilled, enhancing its performance.[9] Second, the AngioJet (Boston Scientific Inc., Marlborough, MA) is an over-the-wire percutaneous rheolytic thrombectomy device that utilizes high-pressure saline jets to create a low-pressure area at the catheter tip. This method generates a strong vacuum, drawing thrombus into the catheter to be fragmented and removed. Although heparin is required, thrombolytic agents are unnecessary for this device to be effective.[10] Third, the Cleaner Rotational Thrombectomy system (Argon Medical Devices Inc., Plano, TX) is a self-directed device that is manufactured with two sinusoidal wire amplitudes (9 and 15 mm), each delivering 4000 rpm of rotational velocity. The large rotational diameter renders excellent wall contact in enlarged or aneurysmal AVF. It also has a side port for easy instillation of saline, contrast, or tPA.[11] To date, no rotational thrombectomy device has proven superiority; however, their use seems to offer improved efficiency with high immediate success and secondary patency rates (without improvement in long-term patency).[12]

6. Confirm access clearance: Confirmation of a cleared access can be ascertained either by gently pulsing contrast into the fistula under fluoroscopy or by direct ultrasound visualization. Infused contrast also exposes any culprit or potentially hemodynamically significant stenoses.

7. Treat culprit stenoses: Once the fistula body and main venous outflow pathway are cleared of thrombus, PTA is then performed to treat stenoses and ensure the venous outflow pathway is sufficiently patent prior to restoration of blood flow. Furthermore, PTA allows for maceration of any residual laminar thrombus missed during the mechanical thromboaspiration.

8. Catheterization of the feeding artery: Attention is then directed toward the arterial inflow, and access is gained in the retrograde direction. We do not aspirate the arterial plug in AVFs because the blunt end of the angulated catheter is likely to increase the risk of distal arterial embolization. (Arterial limb thromboaspiration is reserved for loop AVGs with a significantly lengthy arterial inflow segment.) A guidewire directed diagnostic catheter is navigated into the upstream (feeding) artery, and imaging is obtained to both confirm adequate arterial inflow and to rule out distal arterial emboli.

9. Restore blood flow: An embolectomy catheter is then utilized to retrieve the arterial plug, which is macerated between the opposing vascular sheaths. With blood flow re-established, we can troubleshoot for contributors to the original thrombosis or consequences of our declot procedure.

10. Rule out downstream arterial emboli: It is imperative to image the downstream arterial tree for inadvertent arterial emboli as well as palpate the distal arterial pulses. Even asymptomatic emboli are considered pathologic and must be removed (by embolectomy catheter or back-bleeding) or lysed (by direct tPA injection).

11. Inspect the access: Finally, we inspect the entire access circuit, from feeding artery to central venous circulation, for any residual stenosis or retained thrombus. Although angioplasty is our first-line therapy for significant stenoses, stent placement is considered for resistant lesions (despite high-pressure balloon PTA), immediate and significant elastic recoil (despite prolonged and repeated PTA), or acute venous rupture refractory to balloon tamponade. Residual thrombus is cleared using an embolectomy catheter or macerated via PTA. Confirmatory imaging completes the rapid fistula declot.

References and Suggested Readings

1. Ito Y, Sato T, Okada R, et al. Comparison of clinical effectiveness between surgical and endovascular treatment for thrombotic obstruction in hemodialysis access. *J Vasc Access.* 2011;12(1):63–66.

2. Aragoncillo I, Amezquita Y, Caldes S, et al. The impact of access blood flow surveillance on reduction of thrombosis in native arteriovenous fistula: A randomized clinical trial. *J Vasc Access.* 2016;17(1):13–19.

3. Brunet P, Gondouin B, Duval-Sabatier A, et al. Does uremia cause vascular dysfunction. *Kidney Blood Pressure Res.* 2011;34:284–290.

4. Beathard GA, Litchfield T. Effectiveness and safety of dialysis vascular access procedures performed by interventional nephrologists. *Kidney Int.* 2004;66(4):1622–1632.

5. Bittl JA. Catheter interventions for hemodialysis fistulas and grafts. *JACC Cardiovasc Interv.* 2010;3(1):1–11.

6. Turmel-Rodrigues L, Raynaud A, Louail B, Beyssen B, Sapoval M. Manual catheter-directed aspiration and other thrombectomy techniques for declotting native fistulas for hemodialysis. *J Vasc Interv Radiol.* 2001;12:1365–1371.

7. Nikam MD, Ritchie J, Jayanti A, et al. Acute arteriovenous access failure: Long-term outcomes of endovascular salvage and assessment of co-variates affecting patency. *Nephron.* 2005;129:241–246.

8. Shatsky JB, Berns JS, Clark TW, et al. Single-center experience with the Arrow-Trerotola Percutaneous Thrombectomy Device in the management of thrombosed native dialysis fistulas. *J Vasc Interv Radiol.* 2005;16:1605–1611.

9. Patane D, Messina M, Morale W, et al. Improving the effectiveness of the Trerotola Percutaneous Thrombectomy Device in thrombosed dialysis arteriovenous fistulas. *J Vasc Access.* 2010;11(4):360–361.

10. Maleux G, De Coster B, Laenen A, et al. Percutaneous rheolytic thrombectomy of thrombosed autogenous dialysis fistulas: Technical results, clinical outcome and factors influencing patency. *J Endovasc Ther.* 2015;22(1):80–86.

11. Kojsoy C, Fatih Yilmaz M, Serdar Basbug H, et al. Pharmacomechanical thrombolysis of symptomatic acute and subacute deep vein thrombosis with a rotational thrombectomy device. *J Vasc Interv Radiol.* 2014;25(12):1895–1900.

12. Yang CC, Yang CW, Wen SC, Wu CC. Comparisons of clinical outcomes for thrombectomy devices with different mechanisms in hemodialysis arteriovenous fistulas. *Catheter Cardiovas Interv* 2012;80(6):1035–1041.

CHAPTER 50

Endovascular Options for Nonmaturing Fistulas due to Collateral Flow

Jayesh M. Soni

Brief Description

Of available hemodialysis accesses, the surgically created fistula is the ideal access type, with the best 4- and 5-year patency rates, and requiring minimal intervention compared to other access types.[1] An ideal access is one that delivers an appropriate flow rate for dialysis, has a long useful life, and has a low rate of complications, including infection, stenosis, thrombosis, aneurysm, and limb ischemia. Patients should have a functional permanent access at the time of dialysis initiation. Following the rule of 6's as per NKF DOQI guidelines, a functional access should yield a flow rate of at least 600 ml/minute, should be less than 6 mm below the surface of the skin, and should have a minimal diameter of 6 mm.

The surgically created fistula needs to mature before it can be used and this typically takes 8–12 weeks. Fistula maturation time is dependent on the size and anatomic qualities of the venous and arterial components of the fistula.[1] A fistula that fails to mature during this time remains difficult to cannulate and is of insufficient diameter to provide adequate flow for dialysis.

There are multiple causes for failed maturation of an AVF, including a small feeding artery and/or outflow vein of the fistula, central vein occlusion or stenosis, post-surgical flow and pressure derangement, and multiple competing collateral veins.[2] Ideally, the afferent artery of an AVF should measure more than 1.5–2 mm. The chosen outflow vein should measure at least 2–2.5 mm in diameter. When there are multiple competing collateral veins, the possibility of the vein maturing after AVF creation decreases considerably.[2] Collateral veins close to the arterial anastomosis are usually ligated during creation of the fistula. However, collateral veins deeper and/or more distant from the anastomosis are difficult to ligate surgically. Endovascular management of competing collateral veins with embolization promotes maturation of the fistula. Embolization can be performed with either coils or endovascular plugs. Early AVF thrombosis can lead to failed maturation and has similar underlying derangements.

Although competing collateral veins can be surgically ligated, in this chapter we discuss embolization as a technically feasible, safe, and highly efficacious technique to salvage an immature fistula or a fistula that experiences early thrombosis.

Applications of the Technique

1. Salvage of a non-maturing AVF
2. Salvage of a fistula that has experienced an early thrombosis
3. Treatment of an existing fistula with an inadequate flow rate

Challenges of the Procedure

1. A major challenge is the completely occluded venous outflow tract that cannot be traversed by guidewire. In these cases, flow is diverted through one or more collateral veins to the central veins. Once clotted, the native fistula outflow can be very difficult to revascularize.
2. Another challenge is a long stricture or diffuse tapering of the venous outflow tract that does not respond to angioplasty. This can be markedly improved with repeated balloon-assisted maturation and embolization of the competing collaterals.
3. Arterial Insufficiency: Many dialysis patients have atherosclerotic disease, frequently the result of uncontrolled diabetes. This can lead to poor arterial inflow to the fistula. At times, the arterial anastomosis is not amenable to dilatation secondary to tortuous or strictured anatomy.

Potential Pitfalls/Complications

1. There is a risk of occluding the fistula when accessing an immature fistula. This is because of the large size of the sheath relative to the small outflow vein. The sheath can occlude flow and result in thrombosis of the entire outflow vein. Fortunately, this complication is rare. Other complications include local hematoma formation, inadvertent coiling of the outflow vein, pain and erythema at the site of collateral vein embolization, migration of embolized coils, and,

rarely, skin erosion at the site of superficial collateral vein embolization.

2. A hematoma can result from cannulation of the fistula, or more commonly, angioplasty of the immature fistula. In most cases, the hematoma is self-limiting and is controlled simply by application of local pressure and conservative measures. However, on occasion balloon tamponade or placement of a covered stent is necessary to control extravasation.

Steps of the Procedure

1. Initial Examination: Initial physical examination and/or Doppler ultrasound aids in finding the optimal location for access. When an inflow stenosis is suspected, the needle is directed retrograde (toward the arterial anastomosis).

2. Initial Access: Based on ultrasound or physical exam findings, the initial cannulation is directed centrally (toward the venous outflow), peripherally (toward the arterial anastomosis), or a direct antegrade proximal arterial (typically brachial) access is used if the outflow vein is very small. It is advisable to obtain access with a micropuncture set, which is less traumatic and allows for a 0.018-in. guidewire with subsequent placement of the 4 or 5 Fr micropuncture sheath (transitional dilator).

3. Diagnostic Fistulography: The fistulagram can be performed through the 4 or 5 Fr micropuncture sheath. If any endovascular interventions are required, the sheath is upsized as required for the planned intervention. If the initial cannulation is directed retrograde toward the arterial anastomosis, the afferent artery proximal to the arterial anastomosis should be catheterized with a 4 or 5 Fr catheter. From here, optimal imaging of the entire AV fistula may be obtained, including the arterial inflow to the fistula and the arterial anastomosis. Additionally, in cases of distal hypoperfusion/steal syndrome, assessment of the extremity arterial vasculature distal to the fistula can be made. In rare cases in which the catheter cannot be advanced into the feeding artery, the fistulagram is performed by injecting contrast as close as possible to the arterial anastomosis. Manual pressure or balloon occlusion of the fistula can be used to reflux contrast to the arterial anastomosis during digital subtraction angiography.

4. Fistulagram Interpretation: Once the fistulagram is obtained, a detailed study of the feeding artery, arteriovenous anastomosis, and outflow vein is essential to determine the etiology of the immature fistula.[2] There may be an inflow problem, such as a small feeding artery, arterial anastomosis stenosis, low cardiac output, and so forth. Similarly, a small-caliber outflow vein, outflow vein stenosis, central vein stenosis, or multiple outflow veins can all result in the fistula failing to mature. Assessing the entirety of the fistula is crucial because the arterial anastomosis and the juxta-arterial segment stenosis are the cause of failed maturation in approximately 10% of cases.

5. Intervention: If one or more competing collateral veins are identified, embolization should be performed. Embolization of the collateral vein(s) may require a separate access depending on their location and orientation relative to the access. The largest collateral vein should be embolized first, followed by the second largest and so forth. Initially, two or three large competing collateral veins should be embolized in the first intervention. Embolization is performed with either coils or endovascular plugs. The decision is based on the size and location (deep vs. superficial) of the target collateral vein, the size of the catheter or sheath that can be safely advanced to the target vein, and the available inventory. In some patients it is necessary to not only embolize the collateral vein(s), but to also angioplasty a focal stenosis in the outflow vein or the entire outflow vein if it is diffusely small caliber.

6. Post-embolization Fistulagram: After embolization, follow-up fistulography should show complete occlusion of the collateral vein(s). Complete occlusion is often seen with endovascular plugs. However, when coils are used there is frequently minimal flow immediately after placement, but complete occlusion is typically observed on follow-up fistulagrams.

7. Follow-up: All patients should have a repeat fistulagram within 1 month of embolization. The follow-up fistulagram will ascertain the success of the prior embolization, the need for additional embolization, and whether the fistula is properly maturing. On occasion, after the large collateral veins are embolized, other collateral veins may enlarge and require embolization.

Example
See Figure 50.1.

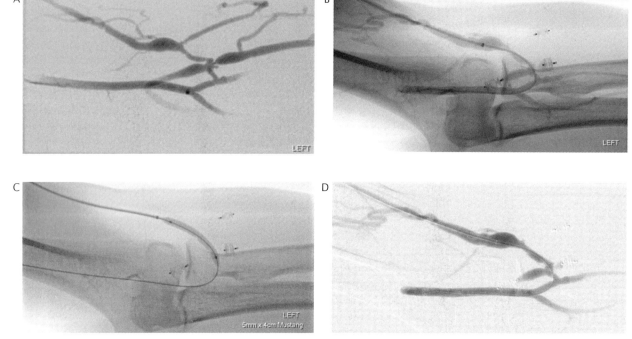

Figure 50.1 (A) Left radial artery-to-antecubital vein AV dialysis fistulogram, which shows small-caliber outflow vein with multiple collateral veins. In this patient, it was difficult to delineate the arterial anastomosis and so brachial arterial access was obtained. (B) After assessing the fistulogram, a second access was obtained in the outflow vein toward the arterial anastomosis and embolization of three collateral veins with Amplatzer plugs was performed. (C) Further angioplasty was performed at arterial anastomosis to improve inflow with a 5-mm balloon catheter. (D) Post embolization fistulogram shows complete occlusion of the embolized collateral veins with excellent flow to outflow vein.

References and Suggested Readings

1. National Kidney Foundation. *2006 Updates: Clinical Practice Guidelines and Recommendations.* New York: National Kidney Foundation; 2006.

2. Nassar GM. Endovascular management of the "failing to mature" arteriovenous fistula. *Tech Vasc Interv Radiol.* 2008;11:175–180.

CHAPTER 51

Percutaneous Creation of Jump Bypass in a Native Arteriovenous Hemodialysis Fistula

Peter Miller, Sabah Butty, and Thomas Casciani

Brief Description

We describe the technique of percutaneous creation of jump bypass grafts in nonmature and failed arteriovenous hemodialysis fistulas based on a case series of 10 patients. Percutaneous intervention has been used to salvage nonmature fistulas, dysfunctional fistulas, and grafts. Frequently, venous outflow stenosis is the major cause of arteriovenous fistula and graft failure. Long-segment and chronically occluded venous outflow stenoses are more difficult to treat percutaneously and may require surgical revision. We describe an endovascular technique creating a percutaneous jump bypass from the cephalic vein to the basilic vein using stent grafts in all patients with excellent immediate results. Limited available follow-up is also reported, including patency of two stent grafts for more than 2 years.

The case example presented in this chapter demonstrates a brachiocephalic fistula with long-segment outflow venous occlusion. Through-and-through guidewire accesses were obtained in the cephalic vein accesses. Another antegrade access was obtained in the basilic vein. The guidewire was then tunneled in a subcutaneous fashion from the retrograde cephalic vein access to the antegrade basilic vein access, allowing re-entry in the outflow for the dialysis conduit via the peel-away sheath. The subcutaneous tunnel, vascular exit site, and vascular re-entry site were balloon dilated. Overlapping Viabahn stent grafts (W.L. Gore & Associates Inc., Flagstaff, AZ) were placed.

Applications of the Technique

The natural history of arteriovenous fistulas and grafts is a gradual stenosis of the venous anastomosis or outflow vein limb. This issue creates the need for lifelong interventions, primarily by angioplasty and stenting of the diseased segments, which ultimately will fail and require creation of a new fistula or graft. There are few recently described percutaneous endovascular techniques for salvage of chronic hemodialysis venous outflow obstruction. Chen et al.[1] were the first to describe percutaneous bypass graft technique to salvage a hemodialysis graft by placing a stent graft (Wallgraft, Boston Scientific, Marlborough, MA) between the venous end of the graft and the basilic vein. They reported only 90-day patency. Heller and Clark[2] reported a percutaneous creation of a venous anastomosis in a native thrombosed immature brachiocephalic fistula with an occluded outflow vein with a parallel vein–vein anastomosis without the use of a stent graft. They reported no long-term results because the patient died. Kuo et al.[3] reported successful salvage of a brachiocephalic dialysis graft by creating a percutaneous jump bypass graft from the cephalic vein to the basilic vein using a stent graft, and they demonstrated 8-month patency. Timpone and Gover[4] reported successful salvage of a native brachiocephalic fistula by percutaneous creation of a jump bypass from the cephalic vein to the brachial vein with a stent graft, and they have reported 9-month patency. We describe our experience with a similar technique of salvaging brachiocephalic fistulas with severe outflow vein stenosis and/or occlusion by placing a jump bypass graft from the patent cephalic vein near the arterial anastomosis to the patent basilic vein.

Challenges of the Procedure

1. It is challenging to create the tunnel between the two connecting veins.
2. Dilating the subcutaneous track to allow insertion of a large sheath for the covered stent requires much effort.

Potential Pitfalls/Complications

1. Brachial plexus nerve injury and brachial artery compression/occlusion if brachial vein is used instead of

basic vein. We chose the basilic vein because such risks are much smaller.

2. Hematoma formation at vessel access sites.
3. Off-label use of Viabahn.
4. Steal syndrome.
5. Infection of the stent graft.
6. Fracture of the stent graft during dialysis access.

Steps of the Procedure

Using modified Seldinger technique, "through-and-through" guidewire access is acquired in the cephalic vein remnant just central to the arterial venous anastomosis. The antegrade access is made with a standard dialysis sheath for eventual upsize, and the second access site is acquired with a 4 or 5 Fr peel-away sheath in the cephalic vein in the retrograde direction at the anticipated location of the extravascular passage of the stent graft ("peripheral anastomosis"). A third access with a peel-away sheath is acquired in the antegrade direction in the basilic vein at the desired site of re-entry for the stent graft ("central anastomosis").

Through-and-through access (0.035-in. Terumo glidewire) is acquired in the cephalic vein accesses by placing the glidewire through the antegrade sheath and externalized out the retrograde sheath. The glidewire is then tunneled in a subcutaneous fashion from the retrograde cephalic vein access to the antegrade basilic vein access, allowing re-entry in the outflow for the dialysis conduit via the peel-away sheath. Using a Cook 4 Fr slip catheter, the glidewire is eventually exchanged for a Lunderquist wire (Cook Medical, Bloomington, IN).

The subcutaneous tunnel, vascular exit site, and vascular re-entry site are balloon dilated (8 mm × 8-cm Dorado, Bard, Tempe, AZ) following placement of a 7 Fr Ansel sheath (Cook Medical) with the tip within the basilic vein outflow tract.

The 7 Fr sheath is exchanged for a larger sheath, varying in sizes up to 12 Fr. Through this access, overlapping stent grafts are placed (Viabahn stent grafts ranging in size from 8 to 13 mm). One to three stent grafts are used per case, and sizes also varied. Most patients require a bypass length of at least 15 cm. Overlapping stent grafts of the same size can be used in some patients, and overlapping stent grafts of varying sizes can also be used in certain situations. The average size of stent grafts used in our experience was 10 mm with average length of 15 cm. For example, one patient required 8-, 10-, and 13-mm overlapping Viabahns. The cephalic vein remnant should be a minimum of 6–8 cm to do the procedure, with a desirable minimum diameter of 6–8 mm. The stent grafts were overlapped by 33%, and it was best if 2 or 3 cm of stent was in the basilic vein. The stent grafts were balloon dilated to full diameter and at times 1 mm past full diameter. The access sites were closed with resorbable suture (4-0 Vicryl) and Dermabond.

Results

Limited follow-up on our 10-patient experience demonstrates an encouraging alternative to abandoning a failing fistula. It is difficult to compare patency rates of our patients given the small number treated. However, the primary patency of grafts was 38.2% at 1 year, and secondary patency was 71.8% at 1 year.[5] With the limited follow-up, 2 of 10 patients had primary patency at 1 year, and likely 2 other patients were lost to follow-up to confirm patency. Seven of 10 patients were patent without reintervention at 3 months, and 4 patients were patent at 6 months. These outcomes are similar to expected outcomes of surgically revised thrombosed grafts. The Dialysis Outcomes Quality Initiative (DOQI) Work Group recommends a primary patency rate of 50% at 6 months and 40% at 1 year for surgically revised thrombosed grafts. In the limited follow-up reported, minimal reinteventions were done to the bypass stent graft. Most repeated interventions were of other stenosis of the native portion of the fistula or nonstented portion of the fistula. Three patients required angioplasty of stenosis of the stent or vein immediately adjacent to the stent. The longest followed patient had a patent stent graft more than 2 years. Of three interventions in the patient to keep his fistula functioning, only one was to treat in-stent stenosis at 12 months. Only 2 of 10 patients had problems within 3 months of bypass: One patient's fistula was taken down because of steal syndrome, and one required angioplasty of a juxta-anastomotic stenosis. Two stent grafts had to be removed because of infection at 5 and 16 months.

Comparison of Jump Bypass Graft Patencies

The following graph compares the jump bypass graft patencies for the 10 patients included in the study. A shift in color denotes intervention required to maintain patency. Events responsible of cessation of fistula use are denoted on the graph. Fadeout of bars indicates continued use of fistula or unknown outcome.

Example

See Figures 51.1–51.8.

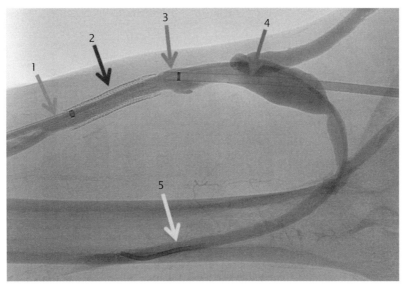

Figure 51.1 Brachiocephalic fistula with chronically stenotic flow limiting cephalic outflow stenosis that had been previously stented (arrow 2). Antegrade access cephalic vein peripheral to occlusion (arrow 4), eventual retrograde access cephalic vein with peel-away sheath (arrow 3), brachial artery (arrow 5), and initial retrograde access for fistulogram (arrow 1).

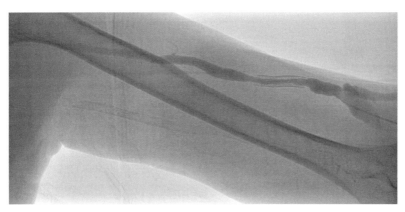

Figure 51.2 Brachiocephalic fistulogram demonstrates poor cephalic outflow.

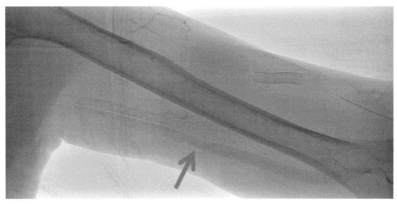

Figure 51.3 Brachiocephalic fistulogram demonstrates patent basilic vein (arrow).

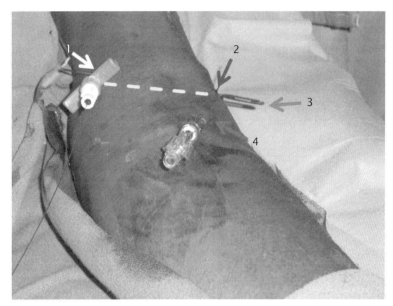

Figure 51.4 Photo demonstrating access sites and tunnel. Peel- away sheath antegrade access into basilic vein (arrow 1), antegrade sheath in cephalic vein peripheral to occlusion/chronically stenotic cephalic vein (arrow 4), site of retrograde cephalic vein access (arrow 2), tunneling device (arrow 3), and subcutaneous tunnel path (white dotted line).

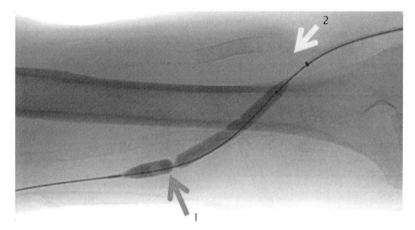

Figure 51.5 Balloon angioplasty of subcutaneous tunnel between cephalic vein (arrow 2) and basilic vein (arrow 1).

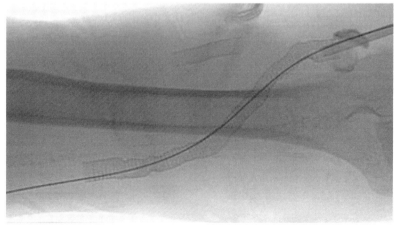

Figure 51.6 Overlapping Viabahn stent grafts between the cephalic and basilic veins.

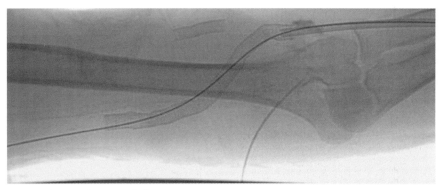

Figure 51.7 Viabahn stent grafts after balloon dilation.

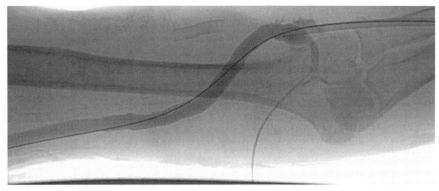

Figure 51.8 Post-bypass fistulogram demonstrates excellent flow through stent graft and basilic outflow vein.

References and Suggested Readings

1. Chen MC, Liang HL, Wu DK, et al. Percutaneous vein graft reanastomosis with use of a covered stent to salvage a thrombosed hemodialysis graft. *J Vasc Interv Radiol.* 2005;16:1385–1389.
2. Heller SL, Clark TW. Percutaneous creation of a venous anastomosis in a native hemodialysis fistula. *J Vasc Interv Radiol.* 2009;20:1371–1375.
3. Kuo MD, Son DH, Miller FJ. Salvage of a failing dialysis graft by percutaneous creation of a jump bypass graft. *J Vasc Interv Radiol.* 2007;8:1054–1058.
4. Timpone VM, Gover DD. Percutaneous creation of a jump bypass graft in a native arteriovenous hemodialysis fistula. *J Vasc Interv Radiol.* 2011;5:734–736.
5. Gibson KD, Gillen DL, Caps MT, et al. Vascular access survival and incidence of revisions: A comparison of prosthetic grafts, simple autogenous fistulas, and venous transposition fistulas from the United States Renal Date System Dialysis Morbidity and Mortality Study. *J Vasc Surg.* 2001;34:694–700.

CHAPTER 52

Using a Glidewire Cheater and Flow Switch to Temporarily Secure Purse-String Sutures

Adam N. Plotnik and Stephen Kee

Brief Description

Following completion of an arteriovenous (AV) graft or fistula intervention, various methods exist by which an interventionalist may achieve hemostasis. Manual compression is the simplest technique but often requires an extended period of time. Many interventionalists will place purse-string sutures at the site of vascular access to achieve hemostasis, with the sutures left in place when the patient leaves the angiography suite. Consequently, these sutures may stay in for an extended period of time and even be present at follow-up interventions many months later or, worse, may get infected. The "glidewire cheater and flow switch" technique is a method by which hemostasis can be achieved and obviates the need for the sutures to be left in place after the patient leaves the angiography suite. When completing the AV graft or fistula intervention, the interventionalist places a purse-string suture at the site of the vascular sheath access without applying a knot. The vascular sheath is then removed, and the two limbs of the sutures are held taught and threaded into a glidewire cheater. Subsequently, a one-way flow switch is then tightened down against the cheater and "cocked off." This apparatus is left in place for 10–15 minutes, allowing enough time to complete the requisite post-procedure paperwork. Following this, the sutures can be loosened by releasing the flow switch, and if hemostasis is achieved, it can be simply removed.

Application of the Technique

1. Following completion of an AV graft or AV fistula intervention, such as a declot procedure.
2. The procedure may be of particular benefit in patients for whom there is questionable follow-up due to patient social factors.

Challenges of the Procedure

1. Once an appropriately placed purse-string suture has been placed at the vascular sheath access site, the procedure is relatively straightforward.

Potential Pitfalls/Complications

1. Poorly placed purse-string suture that does not allow for adequate hemostasis with sutures held taught and locked with the one-way flow switch.
2. A suture knot that is tied before placing the glidewire cheater and one-way flow switch.

Steps of the Procedure

1. Following completion of an AV graft or AV fistula intervention, a purse-string suture is placed surrounding both the vascular sheaths as per standard technique.
2. With the vascular sheath still left in place, a glidewire cheater together with a one-way flow switch are placed over the ends of the suture. Note that to allow for easy removal of the suture at the end of the procedure, it is important not to tie a knot prior to placing the glidewire cheater and one-way flow switch.
3. The vascular sheath is then removed. With the ends of the purse-string suture held taught, the glidewire cheater together with the one-way flow switch are then advanced to the vascular access site, and the purse-string suture is then locked by closing the flow switch.
4. The temporarily locked purse-string suture is then left in place for approximately 10–15 minutes, at which time the interventionalist may complete the requisite post-procedure paperwork.
5. Following this, the one-way flow switch is unlocked and the purse-string suture loosened. If hemostasis

is achieved, the glidewire cheater and one-way flow switch together with the purse-string suture are gently removed, and the patient leaves the angiography suite without any suture in place.

6. If hemostasis is not achieved following this period, the interventionalist may again pull taught the purse-string suture and lock it in place with the glidewire cheater and one-way flow switch and then wait for another 10–15 minutes before repeating step 5.

Example

See Figures 52.1–52.4.

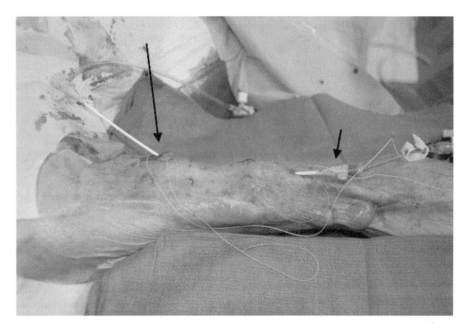

Figure 52.1 Following completion of the AV graft intervention, purse-string sutures have been placed around the 6 Fr vascular sheath toward the venous outflow limb (short arrow) and around the 6 Fr vascular sheath toward the arterial inflow (long arrow).

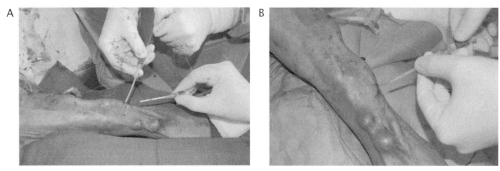

Figure 52.2 After the vascular access sheath used to access the venous outflow limb has been removed (A), the purse-string suture is held taught as the glidewire cheater together with the one-way flow switch are advanced toward the vascular sheath access site (B).

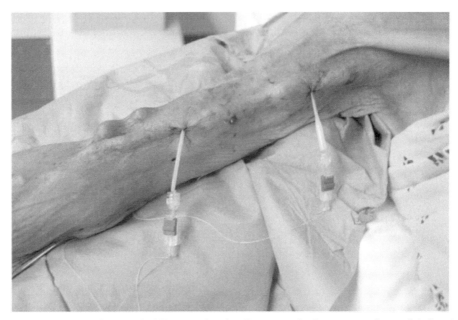

Figure 52.3 With the glidewire cheater flush against the vascular sheath access site, the one-way flow switch then locks the purse-string suture allowing for hemostasis. This is left in place for 10–15 minutes.

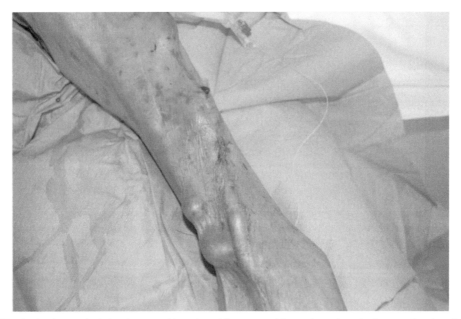

Figure 52.4 After 15 minutes, hemostasis has been achieved and the purse-string sutures from both vascular sheath access sites have been removed.

Filter Placement and Retrieval

CHAPTER 53

Deploying a Straight Conical Filter

S. Lowell Kahn

Brief Description

Placement of inferior vena cava (IVC) filters is among the most common medical procedures, with more than 265,000 placed annually.[1] Absolute indications for their placement include acute proximal deep venous thrombosis (DVT) and pulmonary embolism (PE) in patients who have an absolute contraindication to anticoagulation and patients with recurrent thromboembolism despite adequate anticoagulation. Filters are also commonly used in patients in whom further embolization would be catastrophic (e.g., patients with poor cardiac reserve and/or massive PE).[2-5] Despite the high prevalence of IVC filters, their use remains controversial given their questionable benefit and known potential complications. Although multiple studies report a decrease in PE after filter placement, there are no definitive data to suggest that filters decrease PE-related death.[2,6,7]

To illustrate this point, the large PREPIC1 study randomized patients with proximal DVT to anticoagulation alone or anticoagulation plus filter placement and showed a lower rate of PE in the filter cohort in the short term, but at 2 years there was no significant difference in survival or symptomatic PE between the two groups.[2,8] Similarly, a delayed 8-year follow-up of these patients again showed fewer PE events in the filter cohort but an increased rate of DVT and no difference in survival between the two groups.[2,9] Similarly, the PRECIP2 study randomized patients with severe PE to anticoagulation alone and to anticoagulation with placement of a filter. The results of this study again showed no significant benefit with placement of a filter.[2,10]

In contrast, studies with data derived from the National Inpatient Sample have shown a decrease in mortality associated with filter placement in patients undergoing thrombolytic treatment.[2,7,10]

Although the survival benefit is unknown, it has been shown that filters decrease the incidence of PE in the short term. Unfortunately, this comes at the expense of known complications, the most important being DVT, which is most commonly seen in patients for whom anticoagulation is contraindicated.[2,11] Although rare, filter migration/embolization, strut fracture, caval thrombosis, and caval penetration are also well-known risks.[12,13] These risks in conjunction with the controversial increased use of prophylactic filters in the trauma, orthopedic, bariatric, and neurosurgery populations have prompted significant interest in the use of retrievable filters.[14-17] In August 2010, the US Food and Drug Administration released an advisory encouraging providers to remove retrievable filters when clinically indicated.[18]

Retrievable filters confer the benefit of a reduction in PE with avoidance of the long-term filter-associated complications. Unfortunately, retrieval rates of these filters remain unacceptably low, with a reported average of only 34%.[19] Interestingly, this is most commonly due to physician oversight and patient noncompliance.[20-24] When retrieval attempts do fail, anatomic considerations (deployment in an angled segment of the IVC), dwell time, and filter positioning are commonly cited as causative factors. Tilting of the filter can lead to the hook becoming embedded in the caval wall, a factor that is considered the most predictive for a failed retrieval attempt.[20,25,26] Many of the newer filters are designed to be self-straightening to prevent tilt, but to date, this has not resulted in improved retrieval rates.[27]

This chapter discusses simple techniques to prevent conical filter tilting and enhance retrieval. For all filter placements, we advise placement in a straight segment of the IVC, even if this requires placing the apex lower than the level of the renal veins. In 2012, Knott et al.[28] described straight femoral filter deployment achieved through advancement of an Amplatz wire (Cook Medical Inc., Bloomington, IN) through the side port of a Tuohy-Borst adapter on the older delivery platform of the Celect filter (Cook Medical Inc., Bloomington, IN). This technique is referred to as the *buddy wire technique* and is described in detail later. A second method, the *jugular sheath deployment technique*, involves deployment of a filter with continuous traction while the apex remains within the delivery sheath. Finally, the *femoral modified delivery technique* involves manually shaping the delivery shaft of the filter to counter the natural angle of the common iliac veins relative to the IVC. All three techniques are easy to learn and reliable for the deployment of a straight filter.

Applications of the Technique

Buddy Wire Technique

1. This technique is remarkably effective but, unfortunately, has become largely obsolete because of a change in the design of the Cook filter delivery systems. The original delivery system of the Celect filter as well as the Günther Tulip filter (Cook Medical Inc., Bloomington, IN) had a Tuohy-Borst adapter that allowed passage of a stiff wire through the side arm immediately adjacent to the filter delivery shaft from a femoral approach after the filter was unsheathed but prior to its release. The stiff wire automatically centered the delivery system along the long axis of the IVC. The new delivery system of both filters lacks a Tuohy-Borst adapter, and the old delivery platform was discontinued in January 2016. In theory, the operator could place a large, long sheath (e.g., 12 Fr × 45 cm) at the beginning of the case through which the delivery system of any of the conical filter systems and a stiff buddy wire could be advanced side by side. As before, the stiff wire would maintain a straight position of the 12 Fr sheath and hence any filter delivery system advanced coaxially through it. Although likely feasible, the added time and expense of doing this would be justified only in a rare circumstance with a particularly tortuous IVC.

Jugular Sheath Deployment Technique

1. This technique is solely for use with the Celect and Tulip filters because it requires the filter to be attached to the delivery system via the hook. Other conical filters, such as the Option (Rex Medical, Conshohocken, PA) and Denali (Bard, Tempe, AZ), are deployed via a simple pin-pull method and are therefore not compatible with this technique.

Femoral Modified Delivery Technique

1. This technique is solely for use with the Celect and Tulip filters because it requires bending the metal shaft of the delivery platform. The pin-pull deployment system of other conical filters is not amenable to this technique.

Challenges of the Procedure

Buddy Wire Technique

1. No specific challenges have been encountered.

Jugular Sheath Deployment Technique

1. No specific challenges have been encountered.

Femoral Modified Delivery Technique

1. Choosing the location (distance from the tip) and amount of angulation to place in the delivery shaft can be challenging. In the author's experience, 15–30 degrees of angulation positioned 10–20 cm from the tip is ideal.

Potential Pitfalls/Complications

Buddy Wire Technique

1. Although unlikely, it is important that the "buddy wire" does not entangle the filter. Removal of the wire after filter deployment should be performed under live fluoroscopy to ensure that the filter is not inadvertently dislodged during removal of the wire and delivery system.

Jugular Sheath Deployment Technique

1. Although typically released on the first attempt, occasionally the release mechanism will re-engage the hook of the filter after being fired. This could result in inadvertent removal/dislodgment of the filter when removing the delivery shaft from the sheath. As with all filter deployments, continuous live fluoroscopy is advised to confirm proper release and deployment.

Femoral Modified Delivery Technique

1. It is possible that excessive bending of the delivery shaft could compromise the function of the delivery system and result in the inability to release the filter. Given that the unsheathed femoral filter cannot be resheathed, this could obviously present a problem. Based on the author's experience, focal sharp bending of the delivery shaft beyond 30 degrees should be avoided.

Steps of the Procedure

Buddy Wire Technique

1. Using the Seldinger technique, a long (e.g., 45 cm) 12 Fr sheath should be advanced to the IVC from a jugular or femoral approach over a stiff Amplatz wire.
2. Once the tip of the sheath lies near the intended location for the filter, the dilator is removed and a second stiff Amplatz wire is placed.
3. IVC venography is performed directly though the 12 Fr sheath or through a flush catheter advanced over one of the two Amplatz wires to denote the location of the renal veins and assess the size of the IVC.
4. Over one of the two Amplatz wires, the delivery sheath of the filter is advanced.
5. Maintaining the second Amplatz wire as a "buddy wire," the filter is deployed per the manufacturer's instructions for use (IFU). The buddy wire ensures

that the delivery platform is maintained closely along the center axis of the IVC.

6. Final venography is obtained, and the sheath is removed.

Jugular Sheath Deployment Technique (Cook Celect and Tulip Filters)

1. Using the Seldinger technique, the delivery sheath of the Cook Celect or Tulip filter should be advanced to the IVC from a jugular approach.
2. IVC venography is performed directly through the sheath or through a flush catheter advanced through the delivery sheath to denote the location of the renal veins and assess the size of the IVC.
3. The filter is advanced to its intended level.
4. The filter is unsheathed until just the tip of the filter remains in the sheath. The legs of the filter are fully expanded with wall apposition to the IVC.
5. Back traction is maintained on the filter while the tip remains in the sheath. The combination of the back traction and the tip placement in the sheath maintains a straight orientation of the filter. The filter is released per the manufacturer's IFU.
6. Final venography is obtained, and the sheath is removed.

Femoral Modified Delivery Technique (Cook Celect and Tulip Filters)

1. The IVC is catheterized from a femoral approach.
2. Diagnostic IVC venography is obtained. In addition to the location of the renal veins and the size of the IVC, the degree of angulation of the IVC particularly in relation to the common iliac vein is studied.
3. On the back table, the delivery shaft of the filter is manually shaped to roughly the same degree of the IVC relative to the common iliac vein from the side on which the filter is to be advanced. For the majority of cases, this angle is between 15 and 30 degrees. The bend should be placed at a distance from the tip that approximates the distance between the iliac vein confluence and the anticipated filter location (usually 10–20 cm).
4. The sheath is advanced with its dilator over a wire beyond the site of intended filter deployment. The dilator and wire are removed.
5. The modified filter is inserted into the sheath.
6. For the Celect filter (which is difficult to rotate once unsheathed because of expansion of the secondary struts), the filter shaft is rotated within the sheath to orient the filter properly along the long axis of the IVC before the filter is unsheathed. For the Tulip filter, rotation to orient the filter along the long axis of the IVC is more easily achieved after it has been unsheathed.
7. With the filter properly oriented, release is performed per the manufacturer's IFU.
8. Final venography is obtained, and the sheath is removed.

Example

See Figures 53.1 and 53.2.

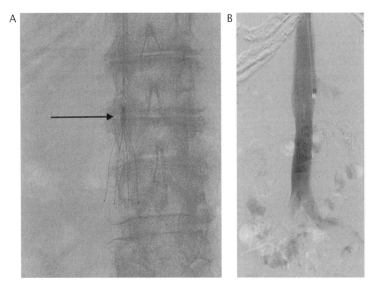

Figure 53.1 Jugular sheath deployment technique. A Cook Celect jugular filter is positioned at an infrarenal location in the IVC. The filter is unsheathed, allowing the primary and secondary struts to expand. The hooks engage the caval wall. (A) With back traction on the delivery shaft, the filter tip is maintained within the delivery sheath tip (arrow) during delivery, thereby preventing tilt. (B) After deployment, digital subtraction angiography shows optimal straight filter deployment.

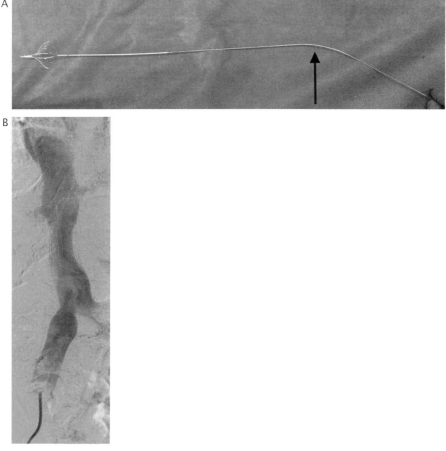

Figure 53.2 Femoral modified delivery technique. (A) The delivery shaft of the Cook Celect femoral filter is manually curved (arrow) on the back table. The curve on the delivery shaft allows rotation and centering of the filter prior to unsheathing. (B) After deployment, the filter deploys in perfect alignment with the long axis of the IVC.

References and Suggested Readings

1. Smouse B, Johar A. Is market growth of vena cava filters justified? A review of indications, use, and market analysis. *Endovascular Today.* 2010;2:74–77.
2. Lip GYH, Hull RD. Overview of the treatment of lower extremity deep vein thrombosis (DVT). http://www.uptodate.com/contents/overview-of-the-treatment-of-lower-extremity-deep-vein-thrombosis-dvt.
3. Guyatt GH, Akl EA, Crowther M, Gutterman DD, Schünemann HJ. Antithrombotic therapy and prevention of thrombosis, 9th ed: American College of Chest Physicians evidence-based clinical practice guidelines. *Chest.* 2012;141(Suppl):7S–47S.
4. Rogers FB, Cipolle MD, Velmahos G, Rozycki G, Luchette FA. Practice management guidelines for the prevention of venous thromboembolism in trauma patients: The EAST practice management guidelines work group. *J Trauma* 2002;53:142–164.
5. Kaufman JA, Kinney TB, Streiff MB, et al. Guidelines for the use of retrievable and convertible vena cava filters: Report from the Society of Interventional Radiology multidisciplinary consensus conference. *J Vasc Interv Radiol.* 2006;17:449–459.
6. Muriel A, Jiménez D, Aujesky D, et al. Survival effects of inferior vena cava filter in patients with acute symptomatic venous thromboembolism and a significant bleeding risk. *J Am Coll Cardiol.* 2014;63:1675.
7. Stein PD, Matta F. Vena cava filters in unstable elderly patients with acute pulmonary embolism. *Am J Med.* 2014;127:222.
8. Decousus H, Leizorovicz A, Parent F, et al. A clinical trial of vena caval filters in the prevention of pulmonary embolism in patients with proximal deep-vein thrombosis: Prévention du Risque d'Embolie Pulmonaire par Interruption Cave Study Group. *N Engl J Med.* 1998;338:409.
9. PREPIC Study Group. Eight-year follow-up of patients with permanent vena cava filters in the prevention of pulmonary embolism: The PREPIC (Prevention du Risque d'Embolie Pulmonaire par Interruption Cave) randomized study. *Circulation.* 2005;112:416.
10. Stein PD, Matta F, Keyes DC, Willyerd GL. Impact of vena cava filters on in-hospital case fatality rate from pulmonary embolism. *Am J Med.* 2012;125:478.
11. Streiff MB. Vena caval filters: A comprehensive review. *Blood.* 2000;95:3669.
12. Shang EK, Nathan DP, Carpenter JP, Fairman RM, Jackson BM. Delayed complications of inferior vena cava filters: Case report and literature review. *Vasc Endovascular Surg.* 2011;45:290–294.
13. Sarani B, Chun A, Venbrux A. Role of optional (retrievable) IVC filters in surgical patients at risk for venous thromboembolic disease. *J Am Coll Surg.* 2005;201:957–964.

14. Rectenwald JE. Vena cava filters: Uses and abuses. *Semin Vasc Surg*. 2005;18:166–175.

15. Tschoe M, Kim HS, Brotman DJ, Streiff MB. Retrievable vena cava filters: A clinical review. *J Hosp Med*. 2009;4: 441–448.

16. Yunus TE, Tariq N, Callahan RE, et al. Changes in inferior vena cava filter placement over the past decade at a large community-based academic health center. *J Vasc Surg*. 2008;47:157–165.

17. Aziz F, Spate K, Wong J, Aruny J, Sumpio B. Changing patterns in the use of inferior vena cava filters: Review of a single center experience. *J Am Coll Surg*. 2007;205:564–569.

18. US Food and Drug Administration (FDA). Safety advisory. http://www.fda.gov/Safety/MedWatch/SafetyInformation/SafetyAlertsforHumanMedicalProducts/ucm221707.htm.

19. Angel LF, Tapson V, Galgon RE, Restrepo MI, Kaufman J. Systematic review of the use of retrievable inferior vena cava filters. *J Vasc Interv Radiol*. 2011;22:1522–1530.

20. Avgerinos ED, Bath J, Stevens J, et al. Technical and patient-related characteristics associated with challenging retrieval of inferior vena cava filters. *Eur J Vasc Endovasc Surg*. 2013;46(3):353–359.

21. Zakhary EM, Elmore JR, Galt SW, Franklin DP. Optional filters in trauma patient: Can retrieval rates be improved? *Ann Vasc Surg*. 2008;22:627–634.

22. Irwin E, Byrnes M, Schultz S, et al. A systematic method for follow-up improves removal rates for retrievable inferior vena cava filters in a trauma patient population. *J Trauma*. 2010;69:866–869.

23. Gasparis AP, Spentzouris G, Meisner RJ, Elitharp D, Labropoulos N, Tassiopoulos A. Improving retrieval rates of temporary inferior vena cava filters. *J Vasc Surg*. 2011;54:34s–38s.

24. Lucas DJ, Dunne JR, Rodriguez CJ, et al. Dedicated tracking of patients with retrievable inferior vena cava filters improves retrieval rates. *Am Surg*. 2012;78:870–874.

25. Marquess JS, Burke CT, Beecham AH, et al. Factors associated with failed retrieval of the Günther Tulip inferior vena cava filter. *J Vasc Interv Radiol*. 2008;19:1321–1327.

26. Hermsen JL, Ibele AR, Faucher LD, Nale JK, Schurr MJ, Kudsk KA. Retrievable inferior vena cava filters in high-risk trauma and surgical patients: Factors influencing successful removal. *World J Surg*. 2008;32:1444–1449.

27. Shelgikar C, Mohebali J, Sarfati MR, Mueller MT, Kinikini DV, Kraiss LW. A design modification to minimize tilting of an inferior vena cava filter does not deliver a clinical benefit. *J Vasc Surg*. 2010;52:920–924.

28. Knott EM, Beacham B, Fry WR. New technique to prevent tilt during inferior vena cava placement. *J Vasc Surg*. 2012;55:869–871.

CHAPTER 54

Removing the Angled Inferior Vena Cava Filter with an Embedded Hook: The "Hangman" Technique

Adam N. Plotnik and Stephen Kee

Brief Description

Multiple advanced techniques for the retrieval of difficult inferior vena cava (IVC) filters have been published in the literature,[1-8] most of which describe mechanical methods to disrupt the fibrous capsule in cases in which the filter hook or struts have become embedded in the IVC wall. Despite reported high success rates, these techniques often require multiple venous access sites or the use of specialist equipment. The "hangman" technique is a modified "loop snare" technique that requires only a single venous access and uses standard interventional equipment. The loop snare technique, initially described by Rubenstein et al.,[9] involves passing a wire between at least two filter legs and then snaring it superiorly to create a loop through the filter struts, which engages the filter for retrieval. This method is particularly effective when filter retrieval using standard technique is not possible due to severe filter tilt; however, it is limited when the hook becomes embedded in the wall. Use of this technique with an embedded hook can result in more severe tilting of the filter and in wall perforation with severe pain. It may also lead to a situation in which the filter is no longer retrievable using endovascular techniques. The Hangman technique modifies the loop snare technique by passing the wire loop between the filter neck and IVC wall, as opposed to the filter struts.[10] Through a 14 Fr sheath via a right internal jugular approach, a reverse curve catheter is advanced to the filter and a glidewire is introduced between the filter neck and IVC wall. The leading end of the glidewire is then snared, and with cranial tension applied on both the leading end and trailing end of the wire, the embedded filter hook is released from the IVC wall. The filter hook is then snared and the sheath advanced for removal of the filter as per standard technique.

When applying tension on the looped wire, the embedded hook is slowly "dissected" off the wall. By applying downward force to the 14 Fr sheath while applying wire tension, the hook can be engaged into the mouth of the sheath. At this point, depending on whether the open edge of the hook faces the looped wire or not, the wire will either engage the hook, at which stage the filter is easily withdrawn, or slip off the hook and become disengaged. Even if the latter event occurs, the hook of the filter should still be in the distal aspect of the sheath. Careful reintroduction of the snare will allow the filter to be resnared inside the sheath and then removed.

Depending on the width of the individual IVC, it may be necessary to combine the reverse curve catheter with a shaped sheath/guide in order to manipulate the tip of the catheter to the location of the space between the neck of the filter and the caval wall.

Application of the Technique

1. Prolonged IVC filter retrieval whereby standard and more advanced retrieval techniques have failed.
2. Severely tilted IVC filter, especially when the filter hook has become embedded in the cava wall, identified on pre-procedural imaging.
3. With minimal experience, this technique is introduced as a first-line option when a simple retrieval fails.

Challenges of the Technique

1. Advancing the wire in the space demarcated by the filter neck, the embedded filter hook, and the IVC wall: If the wire is advanced between the filter struts, then the tradition loop snare technique results, which is most often ineffective in retrieving IVC filters with embedded filter hooks.

Potential Pitfalls/Complications

1. Traumatic IVC injury: During the release of the embedded filter hook, it is feasibly possible to cause IVC injury, such as IVC intussusception or tear. In practice, however, this should not occur because the

wire is "dissecting" the hook from the wall, even in cases of significant upward force applied to the wire.

2. Thrombus within the filter: As per standard recommendation, substantial filling defects within the filter may present an immediate risk of pulmonary embolus during filter retrieval.[11]

Steps of the Procedure

1. Access the right internal jugular vein under ultrasound guidance with a micropuncture kit as per standard technique. Following requisite IVC venogram and failed standard retrieval techniques, a 14 Fr 45-cm sheath (special order; Cook Medical Inc., Bloomington, IN) is placed via a right internal jugular venous access and advanced to the filter.

2. Through the 14 Fr sheath, a 5 Fr reverse curve catheter (SOS Omni Selective Catheter; AngioDynamics, Latham, NY) is advance to the filter, but not between the filter struts, with the leading end terminating near the filter neck.

3. An angled 0.035-in. glidewire is then introduced through the reverse curve catheter and guided into the space between the filter neck, the embedded filter hook, and the IVC wall.

4. A snare (e.g., 25-mm GooseNeck [Medtronic, Minneapolis, MN] or En Snare [Merit Medical, South Jordan, UT]) is then placed through the 14 Fr sheath, and the leading end of the Glidewire (Terumo, Somerset, NJ) is snared and withdrawn through the sheath, thereby creating a loop snare with the Glidewire in the space demarcated by the filter neck, the embedded filter hook, and the IVC wall.

5. The reverse curve catheter is then withdrawn and upward (cranial) force is applied to both the leading end and the trailing end of the wire (i.e., the loop snare), with simultaneous downward (caudal) force applied to the 14 Fr vascular sheath. This results in the release of the embedded IVC filter hook from the IVC wall.

6. Snare the filter hook: During the release of the embedded IVC filter hook, the loop snare glidewire may in fact snare the filter hook. In such cases, the 14 Fr sheath is simply advanced and the filter is retrieved as per standard technique. If the loop snare glidewire slips past the filter hook during its release, the hook is in the sheath and can be subsequently snared via a snare placed through the 14 Fr sheath.

7. A venogram is performed immediately following filter retrieval, via the 14 Fr sheath.

Example

See Figure 54.1–54.6.

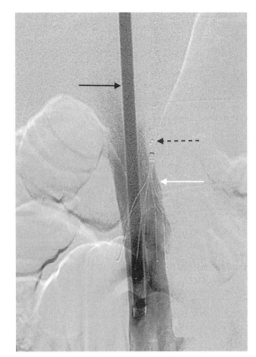

Figure 54.1 Venogram obtained before IVC filter retrieval via a 14 Fr sheath (black arrow) demonstrates a Cook Celect retrievable IVC filter with significant lateral tilt and an embedded filter hook (dashed arrow). Note the contrast opacified space demarcated by the filter neck, the embedded filter hook, and the IVC wall (white arrow).

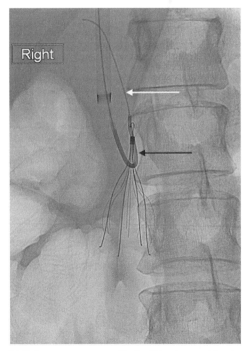

Figure 54.2 A reverse curve catheter (black arrow) is placed adjacent to the filter, in the space between filter neck and the IVC wall. The leading end of an angled 0.035-in. Glidewire (white arrow) is then advanced through the reverse curve catheter.

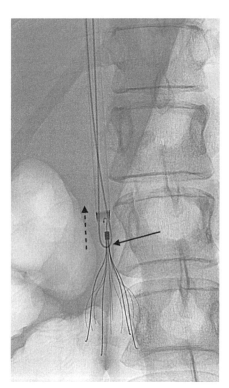

Figure 54.3 The leading end of the wire is snared and withdrawn through the sheath, creating a loop snare around the filter neck (black arrow), and the reverse curve catheter is removed. Tension is then applied cranially on the snared wire (dashed arrow) as gentle caudal force is applied to the 14 Fr sheath.

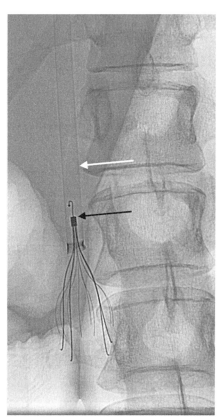

Figure 54.4 The snared wire slipped past the embedded filter hook as it was released from the IVC wall. Simultaneous downward (caudal) force on the 14 Fr sheath resulted in the filter neck and hook (black arrow) ending up within the lumen of the 14 Fr sheath (white arrow).

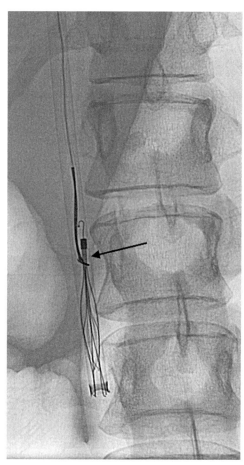

Figure 54.5 The filter neck is then snared (arrow) within the 14 Fr sheath, with the filter subsequently removed.

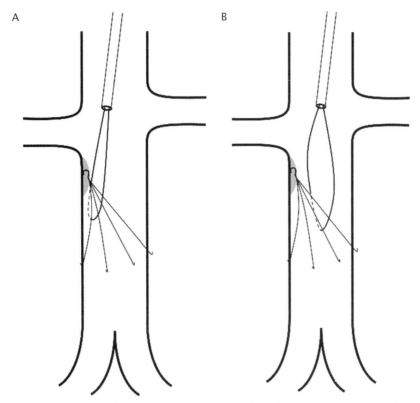

Figure 54.6 Schematic representation of an IVC containing a tilted conical-type IVC filter with an embedded hook secondary to a fibrous capsule (gray shading). Comparison of the (A) hangman technique, in which the wire is advanced between the filter neck and the IVC wall just beneath the embedded hook, with the (B) original loop snare technique,[10] in which the wire is advanced through the filter struts.

Source: Images reproduced with permission from Al-Hakim R, et al. The hangman technique: A modified loop snare technique for the retrieval of inferior vena cava filters with embedded hooks. *J Vasc Interv Radiol.* 2015;26(1):107–110.

References and Suggested Readings

1. Stavropoulos SW, Dixon RG, Burke CT, et al. Embedded inferior vena cava filter removal: Use of endobronchial forceps. *J Vasc Interv Radiol.* 2008;19(9):1297–1301.

2. Lynch FC. Balloon-assisted removal of tilted inferior vena cava filters with embedded tips. *J Vasc Interv Radiol.* 2009;20(9):1210–1214.

3. Kuo WT, Odegaard JI, Louie JD, et al. Photothermal ablation with the excimer laser sheath technique for embedded inferior vena cava filter removal: Initial results from a prospective study. *J Vasc Interv Radiol.* 2011;22(6):813–823.

4. Kuo WT, Cupp JS, Louie JD, et al. Complex retrieval of embedded IVC filters: Alternative techniques and histologic tissue analysis. *Cardiovasc Intervent Radiol.* 2012;35(3):588–597.

5. Kuo WT, Bostaph AS, Loh CT, Frisoli JK, Kee ST. Retrieval of trapped Gunther Tulip inferior vena cava filters: Snare-over-guide wire loop technique. *J Vasc Interv Rad.* 2006;17(11 Pt 1):1845–1849.

6. Kassavin DS, Constantinopoulos G. Cone over guide wire technique for difficult IVC filter retrieval. *Cardiovasc Intervent Radiol.* 2011;34(3):664–666.

7. Iliescu B, Haskal ZJ. Advanced techniques for removal of retrievable inferior vena cava filters. *Cardiovasc Intervent Radiol.* 2012;35(4):741–750.

8. Esparaz AM, Ryu RK, Gupta R, Resnick SA, Salem R, Lewandowski RJ. Fibrin cap disruption: An adjunctive technique for inferior vena cava filter retrieval. *J Vasc Interv. Radiol.* 2012;23(9):1233–1235.

9. Rubenstein L, Chun AK, Chew M, Binkert CA. Loop-snare technique for difficult inferior vena cava filter retrievals. *J Vasc Interv Radiol.* 2007;18(10):1315–1318.

10. Al-Hakim R, McWilliams JP, Derry W, Kee ST. The hangman technique: A modified loop snare technique for the retrieval of inferior vena cava filters with embedded hooks. *J Vasc Interv Radiol.* 2015;26(1):107–110.

11. Kaufman JA, Kinney TB, Streiff MB, et al. Guidelines for the use of retrievable and convertible vena cava filters: Report from the Society of Interventional Radiology multidisciplinary consensus conference. *J Vasc Interv Radiol.* 2006;17(3):449–459.

CHAPTER 55

Femoral Flip Technique for Removal of the G2 Filter

Adam N. Plotnik and Stephen Kee

Brief Description

The purpose of temporary retrievable inferior vena cava (IVC) filters is to provide protection from pulmonary emboli while the patient is at risk while simultaneously avoiding the long-term complications that result from permanent filters, such as the Greenfield (Boston Scientific Inc., Marlborough, MA). In addition to the complications of filter fracture and caval penetration, there is an increasing incidence of recurrent deep vein thrombosis and caval occlusion following filter placement;[1] therefore, whenever possible, retrieval of IVC filters should be attempted. The "femoral flip" technique may be employed for difficult G2 IVC filter (Bard, Tempe, AZ) retrievals where standard techniques have failed, usually due to either one of the legs or the hook becoming embedded in the wall. This is a relatively rare occurrence because the G2 filters tend to lie in a favorable orientation in the IVC, with retrieval rates reported up to 97.7%.[2] After performing the requisite IVC venogram via an internal jugular approach and failure of standard retrieval techniques, a snare is placed around a leg of the G2 IVC filter. Upward (cranial) pressure is then employed until the G2 filter flips, with the filter hook now positioned caudally. Through a sheath via a femoral venous access, the filter is now snared or retrieved using the standard Bard Recovery Cone retrieval system.

Application of the Technique

1. Tilted G2 IVC filter with hook embedded into the wall of the IVC that is not retrieved by standard technique.

Challenges of the Procedure

1. Filter tilt: The interventionalist will need to place considerable upward (cranial) force on the G2 filter once the leg has been snared. Insufficient force will result in incomplete filter flip. If this occurs, one can place a snare within a right femoral access sheath, snare one of the filter legs, and, with downward (caudal) force, complete the full rotational flip of the filter.

Potential Pitfalls/Complications

1. Traumatic caval injury: Although the technique appears to be quite "aggressive," the G2 IVC filter is flexible and fairly soft, and in the authors' experience, IVC traumatic injury is rare. However, this technique should not be used with other "stiffer" IVC filters.
2. Fractured G2 filter strut: Again, due to the flexibility of the G2 filter, this is an unlikely but potential complication of the technique.
3. Thrombus within the filter: As per standard recommendation, substantial filling defects within the filter may present an immediate risk of pulmonary embolus during filter retrieval.[3]

Steps of the Procedure

1. Access the right internal jugular vein under ultrasound guidance with a micropuncture kit as per standard technique. Following requisite IVC venogram and failed standard retrieval techniques, a snare (e.g., 25-mm GooseNeck [Medtronic Inc., Minneapolis, MN] or En Snare [Merit Medical Systems Inc., South Jordan, UT]) is placed through a 10 Fr sheath via a right internal jugular venous access and advanced to the filter.
2. Snare leg of G2 filter: Using the snare, grab one of the legs of the G2 filter and apply upward (cranial) pulling force until the filter begins to tilt. An alternative to grabbing a filter leg with a standard snare (e.g., 25-mm GooseNeck or En Snare) may be employing a loop snare method with the use of a reverse curve catheter (Sos Omni, AngioDynamics Inc., Latham, NY) through the G2 filter leg and then passing a Glidewire (Terumo, Somerset, NJ) through this catheter and snaring the Glidewire via the sheath.
3. Filter flip: With continued sustained upward (cranial) force, the G2 filter will invert itself in the IVC. This is due to the flexibility and relative softness of the G2 filter.
4. Snare filter from groin: Access the right common femoral vein under ultrasound guidance with

micropuncture kit as per standard technique and place a 12 Fr sheath. Through this sheath, place either another snare (e.g., 25-mm GooseNeck or En Snare) or the standard Bard Recovery Cone retrieval system, and retrieve the G2 filter through the groin sheath.

5. Incomplete filter flip: If the G2 filter has been incompletely flipped lying horizontal in the IVC, the snare placed within the groin sheath can grab one of the filter legs and continue downward force to complete the full rotational flip of the filter. Following this, continue with step 4.

6. Venogram: Perform post-procedure venogram to confirm total removal of filter and exclude any IVC trauma or thrombus.

Example

See Figures 55.1–55.5.

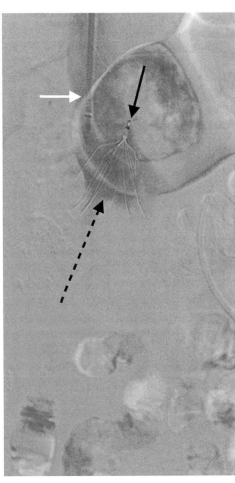

Figure 55.1 Initial IVC venogram. Following right internal jugular access, a 7 Fr sheath (white arrow) is advanced into the IVC and a cavogram performed. The G2 filter is tilted with hook embedded in the wall (black arrow). It is also noted that the G2 filter contains no thrombus to prohibit filter retrieval (dashed arrow).

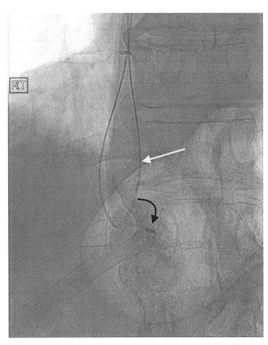

Figure 55.2 Snare G2 filter leg. A loop snare (white arrow) is then placed through the indwelling sheath and is hooked around one of the legs of the G2 filter. Upward force is then applied to the snare surrounding the G2 filter leg, with resultant tilting of the entire filter (black arrow).

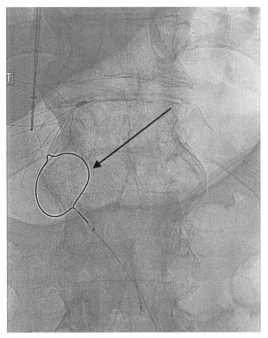

Figure 55.3 Incomplete filter flip. Following sustained upward (cranial) force, the G2 filter has flipped 90 degrees. Consequently, a second snare (arrow) is placed via a common femoral venous access in order to grab a filter leg and complete the filter flip.

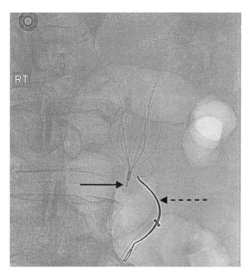

Figure 55.4 Complete filter flip. With a G2 filter leg grabbed by the second snare (dashed arrow), sustained downward (caudal) force is applied until the full 180-degrees rotational flip of the G2 IVC filter has been achieved. Note that the filter hook (black arrow) is now facing caudally, aiding standard retrieval via a femoral approach.

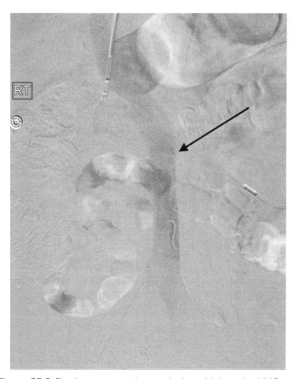

Figure 55.5 Final venogram demonstrates widely patent IVC with no evidence of traumatic sequelae, thrombus, or retained filter struts (arrow).

References and Suggested Readings

1. Decousus H, Leizorovicz A, Parent F, et al. A clinical trial of vena caval filters in the prevention of pulmonary embolism in patients with proximal deep-vein thrombosis: Prevention du Risque d'Embolie Pulmonaire par Interruption Cave Study Group. *N Engl J Med.* 1998;338(7):409–415.
2. Lynch FC, Kekulawela S. Removal of the G2 filter: Differences between implantation times greater and less than 180 days. *J Vasc Interv Radiol.* 2009;20(9):1200–1209.
3. Kaufman JA, Kinney TB, Streiff MB, et al. Guidelines for the use of retrievable and convertible vena cava filters: Report from the Society of Interventional Radiology multidisciplinary consensus conference. *J Vasc Interv Radiol.* 2006;17(3):449–459.

CHAPTER 56

Femoral Retrieval of Conical Filters

Mikin V. Patel and Steven Zangan

Brief Description

Inferior vena cava (IVC) filters are a safe, effective treatment option for the prevention of pulmonary embolism in patients who either have contraindication to or fail anticoagulation. However, filters pose long-term risk, such as IVC thrombosis, deep vein thrombosis, penetration of the IVC wall, filter fracture, and filter migration. For these reasons, interventionalists should attempt to retrieve IVC filters when they are no longer needed, and safe retrieval is possible. For conical filters, a hook on the cranial end of the device can typically be snared from a jugular approach, a sheath can be advanced over the struts, and the filter can be removed. Although the majority of filters can be retrieved without difficulty, certain situations can make filter retrieval challenging. Occlusion of the internal jugular veins, subclavian veins, brachiocephalic veins, and superior vena cava precludes the conventional approach to filter removal, and advanced techniques need to be employed. One such technique to retrieve the filter from a femoral approach is as follows. A right femoral sheath is placed, and a snare is advanced to a position cranial to the IVC filter. The snare is then opened and used to encircle the struts of the filter. The snare is then slowly closed to pull the struts together, and a sheath is advanced over the device. If the device geometry allows, the filter can then be removed via the right femoral vein. Otherwise, a left femoral sheath can be inserted with a snare, which is then used to capture the cranial end of the filter and remove the device. Additional options to consider in situations with limited superior access include sharp recanalization of the occluded segment followed by conventional filter retrieval or placement of an Optease filter (Cordis Corp. , Milpitas, CA) if the presence of central venous occlusion was known beforehand.

Applications of the Technique

1. Retrieval of conical IVC filters in patients with central venous occlusion preventing access through the internal jugular, subclavian, brachiocephalic veins or superior vena cava.

Challenges of the Procedure

1. The filter must be positioned such that an opened snare can be passed over the apex and struts. A tilted filter apex abutting the vena cava wall may be difficult to capture within the snare.
2. The IVC filter geometry may be such that, when partially sheathed, the struts may flare outwards so that they cannot be completely sheathed. This challenge can be overcome by introducing a contralateral femoral sheath and removing the filter from the "conventional" approach.

Potential Pitfalls/Complications

1. The IVC filter may disengage from the snare at any point during the retrieval process and may migrate.

Steps of the Procedure

1. The femoral vein is accessed, and a vascular sheath is placed (9 Fr or larger).
2. An angiographic catheter is advanced into the IVC, and vena cavagram is performed to verify the filter is free of significant embolus.
3. A 25-mm GooseNeck snare (Medtronic Inc, Minneapolis, MN) is placed through the sheath, and the tip of the snare is passed above the filter apex.
4. The snare is opened, and the loop is pulled down to encircle the struts.
5. The snare is slowly closed to collapse the filter struts.
6. The closed filter is retracted into the iliac vein, and the sheath is advanced over the collapsed struts.
7. If the struts cannot be completely collapsed into the sheath, a contralateral sheath is inserted. An 8 Fr Balkan sheath (Cook Medical Inc, Bloomington, IN) can be used to traverse the confluence of the common iliac veins and reach the cranial end of the filter device.
8. A 25-mm GooseNeck snare is placed through the contralateral sheath, and the hook at the apex of the filter is snared.
9. The sheath is advanced over the filter in the "conventional" fashion.
10. The IVC filter is then removed.

Example

See Figures 56.1–56.5.

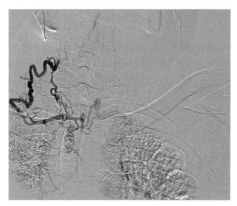

Figure 56.1 Digital subtraction angiography image in a cervical vein. A small cervical collateral vein was accessed using a micropuncture kit. Bilateral internal jugular, external jugular, and subclavian veins are occluded, and multiple collateral vessels are noted.

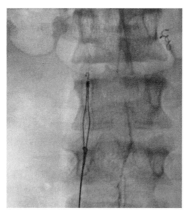

Figure 56.2 Fluoroscopic image in the IVC. After normal cavagram, a 25-mm Amplatz GooseNeck snare is advanced over the cranial aspect of the IVC filter. The loop is then opened and retracted to encircle and collapse the struts of the filter.

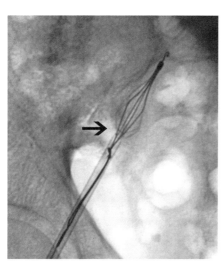

Figure 56.3 The struts of the IVC filter are collapsed and retracted into a 9 Fr sheath in the right iliac vein. The filter can then be removed using the femoral approach. In this case, the geometry of the filter was such that the struts did not completely collapse into the sheath (arrow).

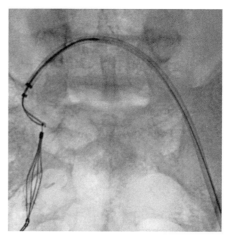

Figure 56.4 The IVC filter could not be fully retracted into the 9 Fr sheath. An 8 Fr Balkan sheath was placed in the left femoral vein and advanced into the right iliac vein. A 25-mm snare is advanced through the 8 Fr sheath and used to capture the cranial hook on the IVC filter.

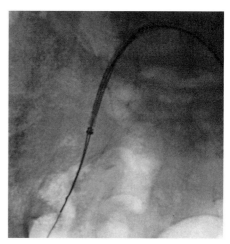

Figure 56.5 The snared IVC filter is fully retracted into the 8 Fr Balkan sheath.

References and Suggested Readings

1. Van Ha TG, Keblinskas D, Funaki B, et al. Removal of Gunther Tulip vena cava filter through femoral vein approach. *J Vasc Interv Radiol.* 2005;16:391–394.
2. Al-Hakim R, Kee ST, Olinger K. Inferior vena cava filter retrieval: Effectiveness and complications of routine and advanced techniques. *J Vasc Interv Radiol.* 2014;25:933–939.

CHAPTER 57

Laser Sheath Assisted Filter Removal

Mohammad Arabi

Brief Description

Laser sheath assisted filter removal may be used for difficult retrieval of chronically embedded inferior vena cava (IVC) filters that failed standard or advanced retrieval techniques.[1-3] This technique entails controlled photothermal ablation of the endothelium surrounding the filter struts using a GlideLight laser-tipped sheath (Spectranetics Corp., Colorado Springs, CO) powered by a 308-nm xenon chloride excimer laser generator (CVX-300, Spectranetics). The 308-nm laser light penetrates only 100 μm into vascular tissue and results in disintegration of the target tissues into particles less than 5 μm.[1] This technique has been long used for extraction of pacemaker leads[4,5] and has recently been extrapolated to filter removal because it minimizes the forces applied during difficult retrieval procedures and allows for removal of permanent filter devices. In addition to requiring less force for filter retrieval, laser sheath assisted removal helps reduce the total fluoroscopic time needed to complete the procedure.

Applications of the Technique

1. Failed retrieval of optional filters using standard or advanced removal techniques.
2. Retrieval of permanent filters to minimize filter-related thrombosis and subsequent morbidity and to eliminate the need for lifelong anticoagulation.
3. Retrieval of chronically embedded filters complicated by IVC thrombosis.

Challenges of the Procedure

1. Tilted filters must be properly captured and engaged by the sheath to allow for controlled ablation of the endothelium.
2. Excessive force application during filter removal may result in sheath tip damage that may require sheath replacement.
3. Laser ablation may be required from both the cranial and caudal aspects of the biconical filters through jugular and femoral access.
4. Laser ablation may be required for the whole length of the filter.

5. Additional devices, such as rigid or flexible forceps, may still be required to further dissect the filter from the wall.

Potential Pitfalls/Complications

1. Increased risk of hemorrhage: Dissection of chronically and deeply incorporated filter struts from the surrounding endothelium increases the risk of hemorrhage. The force applied during the retrieval procedure may result in shearing of the IVC with subsequent major/minor bleeding or pseudoaneurysm formation. Availability of large (up to 24 mm) compliant balloons and stent grafts is important to manage potential bleeding complications.
2. IVC stenosis: Filter retractions during removal may result in IVC wall collapse and stenosis that may require post-removal angioplasty to maintain patency and prevent thrombosis.
3. IVC thrombosis: Flow stagnation during filter removal may lead to caval thrombosis. Proper intraprocedural anticoagulation is required.

Procedural Steps

1. Sedation: The procedure can be painful due to significant forces applied during filter removal. Although the procedure may be done under moderate sedation, general anesthesia may be required if pain cannot be managed with sedation.
2. Venous access: A femoral or jugular access is obtained using a 14 Fr sheath. This can accommodate the 12 Fr laser sheath and allows for intermittent contrast injections during retrieval. Filter dissection with the laser sheath may be required from both accesses.
3. The filter is first engaged using a snare or a cone device, and retrieval is initially attempted using standard techniques. If device removal is deemed not possible, then the laser sheath is to be used.
4. The 12 Fr laser sheath, which has a 50-cm working length calibrated to deliver 60 mJ/mm^2, is then inserted through the outer sheath to the level of the filter.

5. Once the filter is captured using a snare, the sheath is advanced gradually while retracting the filter device into it. Once resistance is met, the laser sheath is activated intermittently to ablate the tissue immediately facing the tip of the sheath. Sheath advancement should be slow to allow efficient tissue ablation.

6. Alternate with advancing the sheath to collapse the filter with and without activation of laser until filter is disengaged and retrieved into the sheath.

7. Perform venogram to check for potential complications, such as active extravasation, pseudoaneurysm, stenosis, or thrombosis.

8. Send the filter for histologic evaluation of the attached tissues to check for the extent of the diathermy effects on the endothelium.

Example
See Figure 57.1.

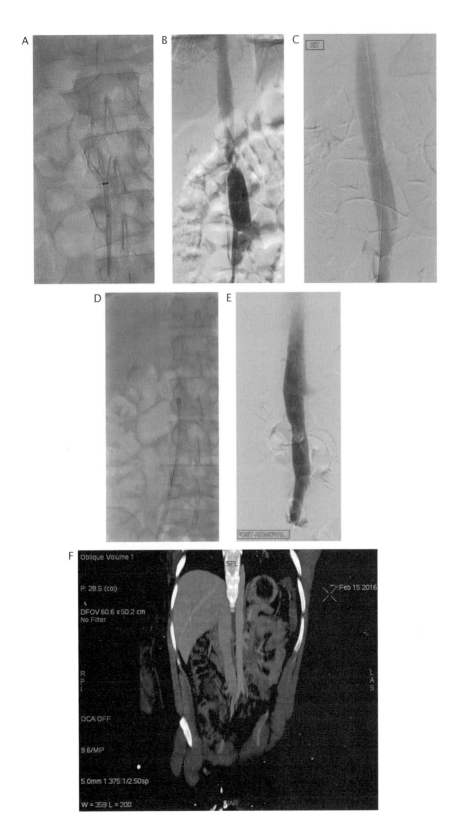

Figure 57.1 A 23-year-old trauma patient who had an IVC filter placed for prophylaxis prior to orthopedic surgery. The filter remained in place for 6 month. (A) Radiograph shows a partially collapsed Optease filter during the initial retrieval attempt. The filter could not be retrieved, despite excessive force application. (B) Post unsuccessful removal attempt venography shows a high-grade stenosis due to IVC collapse during the retrieval procedure. (C) Post balloon angioplasty venography shows patent IVC and resolution of the stenosis. (D) In a different session, a 12 Fr GlideLight laser sheath was introduced through a 14 Fr outer sheath and intermittently activated to gradually collapse the filter. (E) Post removal venography shows a residual filling defect that may represent a fibrin sheath or acute thrombus. The total fluoroscopy time for laser sheath assisted removal was 3.3 minutes. The patient was prescribed enoxaparin 40 mg daily for 2 weeks, (F) Coronal reconstruction of a computed tomography scan of the abdomen 2 months later shows complete resolution of the filling defect with no residual stenosis.

References and Suggested Readings

1. Kuo WT, Odegaard JI, Louie JD, et al. Photothermal ablation with the excimer laser sheath technique for embedded inferior vena cava filter removal: Initial results from a prospective study. *J Vasc Interv Radiol.* 2011;22:813–823.
2. Kuo WT, Odegaard JI, Rosenberg JK, Hofmann LV. Excimer laser-assisted removal of embedded inferior vena cava filters: A single-center prospective study. *Circ Cardiovasc Interv.* 2013;6:560–566.
3. Saito N, Shimamoto T, Takeda T, et al. Excimer laser-assisted retrieval of Gunther Tulip vena cava filters: A pilot study in a canine model. *J Vasc Interv Radiol.* 2010;21:719–724.
4. Hakmi S, Pecha S, Sill B, et al. Initial experience of pacemaker and implantable cardioverter defibrillator lead extraction with the new GlideLight 80 Hz laser sheaths. *Interact Cardiovasc Thorac Surg.* 2014;18:56–60.
5. Wilkoff BL, Byrd CL, Love CJ, et al. Pacemaker lead extraction with the laser sheath: Results of the Pacing Lead Extraction with the Excimer Sheath (PLEXES) trial. *J Am Coll Cardiol.* 1999;33:1671–1676.

Miscellaneous Catheterization, Wire, and Embolization Techniques

3. Type III aortic arch: This may make accessing the descending aorta difficult. Deep inspiration elongates the thoracic aorta, facilitating this step of the procedure. The 1.5-mm "J" Glidewire (Terumo) is our wire of choice because the tip design allows easy access to the descending aorta in most cases. As an alternative, a pigtail catheter can be used at the level of the aortic arch, facing the descending aorta, and a wire is pushed to uncoil the pigtail and to enter the descending aorta ("whip maneuver").

4. Tall patients: In patients taller than 6 feet 2 inches, the Jacky radial catheter, which is 110 cm in length, may not reach the celiac axis. In this case, a 125-cm direction catheter can be used to catheterize any visceral branches. In most patients shorter than 5 feet 10 inches, a 110-cm sheath will reach the common iliac arteries. If additional length is needed, a 125-cm guiding catheter can be used through a long sheath. Ensure that balloon and stent systems have 135-cm shafts and 6 Fr compatibility.[8]

5. Staff training: To perform radial artery access successfully, it is crucial to have all team members fully involved and well trained; including nurses in the preparation and recovery area, procedure nurses, and technologists. Making everyone aware of the benefits and potential risks associated with the procedure increases staff engagement and improves outcomes.

Potential Pitfalls/Complications

1. Spasm or need for a larger sheath: Some radial arteries can accommodate up to a 7 Fr (3.1 mm) long length sheath if needed. Only use hydrophilic sheaths. The most severe spasm usually occurs when withdrawing a long sheath after an extended period of time.[17] Consider increasing patient sedation, and administer sublingual nitroglycerine. Maximize usage of anticoagulation with heparin and vasodilator agents based on activated clotting time (ACT) and blood pressure. Pull back in a gentle continuous manner near the skin entry site, which limits catheter vibration.[8] Applying a blood pressure cuff over the area of spasm to 40 mmHg greater than systolic blood pressure (SBP), which is then deflated rapidly, and using warm compresses can be helpful. Nitroglycerine can be injected subcutaneously if there is a focal area of spasm. In extreme cases, consider general anesthesia and/or axillary nerve block.

2. Catheterization of the left internal mammary artery (IMA): When obtaining access into the descending thoracic aorta, the wire and catheter can inadvertently enter the IMA and follow its normal caudal pathway similar to the descending aorta. In this case, the catheter will be located more laterally than expected, and the operator might experience some resistance as the artery narrows distally or the catheter tip engages some branches of the IMA. If either of these happen, gentle hand contrast injection should be performed to confirm proper location.

3. Radial artery occlusion (RAO): This is rare with proper heparinization and use of the patent hemostasis concept. RAO is usually identified in the postoperative area after the compression band is removed and a weak or absent radial pulse is noted. If ischemic changes are noted on the hand, one should look for the ulnar pulse. If this is also absent, there is likely a brachial artery problem. If the hand is not ischemic and the ulnar pulse is present, consider RAO. *Note*: 90% of RAOs will still have a radial pulse due to the water hammer effect, but the pulse may feel weaker. Consider antegrade recanalization of the radial artery and 3–6 months of anticoagulation.

4. Pseudoaneurysms: If identified, treat with compression after performing ultrasound to ensure there is no clot within the pseudoaneurysm that could embolize distally. This can also be treated with direct thrombin injection if unresolved with compression.

5. Radial artery rupture: Risk is decreased with an initial sheath angiogram, direct wire visualization, and keen attention to tactile wire resistance. If it occurs, maintaining wire access, 3- or 4-mm balloon inflation, and immediately applying a compressive wrap are the necessary steps to decrease the chance of hematoma, which can lead to compartment syndrome. Evaluate and treat forearm hematomas based on the EASY Hematoma Classification.[18,19]

Steps of the Procedure

1. Preoperative evaluation: Start with Allen's test if oximetry pulse wave detector and monitor are not available. Because it is more sensitive than Allen's test, Barbeau's test may be used instead if the necessary equipment and supplies are available. *Barbeau's test*: Place the oximetry probe on the index finger. Use manual pressure to occlude the radial and ulnar arteries. Next, release pressure from the ulnar artery while keeping the radial artery compression. A recognizable waveform should return. As long as you have a Barbeau's type A, B, or C waveform, you can proceed to ultrasound evaluation. If you have a type D waveform, TRA from the chosen wrist is contraindicated. To measure the diameter of the radial artery, use a high-frequency ultrasound probe 1 or 2 cm proximal to the styloid process. First, ensure that the artery is compressible (patent) and free of significant calcification (echogenicity). Use minimal probe pressure because this can cause anteroposterior (AP) (inner-to-inner wall diameter) size underestimation. We consider a radial artery less than 2 mm to be a relative contraindication for

TRA if the radial sheath is larger than 5 Fr. Take this opportunity to scan 10–20 cm up the radial artery, looking for vascular loops or tortuosity. Important to mention that the slender sheath technology will probably provide an opportunity to use smaller outer diameter sheaths in smaller AP radial arteries (5 Fr slender sheath would be compatible with a radial artery larger than 1.6 mm).

2. Patient preparation: Position the patient with left arm abduction at 75–90 degrees. The abducted position enables matching of the angiography table to the procedure table, creating a large, efficient work surface. Place a radiation shield between the interventionalist and the patient to reduce scattered radiation dose. The wrist should be slightly hyperextended on top of a folded sterile towel and the fingers taped.

3. Sheath insertion: Prealign and collimate the intensifier over the forearm. Use ultrasound guidance to locate the radial artery 1 or 2 cm proximal to the styloid process. Anesthetize with 0.5–1 ml of lidocaine. In patients with a minimal amount of soft tissues around the radial artery, the lidocaine may be used not only as a local anesthetic but also as a cushion (creation of extra space) between the skin and the artery. Preferably, single wall puncture of the radial artery is performed under ultrasound visualization at a 30- to 45-degree angle using a short 21 gauge radial needle bevel up. Advance the 0.021-in. wire under fluoroscopy. Remove the needle and hold pressure (preventing rapid hematoma development); advance the hydrophilic sheath without skin nick, as mentioned previously. Secure the sheath with an adhesive dressing because hydrophilic radial access sheaths can easily be displaced. Confirm blood return and administer 200 μg of nitroglycerine (NTG) (if SBP >100 mmHg) via the sheath. We typically give heparin through a peripheral venous access. We loosely use 50 U/kg and typically give 2000–3000 units for average body weight followed by an additional 1000 units every 30 minutes for the duration in case the procedure lasts more than 60 minutes. If more than 2 hours, we check ACT levels and dose accordingly. Initial forearm angiography is performed with gentle hand injection of 6–8 ml 50% dilute contrast under digital subtraction angiography until the radial palmar arch filling retrograde from the ulnar or interosseous artery behind the sheath hub. For upper abdominal interventions, load the 110-cm 5 Fr Jacky radial catheter and lead with the 1.5-mm J Glidewire, breaking the table as you advance centrally. Advance the guidewire and catheter only under fluoroscopy. Level your angiography table to the height of your procedure table. Navigate the left subclavian and the descending aorta, and select the desired vessel. Remember that the Jacky radial catheter is a flush diagnostic catheter (two side holes at the tip) and is

excellent for power injection. If you need to place a long sheath, consider a second 200-μg NTG prior to placement. We do not routinely use calcium channel blockade. Typically, a 130-cm-long microcatheter system is sufficient for hepatic, gastroduodenal, and renal procedures, except if the patient is more than 6 feet 2 inches tall. A 150-cm-long microcatheter should be selected in taller patients, as well as for splenic, superior mesenteric, and inferior mesenteric artery catheterization and endoleak procedures.

4. Sheath removal: At the end of the procedure, remove the Jacky catheter over the 0.035-in. wire in order to protect the tip as it is pulled back around the aortic arch. These wires and catheters are long, and there is a tendency to grab both at the back end and pull. This creates a guitar string effect causing catheter shaft vibration, which can induce radial artery spasm. Avoid this by keeping two fingers close to the sheath as the catheter is pulled back. Because continuous infusion through the sheath is not used, aspirate any potential clot from the sheath and give an additional 200 μg NTG via the sheath. Acquire forearm arteriogram to confirm retrograde palmar arch filling via a patent ulnar artery. Slip a 4 × 4 gauze under the sheath until it abuts the skin entry site. Apply the TR Band (Terumo) with the green marker over the radial entry site. Inject 15 ml of air and remove the syringe. Rapid syringe connect/disconnect maintains the valve seal. Pull the sheath and observe. Now empty the syringe and reconnect. Withdraw 1 ml at a time and check for bleeding. Do this until a jet of blood is observed or there is 10 ml of air remaining in the TR Band balloon (whichever occurs first) and then stop. If you encounter bleeding during deflation, stop and add 2 ml air back. During the hemostasis period, capillary refill is checked along with pulse oximetry: Manually occlude the ulnar artery and check the waveform (reversed Barbeau's test). If present, you have finished, if not, deflate 1 ml of air and re-evaluate the plethysmograph during ulnar occlusion (reversed Barbeau's test). The goal is to achieve patent hemostasis (enough compression to prevent bleeding through the arteriotomy but not so much that it could result in occlusion of the radial artery).[14] Remove the gauze and write the time and amount of air on a sticker and apply it on the syringe. Then place the syringe in the patient's hand and ask him or her to hold it until it is delivered to the recovery area nurse.

5. Recovery area: Monitor for bleeding and assess index finger pulse oximetry, hand color, and capillary refill. After 1 hour of observation, deflation can be started, and 2 or 3 ml of air should be removed every 15 minutes. If bleeding occurs, add back 2 ml and begin again after 45 minutes. Upon complete deflation, remove the band and apply a sterile

dressing. If no bleeding after 30 minutes, the patient can be safely discharged. Minimal bruising and tenderness for 2 or 3 days are the most common post-procedure findings. An alternative protocol that we are currently testing is to observe for 15 minutes after the patent hemostasis is obtained with the TR Band and then deflate the balloon over a period

of 30 minutes and observe for an additional 15 minutes. The goal is to discharge the patient home or to the floor in 1 hour.

Example
See Figures 58.1–58.4.

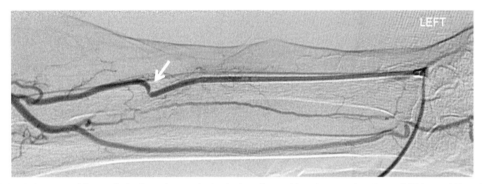

Figure 58.1 Initial arteriogram of the radial artery demonstrates tortuosity and focal narrowing (arrow). This could lead to difficulty advancing the wire and catheter blindly. Under real-time fluoroscopy, a micro-guidewire, followed by a microcatheter, is typically sufficient to straighten the artery. Then, coaxially, a 4 or 5 Fr diagnostic catheter is advanced without complications.

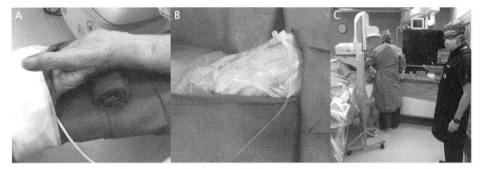

Figure 58.2 (A) Left arm in 90-degree abduction. Note the wrist slightly hyperextended on top of a folded sterile towel and the fingers taped. This helps better expose the radial artery, facilitating needle puncture. (B) After access is obtained, a dressing is used to secure the sheath in place because the hydrophilic coat can lead to accidental sheath withdrawal and loss of the access. (C) Room setup. Note the back table aligned and in continuity with the patient's abducted arm. This provides a satisfactory working area, where wires and catheters can be manipulated.

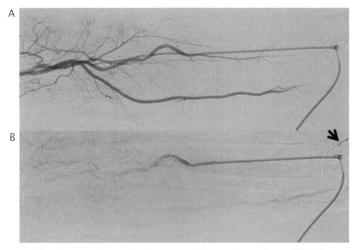

Figure 58.3 (A) Initial arteriogram of the forearm demonstrating normal vascular anatomy. (B) Late acquisition showing retrograde filling of the distal radial artery (arrow), confirming patent palmar arch.

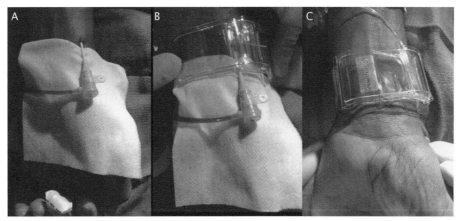

Figure 58.4 (A) A 4 × 4-in. gauze is placed underneath the sheath to absolve potential bleeding. (B) Application of the TR Band around the wrist. Note the marking dot immediately on top of the skin puncture site. (C) Once the band is inflated and no bleeding is present, the gauze can be removed. At this point, the patient is transferred to the recovery area.

References and Suggested Readings

1. Peterson ED, Dai D, DeLong ER, et al. Contemporary mortality risk prediction for percutaneous coronary interventions: Results from 588,398 procedures in the National Cardiovascular Data Registry. *J Am Coll Cardiol.* 2010;55:1923–1932.

2. Agostoni P, Biondi-Zoccai GG, de Benedictis ML, et al. Coronary diagnostic and interventional procedures: Systematic overview and meta-analysis of randomized trials. *J Am Coll Cardiol.* 2004;44:349–356.

3. Chase AJ, Fretz EB, Warburton WP, et al. Association of the arterial access site at angioplasty with transfusion and mortality: The M.O.R.T.A.L study (Mortality Benefit of Reduced Transfusion After Percutaneous Coronary Intervention via the Arm or Leg). *Heart.* 2008;94:1019–1025.

4. Kiemeneij F, Laarman GJ, Odekerken D, et al. A randomized comparison of percutaneous transluminal coronary angioplasty by the radial, brachial and femoral approaches: The ACCESS study. *J Am Coll Cardiol.* 1997;29:1269–1275.

5. Lo T S, Nolan J, Fountzopoulos E, et al. Radial artery anomaly and its influence on transradial coronary procedural outcome. *Heart.* 2009;95:410–415.

6. Barbeau GR, Arsenault F, Dugas L, Simard S, Lariviere M. Evaluation of the ulnopalmar arterial arches with pulse oximetry and plethysmography: Comparison with the Allen's test in 1010 patients. *Am Heart J.* 2004;147:489–493.

7. Pancholy SP, Coppoa J, Patel T, Roke-Thomas M. Prevention of Radial Artery Occlusion: Patent Hemostasis Evaluation Trial (PROPHET study): A randomized comparison of traditional versus patency documented hemostasis after transradial catheterization. *Catheter Cardiovasc Interv.* 2008;9:335–340.

8. Sanghvi KA. Ten critical lessons for performing transradial catheterization. *Endovascular Today.* 2014;3:62–67.

9. Campeau L. Percutaneous radial artery approach for coronary angiography. *Cathet Cardiovasc Diagn.* 1989;16:3–7.

10. Cooper CJ, El-Shiekh RA, Cohen DJ, et al. Effect of transradial access on quality of life and cost of cardiac catheterization: A randomized comparison. *Am Heart J.* 1999;138:430–436.

11. Benamer H, Louvard Y, Sanmartin M, et al. A multicentre comparison of transradial and transfemoral approaches for coronary angiography and PTCA in obese patients: The TROP registry. *EuroIntervention.* 2007;3:327–332.

12. Fishman AM, Swinburne NC, Patel RS. A technical guide describing the use of transradial access technique for endovascular interventions. *Tech Vasc Interv Radiol.* 2015;6:58–65.

13. Resnick NJ, Edward K, Patel RS, et al. Uterine artery embolization using a transradial approach: Initial experience and technique. *J Vasc Interv Radiol.* 2014;3:443–447.

14. Etxegoien N, Rhyne D, Kedev S, et al. The transradial approach for carotid artery stenting. *Cathet Cardiovasc Interv.* 2012; 80(7):1081–1087.

15. Ostojić Z, Bulum J, Ernst A, Strozzi M, Marić-Bešić K. Frequency of radial artery anatomic variations in patients undergoing transradial heart catheterization. *Acta Clin Croat.* 2015;54(1):65–72.

16. Numasawa Y, Kawamura A, Kohsaka S, et al. Anatomical variations affect radial artery spasm and procedural achievement of transradial cardiac catheterization. *Heart Vessels.* 2014;29(1):49–57.

17. Rathore S, Stables RH, Pauriah M, et al. Impact of length and hydrophilic coating of the introducer sheath on radial artery spasm during transradial coronary intervention: A randomized study. *JACC Cardiovasc Interv.* 2010;3:475–483.

18. Bertrand OE. Acute forearm muscle swelling post transradial catheterization and compartment syndrome: Prevention is better than treatment! *Catheter Cardiovasc Interv.* 2010;75: 366–368.

19. Caputo RP. Avoiding and managing forearm hematomas. *Cardiol Interv Today.* 2011;3:55–58.

CHAPTER 59

Slow and Steady Method for Advancing Devices Through Tight or Tortuous Anatomy

Robert Evans Heithaus, Almas Syed, and Chet R. Rees

Brief Description

Advancing vascular sheaths, catheters, balloons, stent grafts, or drainage catheters can prove difficult in tight or tortuous anatomy, leading to prolonged procedure and fluoroscopy time. Understanding the physical principles of kinetic versus static friction can help the operator overcome these difficulties. The application of slow, steady force of a lower magnitude may result in more successful advancement of the device with reduction of pain and complications due to tissue tearing.

Overcoming the static forces of friction (i.e., the force that is required to start an object in motion) requires a greater magnitude of force compared to the kinetic forces of friction (i.e., the force that is required to keep an objection in motion). Static forces of friction can result in catheter or device kinking, particularly in tight or tortuous anatomy. By applying steady force of lower magnitude, the effects of both static and kinetic friction are overcome without catheter or device kinking that can occur when applying a large amount of force multiple times. This will ultimately result in less friction and thus less pain and difficulty passing a device or catheter.

Applications of the Technique

1. Difficult passage of biliary catheter.
2. Difficult passage of nephrostomy catheter.
3. Percutaneous drainage catheter that is difficult to pass through different fascial planes.
4. Passage of a balloon or stent graft through stenotic vasculature.
5. Removal of permcaths, T-tubes, ureteral stents, peripherally inserted central catheters, or foreign bodies.

Challenges of the Procedure

1. Overcoming the desire to force a catheter or device into place, making multiple attempts.
2. Need for rapid procedural completion and turnover.
3. Need for larger drainage catheter.

Potential Pitfalls/Complications

1. Increase radiation exposure if the use of intermittent fluoroscopy is not instituted by the operator.

Steps of the Procedure

1. Obtain access to the organ system of interest with a guidewire of appropriate stiffness.
2. Using the Seldinger technique, advance the device, drain, balloon, or catheter of interest.
3. When difficulty passing the object is encountered, apply a low to intermediate level of constant force to the device. Do not stop applying force because you will have to again overcome the static forces of friction.
4. Use intermittent fluoroscopy to visualize device advancement if needed.
5. Continue to apply a steady level of force over several minutes to slowly advance the device or catheter.

Example

See Figure 59.1.

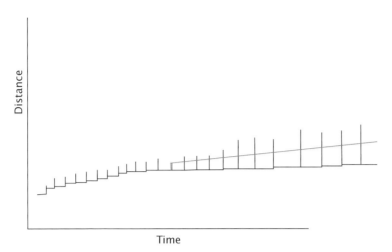

Figure 59.1 Operators often apply repetitive forceful thrusts when advancing catheters and sheaths through tissues with high friction (black spikes), resulting in sudden incremental advances as shown. The high force and repeated to-and-fro motion of the tissues can lead to pain and injury. The pale line depicts the use of steady, constant force of lower magnitude, which results in smooth motion of the catheter. This can improve successful advancement while reducing pain and complications.

CHAPTER 60

End of the Road: Bailout Techniques for the Short Wire

S. Lowell Kahn

Brief Description

Guidewires for peripheral interventions come in a variety of lengths for the 0.035/0.038-, 0.018-, and 0.014-in. platforms. Common lengths include 75/80, 145, 180, 200, 260, 300, and 330 cm. Whereas a navigation wire need only be slightly longer than the catheter in use, guidewires over which exchanges are necessary for intervention need to be considerably longer. As a general rule, a guidewire should be long enough to be passed sufficiently beyond the treatment zone (e.g., occlusion) to facilitate adequate support with enough wire external to the patient to allow for any desired catheter or balloon use/exchange (e.g., 150 cm for a typical tibial balloon).

Unfortunately, despite the best efforts at planning, it is not uncommon for an interventionalist to realize that there is insufficient wire to perform the task at hand. If catheterization of a vessel or traversal of occlusion is difficult, sacrificing wire access for a catheter exchange is unacceptable.

This chapter presents three bailout techniques that may be employed in short wire scenarios. Each technique should be performed cautiously and with live fluoroscopy where necessary to prevent untoward complications.

The first technique, the *back end of the wire technique*, is a method for removing a catheter or device when there is insufficient wire external to the patient to facilitate the removal without compromising access. During this technique, the catheter (device) to be removed is retracted until the back end of the wire is flush with the hub of the catheter. The back end of a second wire is then placed into the hub against the back end of the wire in the patient. The catheter (device) is safely removed by pinning the second wire (preventing the primary wire from pulling out) and sliding the catheter (device) over the second wire.

The second technique, the *short wire advancement technique*, is a method for advancing a catheter or device a short distance when the wire is not present at the hub to be pinned. This technique must be performed on a limited basis and with caution given the potential risks of a complication. With this technique, the wire tip is carefully placed in either a small-caliber side branch or in the subintimal space where there is clear resistance to forward advancement of the wire. With continual fluoroscopy performed both distally near the wire tip and proximally near the sheath, the catheter (device) is slowly advanced until wire exits the hub, at which point standard advancement is performed.

The final technique, the *physician-modified rapid exchange technique*, involves the creation of a rapid exchange catheter that can be advanced over a short wire and subsequently used to exchange the short wire for a longer wire. A small side hole is cut in a standard angiography catheter a short distance (e.g., 20 cm) from the tip of the catheter. This catheter is then advanced over the wire, bringing the back end of the wire through the side hole rather than the hub of the catheter. The catheter is then advanced to the wire tip, and the wire is exchanged for a longer wire.

Applications of the Technique

Back End of the Wire Technique
1. Removal of a catheter or device when there is insufficient wire external to the patient.

Short Wire Advancement Technique
1. Advancement of catheter or device to an intended target when there is insufficient wire external to the patient to load and advance the catheter or device.

Physician-Modified Rapid Exchange Technique
1. Exchange of a short wire for a longer wire when there is insufficient wire to allow advancement of the catheter necessary for the exchange.

Challenges of the Procedure

Back End of the Wire Technique
1. During this procedure, mating the back ends of the two wires in the hub can be moderately challenging because there is a tendency for the back end of the second wire to pass side by side the back end of

the primary wire within the widened hub. When this occurs, we retract the catheter or device back slightly so that the primary wire is truly in the catheter (device) lumen rather than the hub. The back end of the second wire is then placed against the primary wire.

Short Wire Advancement Technique

1. It can be difficult to find a small side branch or subintimal wire placement suitable for this technique. Specifically, this technique is the most risky, and it is imperative that the wire does not advance forward as the catheter or device is advanced. Forward advancement of the wire could lead to a lost wire (retained foreign body) or vascular injury.

Physician-Modified Rapid Exchange Technique

1. Although this technique is fairly easy to perform, a rapid exchange platform lacks the support of a wire brought through the end hole of a catheter. Therefore, advancing a catheter with this technique through tortuous or tight anatomy may be challenging.

Potential Pitfalls/Complications

Back End of the Wire Technique

1. Although highly unlikely, care must be taken not to push the primary wire into the patient. The goal is simply to pin the primary wire with the back end of the second wire while the catheter is removed.

Short Wire Advancement Technique

1. Vessel dissection or bleeding is possible if too much forward pressure is placed on the catheter (and hence the wire). Slow forward advancement under continuous fluoroscopy is advised.

2. In addition to the risk of vessel injury, this technique carries a risk of losing a wire in the patient. For this reason, we advise that it be performed with fluoroscopy with attention paid to both distal and proximal ends of the wire to ensure that the proximal end of the wire does not get pushed into the sheath or the patient.

Physician-Modified Rapid Exchange Technique

1. Creating a side hole in a standard catheter carries the risk of compromising the structural integrity of the catheter. Therefore, the hole should be made as small as possible to allow passage of the wire, and the catheter should be inspected carefully before inserting it into the patient. If the structural integrity were compromised, the catheter could break, necessitating extraction of the catheter tip from the patient.

Steps of the Procedure

Back End of the Wire Technique

1. After identifying that there is insufficient wire to exchange the catheter (device) in place, the catheter (device) is retracted such that wire is located at the transition between the hub and the lumen of the catheter (device).

2. The back end of the second wire is then brought end to end with the back end of the primary wire. We prefer a stiff wire e.g., Rosen (Cook Medical Inc., Bloomington, IN) and Amplatz (Boston Scientific Inc., Marlborough, MA) as our second wire. Care is made that the two ends of the wire are firmly abutting one another. If necessary, the catheter (device) can be pulled back slightly further to allow the second wire to advance beyond the hub into the lumen of the catheter (device).

3. The second wire is then pinned as though it is simply an extension of the primary wire.

4. While pinned, the catheter (device) is retracted over both wires. Intermittent fluoroscopy is used to confirm that the tip of the primary wire has not moved.

5. Additional interventions are then performed. To avoid having to use this technique a second time, a short catheter (long enough to reach the wire end) can be placed (with the short wire advancement technique if necessary) to allow exchange for a longer wire prior to additional interventions.

Short Wire Advancement Technique

1. This technique is riskier than the other techniques, and its use is advised on a limited and cautious basis with judicious use of fluoroscopy.

2. The wire in use is either navigated into a small side branch or carefully buckled within a tight subintimal space.

3. Gentle forward pressure is then placed on the wire to confirm that there is resistance to advancement.

4. The catheter (device) to be advanced over the wire is flushed, and the wire is wet again immediately prior to placing the catheter (device) to minimize friction with the wire.

5. The catheter (device) that is to be advanced over the wire is placed on the wire and advanced until the hub of the catheter (device) is flush with the back end of the wire.

6. Further advancement is then performed cautiously until the catheter (device) reaches the intended target or until the wire presents itself at the hub, at which point the wire is pinned in standard fashion. This is done with live fluoroscopy performed at both the wire tip and the sheath to confirm that the wire is not moving. We advise spinning of the catheter (device) to minimize friction of the catheter (device) relative to the wire.

7. If the wire tip advances any significant distance, the technique is aborted and the catheter is removed. To prevent wire dislodgment, the back end of the wire technique can be applied as needed to maintain wire position.

Physician-Modified Rapid Exchange Technique

1. If a short wire is optimally placed but there is insufficient wire external to the patient to advance the desired catheter (device) to the target, this technique can be employed to exchange for a longer wire.
2. A 100-cm hockey stick catheter (e.g., Kumpe, Cook Medical) is usually sufficient for most exchanges. Shorter or longer catheters can be used as needed.
3. The catheter is kinked approximately 20 cm from the tip of the catheter. This distance can be adjusted as needed.
4. At the point where the catheter is kinked, the catheter is cut with scissors or a number 11 blade on one side. This may require some practice, but the goal is to create a side hole 20 cm proximal to the tip that is of adequate size to pass the wire (typically 0.035 in.).
5. Once the side hole is created, it is assessed for adequate size by passing a wire carefully through the side hole on the back table.
6. The modified catheter is then loaded on the wire. As the wire approaches the side hole, the catheter is bent to favor the back end of the wire to exit through the side hole.
7. Once the back end of the wire reaches the side hole, the wire is pinned, and the catheter can be advanced as a rapid exchange system.
8. Once the catheter reaches the end of the wire, the short wire may be removed.
9. An exchange length wire can then be placed through the catheter, and the catheter is removed.

Example
See Figures 60.1 and 60.2.

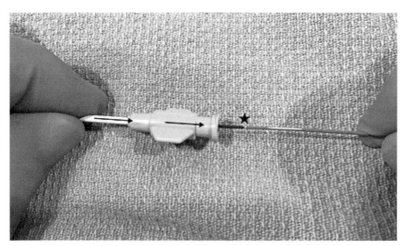

Figure 60.1 Back end of the wire technique. The wire is too short for exchange, but the wire tip is in an ideal location. The back end of a Fixed Core Wire Guide (Cook Medical) is brought end-to-end (star) with the back end of the Glidewire (Terumo, Somerset, NJ) that is in the catheter. Maintaining wire position, the catheter can now be removed (arrows) over the two wires.

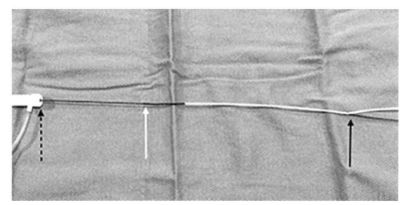

Figure 60.2 Physician-modified rapid exchange technique. A short wire is in optimal position and needs to be exchanged for a longer wire. A Kumpe catheter has been modified with a side hole created (black arrow) approximately 20 cm proximal to the end. The Kumpe catheter is then loaded over the wire (white arrow), which is subsequently passed through the side hole (black arrow) and then advanced through the sheath (dashed arrow). Upon reaching the target, the short wire is removed and exchanged for a longer wire as needed.

CHAPTER 61

Balloon Anchor Techniques for Sheath, Guide Catheter, and Stent Advancement and to Facilitate Chronic Total Occlusion Traversal

S. Lowell Kahn

Brief Description

Advancement of a sheath or guide catheter into a small, diseased or angled branch vessel such as the superior mesenteric artery or renal artery can be difficult. Similarly, there are times when placement of a sheath up and over a sharply angulated aortic bifurcation can present a challenge. Obtaining a sheath position at or beyond a stenotic or occlusive lesion may be critical for delivering a stent, particularly with the inherent risk of dislodgment associated with balloon-expandable stents. Planning an access in close proximity to the lesion and one that minimizes angulation is undoubtedly helpful. In addition, selecting a shaped, hydrophilic, and braided guide catheter or sheath (e.g., Flexor, Cook Medical Inc., Bloomington, IN) as well as pre-dilating a target lesion are important strategies.

Despite these measures, there are times when delivery of the sheath to its desired position remains difficult. This chapter briefly discusses the utility of balloons as an anchor to advance a sheath or stent to a target location. The use of balloons as anchors has been described most commonly in the coronary vasculature, but it nonetheless can have an important role in peripheral and visceral applications.[1–9] Anchoring a balloon has also been described in the neurointerventional literature as a means for stenting and embolization as well as eliminating redundancy (looping) of a wire in a large aneurysm.[10–12]

The *standard balloon anchor technique* is very commonly employed and simply involves inflation of a balloon distal to the sheath or guide catheter and using the stability of the balloon to provide traction for sheath or guide catheter advancement.[5,13] It is commonly performed with the balloon located immediately beyond the sheath or guide catheter, and the sheath or guide catheter is advanced over the balloon as it is deflated. This minimizes the free edge of the sheath or guide catheter and provides for a more smooth advancement. The technique is highly effective for

sheath advancement, frequently superior to advancement of the sheath with the dilator in place.

This standard technique has been modified whereby a buddy wire system functions as the anchor, herein described as the *buddy wire balloon anchor technique*. One iteration of this was first described by Fujita et al.[3] in 2003 and involves placement of a buddy wire into a small side branch of the target vessel. Over the buddy wire, a small balloon is advanced and inflated, providing support for further advancement of the sheath, guide catheter, or stent over the primary wire in the target vessel. This technique has proven useful in the coronary vasculature,[3,4,7] but it has potential application elsewhere in the body, particularly in the mesenteric vasculature. Similarly, placement of the balloon over a buddy wire located distally in the target vessel is also possible and provides stability for sheath, guide catheter, or stent delivery as needed.

Finally, a balloon anchor can be placed proximal to a chronic total occlusion (CTO) and used to provide guidewire support for crossing of a CTO.[8,14] In this chapter, this technique is referred to as the *anchor balloon CTO crossing technique*.

Applications of the Technique

Standard and Buddy Wire Balloon Anchor Techniques

1. Delivery of a sheath, guide catheter, and/or stent in tight or tortuous vascular anatomy.

Anchor Balloon CTO Crossing Technique

1. Traversal of CTOs where added guidewire support is necessary for success and intraluminal recanalization is desirable. Use of a balloon not only provides added support but also by nature will center a wire on the proximal cap of a CTO. In so doing, this increases

the chance that the wire will traverse the CTO intraluminal as opposed to subintimal. In small vessels (e.g., tibial arteries) in which re-entry from the subintimal plane may be difficult, this confers an advantage.

Challenges of the Procedure

1. With all of the balloon anchor techniques, delivery of the anchor balloon may present a challenge. In these situations, use of the smallest possible balloon diameter that allows vessel wall apposition and hence friction is advised. We commonly employ 0.014- or 0.018-in. balloons because of their low profile. Also, the use of short balloons for all of these interventions is preferable.

Potential Pitfalls/Complications

1. Use of an anchor balloon carries inherent risk of vascular injury and may result in endothelial denudation, intimal tears, neointimal proliferation with accelerated atherosclerosis, dissection, or plaque rupture.[15]

Steps of the Procedure

Standard Balloon Anchor Technique

1. The sheath or guide catheter is advanced as close as possible to the intended location.
2. The target vessel is catheterized with standard wire and catheter technique.
3. Wire access adequately beyond the intended sheath or guide catheter location is obtained.
4. Over the wire, a short low-profile balloon of appropriate diameter (equal to or one size larger than the target vessel) is advanced into the vessel at or beyond the desired location of the sheath or guide catheter.
5. The balloon is inflated to a low pressure (just high enough to allow apposition of the balloon to the vessel wall). If a 0.035-in. balloon will not deliver, downsize to a 0.014- or 0.018-in. platform to obtain a lower profile.
6. At this point, the sheath or guide catheter can be advanced carefully while gentle back traction is applied to the anchor balloon. Care must be taken that the free edge of the sheath or guide catheter (which is not tapered fully to the balloon catheter) does not injure the vessel (dissection) or result in embolization (plaque dislodgement).
7. *Optional*: We commonly place the balloon immediately beyond the tip of the sheath or guide catheter. The assistant deflates the balloon while the operator advances the sheath or guide catheter over the deflating balloon. This strategy of "paying the sheath/

guide catheter off of the balloon" is highly effective and arguably safer because it minimizes the free edge of the sheath or guide catheter.
8. After the sheath or guide catheter reaches its desired location, the procedure is continued as intended.

Buddy Wire Balloon Anchor Technique

1. The sheath or guide catheter is advanced as close as possible to the intended location.
2. The target vessel is catheterized with standard wire and catheter technique.
3. Wire access adequately beyond the intended sheath, guide catheter, or stent location is obtained.
4. A second buddy wire is advanced into the target vessel and is either advanced adjacent to the primary wire distal to the intended sheath, guide catheter, or stent location (scenario 1) or is steered into a small side branch (scenario 2) in conjunction with a microcatheter.
5. Over the buddy wire, a small low-profile balloon (0.014- or 0.018-in. platform) is placed either distally within the target vessel (scenario 1) or into the side branch (scenario 2). The anchor balloon diameter need only match or slightly exceed the diameter of the vessel.
6. The balloon on the buddy wire is inflated as the anchor to a low pressure that allows apposition to the vessel wall.
7. The sheath, guide catheter, and/or stent is then carefully advanced over the primary wire with gentle traction applied to the anchor balloon.
8. After the sheath, guide catheter, and/or stent reaches the desired location, the procedure is continued as intended.

Anchor Balloon CTO Crossing Technique

1. The guidewire is advanced to the proximal cap of a CTO.
2. Over the guidewire, a balloon is advanced immediately adjacent to the proximal cap of the CTO.
3. If possible, the sheath or guide catheter should be advanced (possibly with utilization of the standard balloon anchor technique) close to the balloon to provide maximal support. The anchor balloon diameter need only match or slightly exceed the diameter of the vessel.
4. The balloon is inflated adjacent to the CTO to a low pressure that allows apposition to the vessel wall.
5. With the balloon inflated, an appropriately selected crossing wire is advanced through the balloon lumen and used to traverse the CTO. Utilization of this technique not only will provide exceptional wire support but also optimizes the chances of the wire remaining within the true lumen.
6. Once the wire successfully traverses the CTO, the balloon is deflated and the procedure is continued.

7. *Optional*: Balloon catheters are inherently rigid with increased longitudinal stability. As such, they often function well as a crossing catheter in tight lesions and may obviate the need for a crossing catheter.

Example

See Figures 61.1–61.6.

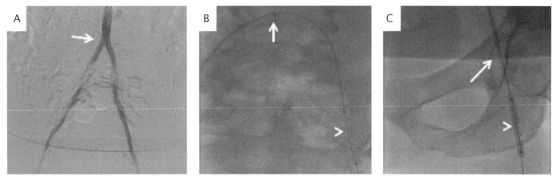

Figure 61.1 A patient presented with severe left superficial femoral artery disease. (A) A sharply angulated aortic bifurcation (arrow) was observed on abdominal aortography. (B) A 6 Fr × 45-cm sheath (arrow) would not advance over the aortic bifurcation. Therefore, a balloon (arrowhead) was advanced to the proximal left superficial femoral artery. (C) With the balloon inflated (arrowhead), the 6 Fr sheath (arrow) was easily advanced to the contralateral left common femoral artery.

Source: From Mahmood A, et al. Applications of the distal anchoring technique in coronary and peripheral interventions. *J Invasive Cardiol.* 2011;23(7):289–292. Reprinted with permission from HMP Communications.

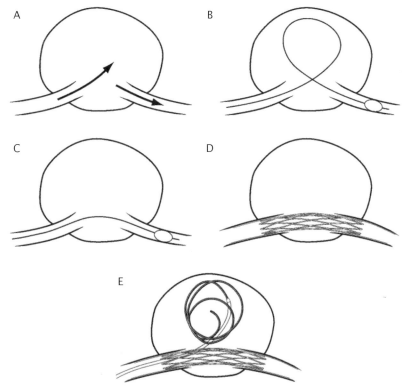

Figure 61.2 Standard balloon anchor technique. Schematic demonstrating the use of a balloon catheter as an anchor for the treatment of a cerebral aneurysm. (A) As one catheterizes the aneurysm, the angulation of the inflow and outflow vessels predisposes the catheter to redundant looping and makes distal catheterization in the outflow vessel difficult. Catheterization beyond the vessel is obtained, but redundant looping within the aneurysm makes additional treatment difficult. (B) A balloon is advanced to the outflow vessel and inflated. (C) With the balloon inflated, traction is applied to the balloon catheter to reduce the loop. With straight catheterization, a stent is deployed across the neck of the aneurysm (D), which allows embolization of the aneurysm while preserving blood flow in the parent vessel (E).

Source: From Snyder KV, et al. The balloon anchor technique: A novel technique for distal access through a giant aneurysm. *J Neurointerv Surg.* 2010;2(4):363–367. Courtesy BMJ Publishing Inc.

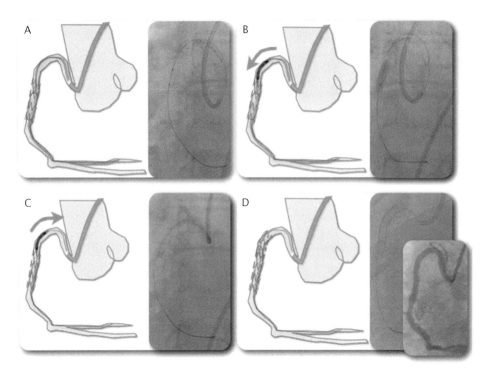

Figure 61.3 Buddy wire balloon anchor technique. Schematic demonstrates existing stent in the right coronary artery. The stent has restenosed and requires angioplasty and proximal stent extension. A guide catheter provides support at the vessel ostium, but delivery of a proximal stent is not possible. Two wires are therefore threaded into the right coronary artery. (A) A balloon is inflated over the first and used for traction and support of the system. (B) Over an adjacent wire, a new stent is delivered to the appropriate position. (C) Once the stent is in place, the balloon is deflated and the second wire is removed (so as not to become trapped behind the new stent). (D) The new stent is deployed. Although the buddy wire anchor technique is described in the coronary literature, this technique could be extrapolated for use elsewhere in the body, namely the mesenteric vasculature (e.g., SMA).

Source: From Surmely JF, Cook S. Variation on the anchor balloon technique for difficult stent delivery. *Kardiovaskuläre Medizin* 2007;10:397–399. Courtesy Kardiovaskulare Medizin/EMH Swiss Medical Publishers.

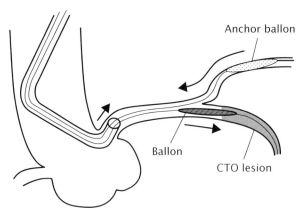

Figure 61.4 Buddy wire balloon anchor technique. A guide catheter is placed at the ostium of the coronary artery to be treated. An anchor balloon can be placed and inflated in a side branch (marginal artery). A second wire is then advanced across the chronic total occlusion (CTO) to be treated, and repair can be performed with placement of a stent. The anchor balloon provides exceptional support for traversal and stenting of the CTO. Although the buddy wire anchor technique is described in the coronary literature, this technique could be extrapolated for use elsewhere in the body, namely the mesenteric vasculature (e.g., SMA).

Source: From Fujita S, et al. New technique for superior guiding catheter support during advancement of a balloon in coronary angioplasty: The anchor technique. *Catheter Cardiovasc Interv.* 2003;59:482–488. Courtesy Wiley InterScience.

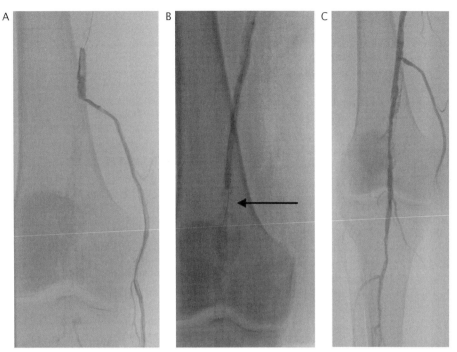

Figure 61.5 Anchor balloon CTO crossing technique. A 78-year-old female with digital ulceration of the right foot. (A) Preliminary angiogram shows abrupt occlusion of the proximal popliteal artery. A true lumen revascularization was desired to avoid stenting that would likely be required with a subintimal approach. With a catheter and wire, the wire continued to deflect into the subintimal space (not shown). Therefore, a balloon was advanced and inflated immediately abutting the occlusion. (B) This provided the support to allow passage of a straight Glidewire (arrow) (Terumo, Somerset, NJ) through the occlusion. (C) Final arteriogram after angioplasty with a drug-eluting balloon reveals a recanalized popliteal artery.

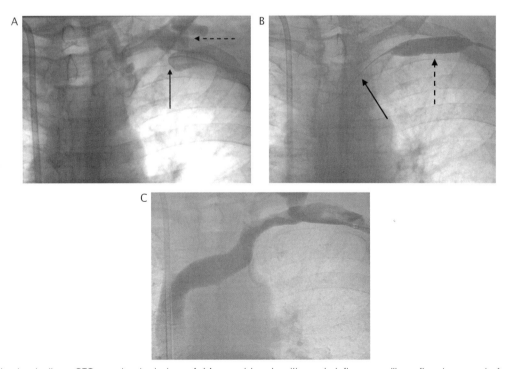

Figure 61.6 Anchor balloon CTO crossing technique. A 64-year-old male with acute left arm swelling after placement of a left upper extremity arteriovenous fistula. (A) Central venogram reveals incidental findings of thoracic outlet syndrome with a focal occlusion of the left subclavian vein (solid arrow). Collateral veins (dashed arrow) are appreciated superiorly. A long 7 Fr sheath was advanced to the occlusion. Although short, the occlusion proved to be very difficult to traverse despite excellent sheath support. Multiple wires and catheters were attempted, including use of the back end of a Glidewire. Despite these maneuvers, the catheter continued to deflect away from the occlusion. (B) A 10-mm balloon (dashed arrow) was inflated immediately adjacent to the occlusion to provide support. The back end of a Glidewire (solid arrow) was advanced a short distance beyond the occlusion. The balloon was deflated, a Kumpe catheter (Cook Medical Inc., Bloomington, IN) was advanced to the tip of the Glidewire, and the Glidewire was removed and flipped to its standard configuration before being used to catheterize the inferior vena cava. (C) The occlusion was then angioplastied, obtaining patency prior to performance of a first rib resection the following day.

References and Suggested Readings

1. Worley SJ. How to use balloons as anchors to facilitate cannulation of the coronary sinus left ventricular lead placement and to regain lost coronary sinus left ventricular lead placement and to regain lost coronary sinus or target vein access. *Heart Rhythm.* 2009;6(8):1242–1246.

2. Surmely JF, Cook S. Variation on the anchor balloon technique for difficult stent delivery. *Kardiovaskuläre Medizin.* 2007;10:397–399.

3. Fujita S, Tamai H, Kyo E, et al. New technique for superior guiding catheter support during advancement of a balloon in coronary angioplasty: The anchor technique. *Catheter Cardiovasc Interv.* 2003;59:482–488.

4. Hirokami M, Saito S, Muto H. Anchoring technique to improve guiding catheter support in coronary angioplasty of chronic total occlusions. *Catheter Cardiovasc Interv.* 2006;67:366–371.

5. Mahmood A, Banerjee S, Brilakis ES, et al. Applications of the distal anchoring technique in coronary and peripheral interventions. *J Invasive Cardiol.* 2011;23:289–292.

6. Pervaiz M, Laham R. Distal anchoring technique: Yet another weapon for successful intervention. *J Invasive Cardiol.* 2011;23:293–294.

7. Di Mario C, Ramasami N. Techniques to enhance guide catheter support. *Catheter Cardiovasc Interv.* 2008;72:505–512.

8. Goswami R. The anchor balloon technique for difficult chronic total occlusions. *Cath Lab Digest.* 2013;21(6).

9. Grantham JA, Marso SP, Spertus J, House J, Holmes DR, Rutherford BD. Chronic total occlusion angioplasty in the United States. *J Am Coll Cardiol Interv.* 2009;2;479–486.

10. Snyder KV, Natarajan SK, Hauck EF, et al. The balloon anchor technique: A novel technique for distal access through a giant aneurysm. *J Neurointerv Surg.* 2010;2(4):363–367.

11. Edwards L, Kota G, Morris PP. The sea anchor technique: A novel method to aid in stent-assisted embolization of giant cerebral aneurysms. *J Neurointerv Surg.* 2013;5(6):e39.

12. Ding D, Starke RM, Evans AJ, Jensen ME, Liu KC. Balloon anchor technique for pipeline embolization device deployment across the neck of a giant intracranial aneurysm. *J Cerebrovasc Endovasc Neurosurg.* 2014;16(2):125–130.

13. Prieto LR, Bellotti CA. Balloon-assisted techniques for advancing long sheaths through difficult anatomy. *Pediatr Cardiol.* 2013;34(5):1125–1129.

14. Aerden D, Debing E, Van den Brande P. Intraluminal crossing of near-impenetrable occlusions by balloon-assisted battering ram technique. *Vasc Endovascular Surg.* 2013;47(5):383–386.

15. Pervaiz M, Laham R. Distal anchoring technique: Yet another weapon for successful intervention. *J Invasive Cardiol.* 2011;23:293–294.

CHAPTER 62

Catheter Modification Techniques for Venous Sampling

S. Lowell Kahn

Brief Description

Venous sampling is critically important in the diagnosis and localization of pituitary, parathyroid, renal, adrenal, and ovarian endocrine tumors and conditions. Catheterization of smaller veins can present a challenge and may be responsible for technical failures, particularly with adrenal vein,[1-4] parathyroid,[5] and inferior petrosal sinus[6] venous sampling. Beyond the inherent challenges of catheterization posed by small veins, obtaining adequate blood samples can be difficult because the return of blood from a small vein may be exceedingly slow.

Commonly, the size of the 4 or 5 Fr diagnostic catheter employed for sampling may closely approximate the diameter of the vein to be sampled. In addition to the risk of venous injury or obstruction, insertion and aspiration on such a catheter may collapse the vein being sampled. Furthermore, it is well known from Poiseuille's law that flow is reduced exponentially with a decrease in the radius and increase in length of the conduit.[7] Therefore, utilization of a microcatheter is typically of no benefit.

This chapter discusses techniques to enhance the return of venous blood flow from a diagnostic catheter in a small vein. First, we present our preferred *catheter cutting technique* to improve venous return through a modification of the tip and the addition of side holes. Second, we present a *microwire technique* described by Buckley et al.,[8] whereby a 0.014- or 0.018-in. wire is placed through a 0.035-in. catheter. This technique improves venous return via stabilizing and centering the catheter and preventing vessel collapse with aspiration. Finally, an *optimal aspiration technique* is described.

The three techniques described herein are applicable to all venous sampling, but they are particularly beneficial when sampling small-caliber veins. As such, their employment has enhanced our technical success rates and reduced our procedure times for the most challenging cases.

Applications of the Technique

1. All of the described techniques may be utilized for any type of venous sampling, but they are most beneficial when obtaining blood from small veins.

Challenges of the Procedure

1. The catheter cutting technique is not particularly challenging per se. However, this technique does carry an inherent risk of compromising the structural integrity of the catheter and must be performed judiciously to avoid inadvertent catheter fragmentation within a patient.
2. Catheterization of small veins is inherently challenging and prone to error or injury/thrombosis of the vein. This is particularly well described for catheterization of the right adrenal vein.[3] Optimal catheter selection and technique (not discussed in this chapter) are both imperative.

Potential Pitfalls/Complications

1. As mentioned previously, the catheter cutting technique carries a risk of compromising the structural integrity of the catheter and could lead to fragmentation within the patient. Although a small catheter fragment in the venous circulation would likely be of little consequence, there are nonetheless embolic and infectious risks associated with this complication. A catheter should be carefully inspected prior to inserting it into the patient.
2. The microwire technique is described in detail later, but it involves advancing a small wire more deeply into a small vein. Consequently, there exist risks of vessel dissection, perforation, and thrombosis with this method.

Steps of the Procedure

Catheter Cutting Technique

1. A Hole Punch (Cook Medical Inc., Bloomington, IN) is used to make several holes (two to four) in the catheter over the first 10 mm from the catheter tip.
2. Next, two "V"-shaped incisions are made with a number 11 blade at the tip of the catheter on opposite sides from one another.

Microwire Technique

1. A Tuohy–Borst adapter (Cook Medical) is attached to the back end of the diagnostic catheter. A Flow Switch (Merit Medical Systems Inc., South Jordan, UT) is attached to the side arm of the Tuohy–Borst adapter.
2. A 0.014- or 0.018-in. wire with an atraumatic tip is inserted through the Tuohy–Borst adapter and into the catheter.
3. The catheter is used to select the vein to be sampled.
4. If needed, a contrast injection may be performed through the side arm to confirm appropriate catheter position.
5. The wire is advanced a short distance into the vein (usually 4 or 5 cm).

6. Sampling is then performed through the side arm of the Tuohy–Borst adapter. The presence of the wire provides several benefits. First, the wire prevents catheter dislodgment, thereby improving stability. This is particularly beneficial when sampling veins that are inherently difficult to catheterize and stabilize the catheter (e.g., the right adrenal vein). Second, the wire forces the catheter tip to a more parallel position relative to the vessel wall, thereby decreasing side wall apposition. Finally, the wire itself decreases collapse of the vein during aspiration.

Optimal Aspiration Technique

1. Return of blood flow may be tedious. At our institution, we have found that gentle, slow, and intermittent aspiration optimizes return.
2. Hanging the hub of the catheter to the side and below the patient creates a pressure differential and therefore favors the return of blood. Often with this method, aspiration is not necessary because a continual drip will provide adequate blood for sampling.

Example

See Figures 62.1–62.4.

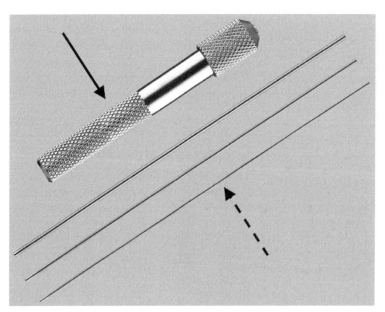

Figure 62.1 Catheter cutting technique. A Hole Punch system is seen with the handle (solid arrow) and multiple different size hole punches (dashed arrow). Multiple side holes will facilitate optimal aspiration. The holes should be present only at the tip to prevent erroneous sampling from outside of the target vein.

Source: Adapted with permission from Cook Medical (https://www.cookmedical.com).

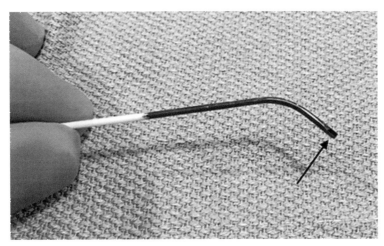

Figure 62.2 Catheter cutting technique. A "V"-shaped incision (arrow) has been made with a number 11 blade at the tip of a Kumpe catheter (Cook Medical). Cutting the catheter in this manner facilitates easier aspiration in a small vein.

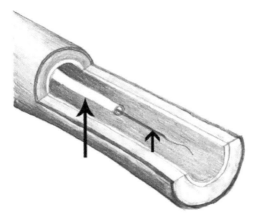

Figure 62.3 Microwire technique. Schematic demonstrates the tip of a 0.035-in. sampling catheter (long arrow) within the lumen of the vein being sampled. Note the microwire (short arrow) extending distal to the catheter. At the hub of the catheter, a Tuohy–Borst adapter is placed and sampling is obtained through the side port of the Tuohy–Borst adapter. The presence of the microwire stabilizes the catheterization and also helps center the catheter within the vein to facilitate a more effective aspiration.

Source: From Buckley O., et al. A novel technique in selective venous sampling in the localization of parathyroid tumours utilizing a micro-wire and standardized catheter. *Eur. Radiol.* 2007;17(4):1125–1127. Courtesy Springer-Verlag.

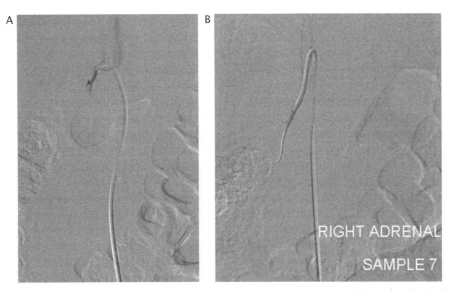

Figure 62.4 (A) Digital subtraction angiography in the right adrenal vein performed through a Cobra 2 catheter (AngioDynamics Inc., Latham, NY) shows branching right adrenal vein. The support was suboptimal, so the catheter was exchanged for more stable catheterization with a Mikaelsson catheter (AngioDynamics). (B) A 0.014-in. wire was advanced deeper into the right adrenal vein for centering and greater catheter support during sampling.

Source: Images courtesy George Hartnell, MD.

References and Suggested Readings

1. Kahn SL, Angle JF. Adrenal vein sampling. *Tech Vasc Interv Radiol.* 2010;13:110–125.

2. Daunt N. Adrenal vein sampling: How to make it quick, easy, and successful. *Radiographics.* 2005;25:S143–S158.

3. Nwariaku FE, Miller BS, Auchus R, et al.: Primary hyperaldosteronism: Effect of adrenal vein sampling on surgical outcome. *Arch Surg.* 2006;141:497–502.

4. Carr CE, Cope C, Cohen DL, et al. Comparison of sequential versus simultaneous methods of adrenal venous sampling. *J Vasc Interv Radiol.* 2004;15:1245–1250.

5. Jones JJ, Brunaud L, Dowd CF, et al. Accuracy of selective venous sampling for intact parathyroid hormone in difficult patients with recurrent or persistent hyperparathyroidism. *Surgery.* 2002;132:944–950.

6. Deipolyi A, Karaosmanoğlu A, Habito C, et al. The role of bilateral inferior petrosal sinus sampling in the diagnostic evaluation of Cushing syndrome. *Diagn Interv Radiol.* 2012;18(1):132–138.

7. Sutera S. The history of Poiseuille's law. *Annu Rev Fluid Mech.* 1993;25:1–19.

8. Buckley O, Brien JO, Doody O, Torreggiani WC. A novel technique in selective venous sampling in the localization of parathyroid tumours utilizing a micro-wire and standardized catheter. *Eur Radiology.* 2007;17(4):1125–1127.

Techniques for Forming Large Reverse Curve Catheters

S. Lowell Kahn

Brief Description

Reverse curve catheters facilitate catheterization of vessels angled oppositely from the point of access. Most commonly, they are used to access caudally angulated vessels from a femoral approach. An array of these catheters exists, and their utilization greatly expands the options for intervention from any single access. Once formed, the catheters are gently advanced forward until their tip engages the vessel of interest, typically confirmed with an injection of contrast under live fluoroscopy. Engagement of the vessel is then performed by advancing a guidewire into the vessel of interest and retracting the catheter to seat the tip more distally within the vessel, providing a stable access. The tip can also be seated by continually injecting saline or contrast while retracting the catheter. The injection of fluid prevents the tip from traumatic engagement of the vessel wall resulting in dissection.

A variety of reverse curve catheters and guide catheters are available on the market. Virtually all are available in 4 and 5 Fr sizes and vary by the size and configuration of their curvature as well as the orientation of their tip. The Sos series of catheters are produced by multiple manufacturers and are the most frequently employed reverse curve catheters with broad applications in visceral, renal, pelvic, and venous applications. These catheters have a fairly tight curve and are therefore readily formed in the aorta and inferior vena cava (IVC) with little difficulty. Larger catheters, such as the Simmons Sidewinder series of catheters have similar applications, but they offer a deeper (more stable) catheterization of their target vessel. This is particularly helpful with the catheterization of sharply (acutely) angulated vessels.

Smaller reverse curve catheters with a tight curve (e.g., Sos) are readily formed in most vessels by simple withdrawal of the guidewire followed by advancement within the aorta or IVC. Slight twisting of the catheter during advancement aids in its formation. Larger catheters (e.g., Simmons Sidewinder) can be more difficult to form, particularly within smaller vessels, the lumen of which may be of similar or lesser size than the diameter of the catheter curve. Care must be taken when forming large reverse curve catheters to avoid vessel dissection or plaque embolization.

This chapter reviews four techniques for forming large reverse curve catheters. The first method, referred to as the *aortic valve technique*, is a simple way to form the catheter by deflecting it off of the aortic valve. The *side branch technique* involves catheterization of an aortic or caval branch and using this as anchor for the tip while the catheter is advanced forward and formed. The *aortic bifurcation or iliac vein confluence technique* describes up-and-over catheterization of the contralateral femoral vasculature with placement of a wire. With the catheter brought partially over the aortic bifurcation or iliac vein confluence, it is formed by advancing the catheter with the wire tip retracted to the apex of the catheter curve. Finally, the *Cope suture technique* was described by Dr. Constantine Cope in 1986 and employs use of a suture anchored to the tip of the catheter by a tightly fitting guidewire.[1] Once the catheter is in position, the catheter is formed by pulling on the suture, which retracts the tip. The suture is then easily removed after the guidewire is withdrawn. These techniques have their individual merits, and all are readily performed with little practice.

Applications of the Technique

1. Formation of large reverse curve catheters in the aorta or IVC.
2. Creation of a Waltman loop with this technique is described in the literature as well.[2]

Challenges of the Procedure

Aortic Valve Technique

1. The catheter can buckle through the aortic valve during this maneuver. This is typically of little consequence if recognized properly.

Side Branch Technique

1. No specific challenges are encountered with this technique other than it does require catheterization of a suitable aortic side branch with a smaller angled or reverse curve catheter.

Aortic Bifurcation or Iliac Vein Confluence Technique

1. As with the side branch technique, there are no specific challenges other than obtaining up-and-over wire access to the contralateral femoral artery or vein. This obviously requires contralateral iliac patency and may be difficult with a severely angled and/or plaque-laden bifurcation.

Cope Suture Technique

1. A particularly narrow (e.g., <15 mm) aorta or IVC could make performance of this technique challenging because the tip may have difficulty deflecting inferiorly when tension is applied to the suture.
2. Proper positioning of the wire is imperative because the floppy end should be positioned only 2–3 cm beyond the catheter tip. If the stiff portion extends well beyond the tip, the maneuver will not work.

Potential Pitfalls/Complications

Aortic Valve Technique

1. Use of the arch and great vessels for catheter formation carries a small risk. Although not studied specifically for this purpose, there is roughly a 1.3% risk of stroke with cerebral angiography, and this risk is higher for patients older than age 55 years.[3]
2. There is a small risk of injury to the valve itself or to the left or right coronary ostia.
3. The catheter and wire can enter the left ventricle with the potential for cardiac injury or arrhythmia. Use of this technique requires continuous fluoroscopy and hemodynamic monitoring.

Side Branch Technique

1. There are few risks related to this procedure other than the aforementioned stroke risk if one of the great vessels is used and a minimal risk of trauma to the side branch selected.

Aortic Bifurcation or Iliac Vein Confluence Technique

1. There are no unique risks to this technique.

Cope Suture Technique

1. There are no unique risks to this technique.

Steps of the Procedure

Aortic Valve Technique (Figure 63.1)

1. A soft-tipped guidewire is advanced to the ascending aorta.
2. The large reverse curve catheter is advanced until the tip of the catheter reaches the aortic valve.
3. The wire is retracted into the shaft of the catheter (proximal to the curve).

4. The catheter is gently rotated and advanced until it forms in the ascending aorta.
5. The guidewire is readvanced just beyond the catheter tip, and the formed catheter is withdrawn to the target vessel. Alternatively, the wire can be removed and the catheter withdrawn during gentle injection of saline or contrast to prevent the catheter from engaging a plaque or causing vessel injury.

Side Branch Technique (Figure 63.2)

1. As stated previously, this technique can be used with any side branch that safely accommodates catheterization with a 4 or 5 Fr catheter. At our institution, we prefer use of the left subclavian artery. The reverse curve catheter is advanced as a unit with a 3 J wire (Cook Medical) or Glidewire (Terumo Medical Corp., Somerset, NJ) extending beyond its tip. The wire will frequently engage the left subclavian artery automatically.
2. The reverse curve catheter is then advanced until the tip engages the branch vessel.
3. The wire is retracted to the apex of the curve, and the catheter and wire are rotated and advanced as a unit until the catheter forms.
4. Once formed, the wire is advanced a short distance beyond the catheter tip, and the catheter is withdrawn to the target vessel of interest. Alternatively, the wire can be removed and the catheter withdrawn during gentle injection of saline or contrast to prevent the catheter engaging a plaque or causing vessel injury.

Aortic Bifurcation or Iliac Vein Confluence Technique (Figure 63.3)

1. A standard angled (e.g., Cobra, Cook Medical) or smaller reverse curve catheter (Sos) is used to engage and obtain up-and-over wire access to the contralateral femoral artery or vein.
2. The initial catheter is exchanged for the large reverse curve catheter, which is advanced over the wire until the apex of the catheter curve lies exactly at the bifurcation or iliac vein confluence. The tip of the catheter should lie a short distance into the contralateral common iliac artery or vein.
3. The wire is retracted to the apex of the catheter curve at the aortic bifurcation or iliac vein confluence.
4. The wire and catheter are advanced as a unit to form the catheter.

Cope Suture Technique (Figure 63.4)

1. On the back table, a Tevdek braided polytetrafluoroethylene-coated suture (Teleflex, Gurnee, IL) is advanced 3–4 cm into the tip of the large reverse curve catheter.
2. The back end of a guidewire (e.g., 3 J) is advanced through the catheter tip to the hub of the catheter.

The floppy part of the wire should extend a short distance (e.g., 2–3 cm) beyond the catheter tip. The wire anchors the Tevdek suture so that it is fixed in place at the catheter tip.

3. The catheter and wire (with the suture on the outside) are placed as a unit into the sheath and advanced to the aorta or IVC.

4. The Tevdek suture is then pulled without moving the guidewire or catheter. This allows the reverse curve to form.

5. Once formed, the suture is removed from the patient by withdrawing the guidewire from the tip of the catheter. The suture is then freed and pulled from the sheath.

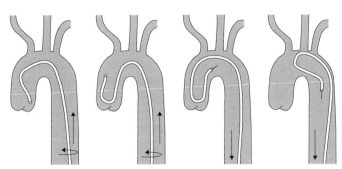

Figure 63.1 Aortic valve technique. A large reverse curve catheter is advanced over a wire until the catheter tip reaches the aortic valve. The guidewire is withdrawn well into the shaft of the catheter, and the catheter is gently rotated and advanced until the reverse curve catheter forms. The catheter can then be used to catheterize the vessel of interest.

Source: From Kadir S. *Diagnostic Angiography*, 1986, p. 74. Courtesy WB Saunders.

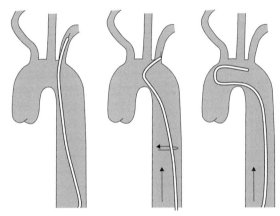

Figure 63.2 Side branch technique. A wire is advanced into the side branch of choice (left subclavian artery shown). With the guidewire in place, the large reverse curve catheter is advanced until the tip barely engages the ostia of the side branch. The wire is withdrawn to the apex of the catheter curve, and the catheter is advanced to form it properly. Occasionally, gentle rotation of the catheter aids in forming the curve.

Source: From Kadir S. *Diagnostic Angiography*, 1986, p. 74. Courtesy WB Saunders.

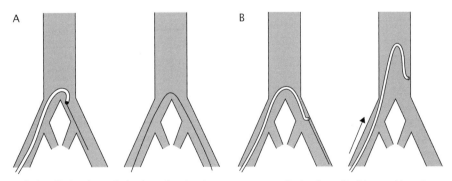

Figure 63.3 (A) An angled catheter (e.g., Cobra) or standard reverse curve catheter (e.g., Sos) is used to advance a wire over the aortic bifurcation or iliac vein confluence to the contralateral femoral artery or vein. (B) Over the wire, the large reverse curve catheter is advanced until the apex of the catheter curve is positioned immediately adjacent to the aortic bifurcation or iliac vein confluence where the tip of the catheter extends a short distance into the tecnralateral common iliac artery or vein. The wire is withdrawn until the tip is positioned at the apex of the catheter curve at the aortic bifurcation or iliac vein confluence. As a unit, the wire and catheter are advanced until the catheter forms.

Source: From Kadir S. *Diagnostic Angiography*, 1986, p. 74. Courtesy WB Saunders.

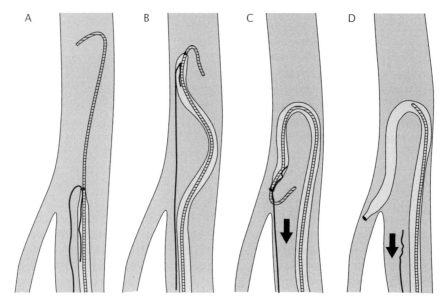

Figure 63.4 Cope suture technique. Outside of the body, a Tevdek suture is advanced a short distance (roughly 3–4 cm) into the tip of the large reverse curve catheter. The back end of a floppy tip guidewire is advanced through the catheter tip and out the hub. A short portion (e.g., 2–3 cm) of the floppy end of the wire extends beyond the catheter tip. The presence of the wire in the catheter creates a tight fit that prevents movement of the Tevdek suture. As a unit, the catheter and wire are placed into the sheath with the Tevdek suture adjacent. The catheter and wire are then advanced into the aorta or IVC. Once in position, the Tevdek suture is pulled while the catheter and wire are fixed in their position. This allows the catheter to form. The suture is then easily removed by pulling the guidewire back into the shaft of the catheter.

Source: From Cope C, et al., eds. *Atlas of Interventional Radiology,* 1990. Courtesy Mosby.

References and Suggested Readings

1. Cope C. Suture technique to reshape the "Sidewinder" catheter curve. *J Intervent Radiol.* 1986;86:63–64.
2. Shlansky-Goldberg R, Cope C. A new twist on the Waltman loop for uterine fibroid embolization. *J Vasc Interv Radiol.* 2001;12(8):997–1000.
3. Willinsky RA, Taylor SM, TerBrugge K, Farb RI, Tomlinson G, Montanera W. Neurologic complications of cerebral angiography: Prospective analysis of 2899 procedures and review of the literature. *Radiology.* 2003;227(2):522–528.

CHAPTER 64

Clearing the Clogged Microcatheter During Particulate Embolization

Roshni A. Parikh and David M. Williams

Brief Description

Embolization with injection of particulates through a microcatheter is routinely used in a variety of settings. If the microcatheter becomes occluded, it can be a challenge to clear the catheter without removing it and thus losing access to the desired location. A standard balloon insufflator offers a solution to this clinical problem.

One atmosphere of pressure equals 760 mmHg, which is approximately six times the arterial blood pressure. Hand compression of a plugged 10-cc syringe exerts approximately 6 atm, that of a 3-cc syringe approximately 10 atm, and that of a 1-cc syringe greater than 15 atm of pressure. Using these fundamentals, the use of manual pressure with a 1-cc syringe can generate up to 100 times the arterial blood pressure. In practice, the pressure on the syringe end of the catheter is damped by intrinsic resistance across the small-caliber catheter. Nevertheless, manual injection can result in overshooting of embolic particles after the resistance in the microcatheter is released, risking nontarget embolization or rupture of a pseudoaneurysm.

This insufflator (e.g., basixTOUCH inflation syringe, Merit Medical Systems Inc., South Jordan, UT) technique exploits the standard balloon insufflator filled with saline. The threaded delivery plunger allows the operator to turn the plunger in small, controlled increments. The needle indicator on the gauge will reflect the rise in pressure proximal to the obstruction in the catheter. When the resistance is overcome, the needle will fall to zero, signaling the operator to stop turning the plunger. The threaded delivery plunger prevents additional volume from being passed through the microcatheter, reducing the risk of nontarget embolization. Once the catheter is unclogged, embolization continues as originally planned.

Applications of the Technique

1. Occlusion of the microcatheter during particulate embolization, when further embolization is desired.
2. Controlled release of residual embolic materials from within the microcatheter.

Challenges of the Procedure

1. Additional radiation exposure to the patient and the operator is expected because direct fluoroscopic guidance is recommended during insufflation.

Potential Pitfalls/Complications

1. Nontarget embolization: Although the use of the balloon insufflator decreases the risk of nontarget embolization, the possibility is still present. Slow plunger revolutions under direct fluoroscopic guidance and close monitoring of the pressure gauge will aid in preventing this complication.

Steps of the Procedure

1. Base catheter and microcatheter selection of the targeted vessel for embolization.
2. Standard initiation of embolization (i.e., particles and gel foam).
3. If the microcatheter becomes clogged, stop advancing more embolic particles into the microcatheter through the syringe.
4. Prepare the balloon insufflator with approximately 30 cc saline.
5. Attach the balloon insufflator to the end of the microcatheter.
6. Under direct fluoroscopic guidance and monitoring of the pressure gauge, slowly turn the insufflator.
7. Continue turning, watching the pressure gauge slowly increase.
8. Stop when the pressure gauge drops to zero, indicating the resistance is overcome and the catheter is unclogged.
9. Disconnect the balloon insufflator.
10. Resume embolization until desired outcome is achieved.

Example

See Figures 64.1–64.3.

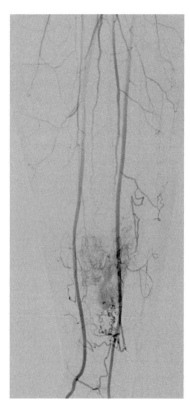

Figure 64.1 Initial left lower extremity angiogram showing a lower leg arteriovenous malformation. This was targeted for embolization.

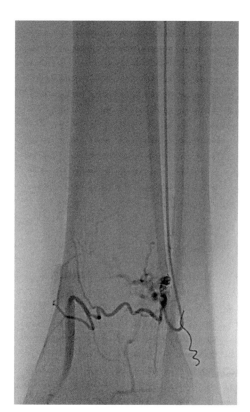

Figure 64.3 Angiogram after using the balloon insufflator to release the obstruction from the microcatheter.

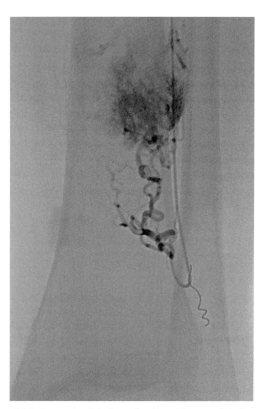

Figure 64.2 Approximately three-fourths of the way into the embolization, the microcatheter becomes occluded.

CHAPTER 65

The Anchor and Scaffold Techniques for Precise Coil Embolization

S. Lowell Kahn

Brief Description

Deploying coils accurately in high-flow vessels can be challenging. Particularly with larger vessels, obtaining the stability to prevent downstream coil migration is of paramount importance. This is particularly true in the embolization of pulmonary arteriovenous malformations (PAVMs), where distal coil migration to the systemic circulation can have disastrous consequences.[1-3] Outside of the pulmonary circulation, the consequences of nontarget coil deployment are serious, including end-organ ischemia and pulmonary embolism.

Although detachable coils/balloons, hydrocoils, and plugs mitigate some of this risk, these devices are costly and not always readily available. Furthermore, there are times when a large plug (e.g., Amplatzer, St. Jude Medical Inc., St. Paul, MN) may not be deliverable to the intended target, necessitating use of coils instead.

This chapter describes two separate techniques to secure coils at their site of deployment. The anchor technique, originally described by White et al.,[4] involves deploying a short segment of the coil in a small side branch and subsequently allowing the remainder of the coil to herniate into the target vessel, where the remainder of the coil is tightly compacted with a weaving technique.

The scaffold technique is also described by White et al.[4] and involves placement of one or more oversized rigid coils in the target vessel first. The high radial strength and oversizing of these coils create a stable scaffold that is unlikely to migrate. Softer coils are then tightly packed within the scaffold to obtain fulminant hemostasis.

These techniques are readily learned, inexpensive, and require no additional equipment beyond standard coils.

Applications of the Techniques

1. Embolization of PAVMs.
2. Embolization of visceral AVMs and arteriovenous fistulae.

3. Any embolization procedure in which distal coil migration could have adverse consequences (e.g., end-organ ischemia).

Challenges of the Procedure

Anchor Technique

1. Finding a suitable side branch in close proximity to the desired coil location is not always possible.
2. With the anchor technique, we attempt to place roughly 2 cm into the side branch, and the remainder of the coil is to be deployed in the target vessel. Occasionally, particularly when the side branch is narrow and/or straight, more than the first 2 cm of the coil continues to pass into the side branch rather than the target vessel.

Scaffold Technique

1. With a tenuous vessel catheterization that has poor stability, delivering the more rigid coils used with the scaffold technique can be difficult and carries a risk of lost catheterization. To counter this, we advise use of a coaxial or triaxial system to provide greater stability.

Potential Pitfalls/Complications

Anchor Technique

1. As mentioned previously, with straight or narrow side branches, too much of the coil can deploy in the side branch. This is typically of little consequence and generally corrected by retracting the microcatheter or catheter from the side branch and deploying the remainder of the coil with a weaving technique.
2. The soft platinum coils (e.g., Nester, Cook Medical Inc., Bloomington, IN) that we employ can still embolize in a high-flow vessel despite using the anchor technique. In situations in which this is a higher

risk, deployment of a larger portion of the coil into the side branch may be useful. Also, if feasible, deploying the coils through a balloon occlusion catheter can prevent distal migration. For example, a Fogarty balloon catheter (Edwards Lifesciences Corp., Irvine, CA) can be inflated in the main vessel, and through the lumen of the Fogarty catheter, a microcatheter can be used to catheterize the side branch and carry out the anchor technique. Use of an occlusion balloon is particularly helpful with larger vessel embolizations.

Scaffold Technique

1. The rigid scaffold coils have considerably higher radial force than their platinum counterparts. Although beneficial for scaffolding and providing traction to prevent migration, oversizing of these coils carries a risk of vessel erosion over time, particularly for thin-walled vessels such as the pulmonary arteries.
2. As mentioned previously, the rigid coils used for the scaffold can cause the catheter to disengage from the target vessel during delivery with consequent loss of access.

Steps of the Procedure

Anchor Technique

1. Secure catheterization of the target vessel is obtained with standard wire and catheter technique. For both techniques, we advise use of a coaxial or triaxial combination, depending on the target vessel location and size as well as the desired coils (e.g., 0.018- vs. 0.035-in. compatible). The selection of sheath, ± guiding catheter, catheter, and microcatheter, should be optimized for vessel stability. Given the frequently small size of side branches and the wide array of coil diameters available on a 0.018-in. platform, we typically employ use of a microcatheter.
2. The selected side branch vessel is catheterized. The selected side branch must be in close proximity to the desired target for the coil plug.

3. The first 2 cm of the coil is deployed into the side branch under fluoroscopic guidance. At our institution, we typically utilize a soft platinum coil (e.g., Nester) for this technique.
4. The remainder of the coil is deployed in the target vessel adjacent to the side branch. A weaving technique is utilized to tightly compact the coil plug.
5. Additional coils are deployed as needed to obtain hemostasis.

Scaffold Technique

1. Secure catheterization of the target vessel is obtained with standard wire and catheter technique in an identical manner as described in step 1 for the anchor technique.
2. One or more scaffold coils are deployed per the manufacturer's instructions for use at the desired target for embolization. The scaffold coil should be a rigid stainless-steel or similar platform (e.g., MReye and Iconel (nickel-based superalloy), Cook Medical). The scaffold should be oversized relative to the vessel to allow for added radial strength and stability. At our institution, we typically oversize by 2 mm or 20% in smaller vessels. It is important to oversize; however, excessive oversizing can prevent the coil from forming or can result in undue stress on the vessel wall.
3. After the scaffold is formed, a tight pack of softer coils (e.g., Nester) are deployed and interwoven with the scaffold coil(s). A gentle weaving motion with the catheter (as performed with the anchor technique) is useful for tightly packing the coils. The soft coils are added until the desired hemostasis is obtained, recognizing that complete stasis is often delayed until thrombosis occurs.

Example

See Figures 65.1 and 65.2.

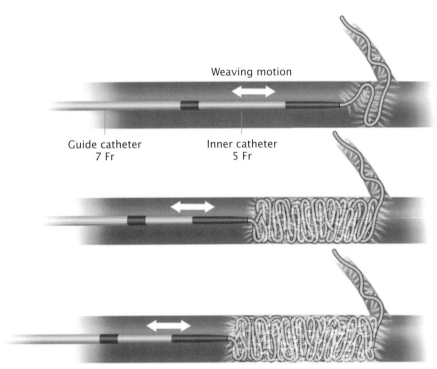

Figure 65.1 A side branch immediately adjacent to the desired coil position in the target vessel has been catheterized. The first 2 cm of a soft platinum-based coil (e.g., Nester) is deployed in the side branch, and the coil naturally herniates into the target vessel. Using a coaxial (or triaxial if a microcatheter is used), a weaving motion of the delivery catheter is performed while the coil is advanced. This facilitates tight packing of the coil as desired for thrombosis and stability.

Source: Image courtesy Cook Medical.

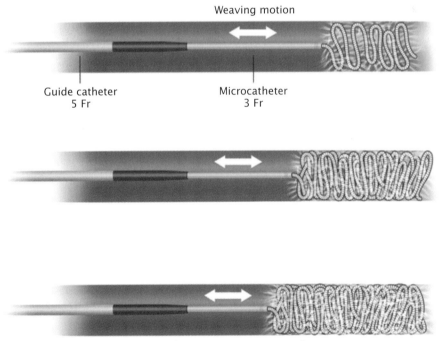

Figure 65.2 One or more rigid, slightly oversized scaffold coils are deployed in the target vessel using a weaving motion, afforded by the presence of the coaxial (or triaxial) system in place. The scaffold coils should be stainless steel or similar (e.g., MReye) to provide optimal radial strength with a high friction coefficient that prevents migration. After placing the scaffold, softer platinum-based coils (e.g., Nester) are carefully deployed with a similar weaving motion whereby the softer coils fill and intertwine with the scaffold coil(s). Compaction is continued to obtain full cross-sectional occlusion of the vessel.

Source: Image courtesy Cook Medical.

References and Suggested Readings

1. Dutton JA, Jackson JE, Hughes JM, et al. Pulmonary arteriovenous malformations: Results of treatment with coil embolization in 53 patients. *AJR Am J Roentgenol.* 1995;165:1119–1125.
2. Lee DW, White RI Jr, Egglin TK, et al. Embolotherapy of large pulmonary arteriovenous malformations: Long-term results. *Ann Thorac Surg.* 1997;64:930–940.
3. Haitjema T, ten Berg JM, Overtoom TT, Ernst JM, Westermann CJ. Unusual complications after embolization of a pulmonary arteriovenous malformation. *Chest* 1996;109:1401–1404.
4. White RI Jr, Lynch-Nyhan A, Terry P, et al. Pulmonary arteriovenous malformations: Techniques and long-term outcome of embolotherapy. *Radiology.* 1988;169:663–669.

CHAPTER 66

Selective Retrograde Thoracic Duct Embolization

Abdulrahman Masrani and Bulent Arslan

Brief Description

Thoracic duct injury is a potential complication of neck surgeries, especially surgeries that include neck dissection. It can present as a lymphatic drainage at the wound site, chylous fistula, chylothorax, chylomediastinum, chylopericardium, lymphocele, persistent lymphorrhea, or secondary lymphedema.[1] This complication is managed with intraoperative repair of the injury if recognized, conservative measures, interventional radiology measures, or surgical re-exploration of the wound with repair.[2] Conservative methods consist of dietary modifications such as fat-free diet or total parenteral nutrition; negative pressure wound; and Octreotide use therapy. Interventional methods include embolization of the thoracic duct either antegrade utilizing abdominal access to the cisterna chyli or retrograde utilizing venous access or percutaneous access to the cervical chyle duct.[2,3] We describe a technique to selectively embolize the injured lymphatic branch of the thoracic duct utilizing coils and Onyx (ev3 Endovascular Inc., Plymouth, MN) instead of embolizing the main duct. This technique eliminates the need for nodal or pedal lymphogram and thus saves time, effort, and reduces expense.

Applications of the Technique

1. Management of iatrogenic or traumatic injury to the lymphatic duct.
2. Difficult catheterization of the cisterna chyli during thoracic duct embolization via abdominal access due to patient obesity and bowel movement.
3. Allergy to Lipiodol, which is used in the nodal or pedal lymphogram to visualize the cisterna chyli.

Challenges of the Procedure

1. Canalizing the confluence of the thoracic duct with the subclavian/brachiocephalic vein.
2. Due to location, the injured branch might be difficult to canalize and embolize.

Potential Pitfalls/Complications

1. Failure to catheterize the confluence of the thoracic duct with the subclavian/brachiocephalic vein.
2. Allergic reaction to Onyx.

Steps of the Procedure

1. Advance a 7 Fr catheter into the axillary vein through the brachial venous access.
2. Advance a 5 Fr SOS-2 catheter (AngioDynamics Inc., Latham, NY) into the brachiocephalic vein.
3. Interrogate the thoracic duct with the 5 F SOS catheter to identify the expected drainage site of the thoracic duct near the internal jugular and subclavian vein confluence.
4. Select a branch vessel and inject small amounts of contrast under fluoroscopy guidance to assess the blood flow within the branch vessel.
5. Selectively catheterize a vessel with no brisk flow that is thought to be the thoracic duct.
6. Advance a 2.1 Fr Echelon microcatheter (Covidien LTD., Plymouth, MN) coaxially through the SOS-2 catheter a few centimeters into the selected vessel.
7. Inject contrast to demonstrate lymphatic branches and confirm that the vessel is the thoracic duct.
8. From this site, perform lymphangiogram to show the extravasation from the injured branch of the thoracic duct.
9. Further advance the microcatheter into the lymphatic system with the guidance of a Synchro 0.014-in. guidewire (Stryker, Fremont, CA).
10. Advance 0.018-in. guidewire to the site of extravasation.
11. At the site of extravasation, deploy two 2 × 4 and two 2 × 8 Concerto detachable mircrocoils (ev3) and then inject 0.1 cc of Onyx.
12. Perform a final lymphangiogram to ensure that there is no persistent extravasation.

Example

See Figures 66.1 and 66.2.

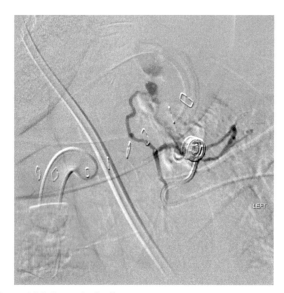

Figure 66.1 Pre-embolization.

References and Suggested Readings

1. Campisi CC, Boccardo F, Piazza C, Campisi C. Evolution of chylous fistula management after neck dissection. *Curr Opin Otolaryngol Head Neck Surg.* 2013;21(2):150–156.
2. Scorza LB, Goldstein BJ, Mahraj RP. Modern management of chylous leak following head and neck surgery: A discussion of percutaneous lymphangiography-guided cannulation and embolization of the thoracic duct. *Otolaryngol Clin North Am.* 2008;41(6):1231–1240, xi.
3. Pieper CC, Schild HH. Direct cervical puncture for retrograde thoracic duct embolization in a postoperative cervical lymphatic fistula. *J Vasc Interv Radiol.* 2015;26(9):1405–1408.

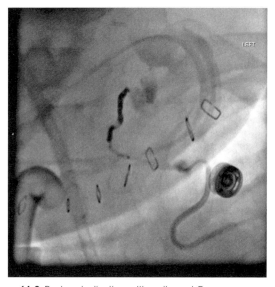

Figure 66.2 Post-embolization with coils and Onyx.

Section VIII

Interventional Oncology and Biopsies

CHAPTER 67

Water Seal Technique for Lung Biopsy

Kazim Narsinh and Thomas Kinney

Brief Description

During percutaneous transthoracic lung biopsy, systemic gas embolism is an infrequent but severe complication. Arterial gas embolism is caused by the entry of gas into the pulmonary vein. There are three proposed mechanisms for this entry. When the biopsy needle tip is positioned within a pulmonary vein, air can enter the pulmonary vein via the needle and become an arterial gas embolus. Alternatively, after the needle is withdrawn, an abnormal communication may have been created between a bronchiole and a pulmonary vein (i.e., a bronchovenous fistula) that can allow air to enter the pulmonary vein. Last, air introduced into the pulmonary arteries can enter the pulmonary veins after incomplete filtration by the pulmonary microvasculature.[1] The introduction of air into the arterial system then obstructs the vessel and induces an inflammatory response, resulting in myocardial or cerebral ischemia that can be fatal.[2] Thus, utmost care must be exercised when performing transthoracic biopsy procedures to minimize risk of gas embolism, even if the patient takes a large breath or becomes more aroused. Scrupulous pre-procedural planning of the biopsy tract can be performed to minimize the risk of creating a bronchovenous fistula. To minimize the risk of introducing air into a pulmonary vein via the biopsy needle, a "water seal technique" can be used to create a hydrostatic column within the introducer needle before the biopsy needle is inserted. Then, if sufficient negative intrathoracic pressure is generated while the needle tip is in a pulmonary vein, saline will enter the pulmonary vein rather than air.

Applications of the Technique

1. Although systemic gas embolism is a rare complication of percutaneous transthoracic lung biopsy, all patients undergoing the procedure are at risk; therefore, this technique should be used during every procedure using a coaxial technique.
2. In any patient who may take large breaths or cough during the procedure, thereby causing large unexpected changes in intrathoracic pressure gradients, use of this technique is especially prudent.

Challenges of the Procedure

1. If multiple needle exchanges are required (e.g., when obtaining multiple core needle biopsies), it can become difficult to (1) withdraw the biopsy needle from the introducer needle with one hand, (2) refill the introducer needle with saline from a syringe using the other hand, and (3) stabilize the introducer needle so that it does not change position. An assistant can help stabilize the introducer needle, if needed.
2. Although scrupulous pre-procedural planning may mitigate the risk of creating a bronchovenous fistula, if one is created, little can be done during or after the procedure to reduce the risk of systemic gas embolism. Use of a water seal technique during the procedure does not mitigate the risk of gas embolism resulting from a bronchovenous fistula.

Potential Pitfalls/Complications

1. Radiologic diagnosis of arterial gas embolism: Prompt recognition of systemic gas embolism is important because simple measures may lead to resolution. Venous gas embolism can be treated with supplemental oxygen administration, intravascular volume expansion, and blood pressure support. If arterial gas embolism is detected by computed tomography (CT), the previously mentioned measures should be pursued, but the patient should be promptly placed in left lateral decubitus or Trendelenberg position in order to keep the left ventricular outflow tract in a dependent position and thereby prevent embolization of the gas into the cerebral or cardiac arteries.
2. Onset of neurologic and cardiac symptoms: Symptoms of cerebrovascular ischemia resulting from gas embolism vary depending on the size of the embolism and the vascular territory affected. Thus, symptomatology may include motor weakness, headache, confusion, seizures, loss of consciousness, hemiparesis, or coma. Myocardial ischemia resulting from gas embolism causes chest pain, characteristic electrocardiographic changes, and elevated serum cardiac biomarkers, similar to the clinical findings expected during episodes of myocardial ischemia attributable

to coronary artery disease. Symptomatic patients, such as those with evidence of cardiopulmonary compromise or neurologic deficits, should receive hyperbaric oxygen therapy, if available. Hyperbaric oxygen therapy reduces air bubble size and increases the arterial oxygen tension, potentially ameliorating ischemia.[3]

Steps of the Procedure

1. Plan the desired trajectory and place introducer needle: Position the patient on the CT examination table. It is useful to practice breath-holding with the patient before beginning the procedure. Then, obtain a scout CT scan to plan the trajectory to the lesion. Sterilize and anesthetize the skin, and then advance the introducer needle (TruGuide, Bard, Tempe, AZ) along the desired trajectory.

2. Create saline seal: Fill a 20-ml syringe with saline, and attach it to a blunt needle or cut-off dilator. Then, with one hand, partially remove the inner stylet of the introducer needle, and use the saline-filled 20-ml syringe in the other hand to quickly fill lumen of the introducer needle with saline before the stylet is completely removed. Then, quickly remove the stylet and insert the biopsy needle (FNA or coring needle) while saline is filling the outer coaxial needle.

3. Maintain saline seal during needle exchanges: After sampling the lesion, remove the FNA/core needle while again filling the outer coaxial introducer needle with saline, and replace the stylet. After filling the introducer needle with saline, the operator will usually see the meniscus of the saline column move in and out of the needle hub with the patient's respirations. If this meniscus drains into the patient, be prepared to quickly instill more saline into the needle so that air does not have an opportunity to enter the thorax through the needle.

Example

See Figures 67.1–67.4.

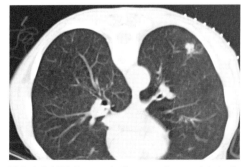

Figure 67.1 Axial CT demonstrating growing nodule in the apicoposterior segment of the left upper lobe.

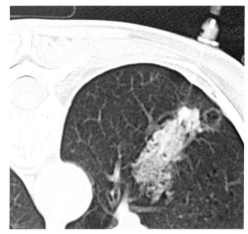

Figure 67.2 Coaxial biopsy set in place. At time of biopsy, the patient coughed and air could be heard entering the needle, which was then covered.

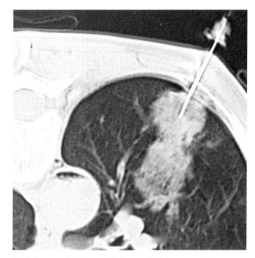

Figure 67.3 Immediate post-biopsy CT shows pulmonary hemorrhage and gas in the aorta.

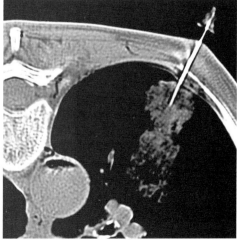

Figure 67.4 Gas embolus in the aorta. The patient had a seizure and recovered without neurologic deficit after hyperbaric oxygen therapy. She was diagnosed with lung adenocarcinoma.

References and Suggested Readings

1. Mansour A, AbdelRaouf S, Qandeel M, Swaidan M. Acute coronary artery air embolism following CT-guided lung biopsy. *Cardiovasc Intervent Radiol.* 2005;28(1):131–134.

2. Muth CM, Shank ES. Gas embolism. *N Engl J Med.* 2000; 342(7):476–482.

3. Blanc P, Boussuges A, Henriette K, Sainty J, Deleflie M. Iatrogenic cerebral air embolism: Importance of an early hyperbaric oxygenation. *Intensive Care Med.* 2002;28(5): 559–563.

CHAPTER 68

Extreme Thoracic Biopsies

William Derry and Scott Genshaft

Introduction

Percutaneous transthoracic biopsy is a commonly used procedure in the diagnosis of intrathoracic pathology. With modern imaging and interventional devices, percutaneous transthoracic biopsy allows access to locations inaccessible by mediastinoscopy or bronchoscopic biopsy. Mediastinal, hilar, and juxtapleural lesions present anatomic challenges that can decrease the chance of safely obtaining tissue and increase complication rates. The use of techniques to displace injury-prone anatomical structures and to open access windows can allow the interventionalist to obtain diagnostic tissue samples from almost all intrathoracic locations.

Pre-procedure Preparation

Percutaneous transthoracic biopsy is a well-established diagnostic method for the assessment of suspicious or indeterminate intrathoracic lesions. Computed tomography (CT) is the most commonly used and preferred imaging modality, but ultrasound can be used in certain situations for large peripheral, pleural-based lesions and some mediastinal masses, allowing real-time visualization and accurate needle placement. Nodules as small as 4 mm can be safely and successful biopsied. As targeted treatments have continued to evolve, sampling of known or highly probable malignant nodules has become necessary to guide treatment. Traditional techniques have included fine needle aspiration and core needle biopsy. Core needle biopsy has a comparable diagnostic accuracy (~95%) and similar complication rates to fine needle aspiration,[1] with a lower false-negative rate.[2] It provides more tissue, allowing for specific diagnostic information, and is superior to fine needle aspiration in providing a specific diagnosis for benign lesions.[3] Our core needle biopsies are typically performed using a 20 gauge automated cutting needle placed through a 19 gauge coaxial introducer needle.

Although there are no absolute contraindications to thoracic biopsy, relative contraindications include coagulopathy, anticoagulant therapy, and significant lung disease such as pulmonary arterial hypertension, respiratory failure, pulmonary fibrosis, or severe chronic obstructive pulmonary disease. These should be appropriately managed and considered prior to proceeding with biopsy.

Periprocedural Considerations

Patient positioning is extremely important in order to maximize success. Access sites close to the costosternal and costovertebral junctions are favored because these sites are least affected by rib motion. A lateral approach is to be avoided, if possible, because the increased motion of the lateral thoracic cage during respiration leads to needle motion that can make targeting the nodule challenging and may in fact enlarge the visceral pleura puncture site. Decubitus positioning should be used infrequently because biopsy of the hyperinflated, non-dependent lung probably increases the risk of a pneumothorax.

Patient cooperation is also vital to a successful biopsy. For this reason, we perform our biopsies under conscious sedation so that the patient can participate in the breath-hold technique. The patient should be instructed to replicate the same small to medium-sized breath prior to an interval scan or needle adjustment, which holds the nodule in place, allowing for more reliable needle tracking. This technique is particularly important when targeting smaller nodules. If the patient cannot hold his or her breath, the needle should be advanced during the same phase of quiet respiration.

Finally, effective local anesthesia at both the skin entry site and pleura improves patient comfort, facilitates proper breath-hold technique, and reduces lung wall motion. The coaxial needle should be introduced until its tip is in the extrapleural fat, at which point local anesthetic should be injected. Adequate pleural anesthesia will prevent any sudden movements or changes in breath-hold when the needle enters the lung. In addition, some believe a large pleural wheal may help seal the pleural puncture site, decreasing the risk of an air leak.

Parenchymal Lesions

For subpleural lesions, the tangential approach is preferred over direct puncture[4] because it creates more needle purchase within the lung parenchyma, thereby improving lesion targeting and reducing the risk of puncturing the visceral pleura more than once. A direct approach to subpleural lesions runs the risk of having the introducer needle slip out of the lung parenchyma and into the pleural space during respiration.

For central and hilar lesions, the peribronchovascular approach involves maintaining a needle trajectory parallel to the bronchi and vessels so as to avoid these structures. In certain situations, intravenous contrast can be administered during the biopsy to help locate vessels that need to be avoided. The needle can then be redirected. Redirecting the needle deep within the chest is difficult because the needle tends to bend at the skin surface, diminishing the degree of needle repositioning within the chest. Shifting the chest wall with one's free hand in the opposite direction of the needle tip direction allows for improved needle steering within the chest.

For lesions that are adjacent to the heart and great vessels, it can be technically challenging to obtain adequate tissue while avoiding serious injury to vital structures. In these cases, it is essential that a tangential approach to the vessel be taken. The needle will then be brushed aside during pulsations, minimizing the risk of vascular puncture. For some difficult locations, such as adjacent to the aortic arch, an out-of-plane approach may be helpful and is facilitated using multiplanar reformatted reconstructions. Angling the needle superiorly while tracking the lesion will provide an avascular clear space posteriorly when core biopsies are taken. Alternatively, lesions abutting the aorta or heart can be displaced by a pneumothorax, facilitating safer biopsy.

Mediastinal Lesions

Depending on the location of target lesions in the mediastinum, there are several techniques that can be used to perform a successful biopsy safely. In most cases, a standard tangential approach to the mediastinal vasculature and pericardium allows for safe biopsy. For some anterior mediastinal lesions, a trans-sternal approach may be most appropriate and is relatively safe and well tolerated with appropriate local anesthesia. Our preferred trans-sternal access is a 10 gauge powered OnControl needle (Teleflex, Research Triangle Park, NC), through which a standard 17 or 19 gauge needle is placed coaxially.

Subcarinal mediastinal masses can also be accessed through the pleural space via an existing or induced pleural effusion after placing the patient in the contralateral decubitus position, allowing the fluid to layer in the posteromedial hemithorax, providing direct access to the target lesion without traversing the lung.

Similarly, an iatrogenic pneumothorax can be used to avoid visceral pleura puncture. Using a blunt-tipped, spring-loaded needle, such as a Veress needle, the procedure is fairly straightforward. After advancing the Veress needle into the pleural space, air is injected to collapse the lung. The mediastinal mass can then be safely biopsied without crossing aerated lung. The air is aspirated after the biopsy to reinflate the lung.

Finally, some middle and posterior mediastinal masses can be safely biopsied via an extrapleural path after injecting saline into the paravertebral space. The extrapleural saline displaces lung laterally, allowing the target lesion to be biopsied without crossing the parietal or visceral pleura.

Post-procedure Care

Important considerations for post-procedure care include pain control, follow-up chest X-rays, dependent positioning, and supplemental oxygen. To reduce the risk of a pneumothorax, avoid both puncturing the visceral pleura more than once and crossing fissures (two layers of visceral pleura). Also consider using an autologous blood patch during the procedure to fill the traversed air space and create a pleural seal. Injecting the patient's own partially clotted blood through the coaxial introducer needle as it is withdrawn is associated with decreased pneumothorax rates, particularly those that require an intervention.[5,6] It is important to remember, however, that a pneumothorax is an expected outcome in certain situations and high-risk patients, and it is therefore more of an inconvenience rather than a complication, as long as it is appropriately treated.

After biopsy, the patient should be decubitus with the biopsied lung down to minimize lung excursion and maintain apposition of the punctured parietal and visceral pleura.[7] Oxygen should be administered by nasal cannula to increase the rate of resorption of any existing pneumothorax[8] because the high nitrogen component of room air is not as well absorbed as oxygen. Upright chest X-rays should be obtained at 1 and 3 hours post biopsy to assess for a new or enlarging pneumothorax that may require pleural catheter placement.[9] The chest X-ray results will ultimately determine the patient's disposition.

Conclusions

Given the increasing utility of percutaneous transthoracic biopsy in the diagnostic algorithm, it is important for interventionalists to feel comfortable obtaining tissue from lesions in all parts of the thorax. We emphasize that a well-planned approach is the most important factor in maximizing yield and preventing complications, particularly when lesions are located in difficult locations. Anticipating complications will allow more effective treatment when they do occur.

Example

See Figures 68.1–68.8.

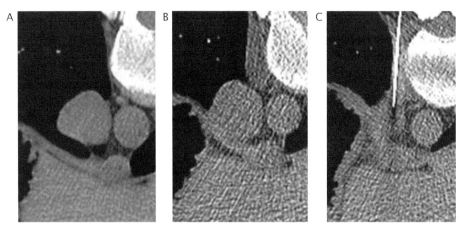

Figure 68.8 (A) Non-contrast CT demonstrates a posterior mediastinal mass adjacent to the descending aorta. (B) Normal saline (50 cc) has been injected into the left paravertebral space. (C) The mass is biopsied via an extrapleural approach through the normal saline in the left paravertebral space.

References and Suggested Readings

1. Charig MJ, Phillips AJ. CT-guided cutting needle biopsy of lung lesions—Safety and efficacy of an out-patient service. *Clin Radiol.* 2000;55(12):964–969.

2. Laurent F, Latrabe V, Vergier B, Michel P. Percutaneous CT-guided biopsy of the lung: Comparison between aspiration and automated cutting needles using a coaxial technique. *Cardiovasc Intervent Radiol.* 2000;23(4):266–272.

3. Greif J, Marmor S, Schwarz Y, Staroselsky AN. Percutaneous core needle biopsy vs. fine needle aspiration in diagnosing benign lung lesions. *Acta Cytol.* 1999;43(5):756–760.

4. Wallace MJ, Krishnamurthy S, Broemeling LD, et al. CT-guided percutaneous fine-needle aspiration biopsy of small (≤1-cm) pulmonary lesions. *Radiology.* 2002;225:823–828.

5. Lang EK, Ghavami R, Schreiner VC, Archibald S, Ramirez J. Autologous blood clot seal to prevent pneumothorax at CT-guided lung biopsy. *Radiology.* 2000;216:93–96.

6. Lee C, Patel V, Suh RD. Autologous blood patch in percutaneous transthoracic core needle biopsy: Clarifying the technique. In: *Radiological Society of North America Scientific Assembly and Annual Meeting Program.* Chicago: Radiological Society of North America; 2006:696.

7. Moore EH, LeBlanc J, Montesi SA, Richardson ML, Shepard JA, McLoud TC. Effects of patient positioning after needle aspiration lung biopsy. *Radiology.* 1991;181:385–387.

8. Moore EH. Percutaneous biopsy in lung cancer. *Semin Roentgenol.* 2005;40:154–170.

9. Gupta S, Hicks ME, Wallace MJ, Ahrar K, Madoff DC, Murthy R. Outpatient management of postbiopsy pneumothorax with small-caliber chest tubes: Factors affecting the need for prolonged drainage and additional interventions. *Cardiovasc Intervent Radiol.* 2008;31:342–348.

CHAPTER 69

Balloon Occlusion Technique During Y90 Radioembolization

Armeen Mahvash and Ravi Murthy

Brief Description

The conventional technique for 90Y microsphere treatment planning involves diagnostic angiography with prophylactic embolization of hepatoenteric collaterals to prevent non-target microsphere administration on the subsequent treatment date. Prophylactic embolization is time-consuming, requires the use of disposable embolic devices, and may result in development of new hepatoenteric collaterals that preclude treatment or cause incomplete treatment. In some instances, embolization is not technically feasible due to anatomy or the size of the collateral vessel. In lieu of prophylactic embolization, the balloon occlusion technique first described by Nakamura et al.[1] may be employed. The technique uses a compliant balloon to temporarily occlude the common hepatic artery to induce reversal of arterial flow in various hepatoenteric collaterals (gastroduodenal, right gastric, supraduodenal, etc.). We generally employ this technique in patients with Michaels type 1 anatomy; however, we have used this technique in patients with variant anatomy. The gastroduodenal artery is not embolized to allow for adequate reversal of arterial flow during the period of balloon occlusion. The technique is employed during both the diagnostic and the treatment session to confirm that flow reversal is complete during angiography. Lack of extrahepatic flow is also confirmed on nuclear medicine technetium-99m (Tc-99) macroaggregated albumin (MAA) single photon emission computed tomography/computed tomography imaging. We generally use a 5.5 Fr over-the-wire Fogarty balloon catheter (Edwards Lifesciences Corp., Irvine, CA); however, similar catheters are available from other manufacturers. The 5.5 Fr catheter will accept a coaxial standard microcatheter to allow for selective administration of the microspheres if desired. Heparin may be administered immediately before balloon occlusion to reduce the risk of thrombus formation in the proximal common hepatic artery.

Applications of the Technique

1. Patients with hepatoenteric vessels that cannot be embolized or safely bypassed.

2. To reduce procedure time by eliminating the need to embolize the hepatoenteric collaterals.

3. Patients with renal insufficiency who may be excluded from treatment due to the volume of contrast needed for adequate angiography and embolization.

Challenges of the Technique

1. Tortuous anatomy that precludes advancement of the balloon catheter to the distal common hepatic artery.

2. High-grade stenosis or occlusion of the celiac axis prevents advancement of the balloon catheter.

3. Lack of adequate reversal of the hepatoenteric collaterals with balloon occlusion. Complete reversal of all hepatoenteric collaterals has been successful in 85% of patients.

Potential Pitfalls/Complications

1. Risk of arterial injury to the common hepatic artery: The balloon catheters are slightly more rigid than standard 5 Fr diagnostic catheters, and advancement in the common hepatic artery may cause arterial injury. Balloon inflation in the common hepatic artery may cause arterial spasm or dissection that precludes treatment. The balloon catheters should be filled with room air or CO_2 to maintain the compliant characteristics of the balloon and to decrease the risk of vascular injury.

2. Risk of exaggeration of extrahepatic arterial supply to subcapsular lesions: In subcapsular lesions with aberrant extrahepatic vascular supply, the extrahepatic arterial flow to the tumor may increase due to the decrease in arterial pressure from the intrahepatic arterial flow. Tumor in the watershed zone between intra- and extrahepatic vascular supply may have incomplete treatment due to accentuated extrahepatic blood supply that has not been embolized.

3. Risk of thrombosis of the proximal common hepatic artery due to occlusion: A stagnant blood column will exist in the proximal common hepatic artery between the celiac trifurcation and the balloon. This area is at

risk for thrombosis if balloon inflation is prolonged. Therefore, temporary anticoagulation may be necessary to minimize the risk of thrombosis. We typically use between 2000 and 5000 IU of heparin during the diagnostic or treatment sessions. If balloon inflation time is only a few minutes for the injection of Tc-99 MAA, then no anticoagulation is necessary.

4. Risk of extrahepatic administration of the microspheres during administration: If unrecognized stasis occurs during microsphere administration and further microspheres are administered, particles may travel to the patent hepatoenteric collaterals.

Steps of the Procedure

1. Review of prior cross-sectional imaging to determine the hepatic arterial anatomy.
2. Standard arterial access with placement of a 5 or 6 Fr short arterial sheath.
3. Standard superior mesenteric and celiac artery angiography should be performed.
4. If the patient has standard Michaels type 1 arterial anatomy, the 5 Fr catheter can be exchanged over a Glidewire (Terumo Medical Corp., Somerset, NJ) for a 4 or 5.5 Fr Fogarty over-the-wire balloon catheter.
5. The distal tip of the balloon catheter should be immediately proximal to the gastroduodenal artery. If the patient has aberrant hepatic arterial supply, these vessels should be embolized to create a single arterial supply to the liver from the common hepatic artery.
6. Common hepatic angiography without balloon inflation is performed. Sites of hepatoenteric collaterals should be noted. Depending on the time of balloon occlusion, heparin may be administered. The balloon is inflated with 0.5–1 cc of CO_2 or room air depending on the balloon type.
7. Repeat common hepatic angiography is performed. The sites of hepatoenteric collaterals should be absent. In our experience, this occurs in 85% of cases.
8. If the plan is to treat the whole liver, then the Tc-99 MAA may be administered from the common hepatic artery.
9. If the plan is to treat in separate sessions or in split doses, a standard microcatheter should be coaxially advanced into the 5.5 Fr balloon catheter to the desired site of treatment in the left or right hepatic arteries. The Tc-99 MAA can then be administered selectively into the location desired. The microcatheter and the balloon catheter can then be removed.
10. On the treatment date, the balloon catheter use depends on the location of treatment. If whole liver treatment is planned, treatment can be done with a 4 or 5.5 Fr balloon catheter from the common hepatic artery with or without a coaxial microcatheter. The resin microspheres can be delivered via the 4 or 5.5 Fr balloon catheter or a coaxial microcatheter. The glass microsphere delivery system requires the use of a coaxial microcatheter due to constraints of the delivery system.
11. If lobar treatment is planned, then the 5.5 Fr balloon catheter is advanced to the distal common hepatic artery and the microcatheter is coaxially advanced to the site of treatment. Treatment is done in the standard fashion after the balloon has been inflated to reverse the hepatoenteric collaterals and angiography confirms reversal of flow/absence of flow in the collateral vessels.

Example

See Figures 69.1–69.5.

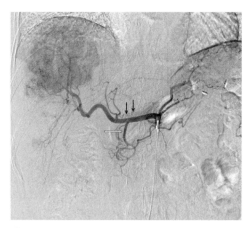

Figure 69.1 Digital subtraction angiography (DSA) of the celiac artery: Angiography demonstrates Michel's type 1 arterial anatomy. The right gastric artery (black arrows) and the gastroduodenal artery (white arrow) demonstrate normal antegrade flow to the stomach and duodenum.

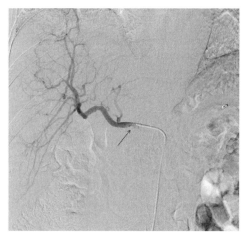

Figure 69.2 DSA of the common hepatic artery with balloon occlusion: The over-the-wire Fogarty catheter is inflated in the distal common hepatic artery. Inflow from the gastroduodenal artery (arrow) is seen at the catheter tip. The right gastric artery is no longer visualized due to reversal of flow. Treatment was administered from the common hepatic artery.

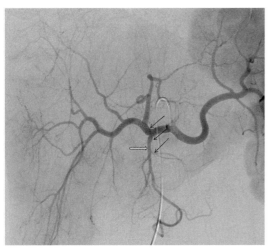

Figure 69.3 DSA of the celiac artery in a different patient: The right gastric artery (black arrows) originates from the proximal left hepatic artery. The gastroduodenal artery (white arrow) demonstrates antegrade flow.

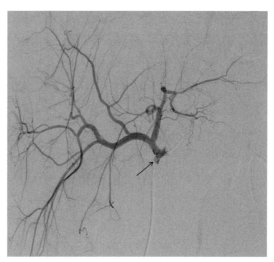

Figure 69.4 DSA of the common hepatic artery with balloon occlusion demonstrates the stump of the gastroduodenal artery (arrow) with retrograde flow. The right gastric artery is no longer visualized due to reversal of flow.

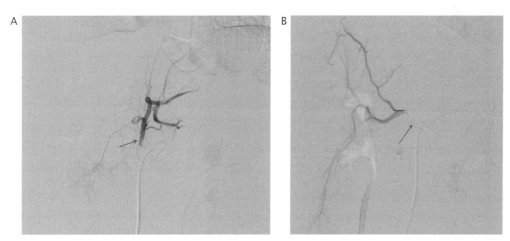

Figure 69.5 (A) DSA of the left hepatic artery via a microcatheter (arrow). Selective treatment was performed from the left hepatic artery. (B) A similar technique was used to selectively treat the right and segment 4A hepatic arteries (arrow).

Reference and Suggested Reading

1. Nakamura H, Tanaka M, Oi H. Hepatic embolization from the common hepatic artery using balloon occlusion technique. *Am J Roentgenol.* 1985;145(1):115–116.

CHAPTER 70

Suprahepatic Catheter Placement for Hydrodissection

Alessandro Gasparetto and John Fritz Angle

Brief Description

Heat injuries of adjacent organs need to be considered when radiofrequency and microwave ablation procedures of hepatocellular carcinoma or hepatic metastases are performed, especially when the target lesion is in a subcapsular portion of the liver. Commonly injured structures include the hepatic flexure of the colon, the small bowel, the stomach, the gallbladder, and the right diaphragm. Hydrodissection can be performed prior to radiofrequency or microwave ablation procedures in which the target lesion is in a subcapsular portion of the liver and adjacent to another structure, particularly the diaphragm. Positioning a catheter between the liver dome and the right diaphragm and injecting fluid or CO_2 in the peritoneal space is a reliable method of creating artificial ascites. This technique creates a fluid layer thick enough to separate the nearby structures from the target lesion in the liver, providing thermal insulation around the ablation area. Moreover, if fluid (rather than CO_2) is used, it improves the sonic window when the target lesion is not visible or only partially visible due to overlapping bowel, lung, or ribs.[1-3]

Applications of the Technique

1. Before microwave or radiofrequency ablation procedures where the target lesion is located in a subcapsular portion of the liver that is adjacent to bowel or diaphragm.
2. Before microwave or radiofrequency ablation procedures under ultrasound guidance where the target lesion is not visible or only partially visible. Typically, these lesions are located in the hepatic dome, where the ribs and lung obscure ultrasound.

Challenges of the Procedure

1. In general, the procedure is easy to perform, safe, and well tolerated. Catheterization of the peritoneal space can be achieved in more than 90% of cases if the patient has not undergone previous right upper quadrant procedures.
2. Previous surgeries, thermal ablations, or transarterial chemoembolizations might result in adhesions. This can make it difficult to place a catheter into the peritoneal space and cause poor separation of the liver from the adjacent organs, increasing the risk for secondary organ injury.[4-6] Changing the position of the patient from supine to decubitus and continuous instillation of fluid or gas during the ablation procedure can improve tissue separation.
3. The peritoneal anatomy sets limits to this procedure: Dome lesions between the coronary ligaments simply cannot be reached by fluid or gas infusion.
4. Tumor infiltrating into a nearby organ cannot be separated by fluid infusion.
5. Patient position and site of infusion affect the distribution of artificial ascites or CO_2. Repositioning the catheter or the patient may help move the thermal shield.

Potential Complications

1. Potential hyperglycemic crisis in diabetic patients after infusion of 5% dextrose solutions.
2. Pain upon injection of CO_2.
3. Peritoneal seeding: Although no direct relation has been proven, the risk of seeding might be increased by the use of artificial ascites because the cooling effect and the presence of free space could facilitate the dissemination of tumor cells in the peritoneal space.
4. Hemoperitoneum: Bleeding can be a complication related to this procedure for two reasons. First, the liquid, washing away the blood during the ablation, might prevent the formation of a clot, especially in patients whose prothrombin time is increased and platelet count is low due to liver disease. Moreover, creating a space between the liver surface and the opposing parietal peritoneum decreases the "tamponade effect."
5. Peritonitis.
6. When CO_2 is used, it can be aspirated to relieve the intra-abdominal pressure and reduce possible complications related to depressed venous return.

Steps of the Procedure

1. The procedure is performed under intravenous conscious sedation because respiratory collaboration from the patient is needed. It should be performed in an interventional radiology suite under ultrasonographic and fluoroscopic guidance. The patient can then be moved to the computed tomography (CT) fluoroscopy room for the ablation procedure.

2. Plan the access between the seventh and eighth right intercostal space along the anterior axillary line. Access into the left lobe from an epigastric approach is reserved for those patients in whom injecting from the right side fails to move away structures from segments II or III or when right side access to the peritoneal space is not possible.

3. Administer 1% lidocaine to the skin at the planned puncture site. Generally, this is along a rib interspace where the entire path of the needle can be seen on longitudinal view with a 12-MHz probe.

4. Under ultrasound guidance, advance a 7-cm 21 gauge needle with echogenic tip (e.g., Micropuncture introducer set by Cook Medical, Bloomington, IN) oriented cranially until the tip of the needle is near the liver capsule. Then ask the patient to inhale to displace the liver inferiorly and to hold his or her breath while the needle is advanced 5 mm into the right lobe of the liver. Then have the patient slowly exhale. The tip of the needle should spontaneously withdraw out of the liver but still remain in the peritoneal space.

5. Quickly insert the 0.018-in. microwire in the needle and gently advance it under fluoroscopy in the peritoneal space adjacent to the liver. Fluoroscopy will confirm if the guidewire is in the peritoneal space. If a guidewire cannot be advanced, it may be in the hepatic parenchyma or the subcapsular space, or it may have withdrawn to the extraperitoneal space. Repeated attempts to very gently advance the guidewire under fluoroscopy as the needle is withdrawn may allow the wire to advance into the peritoneum. It is possible to advance the wire into the pleural space, and fluoroscopy should be used to confirm that the wire stays inferior to the diaphragm.

6. Remove the needle, leaving in the 0.018-in. guidewire. Advance the 3 Fr introducer of the Micropuncture set over the guidewire if CO_2 will be injected. Boluses of CO_2 will be injected using a 60-cc syringe in CT.

7. For more directed infusion of fluid, use a 0.035-in. wire to exchange the introducer with a 5 Fr catheter (e.g., 5 Fr 40-cm KMP Beacon Tip Torcon NB, Cook Medical), and advance its tip between the hepatic dome and the right diaphragm. Placement of a 5 or 6 Fr sheath or direct injection of fluids once the peritoneal space has been selected with the 18 gauge needle have been described as alternatives.[7,8] Placing a 5 Fr catheter instead allows the operator to advance the tip closer to the structure that needs to be separated from the liver and is more stable than a short sheath or needle. Moreover, the use of a catheter does not require monitoring during transportation to the CT fluoroscopy room or during the ablation procedure.

8. Fix the catheter to the skin and start the fluid infusion. Continue a gravity infusion under CT fluoroscopy or ultrasound guidance until a 0.5- to 1-cm fluid layer next to the target lesion is obtained. Usually, 500–1500 ml of fluid or 3–6 liters of CO_2 is enough to create an adequate buffer zone. At the end of the procedure, it is not necessary to aspirate the liquid infused because in most cases it will be completely reabsorbed by the peritoneum within 1 week.[7] If large amounts of CO_2 are injected, some CO_2 can be aspirated to avoid complications related to depressed venous return due to increased pressure in the peritoneal space.[9]

Fluid or Gas Choices

Three different fluids/gasses can be used (for the different characteristics of the fluids/gasses, see Table 70.1):

1. 5% dextrose water solution is preferred due to its non-ionic nature. It should be avoided in diabetic patients because its high rate of absorption from the peritoneum might cause a hyperglycemic state. It also seems to reduce the post-procedural pain and recovery time.[10]

Table 70.1 Characteristics of Fluids That Can Be Instilled in the Peritoneal Cavity

FLUID	INDICATIONS	CONTRAINDICATION	THERMAL INSULATION	SONIC WINDOW
0.9% saline	Microwave Poor sonic window	Radiofrequency	++	↑↑
5% dextrose solution	Microwave Radiofrequency	Diabetes mellitus	++	↑↑
Carbon dioxide	Microwave Radiofrequency		+++	↓↓

2. 0.9% saline water solution is suitable for microwave but it not for radiofrequency ablation procedures because, being an electrolytic solution, it can conduct electricity.

3. CO_2 gas provides better thermal insulation and more rapid distension compared to liquids. Some patients even with heavy conscious sedation report pain during insufflation.

Example
See Figures 70.1–70.4.

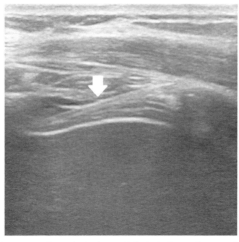

Figure 70.1 The arrow indicates the needle, whose tip, oriented cranially, is in the subcapsular region of the liver parenchyma.

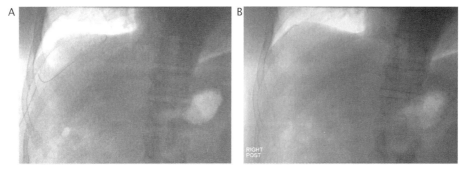

Figure 70.2 (A) A 0.035-in. wire is advanced over the liver dome. (B) A 5 F catheter with the tip in the peritoneal space adjacent to the liver dome is shown.

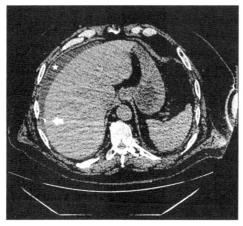

Figure 70.3 The arrow indicates the catheter in the subdiaphragmatic space. Note the approximately 1-cm fluid layer around the liver (star).

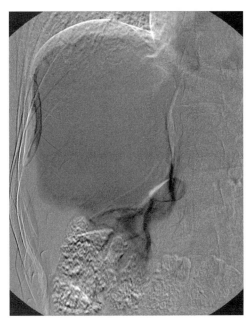

Figure 70.4 Double subtracted angiography image of carbon dioxide diffusion in the peritoneal space.

References and Suggested Readings

1. Minami Y, Kudo M, Kawasaki T, et al. Percutaneous ultrasound-guided radiofrequency ablation with artificial pleural effusion for hepatocellular carcinoma in the hepatic dome. *J Gastroenterol.* 2003;38:1066–1070.
2. Shibata T, Iimuro Y, Ikai I, Hatano E, Yamaoka Y, Konishi J. Percutaneous radiofrequency ablation therapy after intrathoracic saline solution infusion for liver tumor in the hepatic dome. *J Vasc Interv Radiol.* 2002;13:313–315.
3. Lee YR, Rhim H, Kim YS, et al. Intraperitoneal saline infusion during radiofrequency ablation of subcapsular hepatic tumor. *J Vasc Interv Radiol.* 2005;16:753–754.
4. Kang TW, Lee MW, Hye MJ, et al. Percutaneous radiofrequency ablation of hepatic tumours: Factors affecting technical failure of artificial ascites formation using an angiosheath. *Clin Radiol.* 2014;69:1249–1258.
5. Kondo Y, Yoshida H, Shiina S, Tateishi R, Teratani T, Omata M. Artificial ascites technique for percutaneous radiofrequency ablation of liver cancer adjacent to the gastrointestinal tract. *Br J Surg.* 2006;93:1277–1282.
6. Rhim H, Lim HK. Radiofrequency ablation for hepatocellular carcinoma abutting the diaphragm: The value of artificial ascites. *Abdom Imaging.* 2009;34:371–380.
7. Rhim H, Lim HK, Kim YS, Choi D. Percutaneous radiofrequency ablation with artificial ascites for hepatocellular carcinoma in the hepatic dome: Initial experience. *AJR Am J Roentgenol.* 2008;190:91–98.
8. Song I, Rhim H, Lim HK, Kim YS, Choi D. Percutaneous radiofrequency ablation of hepatocellular carcinoma abutting the diaphragm and gastrointestinal tracts with the use of artificial ascites: Safety and technical efficacy in 143 patients. *Eur Radiol.* 2009;19:2630–2640.
9. Raman SS, Aziz D, Chang X, Sayre J, Lassman C, Lu D. Minimizing diaphragmatic injury during radiofrequency ablation: Efficacy of intraabdominal carbon dioxide insufflation. *AJR Am J Roentgenol.* 2004;183(1):197–200.
10. Hinshaw JL, Laeseke PF, Winter TC 3rd, Kliewer MA, Fine JP, Lee FT Jr. Radiofrequency ablation of peripheral liver tumors: Intraperitoneal 5% dextrose in water decreases postprocedural pain. *AJR Am J Roentgenol.* 2006;186:S306–S310.

CHAPTER 71

Percutaneous Thermal Ablation: Hydrodissection and Balloon Displacement to Protect Adjacent Non-Target Critical Structures

Farrah J. Wolf and Jason Iannuccilli

Brief Description

Percutaneous thermal ablation has emerged as a viable minimally invasive option for cancer treatment, whether a patient has been deemed a nonsurgical candidate or wishes to pursue an organ-sparing intervention. Thermal modalities include radiofrequency and microwave ablation as well as cryoablation, utilizing temperatures above 50°–100°C and below –60° to –180°C, respectively. Given that the ablation zone is designed to include the index lesion and a circumferential treatment margin, localized tumor ablation is ideal for patients with impaired hepatic, pulmonary, or renal function. Despite the localized nature of image-guided thermal ablation treatments, soft tissue structures that lie in close proximity (usually <1 cm) to the ablation zone are at risk of inadvertent thermal injury. Thus, several techniques exist to mechanically displace non-target organs, which lie in close proximity to the ablation zone, in a minimally invasive manner.

Applications of the Technique

Prior to the development of percutaneous displacement techniques, the presence of a non-target vital organ or structure within 1–3 cm of the index lesion was considered a contraindication to thermal ablation. The use of percutaneously instilled sterile water to displace bowel adjacent to solid renal tumors prior to ablation was first described by Farrell et al.,[1] who coined the term "hydrodisplacement." Water is a non-ionic medium with relatively low thermal conductivity. Infusion of sterile water between the ablation zone and an adjacent non-target organ effectively decreases heat conduction and prevents further propagation of the ablation zone margin, preventing injury to the adjacent non-target organ (e.g., bowel, which is vulnerable to perforation). The use of dextrose 5% in water (D5W) combined with a small amount of non-ionic contrast material was subsequently described by DeBenedectis et al.[2] By increasing the average Hounsfield units of the hydrodissection fluid to approximately 171, there was improved visualization of the hydrodissection fluid relative to the adjacent organs. Additional displacement techniques have also emerged, including CO_2 gas dissection, antenna/electrode leveraging or torquing, and angioplasty balloon displacement. An angioplasty balloon interposed between the ablation zone and an adjacent non-target organ, when inflated with air, provides thermal protection by means of both physical displacement and thermal insulation. DeBenedectis et al.[2] report a distance of displacement greater than 1 cm as adequate to prevent thermal injury to a non-target organ.

Steps of the Technique

Because image-guided thermal ablation is a minimally invasive procedure, general anesthesia is rarely required, and most procedures are performed under moderate (conscious) sedation. Midazolam (0.5–1 mg/dose) and fentanyl (25–50 µg/dose) are administered intravenously in incremental doses while vital signs and electrocardiogram tracings are continuously monitored by a dedicated nursing staff.

Computed tomography (CT) fluoroscopy is also routinely utilized. Although percutaneous ablation may be performed under real-time ultrasound guidance, CT fluoroscopy is preferred for cases in which displacement techniques will be required.

The steps of the technique are as follows:

1. Initial pre-procedure CT images are obtained, confirming both size and location of the index lesion.
2. Image analysis is performed on a workstation monitor utilizing a software-generated mapping grid for measurement purposes. At this time, the percutaneous access site(s) may be determined as well as the microwave antenna or radiofrequency

electrode trajectory. The number of antennae and electrodes to be used is also determined. With the goal of creating a sufficiently sized ablation zone to encompass the index lesion, and a circumferential 1.0-cm disease-free ablation zone margin (the equivalent of a surgical resection margin), the expected size of the ablation zone is calculated. If a critical organ or structure is located within the planned ablation zone or <1 cm from the ablation zone outer margin, protective measures should be taken. Options to consider include hydrodissection and/or balloon displacement as detailed later. Thus, additional plans should be made on the mapping grid to account for a hydrodissection catheter to be directed between the index lesion and critical structure to be displaced away or for the placement of an air-filled balloon.

3. With the patient positioned in the CT gantry, a laser grid is used to mark the planned percutaneous access sites on the patient's skin based on the previously annotated software-generated mapping grid on the CT workstation.

4. Access sites are prepped and draped in standard sterile fashion. Utilizing a 25 gauge needle, intradermal and subcutaneous 1% lidocaine buffered with bicarbonate is injected to obtain local anesthesia. Based on the planned trajectory for the antenna or electrode, additional targeted local anesthesia is administered via a 22 gauge spinal needle. A CT-fluoroscopic image is then obtained to confirm appropriateness of the anesthetized tract. This is an appropriate time to make adjustments in patient positioning and/or needle trajectory, prior to antenna or electrode insertion.

5. With a number 11 scalpel blade, a small skin nick is made at the access site, adjacent to the spinal needle. The antenna or electrode may then be placed through the skin nick, mimicking the trajectory of the spinal needle, which is then to be removed. The antenna or electrode may be advanced approximately halfway to the index lesion. CT fluoroscopic imaging is then used to confirm positioning, enabling adjustments to be made. The antenna or electrode may then be advanced further into the index lesion, optimally positioned as per the manufacturer's instructions. The previously described process may be repeated until all required antennae or electrodes are in place.

6. If hydrodissection is to be used, a 5 Fr Yueh catheter (Cook Medical Inc., Bloomington, IN), 7 or 15 cm in length, may be placed through an additional skin access site and positioned using CT fluoroscopic guidance. The distal tip of the Yueh catheter should be directed between the index lesion and critical structure to be displaced away. Due to the presence of multiple side holes, three-dimensional displacement is possible. A total of 10 ml contrast material (Omnipaque-350) is then placed in a 500-ml bag of D5W, forming the hydrodissection fluid. This may be instilled in 10- to 20-cc aliquots via the Yueh catheter until there is sufficient displacement of the critical structure from the index lesion (>1 cm as per DeBenedectis et al.[2]), as shown on CT fluoroscopic imaging. Alternatively, the hydrodissection fluid may be hung on an intravenous pole to allow for continuous infusion via the Yueh catheter. Thus, most commonly, the Yueh catheter is left in place throughout the duration of the ablation in case additional fluid needs to be administered due to local diffusion or tracking of the fluid. DeBenedectis et al.[2] report use of an average volume of 285 ml (range, 100–600 ml) of hydrodissection fluid during percutaneous renal mass ablation.

7. If balloon displacement is to be used, via an additional skin access site, local anesthesia may again be obtained using 1% lidocaine buffered with bicarbonate administered via both a 25 gauge needle and a 22 gauge spinal needle. A 0.014/0.018- or 0.035-in. system may be used, with most commonly utilized angioplasty balloons measuring 7–10 × 40 mm. An Accustick 21 gauge needle (Boston Scientific Inc., Marlborough, MA), or alternatively a 19 gauge coaxial needle, may be placed in the desired trajectory through a small skin nick, and the spinal needle then removed, such that the tip of the needle is directed toward the region of intended dissection between the index lesion and critical structure. After removing the inner stylet of the needle, a 0.014- or 0.035-in. wire may be passed into the dissection plane. The angioplasty balloon is then directly placed over the wire and positioned under CT fluoroscopic guidance such that it spans the intended region of mechanical displacement. The balloon, usually a relatively low-pressure balloon, is then inflated with air, enabling it to serve as a thermal barrier during the ablation session.

8. Once the ablation antenna(e) or electrode(s) is in the appropriate position and sufficient hydrodissection and/or balloon displacement is demonstrated fluoroscopically, the generator may then be turned on. Ablation parameters will be determined by the lesion size, number of antennae/electrodes, and manufacturer's recommendations for the given ablation system.

9. At the conclusion of the procedure, the antennae or electrodes may be removed as well as the Yueh catheter and/or angioplasty balloon following deflation. Dry sterile dressings are then placed at the access sites.

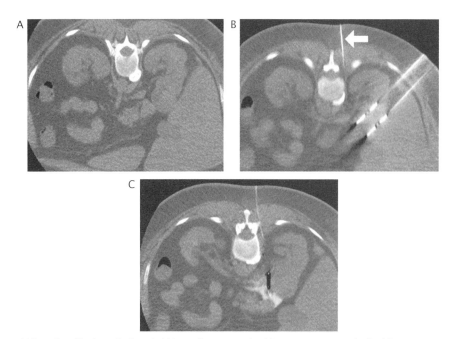

Figure 71.1 A 46-year-old female with stage 3 chronic kidney disease and a biopsy-proven exophytic 4.3-cm upper pole right renal cell carcinoma (A). The patient was deemed a nonsurgical candidate due to poor pulmonary function and medical comorbidities. (B) Under CT fluoroscopic guidance, two BSD 20-cm, LT antennae were placed within the renal mass, and 90 cc of hydrodissection fluid was administered via a 21 gauge AccuStick needle (white arrow) in 20-cc aliquots to separate the adjacent duodenum from the renal mass. Thermal protection of the adjacent renal vein was also achieved by placing an 0.014-in. wire through the AccuStick needle, over which a 7 × 40-mm low-pressure angioplasty balloon was then delivered into the intended dissection plane between the ablation zone and the renal vein. The balloon was then inflated with air to provide both mechanical displacement of the renal vein and insulation to prevent thermal venous injury. (C) Pre-ablation fluoroscopic imaging confirmed adequate displacement of the duodenum from the renal mass and appropriate interposition of the balloon between the ablation zone and the renal vein. A single microwave treatment was then performed at 120 W for 15 minutes. The duodenum and renal vein were successfully protected from inadvertent thermal injury.

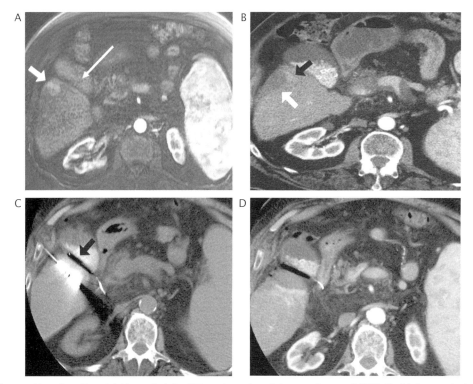

Figure 71.2 A 74-year-old male with a right hepatic lobe 2.7-cm hepatocellular carcinoma (HCC) (A, thick arrow) abutting the gallbladder (thin arrow). Initial CT fluoroscopic guided radiofrequency (RF) ablation was performed with hydrodissection fluid instilled within the gallbladder fossa. However, there was poor accumulation of hydrodissection fluid in the gallbladder fossa, limiting the positioning of the cluster RF electrode and, thus, the size of the ablation zone. (B) Post-ablation 6-week follow-up CT examination demonstrated residual enhancing tumor (black arrow) along the periphery of the ablation zone (white arrow). (C) Thus, repeat RF ablation was performed, this time using an angioplasty balloon (arrow) positioned along the lateral aspect of the gallbladder, to displace the gallbladder and protect it from thermal injury. (D) The RF electrode was then able to be positioned more medially and centrally, successfully treating the residual HCC now encompassed within the ablation zone margin.

References and Suggested Readings

1. Farrell MA, Charboneau JW, Callstrom MR, Readinf CC, Engen DE, Blute ML. Paranephric water instillation: A technique to prevent bowel injury during percutaneous renal radiofrequency ablation. *Am J Roentgenol.* 2003;181:1315–1317.
2. DeBenedectis CM, Beland MD, Dupuy DE, Mayo-Smith WW. Utility of iodinated contrast medium in hydrodissection fluid when performing renal tumor ablation. *J Vasc Interv Radiol.* 2010;21:745–747.
3. Ginat DT, Saad W, Davies M, Walman D, Ertuk E. Bowel displacement for CT-guided tumor radiofrequency ablation: Techniques and anatomic considerations. *J Endourol.* 2009;23:1259–1264.
4. Livraghi T, Solbiati L, Meloni MF, Gazelle GS, Halpern EF, Goldberg SN. Treatment of focal liver tumors with percutaneous radiofrequency ablation: Complications encountered in a multicenter study. *Radiology.* 2003;226:441–451.

CHAPTER 72

Taming Cryoablation for Lung Tumors

Anshuman Bansal and Fereidoun Abtin

Introduction

Percutaneous cryoablation (PC) is a cold-based ablative therapy for primary and secondary lung tumors. Image-guided placement of cryoablation probes precisely into the site of tumor allows minimally invasive tumor debulking in patients who cannot undergo conventional surgical treatment.

Indications

Primary Lung Cancer

1. Lung cancer is the deadliest cancer in both men and women, accounting for 29% of all cancer deaths in the United States.[1-3]
2. Primary surgical resection can be curative in patients with stage I and stage II non-small cell lung cancer (NSCLC). However, up to two-thirds of patients may not be candidates for lobar resection at the time of diagnosis.[4]
3. For these patients, therapeutic options that remain are sublobar resection, radiotherapy, and percutaneous ablation. Sublobar resection has shown higher local recurrence rates than lobar resection and is therefore considered a less favorable treatment. [5,6]

Metastatic Disease to the Lung

1. Patients with oligometastatic disease to the lung in the absence of metastasis outside the lung benefit from metastesectomy.
2. Ablation provides an alternative minimally invasive tumor debulking in patients who are poor surgical candidates.[7,8]

Types of Ablation

1. Multiple thermal-based ablation modalities have been used in the lung. The modalities commonly used are radiofrequency ablation (RFA), microwave ablation, and cryoablation.
2. Radiofrequency ablation and microwave ablation are both heat-based ablative modalities with distinct characteristics. Cryoablation has specific advantages over other thermal ablation modalities.

Advantages of Cryoablation

1. Cryoablation is less painful than heat-based modalities due to the analgesic cooling effect on nerves. This is especially useful in lesions that abut the pleura, which has a rich innervation.[9,10]
2. Cryoablation will preserve collagenous architecture, allowing it to be used near larger airways and blood vessels without as much collateral damage to normal lung. Cryoablation is also less prone to the heat-sink effect compared to radiofrequency ablation.[10]
3. Release of intact cellular proteins from ablated cells allows for the patient to theoretically develop an immunologic response against tumor antigens.
4. Intraprocedural visualization of the ablation zone and expanding ice ball allows for control of ablation.[11]
5. Cryoablation can be used with pacemakers and implantable cardiac devices.

Physics of Cryoablation

1. Joule–Thompson effect
   a. Pressurized argon is channeled into the tip of the probe, where it expands and cools. Heat from the surrounding tissue is absorbed, and the argon is vented back through the probe. When thawing, the opposite effect of heating tissue is obtained with helium.
2. Cell death
   a. Two main mechanisms of cell death occur that vary by the rate of freeze. In areas of rapid freezing closer to the probe tip, intracellular ice formation causes physical damage to the cell organelles and cell membranes, which causes cellular death and rupture. In areas further from the probe where freezing occurs more slowly, ice crystals first form in the extracellular space, drawing water out of the cells due to increased extracellular solute concentration. The increased intracellular solute concentration causes

cell dehydration, enzyme denaturation, and destabilization of the cell membrane.[12]

Patient Selection

1. Lung function
   a. An ideal candidate should have enough lung reserve to be able to tolerate the development of a small amount of intra-alveolar hemorrhage or pleural effusion. There are no lower limits for forced expiratory volume in 1 second (FEV1) or diffusing capacity of the lungs for carbon monoxide (DLCO) in determining which patients can undergo cryoablation; however, severe underlying respiratory disease can be a contraindication. Patients must be able to tolerate supine or prone positioning. Unlike radiotherapy, a patient can undergo multiple cryoablation procedures without a significant decline in pulmonary reserve. Patients with FEV1 <30% are not good cryoablation candidates.
2. Lesion size.
   a. Tumors up to 3 cm in diameter can be treated with multiple probes. At sizes larger than 3 cm, obtaining adequate ablation margins becomes difficult.
3. Lesion location
   a. Lesions in the central lung are more difficult to treat due to the heat sink effect that occurs when trying to cool tissue close to large blood vessels. This feature can be challenging for complete ablation but rewarding because major vessels will be spared from injury.
   b. Cryoablation is better suited for peripheral lesions close to the pleura because it is usually less painful than heat-based ablation.[13,14]
4. Pre-procedural labs
   a. Basic pre-procedural labs, including prothrombin time (PTT), activated PTT, complete blood count with differential count, and basic metabolic panel, should be obtained prior to performing a cryoablation procedure. Uncorrectable coagulopathy is one contraindication to performing the procedure.
   b. International normalized ratio should be corrected to 1.5.
5. Curative versus palliative intent
   a. Some authors believe that a life expectancy of less than 1 year should be considered a relative contraindication to performing the procedure.

Patient Preparation

1. Anesthesia
   a. PC can be performed under moderate sedation using a combination of an intravenous amnestic/anxiolytic such as midazolam and an opioid analgesic such as fentanyl or morphine.
   b. Some practitioners advocate the use of general anesthesia, particularly for patients who are anticipated to hemorrhage, in whom selective intubation and lobar exclusion may be needed.
2. Pre-procedural planning
   a. Margins
      i. There is a synergistic effect of multiple probes such that the ablation zone volume resulting from overlapping multiple probes will be larger than the sum of the ablation volume of each probe separately.
      ii. The visible ice ball should extend 5–7 mm beyond the edge of the tumor to get adequate negative margins. The ablation zone size can be predicted based on manufacturer-provided isotherm maps that define the expected temperature relative to a distance from the probe. A variety of probe sizes are available, the two most common being a 2.4-mm probe and a 1.7-mm probe. Various shaft lengths are available. Ablation probe selection depends on operator preference. Two main manufacturers are available in the United States market.
   b. Trajectory
      i. To minimize the potential for complications, the pleural should be crossed as few times as possible. Crossing fissures in order to reach a target increases the risk of developing a pneumothorax and potential air leak. Whenever possible, a posterior approach is preferable to minimize the bucket handle-type motion of the ribs, which is exaggerated laterally and anteriorly.
   c. Patient positioning
      i. The patient should be positioned in a manner that maximizes comfort and so that the skin access site is easily accessible to the radiologist. Care should be taken to ensure that once the probes are in place, the patient and the probes will clear the computed tomography (CT) gantry during scanning.
   d. Equipment
      i. Argon and helium tank levels should be checked to avoid exhausting the gas during the procedure with subsequent incomplete ablation.
      ii. The probe generator should be checked to ensure functionality prior to skin entry, commonly by running the helium gas followed by a test freeze cycle.
      iii. Each probe will be tested in sterile water prior to placement in order to check for circuit leaks.

3. Intraprocedural monitoring
    a. Patients are placed on continuous electrocardiogram and pulse oximetry. Supplemental oxygen is routinely used.
    b. We use dedicated nursing staff to monitor and administer sedation and a radiologic technologist to operate the CT scanner, ablation generator, and obtain instruments and supplies.

Procedure

1. Initial CT is performed, and the site of entry is marked using a radiopaque marker placed on the skin. Once the skin entry site is confirmed, it is prepared with antiseptic solution and draped with sterile towels. Subcutaneous analgesia is administered using 1% lidocaine. With intermittent scanning as required, a coaxial needle is directed to the endothoracic fascia and parietal pleural surface, where liberal local anesthetic is deposited to achieve pleural anesthesia.

2. Once the trajectory is confirmed using the coaxial needle, a small incision is made adjacent to the coaxial needle, and the tested cryoablation probe is advanced into the subcutaneous tissue. The probe will not be securely anchored until the tip penetrates musculature or through the endothoracic fascia. Sterile towels can be used to support the probe for intermittent scans until the probe is securely anchored.

3. To minimize complications, it is of paramount importance to ensure that the probe trajectory is on target prior to puncturing the pleura. Intermittent CT scans are used to ensure proper targeting. Once the probe tip engages the targeted nodule or mass, it should not be withdrawn. Ideally, the probe "skewers" the targeted lesion and the tip lands 0.5 cm deep to the lesion to ensure a wide ablation margin.

4. Cryoablation and the number of probes should be planned using the maps provided by the vendors, although these maps are the result of ice formation in gel and not true representations of human lung.

5. For smaller lesions up to 1 cm, it is often difficult to penetrate through the lesion, and the best probe placement will be immediately adjacent to the lesion so that the lesion is covered by the widest radius of the ablation zone, which typically occurs 1.5 cm behind the tip of the probe.

6. For lesions larger than 1 cm, multiple probes should be used, with the distance between the shafts of the parallel probes no greater than the radius of the ablation zone for the probes. The 2-1 rule can be followed, with probes placed no more than 1 cm from edge of tumor and no more than 2 cm apart.

7. Once the probes are in position, ablation is started. Because cytotoxic conditions occur in the −20°C isotherm, and the visible ice likely represents the 0°C isotherm, the goal is to achieve at least 5–7 mm of visible ice beyond the edge of the tumor by the completion of the last freeze cycle. Intermittent scans are routinely performed at 2-minute intervals once the ablation cycle begins.

8. Both double-freeze and triple-freeze cycles have been described in lung ablation. The typical cycles used are a double-freeze cycle of 10 min freeze, 8 min thaw, and 10 min freeze or a triple-freeze cycle of 3 min freeze, 3 min thaw, 7 min freeze, 7 min thaw, and 5 min freeze. During the thaw cycles, the generator is set to active thaw where the probe is heated using helium to raise the temperature.[15]

9. In the lung, modified triple-freeze cycle (3 min freeze, 3 min passive thaw, 7 min freeze, 3 min passive thaw, and 10 min freeze) is recommended. The purpose of this protocol is to limit the hemorrhage that can occur during prolonged thaw cycle. Also, no active thaw is performed because there does not seem to be a reason to thaw the ice ball at shaft level, and it is best to leave the cryozone to melt passively from periphery to center.[16]

10. The first freeze cycle will usually produce minimal visible changes on CT scan. Ground-glass opacity in the region surrounding the probe can be seen as early as 2 minutes into the first thaw cycle. This appearance is believed to result from fluid and hemorrhage filling the alveoli surrounding the probe. CT during subsequent freeze cycles will demonstrate hypodense ovals surrounding the probe representing the ice ball.

11. In oblong or sausage-shaped tumors, at the completion of the ablation cycle, the probe can be withdrawn slightly and a second ablation cycle performed to obtain full ice ball coverage. This is possible mostly in chest wall lesions.

12. Once the temperature increases above 0°C, the probe(s) can be removed. The probes can usually be mobilized at a temperature of approximately 10°C. Following probe removal, the patient should be positioned such that the ablation zone is now in the dependent position.

13. A post-ablation scan should be performed to check for complications. If the cryozone has extended into pleura, delayed scan in 10 minutes should be performed to detect pleural hemorrhage and plan for active drainage and management.

14. Post-procedure patients are closely observed, and hemodynamic monitoring should be continued. Chest radiographs should be obtained 1 and 3 or 4 hours after PC to ensure no enlarging or significant pneumothorax, pleural, or parenchymal hemorrhage before discharge.

Complications and Prevention

1. Pneumothorax
   a. This is the most common complication, and it is seen to some degree in almost all patients. The published incidence of pneumothorax ranges between 12% and 62%. Few patients require active intervention; most can be treated conservatively with observation.[17]
   b. The incidence of pneumothorax requiring chest tube placement or aspiration is approximately 10–20%.[10]
   c. Techniques to minimize complication
      i. Once engaged in the pleural, manipulation of the cryoprobe should be kept to a minimum.
      ii. Avoid crossing abnormal lung, particularly emphysematous lung, or areas with large bullae.
      iii. Avoid interlobar fissures.
      iv. Use of conscious sedation is preferred compared to general anesthesia because positive pressure ventilation increases the incidence of pneumothorax.
   d. If a patient has bilateral lesions requiring ablation, sequential cryoablation is recommended to avoid the chance of bilateral pneumothorax.
2. Hemoptysis
   a. Cryoablation has a higher rate of hemoptysis compared to RFA, and in one study, hemoptysis was seen in up to 36.8% of patients undergoing lung cryoablation.[17]
   b. Hemoptysis is mostly self-limited, but precautions should be taken to clear the airways in a time-sensitive manner.
3. Pleural effusion and hemorrhage
   a. Post-procedural pleural effusion is common and usually requires no treatment if the fluid is simple. Thoracotomy tube placement can be done for symptomatic relief.
   b. Hemothorax is a more serious complication and is usually caused by mechanical injury or cryoinjury to the intercostal arteries, other chest wall vessels, or plural veins.
   c. Hemorrhage into the pleural space can be rapidly fatal due to the potentially large volume. Rapidly accumulating pleural fluid on intraprocedural CT scans or follow-up chest radiographs, signs of intra- or post-procedural hypotension, or tachycardia should be treated with prompt intervention, including either transcatheter arterial embolization or operative ligation.
4. Air embolism
   a. This is a serious complication with high morbidity and mortality.
   b. If the patient develops stroke-like symptoms, angina, or an impending feeling of doom, the diagnosis should be suspected. The patient should be placed on high-flow oxygen and in the right lateral decubitus in order to attempt to trap air in the left ventricle and prevent flow of air emboli into the left ventricular outflow tract.
5. Mediastinal and neural injury
   a. Care must be taken with ablation of apical lung and superior sulcus tumors. Ablation of these tumors can cause injury to brachial plexus.
   b. Recurrent laryngeal nerve injury and Horner's syndrome have been reported with mediastinal mass or lymph node ablations. Vigilance and awareness of vulnerable anatomy on CT are needed to prevent these complications.
   c. Ablation of tumors abutting the mediastinum can cause phrenic nerve injury and resultant diaphragmatic palsy.
6. Skin frost
   a. Ice ball proximity to the skin should be monitored with intraprocedural imaging and physical examination. The skin should blanch with normal capillary refill in less than 2 seconds.
   b. Normal saline can be infiltrated in the subcutaneous region to increase tumor margin to the skin.
   c. A warm saline-filled glove or heat pad placed on the skin can prevent frostbite-type injury.

Recovery

1. Following cryoablation, patients need to be observed to ensure safe recovery from sedation and for potential complications.
   a. Patients need to be observed in a post-anesthesia care unit, and frequent monitoring of vital signs and continuous pulse oximetry should be performed.
   b. Chest radiographs should be obtained and reviewed at 1 and 3 or 4 hours to exclude complications, including pneumothorax, pleural effusion or hemorrhage, and pulmonary infiltrates.
   c. At the discretion of the operator, hemoglobin and hematocrit levels can be obtained approximately 3 or 4 hours post procedure to screen for occult hemorrhage.
   d. Post-procedural pain management can include oral analgesics including narcotics. Use of anti-inflammatory agents, such as ibuprofen or ketorolac, is recommended. Suppression of inflammatory response post-ablation for at least 5 days may decrease the pleural-based pain, degree of pleural effusion development, and systemic inflammatory response.
2. In uncomplicated cases, patients can be discharged home 6 hours after ablation.

Follow-Up

1. Post-procedure follow-up includes a phone call post procedure to confirm no early complications; chest X-ray and office visit within 1 week; followed by CT scan and office visit 1, 3, 6, 9, and 12 months post procedure for the first year and every 6 months thereafter. In the first year, the 6- and 12-month CT scans are preferentially replaced with positron emission tomography/CT scan.[18]

Example

See Figures 72.1–72.9.

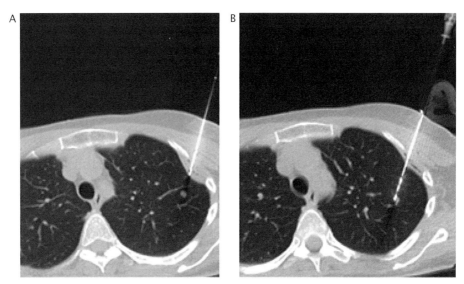

Figure 72.1 (A) Coaxial needle is placed at the endothoracic fascia for injection of lidocaine and pleural anesthesia. (B) Ablation probe is introduced in tandem to the coaxial needle.

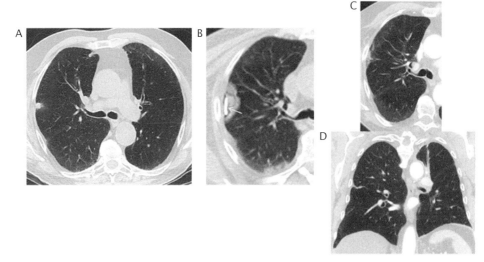

Figure 72.2 (A) 10 mm peripheral right upper lobe primary lung carcinoma. (B) A single PCS -24 probe was placed at the edge of this tumor with the tip extending 0.5 cm beyond the tumor (arrow). (C and D) Post procedure 6 months follow up CT scan demonstrates significant decrease in size of ablation zone with residual scarring.

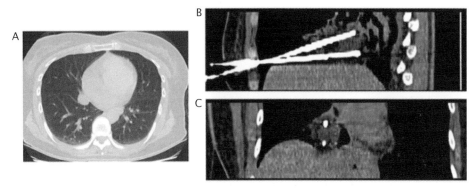

Figure 72.3 (A) Endometrial carcinoma with metastasis to right lower lobe. The metastasis is in close proximity of pericardium and atrial border. (B and C) Sagittal and coronal reconstructions respectively, demonstrate the two cryoprobes which are placed on either side of the tumor and the tumor is pinched or chopsticked on either side. The hypodense ice ball extends between the probes to engulf the tumor.

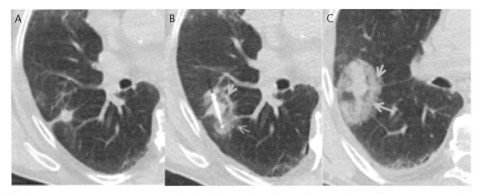

Figure 72.4 (A) A 1.2 cm metachronous lung cancer in right lower lobe. Cryoprobe was placed through the center of tumor. (B) Following three minute of cryoablation and 3 minutes of passive thaw, a hypodense ring is seen surrounding the tumor followed by a denser ring of ground glass and consolidation (arrow). The inner hypodense ring represents the ice and trapped air. The outer denser ring represents melting iceball and hemorrhage. (C) The second freeze cycle for 7 minutes followed by passive thaw for 3 minutes, demonstrate the second layer of trapped air and Ice (arrow) surrounded by melting ice and hemorrhage.

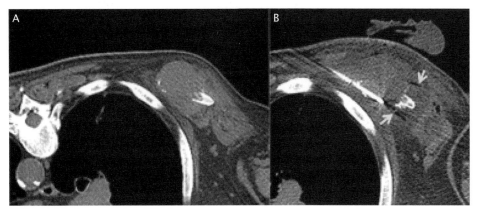

Figure 72.5 (A) Large metastatic tumor to right scapula. (B) Multiple probes were placed with one of the probes seen on this image. An initial cycle of ablation was performed. Then the probes were thawed actively and retracted to perform an overlapping ablation. The probe tracks within the ice ball can be seen (arrow).

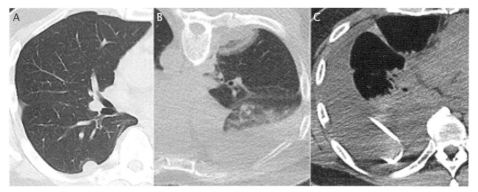

Figure 72.6 (A) Metastatic colon carcinoma to right lower lobe. The metastasis is peripheral and abuts the pleura. (B) At the end of ablation patient is monitored on the scanner for 10 minutes. There is development of moderate effusion. (C) The patient was turned supine to position the tumor in dependent position. A chest tube was placed to drain the pleural fluid and hemorrhage.

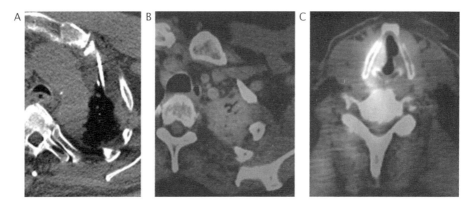

Figure 72.7 (A) Recurrent mesothelioma in the left aorto-pulmonary window. Cryoablation was performed using 2 cryoprobes and the edge of ice ball is seen being carved out by the aorta. The tumor is located along the path of recurrent laryngeal nerve and the sacrifice of this nerve to obtain a complete ablation was discussed with patient. (B) 6 months post ablation fused PET/CT scan demonstrates absence of metabolic activity at the ablation site suggestive of no definite residual tumor. (C) During the same PET/CT scan there is absence of metabolic activity in left vocal suggestive of left sided cord paralysis.

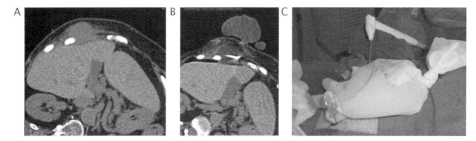

Figure 72.8 (A) Large chest wall tumor extending into the subcutaneous tissue and close to the dermal layer. (B) To obtain adequate cryoablation margin, saline can be injected in the subcutaneous region (arrow). (C) Additionally, placement of sterile glove filled with warmed saline can help decrease the peripheral extension of ice ball into the skin.

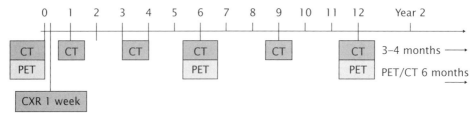

Figure 72.9 Following diagram demonstrates the preferred follow up imaging and office visit schedule. An initial PET/CT scan to assess the extent of disease is performed at baseline. CXR and office visit within 1 week. Followed by CT scan and office visit in 1, 3, 6, 9 and 12 months for first year and every 6 months thereafter. In the first year, the 6 month and 12 month CT scan can be replaced with PET/CT scans.

References and Suggested Readings

1. Jemal A, Taylor M, Ward E, et al. Cancer Statistics 2005. *CA Cancer J Clin.* 2005;55:10–30. [Erratum in: *CA Cancer J Clin* 2005;55:259]

2. Boring CC, Squires TS, Tong T, Montgomery S. Cancer Statistics, 1994. *CA Cancer J Clin.* 1994;44:7–26.

3. American Cancer Society. *Cancer Facts and Figures 2005.* Atlanta, GA. American Cancer Society; 2005.

4. Schiller JH, Harrington D, Belani CP, et al. Comparison of four chemotherapy regimens for advanced non-small-cell lung cancer. *N Engl J Med.* 2002;346(2):92–98.

5. Mery CM, Pappas AN, Bueno R, et al. Similar long-term survival of elderly patients with NSCLC treated with lobectomy or wedge resection within the SEER database. *Chest.* 2005;128:237–245.

6. Burt M, Martini N, Ginsberg RJ. Surgical treatment of lung carcinoma. In: Baue AE, ed. *Glenn's Thoracic and Cardiovascular Surgery.* 6th ed. Stamford, CT: Appleton & Lange; 1996:421–443.

7. Saito Y, Omiya H, Kohno K, et al. Pulmonary metastasectomy for 165 patients with colorectal carcinoma: A prognostic assessment. *J Thorac Cardiovasc Surg.* 2002;124:1007–1013.

8. Mountain CF, McMurtrey MJ, Hermes KE. Surgery for pulmonary metastasis: A 20-year experience. *Ann Thorac Surg.* 1984;38:323–330.

9. Kawamura M, Izumi Y, Tsukada N, et al. Percutaneous cryoablation of small pulmonary tumors under computed tomographic guidance with local anesthesia for nonsurgical candidates. *J Thorac Cardiovasc Surg.* 2006;131:1007–1013.

10. Wang H, Littrup P, Duan Y, et al. Thoracic masses treated with percutaneous cryotherapy: Initial experience with more than 200 procedures. *Radiology.* 2005;235:289–298.

11. Saliken JC, McKinnon JG, Gray R. CT for monitoring cryotherapy. *AJR Am J Roentgenol.* 1996;166:853–855.

12. Gage AA, Baust J. Mechanisms of tissue injury in cryosurgery. *Cryobiology.* 1998;37:171–186.

13. Allaf ME, Varkarakis IM, Bhayani SB, et al: Pain control requirements for percutaneous ablation of renal tumors: Cryoablation versus radiofrequency ablation—Initial observations. *Radiology.* 2005;237:366–370.

14. Abtin F, Suh R, Nasehi L, et al. Percutaneous cryoablation for the treatment of recurrent thymoma: Preliminary safety and efficacy. *J Vasc Interv Radiol.* 2015;26:709–714.

15. Hinshaw JL, Littrup PJ, Durick N, et al. Optimizing the protocol for pulmonary cryoablation: A comparison of a dual- and triple-freeze protocol. *Cardiovasc Intervent Radiol.* 2010;33:1180–1185.

16. Sharma A, Abtin F, Shepard J. Image-guided ablative therapies for lung cancer. *Radiol Clin North Am.* 2012;50(5):975–999.

17. Inoue M, Nakatsuka S, Yashiro H, et al. Percutaneous cryoablation of lung tumors: Feasibility and safety. *J Vasc Interv Radiol.* 2012;23:295–302.

18. Abtin F, Eradat J, Gutierrez A, Lee C, Fishbein M, Suh R. Radiofrequency ablation (RFA) of lung tumors: Imaging features of the post-ablation zone. *Radiographics.* 2012;32(4): 947–969.

CHAPTER 73

Bland Lipiodol-Assisted Thermal Ablation of Renal Cell Carcinoma

S. Lowell Kahn

Brief Description

Surgical resection of renal cell carcinoma (RCC) remains the standard of care given the excellent reported outcomes for early stage disease, with 5-year cancer-specific survival (CSS) rates of 97% for pT1a and 87% for pT1b tumors after nephrectomy.[1,2] Outcomes after partial nephrectomy are equally encouraging, with 5- and 10-year CSS rates of 92% and 80%, respectively, across all stages and 96% and 90%, respectively, for tumors less than 4 cm.[1,3]

Radiofrequency ablation (RFA) and cryoablation are accepted alternative nephron-sparing techniques for nonsurgical candidates. Although the outcomes may be comparable to those of surgery for smaller tumors, the lack of long-term data relegates these methods to secondary therapy by most urologists. Nonetheless, the results of both have been encouraging. A thermoablation meta-analysis performed in 2008 showed local tumor progression rates to be 5.2% after cryoablation and 12.9% after RFA.[1] Progression to metastatic disease occurred in 1% of cryoablation patients and 2.5% of RFA patients.[1] Long-term outcomes after thermal ablation are promising as well. A recent study reviewed the outcomes of RFA on small tumors in patients with T1 RCC over a median follow-up of 6.43 years. Local recurrence was 6.5% with a disease-free survival rate of 88.6% at last follow-up and a 2.2% rate of metastatic disease development.[4]

Unlike the RCC literature, the combination of transarterial embolization prior to RFA is well established for hepatocellular carcinoma. A number of studies have demonstrated a modest benefit of combined therapy versus RFA alone, particularly when treating larger tumors.[5-7] In fact, RFA combined with transarterial chemoembolization is recommended by the Japan Society of Hepatology consensus guidelines for tumors larger than 3 cm.[8] The benefit of embolization prior to RFA likely stems from the fact that lipiodol passes into the peribiliary venous plexus, resulting in a transient local infarction. This in turn reduces the heat sink of local vessels and expands the ablation zone, which is particularly beneficial in treating satellite lesions.[9]

Transarterial embolization prior to thermal ablation for renal cell carcinoma is far less frequent, but it is described in the literature.[10] To date, there are no randomized controlled studies that demonstrate a benefit of combined therapy over RFA or cryoablation alone. However, lipiodol is profoundly radiopaque, and utilization prior to RFA or cryoablation may aid in the visualization of the tumor. At our institution, selective lipiodol embolization prior to thermal ablation of large and/or central renal cell carcinomas has been employed to aid in the visualization of the tumor by computed tomography (CT) during ablation. We have found this technique to be particularly useful in delineating the margins clearly and giving the operator greater confidence in the placement of the ablation probe.

Applications of the Technique

1. Challenging renal cell carcinoma ablation procedures including large tumors, irregularly shaped tumors, and those with central extension in close proximity to collecting system and vascular structures.

Challenges of the Procedure

1. Identification of all feeding branches of the tumor on renal angiography with selective catheterization and lipiodol embolization is imperative. If branches supplying the tumor are not identified and embolized, the operator may falsely assume that the entirety of the tumor is outlined with lipiodol and an incomplete subsequent thermal ablation may result.

Potential Pitfalls/Complications

1. As mentioned previously, incomplete identification of the feeding arteries and hence incomplete uptake of lipiodol throughout the entirety of the tumor may result in inadequate ablation and consequent local recurrence.
2. Although lipiodol is a temporary embolic agent, nephron death occurs within hours of arterial occlusion. Therefore, limitation of the lipiodol infusion solely to the tumor branches is critically important to avoid unnecessary kidney injury.

Steps of the Procedure

1. Pre-procedural cross-sectional CT/CT angiography or magnetic resonance imaging is reviewed to assess for the need for lipiodol prior to thermal ablation. Careful attention is paid to the arterial supply of the tumor, with assessment for any non-renal supplying branches.
2. A renal angiogram is performed with standard femoral access (brachial if the femoral artery is nonaccessible or the renal arteries are sharply angled in a caudal fashion).
3. The main renal artery of the involved kidney is catheterized with standard catheter and wire technique according to the operator's preference.
4. Selective renal arteriography is performed with additional oblique images as necessary to identify all arterial branches to the tumor.
5. Each supplying branch is selectively catheterized and confirmed with angiography.
6. Lipiodol is carefully injected at a slow rate through a microcatheter using a 1- or 3-cc syringe. The infusion can be administered with short, small-volume intermittent injections (i.e., 0.1–0.3 cc) and should be allowed to flow distally between injections to maximize tumoral uptake. The infusion is continued until near stasis is obtained within the branch vessel. This process is repeated carefully for each branch supplying the tumor.
7. A final angiogram is performed in the main renal artery to confirm fulminant embolization of the tumor.
8. Optional: If available, three-dimensional rotational CT may be beneficial in assessing for complete treatment of the tumor.
9. The patient subsequently undergoes CT-guided RFA or cryoablation with the technique performed per the manufacturer's instructions for use. Although it is reasonable to delay the ablation for a short period of time, at our institution, we regularly perform the ablation on the same day as the angiogram.

Example
See Figure 73.1.

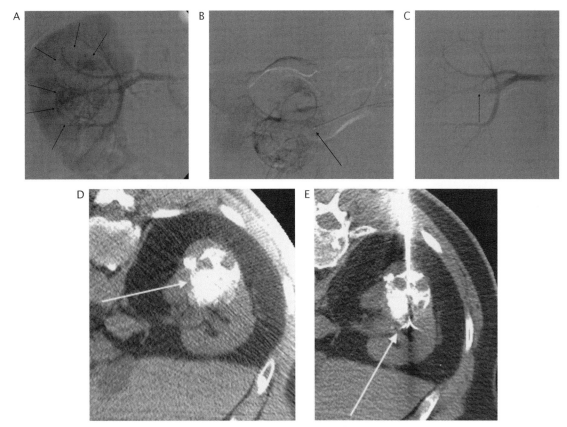

Figure 73.1 A 75-year-old male with a 4.5-cm renal cell carcinoma with central extension. The patient was deemed high risk for surgery and sent for radiofrequency ablation. The patient is disease free at 5 years. (A) A selective arteriogram performed in the main right renal artery through a 5 Fr Simmons 1 catheter (AngioDynamics, Latham, NY) shows a hypervascular mass (arrows) centrally in the right kidney. (B) Multiple third-order branches were identified and selectively embolized through a Renegade HI-FLO (Boston Scientific, Marlborough, MA) microcatheter (arrow). Stasis was subsequently obtained. (C) A final angiogram through the Simmons 1 catheter shows truncation of the mid pole artery (arrow) and virtually absent flow to the tumor. (D) Same-day CT performed with the patient prone shows lipiodol uptake (arrow) throughout the tumor. (E) A 5-cm LeVeen RFA needle (arrow) was used with a RF 3000 Radiofrequency Generator (Boston Scientific) at multiple locations using the lipiodol to plan and guide treatment.

References and Suggested Readings

1. Kunkle DA, Uzzo RG. Cryoablation or radiofrequency ablation of the small renal mass: A meta-analysis. *Cancer.* 2008;113(10):2671–2680.

2. Frank I, Blute ML, Leibovich BC, Cheville JC, Lohse CM, Zincke H. Independent validation of the 2002 American Joint Committee on cancer primary tumor classification for renal cell carcinoma using a large, single institution cohort. J Urol. 2005;173(6):1889–1892.

3. Hafez KS, Fergany AF, Novick AC. Nephron sparing surgery for localized renal cell carcinoma: Impact of tumor size on patient survival, tumor recurrence and TNM staging. *J Urol.* 1999;162(6):1930–1933.

4. Psutka SP, Feldman AS, McDougal WS, et al. Long-term oncologic outcomes after radiofrequency ablation for T1 renal cell carcinoma. *Eur Urol.* 2013;63:486.

5. Wang YB, Chen MH, Yan K, Yang W, Dai Y, Yin SS. Quality of life after radiofrequency ablation combined with transcatheter arterial chemoembolization for hepatocellular carcinoma: Comparison with transcatheter arterial chemoembolization alone. *Qual Life Res.* 2007;16(3):389–397.

6. Morimoto M, Numata K, Kondou M, Nozaki A, Morita S, Tanaka K. Midterm outcomes in patients with intermediate-sized hepatocellular carcinoma: A randomized controlled trial for determining the efficacy of radiofrequency ablation combined with transcatheter arterial chemoembolization. *Cancer.* 2010;116(23):5452–5460.

7. Peng ZW, Chen MS, Liang HH, et al. A case–control study comparing percutaneous radiofrequency ablation alone or combined with transcatheter arterial chemoembolization for hepatocellular carcinoma. *Eur J Surg Oncol.* 2010;36(3): 257–263.

8. The Japan Society of Hepatology. *Consensus-Based Clinical Practice Manual*; Tokyo: Igakushoin; 2007.

9. Kudo M. Local ablation therapy for hepatocellular carcinoma: Current status and future perspectives. *J Gastroenterol.* 2004;39(3):205–214.

10. Gebauer B, Werk M, Lopez-Hanninen E, Felix R, Althaus P. Radiofrequency ablation in combination with embolization in metachronous recurrent renal cancer in solitary kidney after contralateral tumor nephrectomy. *Cardiovasc Intervent Radiol.* 2007;30:644–649.

Section IX

Hepatobiliary Interventions

Optimal Imaging Techniques of the Portal Vasculature During TIPS Creation: Use of the CO_2 Portogram

Hector Ferral

Brief Description

Transjugular intrahepatic portosystemic shunt (TIPS) creation is one of the most complex interventional procedures. It requires skills in imaging, vessel catheterization, guidewire techniques, balloon angioplasty, endovascular stent deployment, and embolization techniques. The key step during this procedure is obtaining access into the portal vein. Several techniques have been described to identify the portal vein during a TIPS procedure. Some authors elect to puncture in a "blind" fashion, based on anatomic landmarks; we do not recommend this approach because it may result in multiple unnecessary, unsuccessful punctures. Our technique of choice is the performance of the "CO_2 portogram," which is an easy, simple technique that provides valuable information regarding the location and anatomy of the portal vein. The CO_2 portogram may be performed with an angiographic catheter wedged in the hepatic vein, with an occlusion balloon inflated within the hepatic vein, or with the transhepatic needle within the liver parenchyma—the so-called "intraparenchymal" injection.

Applications of the Technique

1. During a routine TIPS procedure.

Challenges of the Procedure

1. Knowledge of the use of CO_2; use of careful technique.
2. Having a user-friendly CO_2 delivery system.
3. Avoiding common CO_2 complications.

Potential Pitfalls/Complications

1. In certain cases, the wedge injections will not demonstrate the portal vein, and conversion to the intraparenchymal technique may be necessary.
2. Incomplete opacification of the portal vein.
3. Technical failure.
4. If used improperly, forceful CO_2 injection may result in capsular perforation, which has been described as a fatal complication of the procedure.

Steps of the Procedure

1. Catheterization of either the right or the middle hepatic vein.
2. Advance a multipurpose catheter or occlusion balloon catheter to a wedge position.
3. Confirm proper catheter wedge position with a gentle injection of a small amount of contrast.
4. Once the optimal wedge position is confirmed, connect catheter to the CO_2 delivery system (the Co_2mmander system (AngioAdvancements, Ft. Meyers, FL) is our preference).
5. Carefully purge catheter with CO_2.
6. Inject 15–20 ml of CO_2 in a gentle fashion and obtain a digital subtraction angiography (DSA) run with CO_2 protocol.
7. Perform the CO_2 portogram in the anteroposterior view, and then perform the CO_2 portogram in a slight (15- to 20-degree) left anterior oblique (LAO) view.
8. If the wedge technique fails, perform a routine transhepatic puncture and repeat the previous steps with the catheter or needle within the liver parenchyma.

Example

See Figures 74.1–74.3.

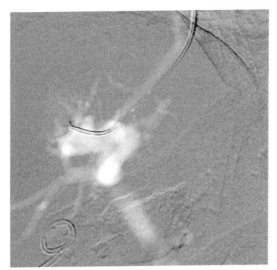

Figure 74.1 DSA CO_2 anteroposterior portogram during a TIPS procedure. A 5 Fr multipurpose catheter has been placed in a wedge position within the right hepatic vein. Note the clear visualization of the right and left branches of the portal vein as well as the main portal vein.

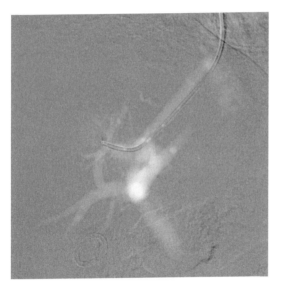

Figure 74.2 DSA CO_2 portogram in a 16-degree LAO view. The importance of the LAO view is to document the relationship between the accessed hepatic vein and the target portal vein. This view will indicate if an anteriorly directed puncture or a posteriorly directed puncture needs to be performed. In this image, the LAO view shows that an anterior puncture needs to be performed.

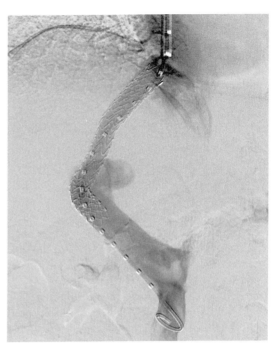

Figure 74.3 The image shows a DSA direct portogram after TIPS completion. The TIPS was completed after two transparenchymal punctures and only 12 minutes of fluoroscopy time.

Reference and Suggested Reading

1. Caridi J. Vascular imaging with carbon dioxide: Confidence in a safe, efficacious, user-friendly system. *Semin Intervent Radiol.* 2015;32:339–342.

CHAPTER 75

Use of Prolapsing Guidewire to Secure Portal Venous Access During the TIPS Procedure

Thomas Kinney and Kazim Narsinh

Brief Description

Perhaps the most critical portion of the transjugular intrahepatic portosystemic shunt (TIPS) procedure involves obtaining secure portal venous access. After positioning a TIPS cannula in the right hepatic vein and advancing a sharp trocar into the right portal vein, one must advance a reliable guidewire from the jugular access site into the main portal vein and subsequently into the splenic or superior mesenteric vein. Unfortunately, advancing a guidewire from the right hepatic vein into the portal venous system can be fraught with unintended challenges. The most common challenge is to advance the guidewire from the right portal vein retrograde into the main portal vein rather than antegrade into the segment 5 or 6 portal vein. Antegrade advancement in the right portal vein typically occurs because of an acute angle of entry into the portal venous system. Use of a guidewire with a long, flexible tip allows one to easily overcome this challenge by initially advancing the wire into the segment 5/6 portal vein and then prolapsing the wire into the larger main portal vein. A movable core guidewire can be used to control the length of the flexible tip. The catheter can then be advanced over the prolapsed wire into the main portal vein, exchanged for a stiff guidewire, and the TIPS set can then be advanced over the stiff guidewire into the main portal vein.

Applications of the Technique

1. An acute angle of entry into the right portal vein can result in preferential selection of the segment 5 or 6 portal vein rather than the main portal vein after advancing a guidewire through the parenchymal tract.
2. Variant TIPS catheterizations (middle hepatic vein to middle portal vein; left hepatic vein to left portal vein), which can result in preferential antegrade advancement of the guidewire within the portal venous system.

Challenges of the Procedure

1. Use of a movable core guidewire allows the operator to control the length of the flexible tip of the guidewire, which can be used to facilitate prolapse of the guidewire into the main portal vein. The movable core, however, should not be advanced when the tip of the wire is in a curved shape because the core can penetrate the outer coil and damage the vessel.
2. If vessel tortuosity is pronounced, the wire can become kinked after prolapsing into the main portal vein. Exchange for a fresh stiff (e.g., Amplatz, Boston Scientific Inc., Marlborough, MA) guidewire is recommended prior to advancing the TIPS set into the main portal vein.

Potential Pitfalls/Complications

1. Injury to the portal vein: A movable core guidewire consists of a fine outer wire and a movable and stiff inner core wire. If the movable wire is advanced while the outer wire is curved or acutely angled, the core wire can penetrate the outer wire and subsequently injure the portal vein. When the guidewire is within a vessel, the core wire should only be advanced when the outer wire is straight.
2. Loss of portal venous access: Once a suitable portal vein branch has been entered, access to the main portal vein should be secured by quickly advancing a guidewire into the splenic or superior mesenteric vein. The liver moves in craniocaudal direction with respiratory motion, and therefore rapid guidewire passage through the needle is important to prevent loss of portal venous access.
3. Increased radiation exposure: Prolapse of the guidewire into the main portal vein cannot be achieved using a stiff guidewire, so an additional wire exchange is required. First, a guidewire with a flexible tip, such as a movable core wire, is prolapsed into

the main portal vein. Then, a catheter is advanced into the main portal vein. Finally, a stiff guidewire is exchanged for the prolapsed wire. The additional wire exchange may slightly increase total radiation exposure during the procedure.

Steps of the Procedure

1. Catheterization of the right hepatic vein and measurement of pressures: This is performed according to standard TIPS technique. After placement of a 10 Fr, 40-cm transjugular sheath, the right hepatic vein can be catheterized using a 5 Fr multipurpose angled catheter (MPA Catheter, Cook Medical, Bloomington, IN). Then, pressure measurements can be obtained in the wedged hepatic vein, free hepatic vein, vena cava, and right atrium.

2. Portal venous imaging and needle access: Multiple techniques have been described to image the portal venous system, including wedged portography with injection of carbon dioxide, percutaneous transhepatic puncture of the portal venous system followed by injection of iodinated contrast, and intravascular ultrasound. Once a suitable target portal vein is identified, the needle is advanced into that portal vein, and aspiration is performed to confirm blood return. Injection of contrast is performed to confirm needle tip position within the portal vein.

3. Main portal vein guidewire access: A movable core guidewire (Coons–Bentson, Cook Medical) or a standard Bentson wire (Cook Medical) is advanced through the parenchymal tract, just into the accessed portal vein branch. The movable core is then withdrawn to elongate the flexible tip. With the movable core withdrawn, the guidewire is advanced into the portal venous system, usually cannulating the segment 5 or 6 portal vein branches located inferiorly. With continued advancement, the guidewire will prolapse into the larger-diameter main portal vein.

4. Exchange of prolapsing guidewire for stiff guidewire: A 5 Fr catheter (MPA Catheter) is advanced into the main portal vein over the prolapsed wire, and then the prolapsed wire is exchanged for a stiff guidewire (Amplatz).

5. TIPS placement: The remaining steps are performed according to standard TIPS technique. The 5 Fr catheter is advanced over the stiff guidewire, and the outer sheath is then advanced into the hepatic parenchyma and portal vein, if possible. The tract is dilated, and a stent of choice is placed (e.g., Viatorr, W. L. Gore & Associates, Flagstaff, AZ) according to standard TIPS technique.

Example
See Figures 75.1–75.3.

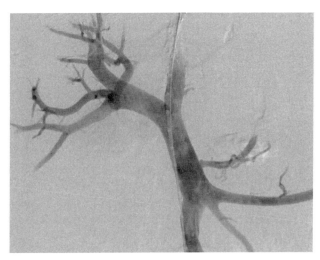

Figure 75.1 Portal venogram demonstrating the relationship between the main portal vein, right portal vein, and segment 5 portal vein.

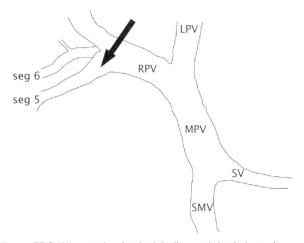

Figure 75.2 If the angle of entry into the portal vein is acute (arrow), the guidewire preferentially cannulates the segment 5 portal vein branch rather than the main portal vein. LPV, left portal vein; MPV, main portal vein; RPV, right portal vein; SMV, superior mesenteric vein; SV, splenic vein.

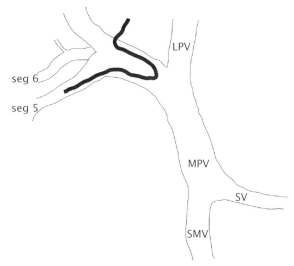

Figure 75.3 A movable core wire with long flexible tip can be used to cannulate the segment 5 portal vein, and the flexible portion of the wire will prolapse into the larger right portal vein and subsequently into the main portal vein (MPV). LPV, left portal vein; SMV, superior mesenteric vein; SV, splenic vein.

CHAPTER 76

Advancing the TIPS Sheath Through a Difficult Cirrhotic Liver: Pay It Forward Off the Balloon

Adam N. Plotnik and Stephen Kee

Brief Description

The "pay it forward off the balloon" technique for advancing the transjugular intrahepatic portosystemic shunt (TIPS) sheath may be employed during a difficult TIPS case when the interventionalist has already accessed the portal vein but cannot get the standard 10 Fr TIPS sheath through the fibrotic tract into the portal vein to thereby allow placement of a standard TIPS covered stent (Viatorr, W. L. Gore & Associates, Flagstaff, AZ). Prior to attempting this technique, most interventionalists will dilate up the intrahepatic tract with a balloon, even up to 10 mm, in order to advance the TIPS sheath. However, in some patients, the fibrotic recoil of the parenchymal hepatic tract can be so severe that this initial maneuver fails. The pay it forward off the balloon technique employs the use of a 6 mm × 4-cm balloon, which is placed through the 10 Fr TIPS sheath and advanced over the wire and across the fibrotic tract into the portal vein. The balloon is inflated to eliminate any possible waist. As the balloon is deflating, the interventionalist advances the 10 Fr TIPS sheath, using the balloon as an "obturator" into the portal vein. The Viatorr stent is then placed, and the TIPS procedure is completed as per standard technique.

Application of the Technique

1. Patients with severely fibrotic livers in whom the fibrotic recoil of the liver is so significant that one cannot advance the standard 10 Fr TIPS sheath into the portal vein, despite pre-dilating the parenchymal tract.
2. Variant TIPS catheterizations (e.g., middle hepatic vein to middle portal vein) in which the passing of the standard 10 Fr TIPS sheath into the portal vein is challenging.

Challenges of the Procedure

1. Occasionally, the angle between the right atrium and the right hepatic vein may be more acute, thereby making the advancement of the sheath over the balloon more challenging. In these circumstances, consider placing a greater curve on the sheath prior to placing it.
2. Considerable back tension is required on the balloon catheter together with the wire when advancing the standard 10 Fr TIPS sheath into the portal vein to avoid kinking of the wire.

Potential Pitfalls/Complications

1. The pay it forward off the balloon technique is successful most of the time; however, there are a few patients with livers that are so severely scarred that this technique is ineffective. In these circumstances, this technique can be used in conjunction with telescoping sheaths (see step 9 in Steps of the Procedure) to aid advancement of the TIPS sheath into the portal vein.

Steps of the Procedure

1. Catheterization of the right hepatic vein: This is performed initially in a manner consistent with standard TIPS technique. After placement of the TIPS sheath (10 Fr) into the right atrium, the right hepatic vein is catheterized (readily performed with a variety of catheters, such as Cobra 2 and Multipurpose).
2. Portal imaging: Wedged portography with either an occlusion balloon or wedged catheter can be performed with CO_2 to confirm portal vein patency and delineate the anatomy for further intervention. In our current practice, we skip this step, relying more on pre-procedural imaging to assess portal vein patency and anatomy in relation to the hepatic vein prior to the TIPS intervention. Moreover, complications such as hepatic capsular rupture and intraperitoneal hemorrhage have been reported during wedge CO_2 portography.[1]
3. Portal vein catheterization: Access of the portal vein from the right hepatic vein is performed using

standard commercially available TIPS needles (e.g., Rosch-Uchida, Cook Medical, Bloomington, IN).

4. Measurement of pressures: As with standard TIPS technique, right atrial and portal pressures should be obtained prior to the placement of a TIPS, most often with a measuring pigtail catheter in the portal vein and the 10 Fr TIPS sheath in the right atrium.

5. Initially attempt routine advancement of the 10 Fr TIPS sheath into the portal vein. When this fails, it is important to retract the TIPS sheath approximately 1 cm from the point of maximum resistance. This is key because there is usually a focal point of narrowing/fibrosis that needs to be balloon dilated and is often at the junction of the parenchymal tract and the portal vein.

6. With an 0.035-in. wire (e.g., Amplatz, Boston Scientific, Marlborough, MA) in the portal vein, a 6 mm × 4-cm balloon (e.g., Rival, Bard, Tempe, AZ) is placed over the wire and through the standard 10 Fr TIPS sheath. This is advanced through the fibrotic parenchymal tract, with the distal end of the balloon just into the portal vein.

7. The balloon is inflated, and a waist is usually identified at the junction of the hepatic parenchymal tract and the portal vein.

8. As the balloon is being gently deflated, forward pressure is placed on the 10 Fr TIPS sheath, which is advanced using the balloon an an "obturator," and into the portal vein.

9. Rarely, the patient's liver is so cirrhotic and scarred that the fibrotic recoil is severe enough to render the previous steps ineffective. In these circumstances, telescoping sheaths can aid the TIPS sheath advancement into the portal vein. A 12 Fr 30-cm sheath is advanced into the right hepatic vein, and then through this the standard 10 Fr TIPS sheath is placed and the previous steps are repeated. The increased stability obtained by having the 12 Fr sheath will overcome the resistance from the fibrotic parenchymal tract and allow the 10 Fr TIPS sheath to advance over the balloon and into the portal vein.

Example

See Figures 76.1–76.3.

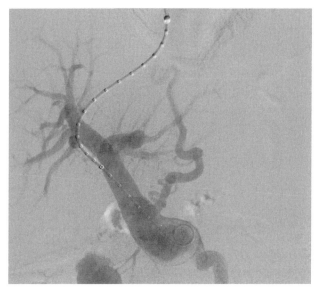

Figure 76.1 Portal venogram. Following successful transjugular intrahepatic access into the portal vein, a marker pigtail catheter is inserted and portal venogram is performed. The 10 Fr TIPS sheath is retracted into the right atrium for pressure measurements. Note is made of a large shunt from the left gastric (coronary) vein.

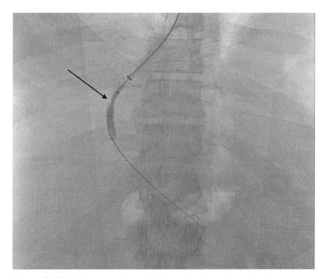

Figure 76.2 A 6 mm × 4-cm balloon has been inserted over the wire and through the 10 Fr TIPS sheath, and it has been advanced across the fibrotic tract into the portal vein. Note the presence of a waist as the balloon is being dilated (arrow).

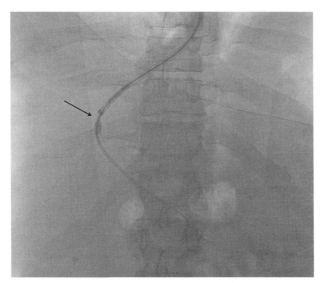

Figure 76.3 As the 6 mm × 4-cm balloon is being deflated, the 10 Fr TIPS sheath is advanced over the balloon, thereby overcoming the fibrotic recoil of the hepatic parenchymal tract.

Reference and Suggested Reading

1. Semba CP, Saperstein L, Nyman U, Dake MD. Hepatic laceration from wedged venography performed before transjugular intrahepatic portosystemic shunt placement. *J Vasc Interv Radiology.* 1996;7(1):143–146.

CHAPTER 77

The Gun-Site and Percutaneous Portocaval Techniques for the Challenging TIPS

S. Lowell Kahn

Brief Description

The transjugular intrahepatic portosystemic shunt (TIPS) was conceived by Josef Rösch in 1969 and became widely accepted with the use of metallic stents in the 1980s.[1] TIPS is indicated for the treatment of refractory variceal bleeding, prevention of recurrent variceal bleeding refractory to conventional medical/endoscopic therapy, refractory ascites, and hepatic hydrothorax.[2–4] Other controversial indications exist as well. Although considered a challenging procedure, TIPS placement has a reported technical success rate greater than 95% and a complication rate less than 5%.[5]

Since its inception, the "Achilles' heel" of the procedure has been catheterization of the portal vein from the systemic venous circulation.[6] Although traditionally performed between the right hepatic vein and the right portal vein, multiple variations exist, including communication between the left, right, and middle hepatic veins and also between the right and left portal veins.[7] Direct portocaval communication (direct intrahepatic portosystemic shunt [DIPS]) is commonly employed as well.[8] The portal vein is most commonly localized using a combination of pre-procedural imaging (and hence landmarks) combined with wedged CO_2 portography. Catheterization of the superior mesenteric artery with delayed portal imaging can also be performed, but this is usually unnecessary. A variety of alternative techniques for portal vein localization are described in the literature. Placing a target such as a wire, catheter, or basket into the portal vasculature is advocated by some.[7,9–11] Use of a recanalized paraumbilical vein to obtain access to the left portal vein and subsequently the right portal vein has been described and is demonstrated in one of the examples in this chapter.[12] Similarly, modern imaging technology can assist localization with the use of intravascular ultrasound (for DIPS placement), cone beam computed tomography (CT), three-dimensional ultrasound, magnetic resonance angiographic guidance, and three-dimensional fluoroscopic guidance.[13–16]

In the majority of TIPS procedures, the portal vein is readily identified with conventional technique and the procedure is completed in no more than 60–90 minutes, if not less.[7] However, there are certain anatomic situations that can make performance of a TIPS procedure difficult. A small cirrhotic liver with an abnormal hepatic to portal venous orientation, thrombosis or cavernous transformation of the portal vasculature, and atrophic or absent (Budd–Chiari) hepatic veins all produce unique challenges for the interventionalist. In such situations, the use of alternative TIPS techniques may be warranted.

In this chapter, two alternative TIPS techniques are discussed to assist with challenging anatomy. The first technique, referred to as the *gun-site technique*, was first described by Haskal et al. in 1996 and has subsequently been described by others.[17,18] The technique is particularly useful in small cirrhotic livers, in which the typical caudal–anterior relationship of the right portal vein relative to the right hepatic vein is not present. In such patients, the right portal vein may lie anterior or even slightly superior and anterior to the right portal vein. The preformed (~30-degree) angle of commercially available TIPS needles (e.g., Haskal and Rosch–Uchida, Cook Medical, Bloomington, IN) is poorly suited for this anatomy. When this orientation exists, access may be impossible (even with aggressive bending of the needle) by conventional technique. In addition, the technique is useful in patients with small or absent hepatic veins (e.g., Budd–Chiari). The gun-site technique is a salvage maneuver for these patients and employs the use of two snares, the first placed in a hepatic vein or inferior vena cava (IVC) from a jugular access (or occasionally the femoral vein if the jugular vein is occluded and the IVC is to be used) and the second placed percutaneously into a portal vein. Once placed, the C-arm is angled to overlap the two snares. If aligned appropriately, an 18 or 21 gauge Chiba (Cook Medical) needle (or needle sheath) can be placed through both snares with subsequent passage of an exchange-length 0.014-, 0.018-, or 0.035-in. wire. The needle is removed, and wire access is now attained from the hepatic vein or IVC to the portal vein. After dilatation, the sheath is advanced from the hepatic vein (or IVC) into the portal vein. Through the sheath and adjacent to the support wire, central catheterization is achieved using a Glidewire (Terumo, Somerset, NJ) and an angled or reverse curve catheter. The TIPS procedure is then completed with standard technique.

The second technique described in this chapter, the *percutaneous portocaval technique*, is well documented in the literature as well.[19–21] This method employs percutaneous simultaneous puncture of a portal vein and the IVC along a single tract under ultrasound guidance. After transgressing the portal vein and reaching the IVC, a wire is threaded into the IVC. The wire tip is snared from an access in the right internal jugular vein (or femoral vein if necessary) and externalized. After balloon dilatation, the sheath is advanced over the wire, where it exits the cava and enters the portal vein. A catheter is advanced through the sheath adjacent to the support wire and used to obtain central catheterization of the main portal vein and subsequently the superior mesenteric or splenic vein. After removing the original wire, the TIPS is completed in standard fashion. As with the gun-site technique, this method is useful in challenging anatomic situations such as Budd–Chiari or in small shrunken livers with atypical hepatic–portal orientations. Other potential applications of both of these techniques are discussed later.

Both techniques require proficient catheter and ultrasound skills, but they require little additional angiographic equipment and are performed successfully with little practice. The addition of both techniques to the interventionalist's repertoire broadens the scope of patients to which TIPS procedures may be offered, potentially as a life-saving intervention.

Applications of the Technique

Gun-Site and Percutaneous Portocaval Techniques

1. Abnormal anatomic relationship of the right portal vein relative to the right hepatic vein.
2. Small or atrophic hepatic veins (Budd–Chiari).
3. Prolonged standard TIPS procedure with multiple unsuccessful portal vein catheterization attempts.
4. Variant TIPS catheterizations (e.g., middle hepatic vein to middle portal vein and left hepatic vein to left portal vein).
5. Occluded jugular veins requiring femoral access for completion of the procedure.

Challenges of the Procedure

Gun-Site Technique

1. Percutaneous access of the right portal vein may be difficult if the vein is small or partially occluded.

2. Percutaneous access to the portal vein in a small cirrhotic liver that is medially displaced secondary to the presence of ascites can pose additional challenges. Where feasible, drainage of the ascites prior to portal vein catheterization is advised. This will also decrease the risk of hemorrhage.
3. Alignment of the snares may require an angulation (typically caudal) of the C-arm that may exceed the manufacturer's limits for the table.
4. Percutaneous needle access through the snares is difficult if the two snares are not similarly oriented such that both form a circular or elliptical orientation.
5. Added radiation exposure to the patient and operator is expected. Passage of the needle under fluoroscopic guidance exposes the operator's hands to excess radiation. If possible, use of leaded undergloves is advised.
6. Once the wire has been grasped at both ends, it can be difficult to avoid kinking of the wire. The wire should be gently retracted by the snare while the opposite end is carefully fed in order to prevent this complication. It may be prudent to utilize a kink-resistant nitinol wire as well.
7. Once access to the portal vein is obtained, typically the catheter is oriented peripherally. It is important to not lose access while reversing the catheter and wire toward the main portal vein. Use of a buddy wire system (discussed later) prevents this from occurring.

Percutaneous Portocaval Technique

1. Identifying a single plane by ultrasound that contains a portal vein and the inferior vena cava can be challenging.
2. Ensuring that the needle passes centrally through the portal vein and IVC is essential for successful completion of the procedure. A cirrhotic liver can make straight passage of a needle difficult. A larger (e.g., 18 gauge) needle allows for a straighter trajectory but increases the risk of bleeding.
3. The trajectory chosen must be free of extrahepatic structures, including pleura and bowel.
4. Once access to the portal vein via the IVC from a jugular or femoral access is obtained, the catheter will be oriented peripherally within the portal vein. Reversing direction with the catheter and wire without losing access to the portal vein is imperative. Use of a buddy wire system (discussed later) is advised.

Potential Pitfalls/Complications

Gun-Site Technique

1. Increased risk of hemorrhage: Access of the portal vein percutaneously increases the risk of hemorrhage

because the liver capsule is violated with two additional needle punctures during this procedure (first for the portal vein catheterization and the second during traversal of the two snares). Coil and/or gelfoam embolization of the tract(s) should be performed after portal vein access has been obtained.

2. If one of the snares is placed in the IVC (rather than the hepatic vein), the risk of hemorrhage increases further with creation of a potentially extrahepatic TIPS between the IVC and portal vein. To reduce this risk, it is advised that the IVC snare be placed in the retrohepatic IVC that extends between 5 and 6.5 cm caudal to the orifice of the right hepatic vein.[17]

3. Increased risk of bowel/gallbladder injury: The angle necessary to traverse the two snares may require a tract that traverses the transverse colon or gallbladder.

4. Increased risk of hepatic injury: The increased punctures required for this procedure pose a mildly increased risk of an iatrogenic fistula creation (typically arterial to biliary) and infection.

5. Access to the portal vasculature can be lost, typically either as a consequence of the wire kinking when snared bidirectionally or while attempting to reverse catheter direction from peripheral to central within the portal vein. Use of a buddy wire system largely obviates this risk.

Percutaneous Portocaval Technique

1. Increased risk of hemorrhage: As with the gun-site technique, a percutaneous puncture itself automatically increases the risk of hemorrhage. Coil and/or gelfoam embolization of the tract should be performed after successful catheterization is obtained.

2. Creation of a portocaval shunt (rather than a portohepatic shunt, as seen with a typical TIPS) predisposes the patient to a higher risk of hemorrhage, particularly if the shunt is created within an extrahepatic segment of the IVC. To mitigate this risk, the targeted IVC should be the retrohepatic IVC, which typically extends between 5 and 6.5 cm caudal to the orifice of the right hepatic vein.[17]

3. As with the gun-site technique, access to the portal vasculature can be inadvertently lost, most commonly while attempting to reverse the catheter direction from peripheral to central within the portal vein. Use of a buddy wire system largely obviates this risk.

Steps of the Procedure

Gun-Site Technique

1. Catheterization of a hepatic vein (usually right) is performed in a manner consistent with standard

TIPS technique. The TIPS sheath (10 Fr) is advanced into the catheterized hepatic vein. *Optional*: If the hepatic veins are not suitable for catheterization, a snare can be delivered to the retrohepatic IVC (within 5–6.5 cm caudal of the right hepatic vein orifice) via either a jugular or a femoral vein access.

2. As with standard TIPS technique, right atrial, free, and wedged hepatic pressures should be obtained to verify the patient is an appropriate TIPS candidate.

3. Wedged portography with either an occlusion balloon or a wedged catheter is performed with CO_2 to confirm portal vein patency and delineate the anatomy for further intervention.

4. The abdomen is prepped and draped in usual sterile fashion. If ascites is present, this should be drained first. Portal vein catheterization is then obtained with an 18 or 21 gauge Chiba (or similar) needle under ultrasound guidance. After access is obtained, a wire is advanced to the central portal vasculature and upsized to a 0.035-in. system with a transitional dilator set (AccuStick Introducer System, Boston Scientific, Marlborough, MA) if a 21 gauge needle and microwire were used. If a sheath is desired, a 6 Fr sheath can be placed, but alternatively, the delivery catheter of the snare can be advanced over a stiff wire without a sheath after appropriate 6 Fr dilator passage. This will reduce the size of the access and reduce the risk of bleeding. A snare (Amplatz GooseNeck [Covidien, Plymouth, MN] or En Snare [Merit Medical Systems Inc., South Jordan, UT]) is then placed under fluoroscopic guidance into the chosen portal vein at the desired site for catheterization (intrahepatic).

5. The C-arm is then angled in a cranial–caudal and oblique (as necessary) orientation in order to align the two snares on top of one another.

6. An 18 or 21 gauge Chiba needle is guided under fluoroscopy through the two snares. The two snares are then sequentially tightened to grasp the needle. *Optional*: Some authors[17] prefer use of a needle sheath (e.g., Yueh Centesis Catheter Needle, Cook Medical Inc., Bloomington, IN) for this step, which allows catheter advancement off of the needle and immediate placement of a 0.035-in. wire.

7. After confirmation that the needle is secured by both snares, an exchange length wire is passed through the needle and the needle is removed. The hepatic vein (or IVC) snare is tightened, and the wire is withdrawn from the jugular (or femoral) access.

8. Tension is now maintained on both ends of the wire from the jugular (or femoral) access and the abdominal exit site. *Optional*: If an exchange length nitinol wire is used (to prevent kinking), the abdominal end (back end) of the wire can be carefully retracted using the abdominal snare (while feeding the end from the prior needle site) to pull it as a loop through

the portal vein sheath because this allows deeper portal vein catheterization. However, if a Glidewire is employed for this step, the Colapinto needle (step 9) can be used with caution to avoid shearing of the wire coating.

9. With firm tension on both ends of the wire, a sheathed Colapinto needle can be advanced over the wire to obtain access to the portal vein. The outer sheath is then carefully advanced over the sheathed needle to the portal vein, again with firm traction on both ends of the wire for maximal support. At this point, the tract (hepatic venous to portal venous or portocaval) should be dilated with an 8-mm balloon. *Note: If a femoral vein access was used, this step will not be possible because of the unsuitable angle for the needle. Also, as stated previously, if a Glidewire is used as the exchange wire, the needle should either not be used or be used very cautiously. Pre-dilatation with a balloon alone and subsequent advancement of the sheath can be performed in lieu of use of the needle.*

10. At this point, the sheath and exchange wire will be directed peripherally in the portal vein, so reversal of direction is necessary. Rather than removing the exchange length wire and attempting reversal with a catheter and Glidewire, we advise maintaining the exchange length wire as a buddy wire (safety wire) to secure the access. Adjacent to the wire and through the sheath, a catheter and Glidewire can be advanced and used to reverse direction in the portal vein to obtain central portomesenteric venous access. This is typically achieved with an angled catheter (Kumpe or Cobra, AngioDynamics Inc., Latham, NY), but occasionally a reverse curve catheter is necessary. The wire is then advanced distally into either the superior mesenteric vein or the splenic vein.

11. At this point, the buddy wire can be removed, and the remainder of the procedure is completed with standard TIPS technique. If a sheath has been used at the lateral abdominal snare location, coil and/or gelfoam embolization of the tract can be performed.

Portocaval Technique

1. Ultrasound of the liver is performed to identify a single plane that identifies the right or left portal vein and the IVC. The left side is regarded as technically easier in most cases, and the puncture will pass from the main left portal vein to the IVC. On the right, the puncture will typically pass through the anterior division of the right portal vein (near the right portal vein itself) to the IVC. A right-sided approach may require an intercostal approach. If ascites is present, this should be drained first to facilitate the puncture and mitigate the risks of bleeding.

2. With both the portal vein and the IVC identified in plane, an 18 gauge Chiba needle or a needle sheath (e.g., Yueh) is inserted under ultrasound guidance percutaneously toward the portal vein. Upon reaching it, contrast is gently injected to confirm portal vein traversal. The needle is then further advanced along the same tract until the IVC is punctured, again verifying placement with a small injection of contrast under fluoroscopy. *Optional*: A balloon can be placed and inflated within the IVC to serve as a target if desired.

3. Access to the jugular vein (or femoral vein if the jugular vein is occluded) is obtained, and a 10 Fr sheath is placed utilizing the Seldinger technique.

4. A snare is advanced to the retrocaval IVC (first 5–6.6 cm caudal to the origin of the right hepatic vein orifice) from the jugular (or femoral) sheath.

5. A 0.035-in. guidewire is threaded through the percutaneous needle into the snare, and the wire is retracted through the jugular (or femoral) sheath.

6. With tension on both ends of the guidewire, the portocaval tract is pre-dilated with an 8-mm balloon. As the balloon deflates, the sheath is advanced from the IVC to the portal vein.

7. As the sheath passes into the portal vein, it will naturally be directed peripherally. Therefore, adjacent to the guidewire (to be used as a buddy wire), an angled catheter (e.g., Kumpe and Cobra) and Glidewire are used to reverse direction and obtain catheterization of the main portal vein and subsequently the superior mesenteric vein or splenic vein. Occasionally, a small reverse curve catheter may be necessary.

8. After access to the superior mesenteric vein or splenic vein is obtained, a stiff wire is placed and the original wire can be removed. The percutaneous tract should be embolized.

9. Over the stiff wire, the remainder of the TIPS procedure is completed with standard technique.

Example

See Figures 77.1–77.3.

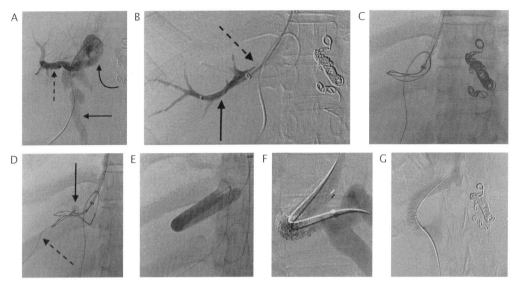

Figure 77.1 Gun-site technique. (A) Catheterization of the right portal vein was obtained using a recanalized paraumbilical vein (solid arrow). Note that the catheter travels anatomically from the recanalized portal vein to the left portal vein (curved arrow), across the portal vein confluence, and ultimately into the right portal vein (dashed arrow). (B) Access has been obtained to the right hepatic vein as well (solid arrow). Note that the delivery sheath has been advanced from a right jugular approach into the right hepatic vein (dashed arrow). (C) Gooseneck snares have been inserted into the right hepatic vein and the right portal vein from their respective accesses. (D) A Chiba needle (solid arrow) has been percutaneously inserted through both snares under fluoroscopic guidance. The inner stylet is removed, and a 300-cm V-18 wire (Boston Scientific) was advanced through the needle (which is subsequently removed). A safety wire (dashed arrow) helps secure access for the right hepatic vein sheath. (E) After wire access is obtained from the right hepatic vein to the right portal vein, the TIPS procedure is continued in the normal fashion. Here, balloon pre-dilatation of the tract is being performed. (F) An anterior–posterior digital subtraction angiography (DSA) image demonstrates final placement of the TIPS. Note the more anterior–posterior orientation of the deployed TIPS. (G) DSA image in a steep cranial oblique demonstrates the TIPS with a more conventional appearance.

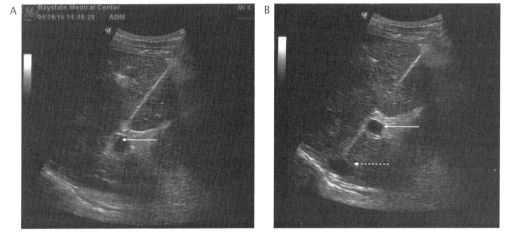

Figure 77.2 Portocaval technique. (A) Ultrasound demonstrates the needle tip (arrow) of a 20-cm needle sheath passing percutaneously through the right portal vein. Contrast was injected under fluoroscopy, confirming the location in the right portal vein. (B) The needle was then further advanced under ultrasound and can be seen traversing the right portal vein (solid white arrow) before reaching the IVC (dashed white arrow).

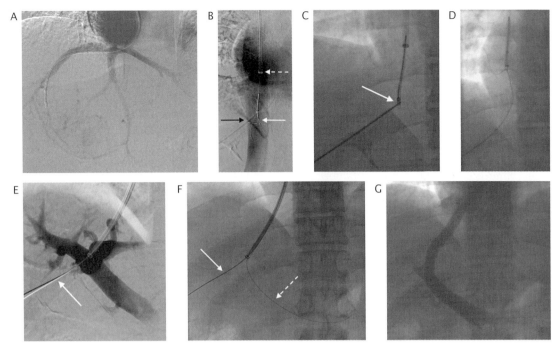

Figure 77.3 Portocaval technique. Fluoroscopic images obtained from the same patient shown in Figure 77.2. (A) CO_2 hepatic venogram reveals an unusual splayed configuration of the hepatic veins. A conventional TIPS had been attempted earlier but was not possible. A 20-cm needle sheath was passed by ultrasound (see Figure 77.2) through the right portal vein and subsequently the IVC. (B) A cavagram through the needle sheath (black arrow) confirmed proper location. The delivery sheath (dashed arrow) of the DIPS is positioned in the right atrium. An En Snare (white arrow) has been positioned in the IVC to capture a wire passed through the needle sheath. (C) The En Snare is used to grasp the needle tip (arrow) before the wire is threaded into the IVC. (D) An Amplatz wire (Cook Medical) is captured by the En Snare and pulled through the jugular sheath. (E) Over the Amplatz wire (which runs percutaneously through the liver and subsequently through the jugular sheath) (arrow), pre-dilatation of the tract is performed with a 4-mm balloon before the sheath is advanced from the IVC to the right portal vein. A portogram through the sheath confirms proper location. (F) The Amplatz wire (solid arrow) is maintained as a safety wire until wire access to the central portal vasculature (dashed arrow) is obtained. (G) Final portography reveals the DIPS extending from the right portal vein to the IVC.

References and Suggested Readings

1. Rösch J, Hanafee WN, Snow H. Transjugular portal venography and radiologic portocaval shunt: An experimental study. *Radiology.* 1969;92(5):1112–1114.

2. Boyer TD, Haskal ZJ. American Association for the Study of Liver Diseases practice guidelines: The role of transjugular intrahepatic portosystemic shunt creation in the management of portal hypertension. *J Vasc Interv Radiol.* 2005;16:615.

3. Spencer EB, Cohen DT, Darcy MD. Safety and efficacy of transjugular intrahepatic portosystemic shunt creation for the treatment of hepatic hydrothorax. *J Vasc Interv Radiol.* 2002;13:385.

4. Shiffman ML, Jeffers L, Hoofnagle JH, et al.: The role of transjugular intrahepatic portosystemic shunt for treatment of portal hypertension and its complications: A conference sponsored by the National Digestive Diseases Advisory Board. *Hepatology.* 1995;22:1591.

5. Haskal ZJ, Martin L, Cardella JF, et al. Quality improvement guidelines for transjugular intrahepatic portosystemic shunts. *J Vasc Interv Radiol.* 2001;12:131–136.

6. Saxon RR, Keller FS. Technical aspects of accessing the portal vein during the TIPS procedure. *J Vasc Interv Radiol.* 1997;8:733–744.

7. Ferral H, Bilbao JI. The difficult transjugular intrahepatic portosystemic shunt: Alternative techniques and "tips" to successful shunt creation. *Semin Intervent Radiol.* 2005;22(4):300–308.

8. Petersen B. Intravascular ultrasound-guided direct intrahepatic portocaval shunt: Description of technique and technical refinements. *J Vasc Interv Radiol.* 2003;14(1):21–32.

9. Teitelbaum GP, Van Allan RJ, Reed RA, Hanks S, Katz MD. Portal venous branch targeting with a platinum-tipped wire to facilitate transjugular intrahepatic portosystemic shunt (TIPS) procedures. *Cardiovasc Intervent Radiol.* 1993; 16:198–200.

10. Warner DL, Owens CA, Hibbeln JF, Ray CE Jr. Indirect localization of the portal vein during a transjugular intrahepatic portosystemic shunt procedure: Placement of a radiopaque marker in the hepatic artery. *J Vasc Interv Radiol.* 1995;6:87–90.

11. Ferro C, Ambrogi C, Perona F, Cianni R, Barile A. Technical and methodologic considerations on a new approach to the transjugular intrahepatic portosystemic shunt. *Radiol Med.* 1993;85(5):653–656.

12. Wenz F, Nemcek AA Jr, Tischler HA, Minor PL, Vogelzang RL. US-guided paraumbilical vein puncture: An adjunct to transjugular intrahepatic portosystemic shunt (TIPS) placement. *J Vasc Interv Radiol.* 1992;3(3):549–551.

13. Bell BM Jr, Cura M, Shaw CJ, Rees CR. Transjugular intrahepatic portosystemic shunt creation using a three-dimensional fluoroscopic guidance system in patients with the Budd–Chiari syndrome. *Proc Bayl Univ Med Cent.* 2015;28(4):484–487.

14. Luo X, Ye L, Zhou X, et al. C-arm cone-beam volume CT in transjugular intrahepatic portosystemic shunt: Initial clinical experience. *Cardiovasc Intervent Radiol.* 2015;38(6): 1627–1631.

15. Muller MF, Siewert B, Stokes KR, et al. MR angiographic guidance for transjugular intrahepatic portosystemic shunt procedures. *J Magn Reson Imaging.* 1994;4:145–150.

16. Rose SC, Pretorius DH, Nelson TR, et al. Adjunctive 3D US for achieving portal vein access during transjugular intrahepatic portosystemic shunt procedures. *J Vasc Interv Radiol.* 2000;11:611–621.

17. Haskal ZJ, Duszak R Jr, Furth EE. Transjugular intrahepatic transcaval portosystemic shunt: The gun-sight approach. *J Vasc Interv Radiol.* 1996;7(1):139–142.

18. Aytekin C, Boyvat F, Firat A, Coskun M, Boyacioglu S. Portocaval shunt creation using the percutaneous transhepatic–transjugular technique. *Abdom Imaging.* 2003;28(2):287–292.

19. Honda M, Baba T, Hashimoto T, Seino N, Gokan T. Ultrasonography-guided percutaneous transhepatic portacaval shunt creation. *Jpn J Radiol.* 2010;28(7):542–546.

20. Boyvat F, Harman A, Ozyer U, Aytekin C, Arat Z. Percutaneous sonographic guidance for TIPS in Budd–Chiari syndrome: Direct simultaneous puncture of the portal vein and inferior vena cava. *AJR Am J Roentgenol.* 2008;191(2):560–564.

21. Boyvat F, Aytekin C, Harman A, Ozin Y. Transjugular intrahepatic portosystemic shunt creation in Budd–Chiari syndrome: Percutaneous ultrasound-guided direct simultaneous puncture of the portal vein and vena cava. *Cardiovasc Intervent Radiol.* 2006;29(5):857–861.

CHAPTER 78

Deployment of Direct Intrahepatic Portocaval Shunt (DIPS) from a Femoral Access

Abdulrahman Masrani and Bulent Arslan

Brief Description

The transjugular intrahepatic portosystemic shunt (TIPS) has been shown to be effective in management of esophageal varices bleeding in patients with liver cirrhosis when endoscopic manuvers fail to control it. Ascites refractory to optimal medical therapy is another indication for TIPS procedure. Occasionally, TIPS cannot be performed due to vascular anatomical difficulties such as occluded central venous access, small hepatic veins, or portal vein occlusion. Direct intrahepatic portocaval shunt (DIPS) can be considered as an alternative option in such circumstances. DIPS is typically performed utilizing jugular access with direct puncture from the inferior vena cava (IVC) to the right portal vein. However, the interventionalist may be challenged by jugular or brachiocephalic veins occlusion. This chapter discusses perfroming DIPS procedure utilizing femoral access in a patient with bilateral occluded brachiocephalic veins and thrombosed right portal vein.

Applications of the Technique

1. Difficult TIPS for patients with refractory esophageal bleeding due to the following anatomical challenges:
    a. Failure of gaining internal jugular access due to occlusion of the central venous system.
    b. Thrombosed right portal vein.

Challenges of the Procedure

1. Accessing portal system from the IVC.
2. Placement of a stent, which requires a 360-degree turn within the liver.
3. In the example dicussed later, recanalization of the main portal vein through the cava to the left portal vein shunt.

Potential Pitfalls/Complications

1. Non-target puncture and hemorrhage while obtaining access to the left portal circulation from the IVC.
2. Ability to track the stent graft system through a 360-degree turn can be difficult; however, this will not be necessary in patients with patent main portal circulation.

Steps of the Procedure

1. Review the abdominal computed tomography (CT) images to identify the relationship between the IVC and the portal veins.
2. Choose the portal vein that is more amenable to access from the femoral approach, which is usually the left portal vein.
3. Obtain access into the IVC through the right femoral vein.
4. Introduce intravascular ultrasound (IVUS) probe through the right groin access sheath.
5. Identify the level of the left portal vein using CT images as a reference for fluoroscopy and IVUS.
6. Puncture the left portal vein directly from the IVC using the Rosch–Uchida portal access needle (Cook Medical Inc., Bloomington, IN).
7. Advance the needle sheath into the portal vein, and confirm blood return from the portal vein.
8. Measure portal and systemic pressures and perform a portogram with simultaneous IVC-gram to identify the length of the stent graft.
9. Advance an Amplatz guidewire (Boston Scientific, Marlborough, MA) through this established route.
10. Dilate this shunt tract using a small-caliber (3 or 4 mm) angioplasty balloon and advancing the 10 Fr Flexor sheath (Cook Medical Inc., Bloomington,

IN) over the balloon into the portal system as the balloon is retracted.

11. Advance the stent graft through the sheath, and deploy it after the sheath is pulled back into the IVC. Deploy a 7 × 59-mm iCAST balloon-expandable stent graft (Atrium, Hudson, NH), or Viator/Viabahn stent grafts (W. L. Gore & Associates Inc., Flagstaff, AZ), depending on the anatomy and the coverage area needed.

12. Repeat angioplasty with larger caliber balloons (8–10 mm) to establish the preferred portosystemic gradient.

13. Perform post-stent deployment hemodynamic measurements and portosystemic venogram.

Example

See Figures 78.1–78.4.

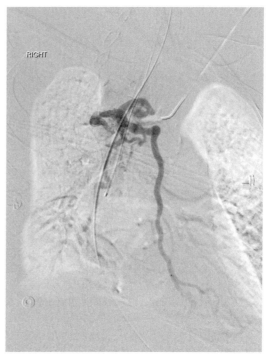

Figure 78.2 Left jugular venogram with multiple failed attempts to reach IVC. Several extraluminal accesses using different chronic occlusion wires and devices were attempted.

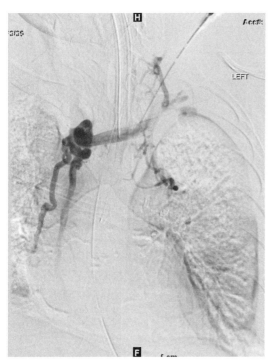

Figure 78.1 Right jugular venogram with multiple failed attempts to reach the IVC. Several extraluminal accesses using different chronic occlusion wires and devices were attempted.

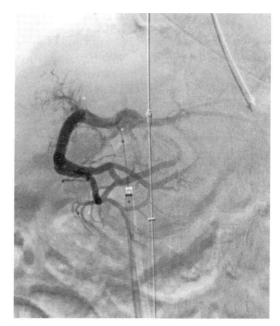

Figure 78.3 Access to the left portal vein (right portal system is atrophic) with Rosh–Ushida system and a left portal venogram.

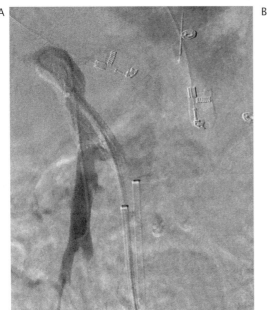 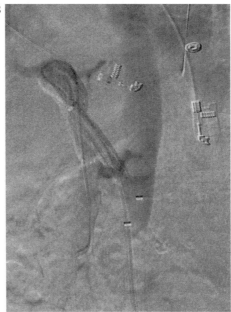

Figure 78.4 Portosystemic venogram from the superior mesenteric vein (SMV) injection, early phase (A) and late phase (B), following placement of two iCAST stents between the left portal vein and the IVC and additional Zilver self-expanding bare stents (Cook Medical) to recanalize the mostly thrombosed main portal vein to the level of the SMV.

References and Suggested Readings

1. Pianta M, Tran N, Given M, Lyon SM. Direct percutaneous portocaval shunt creation for haematemesis: Case report. *Australas Radiol.* 2007;51(Suppl):B328–B330.
2. Loffroy R, Favelier S, Pottecher P, et al. Transjugular intrahepatic portosystemic shunt for acute variceal gastrointestinal bleeding: Indications, techniques and outcomes. *Diagn Interv Imaging.* 2015;96(7-8):745–755.
3. Ward TJ, Techasith T, Louie JD, Hwang GL, Hofmann LV, Sze DY. Emergent salvage direct intrahepatic portocaval shunt procedure for acute variceal hemorrhage. *J Vasc Interv Radiol.* 2015;26(6):829–834.
4. Petersen B, Binkert C. Intravascular ultrasound-guided direct intrahepatic portacaval shunt: Midterm follow-up. *J Vasc Interv Radiol.* 2004;15(9):927–938.
5. Petersen B. Intravascular ultrasound-guided direct intrahepatic portacaval shunt: Description of technique and technical refinements. *J Vasc Interv Radiol.* 2003;14(1):21–32.

CHAPTER 79

Transmesenteric Method of TIPS Placement Using Portal Access via Mini-Laparotomy

Sam McCabe, Christopher Harnain, and Grigory Rozenblit

Brief Description

Transmesenteric portal access via mini-laparotomy may be used as a salvage technique when standard transjugular intrahepatic portosystemic shunt (TIPS) is unsuccessful due to difficult anatomy or portal vein thrombosis. This technique allows for precise determination of both the portal and the hepatic vein branch involved in the TIPS. In distinction to standard technique, the hepatic parenchymal tract is created by a puncture from the portal vein into the hepatic vein. This method usually involves the cooperation of a surgeon, who performs a mini-laparotomy and exposes a small bowel loop in the interventional suite. A mesenteric venous branch is then cannulated, providing direct access to the portal venous system. Simultaneously, a suitable hepatic vein is cannulated via a standard transjugular approach. A biliary stone retrieval basket is then advanced into the selected hepatic vein and opened. The liver parenchyma separating the portal and hepatic veins is traversed with a 20 gauge needle, which is advanced through an angled metal guide cannula and aimed toward the stone retrieval basket under fluoroscopic guidance. A 0.018-in. nitinol guidewire is introduced through the 20 gauge needle from the mesenteric access. The leading end of the guidewire is grasped by the basket and retrieved through the jugular access. The TIPS procedure is then completed with standard technique. Upon completion, the mini-laparotomy is closed by the surgeon.

Applications of the Technique

1. Markedly distorted hepatic vascular anatomy (such as in a very small cirrhotic liver) that is believed to preclude or complicate the standard TIPS procedure.
2. Portal vein thrombosis.
3. Variant TIPS required (e.g., left hepatic vein to left portal vein).
4. Failed standard TIPS procedure.

Challenges of the Procedure

1. The procedure usually requires the assistance and co-operation of a surgeon.
2. Accessing a small mesenteric vein requires some skills not dissimilar to those required for venipuncture. A standard micropuncture access set should be used. If the access is compromised, the vessel can be safely ligated, and any one of the numerous other mesenteric veins can be chosen for an access.
3. Appropriate direction of the metal cannula requires angulation of the C-arm and confirmation in two or more projections.

Potential Pitfalls/Complications

1. Risks of mini-laparotomy: Postoperative ventral hernia and persistent ascites leak through the incision.
2. Theoretical risks of mini-laparotomy: Peritonitis and small bowel injury/perforation.
3. There is essentially no risk of liver capsule puncture or injury to gallbladder, hepatic flexure of colon, or stomach.
4. Inadvertent mesenteric arterial branch catheterization: Small mesenteric arterial branches can be safely ligated without clinical sequelae.

Steps of the Procedure

1. Hepatic vein access: Standard IJ venous access is performed with upsizing to a 10 Fr TIPS sheath allowing eventual placement of a Viatorr endoprosthesis (W. L. Gore & Associates, Flagstaff, AZ). Measurement of the right atrial and free and wedged hepatic vein pressures may be performed at this point, along with wedged CO_2 portography. Following this, a biliary stone retrieval basket in its guiding catheter is positioned in the desired hepatic vein segment and opened.

2. Mini-laparotomy: A 6-cm midline incision is made superior to the umbilicus by the surgeon, and the peritoneal cavity is entered. A small bowel loop is pulled through the incision and placed on a damp surgical sponge. A mesenteric vein branch 2–4 cm from the mesenteric border of the bowel is selected. Transillumination of the mesentery may be helpful in identifying a target vein.

3. Mesenteric vein access: The mesenteric vein branch is accessed with a 21 gauge micropuncture needle, and a 0.018-in. guidewire is advanced toward the portal vein. The position of the guidewire is verified using fluoroscopy. The access is then upsized to a 0.035-in. system, and an 8 Fr sheath is placed. The sheath is affixed to the mesentery with a suture, and the bowel loop is covered with a damp surgical sponge.

4. Liver puncture: Portography is performed by contrast injection through the mesenteric vein sheath. A suitable portal vein branch for TIPS is then selected. A curved metal directional cannula from a transjugular liver biopsy kit is advanced through the mesenteric sheath over a guidewire into the selected portal vein branch. Using fluoroscopy in at least two projections, the cannula is aimed at the stone retrieval basket in the hepatic vein. A 60-cm 20 gauge needle (Chiba or similar) is then advanced through and out of the metal guide cannula into the stone retrieval basket, thus traversing the liver parenchyma between the portal and hepatic veins. The position of the needle inside of the basket is confirmed with gentle attempts to retrieve the basket: If the needle is engaged, the basket cannot be pulled back into its guiding catheter. A 0.018-in. exchange length nitinol wire is then advanced through the 20 gauge needle. The basket is retracted back into its guiding catheter, thus snaring the leading end of the guidewire. The stone retrieval basket is then removed through the jugular access sheath along with the 0.018-in. nitinol wire, giving "through-and-through" access. The 20 gauge needle and directional cannula can then be removed through the mesenteric sheath.

5. Procedure completion: Once through-and-through access is obtained, with control of the 0.018-in. nitinol wire from both mesenteric and jugular access points, the hepatic parenchymal tract can be dilated with a 4-mm 0.018-in. angioplasty balloon. This facilitates passage of a 4 Fr directional catheter (Cobra or similar) from the jugular access into the portal circulation. The 0.018-in. nitinol wire can then be exchanged for a 0.035-in. guidewire, and the mesenteric sheath can be removed and the mini-laparotomy closed. The procedure is then completed using standard techniques.

Example

See Figures 79.1–79.6.

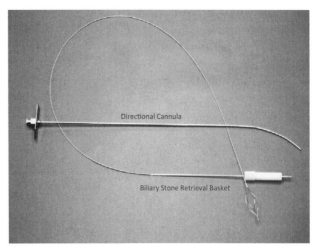

Figure 79.1 A transjugular liver biopsy kit metal directional cannula and a biliary stone retrieval basket are utilized in this technique.

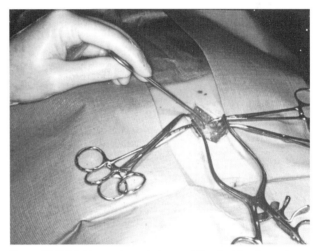

Figure 79.2 Mini-laparotomy. A 6-cm midline incision is made superior to the umbilicus.

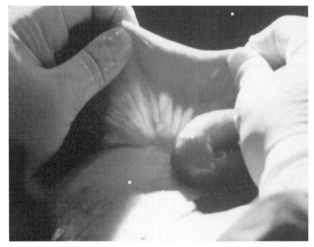

Figure 79.3 A small bowel loop has been pulled through the incision. Transillumination of the mesentery may be helpful in identifying a target vein.

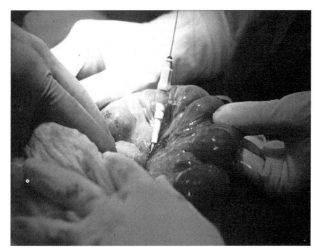

Figure 79.4 Mesenteric vein access. Mini-laparotomy was performed, and the mesenteric vein was accessed with a 21 gauge micropuncture needle. The access needle has been exchanged for a micropuncture catheter over an 0.018-in. guidewire.

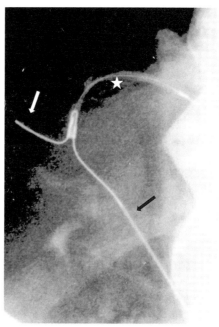

Figure 79.6 A 0.018-in. nitinol guidewire (white arrow) is introduced through the 20 gauge needle (black arrow) from the mesenteric access. The leading end of the guidewire is grasped by the basket and retrieved within its guiding catheter (star) through the systemic venous access. This provides "through-and-through" access, and the procedure can be completed using standard technique.

Reference and Suggested Reading

1. Rozenblit G, DelGuercio LR, Savino JA, et al. Transmesenteric–transfemoral method of intrahepatic portosystemic shunt placement with minilaparotomy. *J Vasc Interv Radiol.* 1996;7: 499–506.

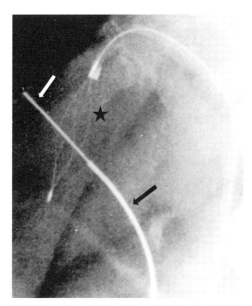

Figure 79.5 A transjugular liver biopsy kit, blunt metal directional cannula (black arrow) has been introduced into the selected portal branch via the mesenteric access. The liver tissue separating the portal and hepatic veins has been traversed with a 20 gauge needle (white arrow), which is advanced through the cannula and directed toward the basket (black star) under fluoroscopic guidance. In this example, the systemic venous system was accessed from the common femoral vein.

CHAPTER 80

Recanalization of Occluded TIPS Using a Transhepatic Percutaneous Technique

Saher S. Sabri

Brief Description

Transjugular intrahepatic portosystemic shunt (TIPS) dysfunction rates have significantly decreased since the introduction of stent grafts.[1,2] However, TIPS occlusion remains a recognized complication, especially when bare-metal stents are used or when the cephalad end of the stent does not extend into the inferior vena cava (IVC). Antegrade recanalization of the occluded TIPS can be routinely achieved using a coaxial or a triaxial sheath system, which provides sufficient stability and pushability to recanalize the TIPS. However, occasionally this cannot be achieved due to the difficult angulation between the IVC and the hepatic vein, poor placement of the initial TIPS short of the IVC, or long-standing occlusion of the TIPS. Retrograde recanalization of the TIPS by transhepatic percutaneous access of the TIPS using a 21 gauge needle can be performed in such situations when antegrade recanalization has failed. Once the wire is passed through the occluded TIPS in a retrograde fashion, the wire can be snared through the antegrade sheath. Once antegrade access into the portal system is achieved, TIPS revision with a stent graft is performed in the standard fashion.

Application of the Technique

1. This technique is applicable when the TIPS is occluded and there is difficulty accessing the TIPS from the jugular approach.
2. Difficulty accessing the TIPS from the jugular approach due to severe angulation at the cephalad end of the TIPS.
3. Recanalization of malpositioned TIPS (e.g., when the TIPS is too long or too short).

Challenges of the Procedure

1. Engaging the cephalad end of the TIPS can be challenging due to the angle between the hepatic vein and the IVC.
2. Retrograde passage of the wire is the most critical and most challenging step.

3. Advancing the 10 Fr sheath into the occluded TIPS over the through-and-through wire may be difficult and can be aided by serial balloon dilatation of the occluded TIPS prior to sheath advancement.

Potential Complications/Pitfalls

1. Increased risk of hemorrhage: Percutaneous access can be limited to 21 gauge needle, which minimizes bleeding complications. If the access is upsized and a sheath is placed to aid in retrograde recanalization, embolization of the transhepatic tract with coils or other embolic material is recommended.
2. Initial retrograde wire access through the percutaneous access needle can be challenging. Aggressive manipulation of the 0.018-in. wire may result in wire shearing. An exchange for a transition dilator is recommended if there is difficulty passing the 0.018-in. wire. Once the transition dilator is advanced into the TIPS, an exchange for a 0.035-in. stiff wire is recommended.
3. If percutaneous access and retrograde recanalization fails, access can be obtained into the caudal (portal) end of the TIPS and a wire is placed in the portal vein. This access will mark the location of the portal vein to aid in creation of a new TIPS.

Steps of the Procedure

1. Access should always be attempted from the jugular approach first.
2. A 10 Fr sheath is placed from the jugular approach into the IVC.
3. A coaxial 6 or 7 Fr sheath (40–70 cm) or a guide catheter is placed through the 10 Fr sheath.
4. A variety of catheters are used initially to catheterize the TIPS. Initially, a multipurpose or a Cobra-shaped catheter can be attempted. A reverse shape catheter (SOS or Simmons) can be used, especially when the IVC is dilated.

5. Antegrade recanalization is attempted with a hydrophilic wire (Glidewire, Terumo, Somerset, NJ). A stiff Glidewire may be needed.

6. If antegrade recanalization fails, transhepatic percutaneous access into the TIPS is attempted.

7. A 15- or 20-cm 21 gauge Chiba needle is advanced under fluoroscopy in the anteroposterior view until it overlies the location of TIPS. The image intensifier is moved to a left anterior oblique projection to determine the anterior–posterior relationship of the needle tip to the TIPS. The needle tip is repositioned until the TIPS is accessed using the Chiba needle.

8. The percutaneous access into the TIPS can be at any level throughout its length. If the cephalad portion of the TIPS can be recanalized but further advancement of the wire and catheter is not achievable despite a coaxial sheath system, then percutaneous access can be obtained into the caudal (portal) end of the TIPS. Otherwise, a more cephalad access is preferred.

9. A stiff 0.018- or 0.014-in wire such as a 300-cm V-18 or V-14 (Boston Scientific, Marlborough, MA) is advanced into the occluded TIPS through the Chiba needle.

10. If there is difficulty in retrograde passage of the wire into the cephalad portion of the TIPS, a transition dilator can be advanced, such as the Stiffened Micropuncture set (Cook Medical Inc., Bloomington, IN) or AccuStick (Boston Scientific). Once the dilator is in place, a 0.035-in. stiff Glidewire is advanced retrograde.

11. A support catheter (e.g., a multipurpose catheter) can be advanced percutaneously to provide pushability for the retrograde wire. A 5 Fr sheath may be needed occasionally.

12. A snare is advanced through the sheath from the jugular approach and placed above the TIPS. The retrograde wire is snared once it exits the cephalad portion of the stent.

13. Once "through-and-through" wire access is established, the occluded TIPS can be balloon dilated with a low-profile balloon (4–8 mm). The antegrade sheath can be advanced over the balloon as it is being deflated.

14. A diagnostic catheter is advanced through the sheath over the through-and-through wire into the TIPS. A second 0.014-in. wire is advanced antegrade into the portal vein. Once this access is established, the retrograde wire is removed.

15. The 0.014-in. wire is exchanged for a stiff 0.035-in. wire (Amplatz, Cook Medical), and the 10 Fr sheath is advanced into the portal vein using the sheath dilator.

16. The occluded TIPS is relined with a new TIPS using a stent graft (Viatorr, W. L. Gore & Associates, Flagstaff, AZ).

17. The percutaneous access can be removed without consequences if the access is through a Chiba needle only. If a catheter or a sheath is placed, embolization of the percutaneous tract is recommended using coils or other embolic material.

Example

See Figures 80.1–80.5.

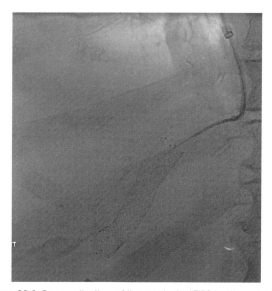

Figure 80.1 Recanalization of the occluded TIPS is attempted through an antegrade access. A triaxial system is in place with a 10 Fr sheath, 6 Fr guide catheter, and a multipurpose 5 Fr catheter. A stiff 0.035in. Glidewire is used to attempt recanalization.

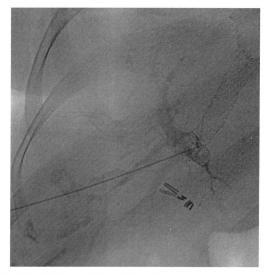

Figure 80.2 Initial access is obtained into the portal end of stent into the main portal vein. Portal venography confirmed patency of the portal vein. A wire will next be advanced into the portal vein to provide a target for a new TIPS if recanalization of the existing TIPS fails.

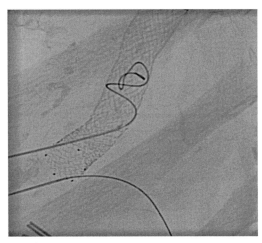

Figure 80.3 A second 21 gauge needle is advanced into the TIPS, and a 0.018-in. wire is advanced into the TIPS in a retrograde fashion. Note that a wire is advanced into the main portal vein through a separate access.

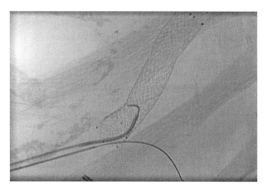

Figure 80.4 The needle was exchanged using a transitional dilator, and eventually a 5 Fr diagnostic catheter and a Glidewire were used to retrograde recanalize the TIPS. Wire access into the main portal vein is maintained through a separate access.

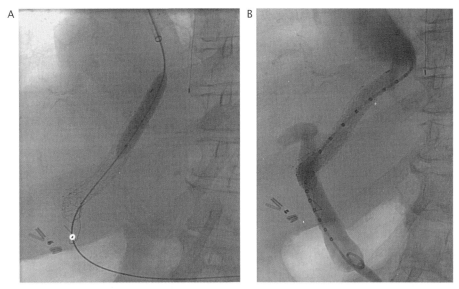

Figure 80.5 After the retrograde wire was snared through the antegrade sheath using a gooseneck snare, the 10 Fr sheath was advanced into the TIPS following balloon dilatation. The through-and-through wire was exchanged for a stiff 0.035-in. Amplatz wire, which was advanced into the portal system. (A) A new TIPS was placed and the balloon dilated. Note a sheared off 0.018-in. wire at the portal end of the stent, which was a result of excessive manipulation. (B) Portal venography showed patency of the new TIPS (Viatorr), with further extension of the new TIPS into the IVC.

References and Suggested Readings

1. Cejna M, Peck-Radosavljevic M, Thurnher S, et al. ePTFE-covered stent-grafts for revision of obstructed transjugular intrahepatic portosystemic shunt. *Cardiovasc Intervent Radiol.* 2002;25(5):365–372.

2. Angermayr B, Cejna M, Koenig F, et al.; Vienna TIPS Study Group. Survival in patients undergoing transjugular intrahepatic portosystemic shunt: ePTFE-covered stentgrafts versus bare stents. *Hepatology.* 2003;38(4):1043–1050.

CHAPTER 81

Adjustable Small-Diameter TIPS

Zubin Irani and Sara Zhao

Brief Description

Transjugular intrahepatic portosystemic shunt (TIPS) was first described by Rosch et al.[1] in 1969, and in 1982, Colopinto et al.[2] described its first clinical application in a patient with cirrhosis and variceal hemorrhage. It was not until 1988 that the first metal-lined shunt was created,[3] and in 1997, the first polytetrafluoroethylene (PTFE)-lined stent was used in humans for shunt revision after stenosis, created by pinning the Gore PTFE (W. L. Gore & Associates, Flagstaff, AZ) graft material between two metal stents.[4] Introduced in 2000, the Viatorr stent graft (Gore) is now the most commonly used device for TIPS.

The Viatorr stent graft is available in 8-, 10-, and 12-mm diameter sizes. One of the major side effects of TIPS creation is hepatic encephalopathy (HE). Current understanding of HE is that bypassing blood flow from hepatic circulation results in buildup of neurotoxins such as ammonia. The rate of post-TIPS HE has been correlated with the degree of portosystemic shunting;[5] therefore, presumably the larger the diameter of the shunt, the higher the risk of HE. In patients with HE, referring clinicians may be hesitant to consult for the procedure due to concern for worsening encephalopathy.

Described here is a technique of primary creation of an adjustable small-diameter TIPS. This allows for graded management of portal hypertension by allowing for subsequent incremental increase in shunt diameter as clinically needed.

In creation of the adjustable TIPS, portal vein access is obtained as per current methods, and after parenchymal tract dilation, a bare-metal balloon-expandable stent is placed within the tract. As a variation, a covered balloon-expandable stent can be placed to span the hepatic outflow end. The self-expanding, covered Viatorr stent is advanced through the balloon-expandable stent and deployed. The shunt can now be dilated to the desired starting diameter; the authors prefer to commence at 6-mm diameter. This can be increased by 1-mm increments until the portosystemic gradient (PSG) is ≤12 mmHg in patients with variceal bleed. For ascites patients, clinical follow-up is performed to guide any further need for shunt dilation, at which point the shunt is adjusted by dilating in 1-mm increments until the desired clinical endpoint is achieved. Primary TIPS creation in this fashion was published by Farsad et al.[6] in 2015. The authors' experience is from cases done between 2007 and 2010 (Table 81.1).

Applications of the Technique

1. Recurrent variceal hemorrhage: The adjustable TIPS diameter should be created such that a PSG of ≤12 mmHg is achieved.
2. Refractory ascites: The adjustable TIPS diameter should be created such that flow through the shunt is not sluggish.
3. Particularly in patients at risk for post-TIPS hepatic encephalopathy, this technique provides the benefit of balancing the risk of overshunting and worsening encephalopathy with the staged management of the previously mentioned indications.

Challenges of the Procedure

1. Placement of the constraining balloon-expandable stent requires some consideration.
   a. The stent needs to be placed within a region of the liver parenchyma that offers some "fixation" and stops stent migration. A small parenchymal track can make correct placement challenging.
   b. When using a bare-metal stent, the Viatorr is sized as per standard, and the constraining stent creates an hourglass configuration of the shunt.
   c. When using a covered balloon-expandable stent, the Viatorr can be sized to land anywhere within this stent and not necessarily back to the hepatic vein–inferior vena cava (IVC) junction. In this approach, the constraining stent is placed at the IVC junction and creates an asymmetric, tapered end to the TIPS shunt.
2. In placing a small-diameter shunt, avoiding thrombosis is also critical. The angiogram should be evaluated to ensure shunt flow is not sluggish; if

Table 81.1 Patient Outcomes in Applying the Adjustable Small-Diameter TIPS Technique

NO. OF PATIENTS	PATENCY RATE AT 5 YEARS (%)	ADJUSTMENT RATE AT 5 YEARS (%)	POST-TIPS HEPATIC ENCEPHALOPATHY RATE AT 90 DAYS (%)
28	73.3	28.6	30.4

this is the case, then the shunt should be dilated by 1 mm and angiogram repeated to look for improved shunt flow.

3. In cases in which clinical response is suboptimal, shunt adjustment can be made. This involves balloon dilation of the shunt typically by 1-mm increments. This "TIPS revision" involves a jugular approach to catheterize the shunt and then the use of a sheath and balloon of the necessary size.

Potential Pitfalls/Complications

1. Standard risks related to TIPS creation apply to this technique (thrombosis, rapidly progressive liver failure, and worsening encephalopathy). In the authors' experience of 28 cases from 2007 to 2010, technical success and complication profile paralleled that of the standard TIPS technique. Table 81.1 outlines outcomes in these patients.

Steps of the Procedure

1. Ultrasound-guided catheterization of the right internal jugular vein is obtained with a micropuncture set.
2. A hydrophilic wire is used to exchange the micropuncture sheath for a 9 or 10 Fr introducer sheath with an end marker.
3. The introducer sheath is guided into the right atrium, and atrial and IVC pressures are measured.
4. The hepatic vein is then catheterized using a 5 Fr diagnostic catheter, the choice of which is operator preference. Hepatic venography and CO_2 wedge portography can be performed at this stage.
5. The TIPS system of choice is then introduced into the hepatic vein.
6. The puncture needle is advanced through the hepatic parenchyma from the right hepatic vein to the right portal vein, and direct portography is performed with CO_2.
7. A stiff guidewire is advanced through the needle into the portal vein.
8. A pigtail catheter is advanced, and portal vein pressure is measured for baseline portosystemic gradient calculation.

9. The parenchymal tract is dilated, and the 10 Fr sheath is advanced into the track at this point to facilitate placement of the constraining balloon-expandable stent.
10. A 6 × 17-mm LD Express balloon-mounted stent (Boston Scientific, Marlborough, MA) is advanced into the parenchymal tract and deployed.
11. The 10 Fr sheath is then advanced through the balloon-expandable stent into the portal vein to facilitate deployment of the Viatorr TIPS stent.
12. The balloon-expandable stent is dilated as needed by 1-mm increments until the desired endpoint is reached (nonsluggish flow through the TIPS in ascites patients or to a PSG ≤12 mmHg in variceal bleed).

Example

See Figures 81.1 and 81.2.

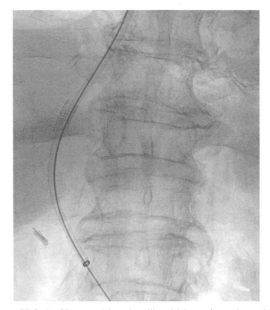

Figure 81.1 An 81-year-old male with a history of cryptogenic cirrhosis and ascites refractory to medical management and a MELD score of 9. Portal decompression was requested. After gaining access to the portal vein via the right hepatic vein using standard technique, a balloon-mounted stent was placed centrally within the hepatic parenchymal tract and dilated to a diameter of 6 mm.

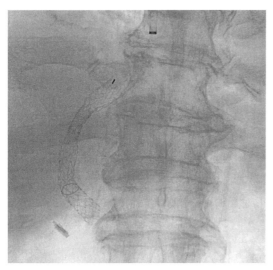

Figure 81.2 Final configuration of an adjustable small-diameter TIPS. The Viatorr stent is deployed through the balloon-mounted stent, and the device is dilated by 1-mm increments until the desire endpoint is reached.

References and Suggested Readings

1. Rosch J, Hanafee WN, Snow H. Transjugular portal venography and radiologic portocaval shunt: An experimental study. *Radiology.* 1969;92(5):1112–1114.
2. Colopinto RF, Stronell RD, Birch SJ, et al. Creation of an intrahepatic portosystemic shunt with a Gruntzig balloon catheter. *Can Med Assoc J.* 1982;126(3):267–268.
3. Richter GM, Palmaz JC, Noldge G, et al. The transjugular intrahepatic portosystemic stent-shunt: A new nonsurgical percutaneous method [in German]. *Radiologe.* 1989;29(8): 406–411.
4. Saxon RR, Timmermans HA, Uchida BT, et al. Stent-grafts for the revision of TIPS stenosis and occlusions: A clinical pilot study. *J Vasc Interv Radiol.* 1997;9(4):539–548.
5. Sarfeh IJ, Rypins EB. Partial versus total portacaval shunt in alcoholic cirrhosis: Results of a prospective, randomized clinical trial. *Ann Surg.* 1994;219(4):353–361.
6. Farsad K, Kolbeck K, Keller F, Barton RE, Kaufman JA. Primary creation of an externally constrained TIPS: A technique to control reduction of the portosystemic gradient. *AJR Am J Roentgenol.* 2015;204:868–871.

CHAPTER 82

Use of a Coda Balloon to Assist Left Renal Vein Sheath Delivery During Balloon-Occluded Retrograde Transvenous Obliteration

S. Lowell Kahn

Brief Description

The concept of obliterating a gastric varix through a transrenal venous approach was first described by Olson et al.[1] in 1984. The idea was revived in the 1990s when Japanese investigators coined the term "balloon-occluded retrograde transvenous obliteration" (BRTO) to describe a novel technique for the treatment of large gastric varices and portosystemic encephalopathy.[2-4] Since its inception, BRTO has gained widespread adoption internationally. The American College of Radiology Appropriateness Criteria Committee on interventional radiology officially recognized BRTO as an alternative to transjugular intrahepatic portosystemic shunt (TIPS) placement in certain anatomic and clinical scenarios for the treatment of gastric varices.[5,6] Although historically reserved for patients who are not TIPS candidates, some institutions are increasingly performing BRTO as first-line therapy for gastric varices with favorable anatomy.[5]

Fundamental to all BRTO procedures is the catheterization of the gastric varix via its drainage through a gastrorenal shunt and its subsequent sclerosis. Although simple in principle, the heterogeneity of gastric variceal anatomy adds a layer of complexity. Understanding the specific variceal anatomy at hand with a clear delineation of the drainage pattern is imperative for safe performance of the procedure. In 2003, Kiyosue et al.[7] drafted a widely accepted anatomic classification system that describes the afferent and efferent venous anatomy of the varix and guides subsequent treatment planning.

The gastrorenal shunt is thought to be an enlarged inferior phrenic vein that has a confluence with the left adrenal vein and drains into the cranial aspect of the left renal vein. Once the gastrorenal shunt is catheterized, it is occluded with a balloon and studied with contrast injections under live fluoroscopy. Additional points of venous drainage (pericardiophrenic, ascending lumbar, etc.) are catheterized when possible and embolized with the goal of isolating the varix from the systemic circulation. Once isolated, the varix is embolized with one of several sclerosants, commonly a sotradecol foam. The sclerosant is allowed to dwell for a variable time to ensure complete thrombosis of the varix.[4,7-12] Multiple variations of this technique are described in the literature and are beyond the scope of this chapter. An excellent review of the BRTO technique is provided by Saad.[13]

Although routinely performed with little difficulty in experienced hands, there exist clinical scenarios and anatomic factors that present technical challenges to the procedure. The BRTO procedure can be performed from a transjugular or transfemoral approach, and there are merits to each.[1,4,7,8] An average gastrorenal shunt is readily occluded with a standard occlusion balloon (e.g., over-the-wire Fogarty thru-lumen Embolectomy catheter [Edwards Lifesciences, Irvine, CA] and Python Catheter [Applied Medical, Rancho Santa Margarita, CA]) that requires between a 5 and 8 Fr sheath. Larger shunts may require a larger sheath size. Irrespective of the access chosen, a common challenge is the delivery of the occlusion balloon to the neck of the gastrorenal shunt to allow occlusion. Two main factors affect this: the angulation of the veins relative to one another and the size of the balloon required to achieve occlusion. Sharp angulation of the vasculature (inferior vena cava (IVC) relative to the left renal vein and left renal vein relative to the shunt) and large draining shunts (requiring large occlusion balloons/sheath sizes) present the greatest challenges. Particularly from the transfemoral approach, delivery of a sheath to the left renal vein is challenging when there is sharp caudal angulation of the left renal vein relative to the IVC. This challenge is compounded when a large shunt mandates delivery of a large balloon and hence larger sheath.

This chapter describes a technique to facilitate delivery of a sheath to the left renal vein from a femoral approach when the caudal angulation of the left renal vein makes catheterization unfavorable. When the renal vein is sharply angulated, the sheath (and catheter/wire) will reflux into the IVC rather than assume the course of the left renal vein. The technique described herein addresses this challenge and involves obtaining a second access through which a large occlusion balloon (e.g., Reliant, Medtronic, Minneapolis, MN) is delivered to the IVC above the confluence of the left renal vein and the IVC. When inflated, the IVC occlusion balloon serves to deflect the catheter and sheath from the other access into the left renal vein. We have used this technique on several occasions with 100% technical success. We believe it is an effective and safe adjunctive procedure that will improve the technical success of a BRTO in challenging anatomy.

Applications of the Technique

1. Obtaining left renal vein catheterization during a BRTO procedure.
2. We have exclusively used this technique in the setting of a BRTO procedure, but in theory, the technique could be used for any of several challenging venous catheterizations:
   a. Left renal vein catheterization for adrenal vein sampling
   b. Left renal vein catheterization for stenting (e.g., nutcracker syndrome)
   c. Left ovarian vein catheterization in the setting of pelvic congestion syndrome
   d. Challenging hepatic venous catheterizations for TIPS or direct intrahepatic portosystemic shunt (DIPS) procedures (e.g., Budd–Chiari) whereby a femoral IVC occlusion balloon is used to divert access into small or partially obliterated hepatic veins
   e. Up-and-over the iliac venous catheterizations (pelvic congestion, etc.)
   f. Other
3. Arterial applications are theoretically possible (difficult aortic side branch catheterizations/interventions), but use of the technique would need to be weighed against the risk of the large arterial sheath size necessary (12 Fr). It might have a role in endovascular aortic aneurysm repair cases that involve fenestrated grafts or snorkels.

Challenges of the Procedure

1. The initial catheterization of the left renal vein is performed prior to inflating the IVC occlusion balloon in the majority of cases. The occlusion balloon is used to facilitate subsequent delivery of the sheath. Occasionally, the initial catheterization of

the left renal vein may be challenging, but usually it is readily accomplished with the appropriate catheter and wire selection.

Potential Pitfalls/Complications

1. IVC injury with consequent hemorrhage could result from overaggressive inflation of the occlusion balloon.
2. IVC occlusion compromises venous return to the heart and can be associated with a drop in blood pressure, tachycardia, and shortness of breath. Inflation of the balloon should be performed for short periods as necessary only.
3. A 12 Fr sheath is typically tolerated well at the femoral vein, but there is an increased risk of bleeding, particularly with coagulopathic patients and/or those with higher central venous pressure.

Steps of the Procedure

1. From a femoral approach (typically right), the left renal vein is catheterized. A variety of catheters are well suited for this application. At our institution, we commonly use an Sos 2 (AngioDynamics, Latham, NY) or Simmons 1 (AngioDynamics Inc., Latham, NY) catheter to pass a Glidewire (Terumo, Somerset, NJ) into a branch of the left renal vein. The Sos 2 or Simmons 1 is then exchanged for a hockey stick catheter, which is spun cranially and used to select the gastrorenal shunt. The Glidewire is exchanged for a stiff wire, and the procedure is continued. Note that there are numerous catheters well suited to catheterize the left renal vein. Many operators prefer use of a hockey stick catheter mounted over a tip deflecting wire. Alternatively, the Cobra series of catheters (AngioDynamics) or any of several reverse curve catheters may be appropriate (e.g., MK1B, AngioDynamics). Regardless of the method chosen, the goal is to obtain stiff wire support in either the left renal vein or preferably the gastrorenal shunt to facilitate subsequent delivery of the support sheath. *Note*: We typically catheterize the left renal vein prior to placing the IVC occlusion balloon. However, if this is difficult, the occlusion balloon can be delivered and inflated first (steps 2–6) to aid the initial catheterization.
2. If the sheath required for delivery of the occlusion balloon fails to advance into the left renal vein, a second access in the femoral vein is obtained. This can be obtained on the same side as the existing access (above or below) or on the contralateral side. In the interest of preventing injury to

the femoral vein, we typically access the contralateral side.

3. At the site of the new access, a 12 Fr sheath is advanced to the IVC using the Seldinger technique.

4. A Reliant (Medtronic, Minneapolis, MN) or Coda (Cook Medical, Bloomington, IN) is advanced through the 12 Fr sheath to a position immediately above the confluence of the left renal vein and the IVC.

5. The required sheath for placement of the occlusion balloon is placed on the support wire in the left renal vein or gastrorenal shunt.

6. The Reliant or Coda IVC occlusion balloon is inflated.

7. The sheath of the variceal occlusion balloon is then advanced over the stiff support wire and deflected by

the IVC occlusion balloon into the left renal vein or gastrorenal shunt. The balloon prevents reflux of the sheath and wire into the IVC.

8. Once stable sheath position is obtained into the left renal vein or preferably the gastrorenal shunt, the IVC occlusion balloon is deflated and removed.

9. The BRTO procedure is then completed in standard fashion. The 12 Fr femoral sheath should be removed once it is no longer required to prevent femoral vein thrombosis.

Example
See Figure 82.1.

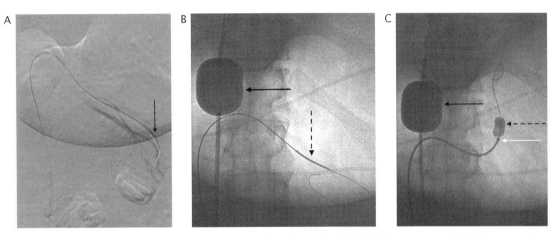

Figure 82.1 A 49-year-old male with alcoholic cirrhosis, encephalopathy, and a high MELD score presented to the emergency room with hemorrhagic gastric varices confirmed by endoscopy. A preliminary computed tomography scan showed anatomy suitable for a BRTO. After stabilization, he was sent to Interventional Radiology for the procedure. (A) The right femoral vein was catheterized and a Cobra 2 catheter (arrow; AngioDynamics, Latham, NY) was used to catheterize the left renal vein, with selective venography demonstrating a sharp caudal angulation of the vein. Despite placement of a stiff support wire, the 6 Fr sheath required for the Fogarty occlusion balloon failed to deliver into the left renal vein. (B) A second access was obtained in the left femoral vein, and a 12 Fr sheath was placed. A Coda balloon (solid arrow) was inflated to maintain the position of a Kumpe catheter (dashed arrow; Cook Medical, Bloomington, IN) in the renal vein while it was used with a Glidewire to catheterize the varix. The Glidewire was subsequently exchanged for a Magic Torque wire (Boston Scientific, Marlborough, MA). (C) The Coda balloon (solid black arrow) is maintained in its inflated state while a 6 Fr Flexor sheath (white arrow; Cook Medical) is advanced into the varix over the Magic Torque wire. Note the Fogarty balloon (dashed black arrow) is then inflated and the BRTO procedure is completed.

References and Suggested Readings

1. Olson E, Yune HY, Klatte EC. Transrenal-vein reflux ethanol sclerosis of gastroesophageal varices. *AJR Am J Roentgenol.* 1984;143(3):627–628.

2. Kawanaka H, Ohta M, Hashizume M, et al. Portosystemic encephalopathy treated with balloon-occluded retrograde transvenous obliteration. *Am J Gastroenterol.* 1995;90(3): 508–510.

3. Iwasaki T, Akahane T, Takahashi N, et al. A case of giant gastric varices successfully treated by arranged balloon-occluded retrograde transvenous obliteration. *Am J Gastroenterol.* 1995;90(3):508–510.

4. Kanagawa H, Mima S, Kouyama H, Gotoh K, Uchida T, Okuda K. Treatment of gastric fundal varices by balloon-occluded retrograde transvenous obliteration. *J Gastroenterol Hepatol.* 1996;11(1):51–58.

5. Saad WE. Balloon-occluded antegrade transvenous obliteration with or without balloon-occluded retrograde transvenous obliteration for the management of gastric varices: Concept and technical applications. *Tech Vasc Interv Radiol.* 2012;15(3): 203–225.

6. Saad WEA, Al-Osaimi AM, Caldwell S, et al.; for the Expert Panel on Interventional Radiology for the American College of Radiology. ACR appropriateness criteria: Radiologic management of gastric varices. https://acsearch.acr.org/docs/70911/Narrative. Accessed July 23, 2012.

7. Kiyosue H, Mori H, Matsumoto S, Yamada Y, Hori Y, Okino Y. Transcatheter obliteration of gastric varices: Part 1. Anatomic classification. *Radiographics.* 2003;23(4):911–920.

8. Kiyosue H, Mori H, Matsumoto S, Yamada Y, Hori Y, Okino Y. Transcatheter obliteration of gastric varices: Part 2.

Strategy and techniques based on hemodynamic features. *Radiographics*. 2003;23(4):921–937.

9. Hirota S, Matsumoto S, Tomita M, Sako M, Kono M. Retrograde transvenous obliteration of gastric varices. *Radiology*. 1999;211(2):349–356.

10. Matsumoto A, Yamauchi H, Inokuchi H. Balloon occluded retrograde transvenous obliteration: A feasible alternative to transjugular intrahepatic portosystemic stent shunt. *Gut*. 2003;52(4):611–612.

11. Kitamoto M, Imamura M, Kamada K, et al. Balloon-occluded retrograde transvenous obliteration of gastric fundal varices with hemorrhage. *AJR Am J Roentgenol*. 2002;178(5): 1167–1174.

12. Shiba M, Higuchi K, Nakamura K, et al. Efficacy and safety of balloon-occluded endoscopic injection sclerotherapy as a prophylactic treatment for high-risk gastric fundal varices: A prospective, randomized, comparative clinical trial. *Gastrointest Endosc*. 2002;56(4):522–528.

13. Saad WEA. Balloon-occluded retrograde transvenous obliteration of gastric varices: Concept, basic techniques, and outcomes. *Semin Intervent Radiol*. 2012;29(2):118–128.

CHAPTER 83

Use of Contrast-Fortified Surgilube for Biliary Drainage in the Setting of Active Leakage

S. Lowell Kahn

Brief Description

Biliary leaks are a common clinical entity that may occur after trauma or surgery. The clinical presentation varies, but classically leaks may present with fever, abdominal pain, abscess, cholangitis, biloma, or secondary biliary cirrhosis due to chronic strictures.[1] Morbidity rates associated with bile leaks range from 22% to 44%, and associated mortality ranges between 8.7% and 39%.[2–6]

In the surgical setting, the major causes of a biliary leak include laparoscopic cholecystectomy, liver transplantation, hepaticojejunostomy, hepatic resection, and common bile duct-to-common bile duct (CBD) anastomoses.[1,7–10] Traumatic bile duct injuries are less common, but they present clinically in a similar fashion. Irrespective of the cause, prompt drainage and diversion is advised given the risks of sepsis, cirrhosis, and abscess formation that may result from an untreated leak.

Endoscopic retrograde cholangiopancreatography (ERCP) is the first choice of treatment for an active biliary leak.[2,11–15] When ERCP allows successful insertion of a biliary stent, closure of the leak is obtained in 75–100% of cases.[1,16,17] Unfortunately, however, technical failure rates may be as high as 46% in the leak setting,[1,7] likely in part because of surgical changes/altered anatomy and edema.

Surgical repair of bile leaks is often attempted, particularly in the setting of large leaks and complete duct transections, but successful repair requires clearance of any associated infections/fluid collections, and delineation of the biliary anatomy with preoperative cholangiography is often essential.[1] Although direct repair of the duct is possible in some cases, others mandate a hepaticojejunostomy to achieve leak exclusion. Injury to intrahepatic ducts may require a hepatic lobectomy.[1,18] Irrespective of the surgical plan, options may be limited by periportal infection, edema, and scarring.[1,7,10,19]

Percutaneous transhepatic cholangiography (PTC) with drain placement (external or internal/external) is increasingly employed either alone or as an adjunct to endoscopy (Rendezvous procedure) or surgery. Early reports of PTC in the nondilated/leaking patient yielded low technical success rates (25%) and high complication rates (21%).[2,14,20] Over time, there has been major improvement in outcomes, with recent reports yielding technical success rates between 90% and 100%, clinical success between 70% and 100%, and major complication rates between 0% and 13%.[2,5,21–27] Although technical success has greatly improved, performance of a PTC on the nondilated system remains technically challenging and is associated with extra needle passes and significantly longer fluoroscopy times.[21,27] Technical challenges arise from needle localization of a small nondilated duct, and the contrast that is injected will pass through the leak rather than distending and opacifying the ducts. Consequently, successful biliary catheterization in this setting often requires a more central puncture, which itself is associated with a higher risk of vascular complications and extrahepatic puncture.[28] Alternative methods including computed tomography-guided puncture, injection through an existing T drain, and injection of the gallbladder are described to aid performance of a PTC in the nondilated patient.[2,21]

This chapter describes the use of contrast-fortified Surgilube (Savage Laboratories Inc., Melville, NY) for biliary opacification in the setting of an active biliary leak. This method was initially described by Dr. Joshua Weintraub at the Society of Interventional Radiology Annual Meeting Potpourri of Pearls session. We have since adopted it in our practice with excellent technical success and no immediate associated complications to date. The admixture of Surgilube and iodinated contrast produces a viscous radiopaque medium that overcomes the limitation of iodinated contrast alone. The viscous nature allows opacification and distention of the biliary system because it is better retained in a leaking biliary system than contrast alone. With adequate biliary opacification and distention, placement of a drain via the initial or a secondary access is more readily attained.

Applications of the Technique

1. Catheterization and subsequent biliary drainage/diversion in the setting of an active bile duct leak, which typically occurs after trauma or surgery: Opacification of the decompressed biliary system is difficult with standard contrast because it leaves the bile ducts quickly when a leak is present. The admixture of Surgilube and contrast yields a viscous, radiopaque medium that more readily opacifies and distends the biliary system.

2. Although not tested, the technique could likely be applied in other situations, such as a nephrostomy or nephroureteral stent placement in the setting of a leaking urinary system.

Challenges of the Procedure

1. The initial catheterization is frequently difficult, even when targeting the central ducts, because the structures are deep and small. Rarely, we have catheterized the gallbladder and subsequently the cystic duct in order to opacify the biliary system for a subsequent access suitable for placement of a drain.

Potential Pitfalls/Complications

1. Catheterization of a peripheral biliary duct as is traditionally performed with a PTC procedure is difficult. Therefore, the initial access (for biliary opacification, not drainage) is often central to improve technical success. A more central access carries an increased risk of bleeding because of the large hilar vessels including the hepatic artery. Also, there is increased risk of an extrahepatic puncture and the potential for injury to adjacent structures (e.g., bowel).

2. Although unlikely, the viscous Surgilube could theoretically impede biliary drainage, thereby initiating or worsening cholangitis or sepsis. However, its water-soluble nature makes this unlikely, and in our practice, we have not appreciated any such issue. Nonetheless, at completion of the procedure, we routinely irrigate the system gently with normal saline to help dissolve the Surgilube.

Steps of the Procedure

1. The contrast and Surgilube mixture is prepared in a bowl on the back table. We typically use an approximately 1:1 ratio of full-strength contrast to Surgilube, but there is no specific ratio that is optimal. The mixture obtained should be tested to ensure that it aspirates into a syringe and injects easily through the biliary access needle. A high Surgilube-to-contrast ratio offers good viscosity and retention in the biliary system but does so at the expense of poor visualization. Similarly, a high contrast-to-Surgilube ratio offers visibility but may leak freely through the biliary defect with poor biliary retention and distention.

2. The initial catheterization of a peripheral biliary duct with a long 21 gauge needle as is commonly performed with a PTC procedure is typically difficult in a decompressed (leaking) state. Therefore, an initial access in a more central location (e.g., left or right hepatic duct vs. common hepatic duct) may be required. The chosen duct is punctured by ultrasound or fluoroscopic guidance. With fluoroscopic guidance, the needle is advanced at or beyond the expected location of a central biliary duct and slowly withdrawn while injecting contrast under collimated, magnified fluoroscopy until a biliary duct is identified.

3. Once needle access is obtained, contrast is injected to delineate the biliary anatomy and confirm the presence and location of the biliary leak. Often, the presence of a biliary leak results in rapid disappearance of contrast from the biliary tree.

4. The contrast-fortified Surgilube is then slowly injected through the needle until the biliary system is adequately opacified and distended to allow secondary access to a peripheral duct. This step must be done with caution in patients with evidence of cholangitis to reduce the risk of sepsis.

5. At a separate intercostal, mid-axillary access, a second long 21 gauge needle is advanced into an opacified peripheral biliary duct (usually right).

6. Once access is obtained, a 0.018-in. nitinol wire is advanced, and the AccuStick Introducer System (Boston Scientific, Marlborough, MA) is used to transition to a 0.035-in. wire platform.

7. *Optional*: After the inner stylet and inner catheter of the triaxial AccuStick system are removed, a Check-Flo (Cook Medical Inc., Bloomington, IN) valve can be placed over the 0.018-in. wire and attached to the outer catheter of the AccuStick system. Using the wire to preserve access, the outer catheter is withdrawn slowly while contrast is injected through the side arm of the Check-Flo valve. This allows the operator to ensure that no major vascular structures were traversed along the tract of the new access. If an arterial or large venous vessel was traversed, a new access should be obtained. If acceptable, the AccuStick system is reassembled with its inner stylet and catheter and again inserted.

8. The procedure is then completed over a stiff 0.035-in. wire, ideally obtaining access beyond the CBD to the duodenum. An external or internal/external drain is placed to provide scaffolding across the biliary leak and optimize diversion of bile away from the biliary leak.

Example

See Figure 83.1.

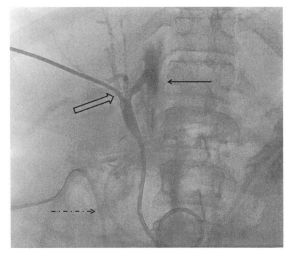

Figure 83.1 A 33-year-old morbidly obese female underwent laparoscopic cholecystectomy that subsequently required an ERCP. The ERCP was complicated by perforation of the CBD and injury to the duodenum. This resulted in a tension pneumoperitoneum, multiple intra-abdominal abscesses, sepsis, and intermittent bleeding requiring surgical intensive care unit admission. Multiple surgical explorations/evacuations and an omental patch were performed with failure of resolution of her biloma and abscesses. PTC shows the drain (open arrow) entering the right hepatic duct centrally in a nondilated system. Contrast injected leaked promptly from the CBD and tracked in a cephalad manner (solid arrow). Contrast-fortified Surgilube was then employed and was retained in the bile ducts, allowing placement of the drain. Incidental note of a percutaneous drain (dashed arrow) positioned at the inferior liver margin.

References and Suggested Readings

1. Popat B, Thakkar D, Deshmukh H, Rathod K. Percutaneous transhepatic biliary drainage in the management of post-surgical biliary leaks. *Indian J Surg.* 2016; first online January 2012.
2. de Jong EA, Moelker A, Leertouwer T, Spronk S, Van Dijk M, van Eijck CHJ. Percutaneous transhepatic biliary drainage in patients with postsurgical bile leakage and nondilated intrahepatic bile ducts. *Dig Surg.* 2013;30:444–450.
3. Buanes T, Waage A, Mjåland O, Solheim K. Bile leak after cholecystectomy significance and treatment: Results from the National Norwegian Cholecystectomy Registry. *Int Surg.* 1996;81:276–279.
4. Lo CM, Fan ST, Liu CL, Lai EC, Wong J. Biliary complications after hepatic resection: Risk factors, management, and outcome. *Arch Surg.* 1998;133:156–161.
5. Kim JH, Ko GY, Sung KB, et al. Bile leak following living donor liver transplantation: Clinical efficacy of percutaneous transhepatic treatment. *Liver Transpl.* 2008;14:1142–1149.
6. Yamashita Y, Hamatsu T, Rikimaru T, et al. Bile leakage after hepatic resection. *Ann Surg.* 2001;233:45–50.
7. Liguory C, Vitale GC, Lefebre JF, Bonnel D, Cornud F. Endoscopic treatment of postoperative biliary fistulae. *Surgery.* 1991;110:779–784.
8. Sherman S, Shaked A, Cryer HM, Goldstein LI, Busuttil RW. Endoscopic management of biliary fistulas complicating liver transplantation and other hepatobiliary operations. *Ann Surg.* 1993;218:167–175.
9. Vaccaro JP, Dorfman GS, Lambiase RE. Treatment of biliary leaks and fistulae by simultaneous percutaneous drainage and diversion. *Cardiovasc Intervent Radiol.* 1991;14:109–112.
10. Kaufman SL, Kadir S, Mitchell SE, et al. Percutaneous transhepatic biliary drainage for bile leaks and fistulas. *AJR Am J Roentgenol.* 1985;144:1055–1058.
11. Akamatsu N, Sugawara Y, Hashimoto D. Biliary reconstruction, its complications and management of biliary complications after adult liver transplantation: A systematic review of the incidence, risk factors and outcome. *Transpl Int.* 2011;24:379–392.
12. Lai EC, Mok FP, Tan ES, et al. Endoscopic biliary drainage for severe acute cholangitis. *N Engl J Med.* 1992;326:1582–1586.
13. Kumar R, Sharma BC, Singh J, Sarin SK. Endoscopic biliary drainage for severe acute cholangitis in biliary obstruction as a result of malignant and benign diseases. *J Gastroenterol Hepatol.* 2004;19:994–997.
14. Teplick SK, Flick P, Brandon JC. Transhepatic cholangiography in patients with suspected biliary disease and nondilated intrahepatic bile ducts. *Gastrointest Radiol.* 1991;16:193–197.
15. McLindon JP, England RE, Martin DF. Causes, clinical features and non-operative management of bile leaks. *Eur Radiol.* 1998;8:1602–1607.
16. Goldin E, Katz E, Wengrower D, et al. Treatment of fistulas of the biliary tract by endoscopic insertion of endoprostheses. *Surg Gynecol Obstet.* 1990;170(5):418–423.
17. Hoffman BJ, Cunningham JT, Marsh WH. Endoscopic management of biliary fistulas with small caliber stents. *Am J Gastroenterol.* 1990;85:705–707.
18. Branum G, Schmitt C, Baillie J, et al. Management of major biliary complications after laparoscopic cholecystectomy. *Ann Surg.* 1993;217:532–541.
19. Smith AC, Schapiro RH, Kelsey PB, Warshaw AL. Successful treatment of nonhealing biliary–cutaneous fistulas with biliary stents. *Gastroenterology.* 1986;90:764–769.
20. Elias E. Cholangiography in the jaundiced patient. *Gut.* 1976;17:801–811.
21. Kuhn JP, Busemann A, Lerch MM, Heidecke CD, Hosten N, Puls R. Percutaneous biliary drainage in patients with nondilated intrahepatic bile ducts compared with patients with dilated intrahepatic bile ducts. *AJR Am J Roentgenol.* 2010;195:851–857.
22. Cozzi G, Severini A, Civelli E, et al. Percutaneous transhepatic biliary drainage in the management of postsurgical biliary leaks in patients with nondilated intrahepatic bile ducts. *Cardiovasc Intervent Radiol.* 2006;29:380–388.
23. Ernst O, Sergent G, Mizrahi D, Delemazure O, L'Herminé C. Biliary leaks: Treatment by means of percutaneous transhepatic biliary drainage. *Radiology.* 1999;211:345–348.
24. Righi D, Franchello A, Ricchiuti A, et al. Safety and efficacy of the percutaneous treatment of bile leaks in hepaticojejunostomy or split-liver transplantation without dilatation of the biliary tree. *Liver Transpl.* 2008;14:611–615.

25. Stampfl U, Hackert T, Radeleff B, et al. Percutaneous management of postoperative bile leaks after upper gastrointestinal surgery. *Cardiovasc Intervent Radiol.* 2011;34:808–815.

26. Aytekin C, Boyvat F, Harman A, Ozyer U, Krakayali H, Haberal M. Percutaneous therapy for anastomotic bile leak in liver-transplant patients with nondilated bile ducts. *Cardiovasc Intervent Radiol.* 2007;30:761–764.

27. Funaki B, Zaleski GX, Straus CA, et al. Percutaneous biliary drainage in patients with nondilated intrahepatic bile ducts. *AJR Am J Roentgenol.* 1999;173:1541–1544.

28. L'Hermine C, Ernst O, Delemazure O, Sergent G. Arterial complications of percutaneous transhepatic biliary drainage. *Cardiovasc Intervent Radiol.* 1996;19:160–164.

CHAPTER 84

Percutaneous Placement of a Temporary Large-Bore Biliary Endoprosthesis

Sam McCabe, Christopher Harnain, and Grigory Rozenblit

Brief Description

Patients with benign common duct biliary strictures often require treatment via bile duct cannulation, intervention, and catheter or stent placement. When endoscopic therapy is not possible due to prior surgical biliary-enteric anastomosis, periampullary duodenal diverticulum, or for any other reason, percutaneous transhepatic intervention is employed. Treatment often requires several sessions, and patients are faced with the discomfort of an indwelling biliary catheter for a protracted time course. In addition, a catheter traversing the skin requires continuous care and may be a portal for infection. Placement of a temporary internal biliary endoprosthesis may improve the patient's experience.

Bare-metal stents are prone to tissue ingrowth and mucosal hypertrophy, becoming incorporated into the bile duct wall. These factors limit bare-metal stent retrieval, which is a serious problem in patients with a long life expectancy. For these reasons, their use is generally not advocated in the treatment of benign biliary strictures.[1] Covered metal stents are resistant to tissue ingrowth; however, they are prone to occlusion and migration. Endoscopic retrieval rates of covered metal stents in place for up to 1 year are as high as 74%.[2] Percutaneous retrieval of covered metal stents, however, is technically demanding and requires either maintaining percutaneous biliary access while the stent is in place or re-establishing access at the time of removal.[3] Commercially available soft plastic biliary stents are only available up to 12 Fr and are prone to migration and occlusion.[4]

This chapter describes construction of a temporary large-bore biliary endoprosthesis from a standard drainage catheter. The pigtail end of a standard biliary tube or drainage catheter is used. The catheter is cut in two a distance above the pigtail determined by the length of the biliary stricture. The pigtail will lie in the intestine, and the trailing end will traverse the stricture. Side holes are cut along the catheter as needed. This endoprosthesis is then positioned, deployed, and tethered to the abdominal wall with an absorbable suture. After the suture dissolves in several months, the catheter is propelled into the intestine by peristalsis and expelled without the need for an additional procedure.

Applications of the Technique

1. Benign common duct biliary stricture of any etiology in patients who are not candidates for endoscopic retrograde cholangiopancreatography or who have previously failed endoscopic management.

Challenges of the Procedure

1. Fashioning an endoprosthesis of proper length requires accurate "bent wire" measurement (described later) or use of a sizing catheter.
2. Accurate positioning of the endoprosthesis is facilitated by use of reference images.

Potential Pitfalls/Complications

1. Placement of a large-bore endoprosthesis may be painful and requires effective sedation and analgesia.
2. Large-bore devices may require occlusion of the percutaneous parenchymal liver access tract after endoprosthesis placement.
3. Malposition of the endoprosthesis: As with any stent, malposition can be avoided by meticulous technique. The operator must ensure that the leading pigtail end of the device is formed within the bowel lumen and also that the body of the stent crosses the stricture before full deployment. The tethering suture may allow the catheter to be retracted if it is advanced too far.

Steps of the Procedure

1. Access: The patient should have established percutaneous transhepatic biliary access. The underlying lesion should be treated with cholangioplasty, stone extraction, or both. A cholangiogram is used as a reference image.

2. Measurement: The distance between the biliary–intestinal junction and the upper end of the stricture can be measured using the bent wire technique. Any guidewire with a stainless-steel core is advanced through a catheter until its leading end reaches the biliary–intestinal junction (either the ampulla of Vater or the surgical anastomosis). At this point, the wire is bent at the catheter's trailing end. The wire is then retracted until its leading end reaches the upper end of the stricture, and the wire is bent again. The distance between the two bends designates the length of the endoprosthesis body. Alternatively, a measuring catheter can be used for this purpose.

3. Endoprosthesis construction: A standard pigtail or biliary drainage catheter of appropriate diameter is used (e.g., 12–16 Fr). The locking string is cut and removed. The catheter is cut transversely according to the length determined in step 2. Measurement should be made from the base of the pigtail and not from the tip of the catheter. Additional side holes are added as needed. A long (at least 70 in.) absorbable suture such as PDS Plus Antibacterial Polydioxanone Monofilament Suture (Ethicon, Bridgewater, NJ) size 1 (182- to 238-day absorption profile) is secured to the trailing end of the endoprosthesis by passing one end through a side hole without knotting the suture. The needle is left attached. The pigtail segment will be the endoprosthesis, and the other piece of the cut catheter will be used as a pusher.

4. Stent assembly: The plastic stiffener supplied with the drainage catheter may be lubricated with sterile Vaseline or bacitracin ointment. The trailing end of the catheter is loaded onto the plastic stiffener, to be used as a pusher. The endoprosthesis is then loaded onto the stiffener.

5. Stent delivery: Care is taken to maintain control of both ends of the trailing suture. The assembly is advanced over a guidewire under fluoroscopic guidance until the trailing end of the endoprosthesis is in the desired location. The guidewire is then removed. The plastic stiffener is carefully removed while the endoprosthesis is kept in place with the pusher. As the stiffener is withdrawn, the pigtail loop of the endoprosthesis should form within the intestinal lumen.

6. Verification of stent position: Cholangiography is performed through the pusher. If the endoprosthesis is patent and well positioned, the pusher can be removed or used for occlusion of the percutaneous parenchymal tract, if needed.

7. Stent anchoring: The trailing suture is stitched to the abdominal wall within the access tract, thereby anchoring the stent in place. A sterile dressing is applied.

Example
See Figures 84.1–84.4.

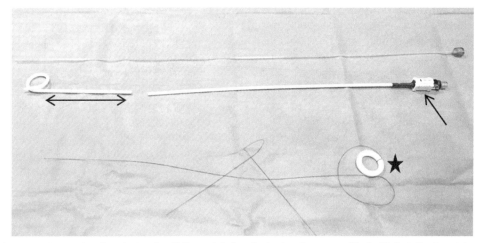

Figure 84.1 Endoprosthesis construction. A standard biliary pigtail catheter has been modified with its tethering string (star) cut and removed. The distance between the biliary–intestinal junction and the upper margin of the stricture was measured, and the catheter has been cut to this length (bidirectional arrow). The Luer lock end of the catheter (arrow) will serve as a pusher during endoprosthesis delivery.

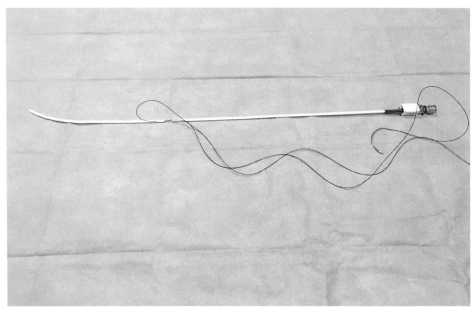

Figure 84.2 Stent assembly. Both pieces of the cut catheter have been loaded onto the plastic stiffener. A size 1 PDS absorbable suture has been passed through the trailing side hole. The assembly is ready for delivery. Care is taken to maintain control of both ends of the suture during device delivery.

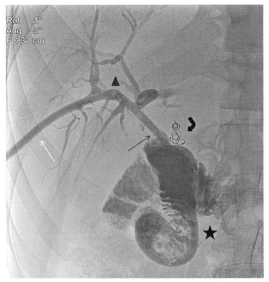

Figure 84.3 A 16 Fr biliary endoprosthesis placement in a 48-year-old male 3 years status post Whipple surgery for pancreatic adenocarcinoma. The patient developed a benign hepaticojejunostomy anastomotic stricture that was treated with cholangioplasty on three separate occasions. Biliary endoprosthesis (star) positioned with pigtail in the jejunum and its shaft traversing the anastomosis (black arrow) and terminating in the right hepatic duct (triangle). Cholangiogram was performed through the pusher (white arrow). Incidental note of embolization coils (curved arrow) used in prior treatment of hepatic artery pseudoaneurysm.

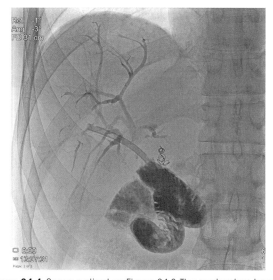

Figure 84.4 Same patient as Figure 84.3. The pusher has been removed, and the endoprosthesis has been sutured to the abdominal wall (not visualized).

References and Suggested Readings

1. Maccioni F, Rossi M, Salvatori FM, et al. Metallic stents in benign biliary strictures: Three-year follow-up. *Cardiovasc Intervent Radiol.* 1992;15:360–366.

2. Deviere, J, Reddy DN, Puspok A, et al. Successful management of benign biliary strictures with fully covered self-expanding metal stents. *Gastroenterology.* 2014;147(2):385–395.

3. Kuo MD, LoPresti DC, Gover DD, Hall LD, Ferrara SL. Intentional retrieval of Viabil stent-grafts from the biliary system. *J Vasc Interv Radiol.* 2006;17:389–397.

4. Lammer J, Hausegger KA, Fluckiger F, et al. Common bile duct obstruction due to malignancy: Treatment with plastic versus metal stents. *Radiology.* 1996;201:167–172.

CHAPTER 85

Method of Increasing Luminal Scaffolding for Biliary Strictures

S. Lowell Kahn

Brief Description

Benign biliary strictures are a common clinical entity encountered by the interventionalist. Balloon dilatation is an acceptable modality of treatment, but restenosis is frequent. Short-term patency is reported between 50% and 90%,[1-5] and long-term patency varies between 56% and 74%.[1,3,6,7] It is well known that benign strictures that are unifocal and short respond considerably better to balloon dilatation than do multifocal and/or long strictures.[4] Protocols for ballooning biliary strictures vary by institution, but most practitioners advocate prolonged inflations with use of a balloon diameter 20% or greater than the bile duct adjacent to the stricture. In addition, the high rate of restenosis mandates that many patients require repeat balloon dilatations. Although variation exists, most interventionalists perform repeat interventions to optimize long-term patency. The interval between dilatation varies between 1 or 2 weeks[1,3,5] and every 3 months.[1,2]

The recoil that follows balloon dilatation of recalcitrant benign biliary strictures presents a treatment challenge. The balloons used for biliary strictures are most commonly between 6 and 12 mm. Unfortunately, the scaffolding provided by the most commonly used 8.5 and 10 Fr internal–external biliary drains has a diameter between 2.8 and 3.3 mm. Therefore, it is commonly the case that despite effective balloon dilatation with full profiling of the balloon, the stricture recoils to the diameter of the drain in place.

It is desirable to have a temporary biliary drain that maintains the biliary duct diameter closer to that attained by the balloon. Some authors advocate the use of large-bore drains that measure between 16 and 18 Fr for this purpose.[1,8] However, large-bore drains are used at the expense of patient comfort as well as the hemorrhagic and biliary risks associated with a larger percutaneous and transhepatic tract.

This chapter presents a single-access dual-drainage catheter technique that we have employed successfully in our practice for more than 6 years. The procedure involves the standard placement of a large drainage catheter (ideally 14 Fr) across the biliary stricture. A second catheter measuring between 5 and 8.5 Fr is advanced through the hub of the 14 Fr drainage catheter and subsequently exits through a proximal hole of the 14 Fr drainage catheter. At the site of the stricture, there is side-by-side placement of the two drainage catheters, providing extra scaffolding (up to 22.5 Fr) despite the 14 Fr percutaneous tract.

This technique is not unique to our institution and has been studied by others. In fact, Gwon et al.[9] reported 100% technical success with a low complication rate in 79 patients using this technique. Clinical success was achieved in 98.7% of patients, with primary patency rates of 96%, 92%, and 91% at 1, 2, and 3 years, respectively. The experience of Gwon et al. is consistent with our own, and we believe that this is an easy, safe, and efficacious procedure that can be performed readily in the angiographic suite.

Applications of the Technique

1. Recalcitrant benign biliary strictures.
2. Recalcitrant benign ureteral strictures.

Challenges of the Procedure

1. At times, we pre-cannulate the proximal side hole of the outer drainage catheter. At other times, we place the outer drainage catheter and subsequently steer a hockey stick catheter and Glidewire (Terumo, Somerset, NJ) through a proximal side hole. This can present a challenge, but typically it is not difficult.

2. Leakage at the hub of the outer drainage catheter: We address drainage of both catheters using a Tuohy–Borst adapter (Cook Medical, Bloomington, IN) or by cutting and clamping the two tubes. This is discussed in detail later. In the former method, the adaptor side arm can be connected to a drainage bag for external drainage or capped for internal drainage.

3. Dislodgement of the second drainage catheter: This is controlled by tightening the Tuohy–Borst catheter so that it is unable to move relative to the outer drainage catheter. The outer drainage catheter is secured (often by suture) to the skin.

Potential Pitfalls/Complications

1. Inadequate biliary drainage: It is important to be mindful of the location of the side holes of both catheters with this technique. At times, we cut additional side holes to ensure drainage on either side of the stricture, particularly if we intend to cap the tubes and allow internal drainage.

Steps of the Procedure

Performance of a standard percutaneous transhepatic cholangiogram (PTC) is completed, obtaining the necessary images and wire access across the stricture. At this point, the operator must decide whether to use the pre-cannulation or post-cannulation method. At our institution, we utilize the post-cannulation method because we have found little difficulty with obtaining access through a proximal side hole after the primary outer drainage catheter is placed. Both methods are discussed here.

Pre-cannulation

1. After obtaining wire access across the stricture, a 23-cm or longer (as needed) 5 Fr or larger sheath is advanced beyond the stricture, and the dilator is removed. The sheath is used to deliver a second wire adjacent to the main support wire. Alternatively, a Dual Lumen Ureteral Catheter (Boston Scientific, Marlborough, MA) can be used in lieu of the sheath. Our preferred primary support wire is an Amplatz Super Stiff guidewire (Boston Scientific).
2. Adjacent to the Amplatz wire, a stiff Glidewire is placed.
3. With dual-wire access, the sheath or dual-lumen catheter is removed.
4. The tract is dilated one size larger (i.e., 16 Fr for a 14 Fr drainage catheter) than the size of the intended primary drainage catheter. We most commonly use a 14 Fr drain, but there are a range of biliary drainage catheters (Cook Medical Inc., Bloomington, IN) from 8.5 to 18 Fr. The practice of overdilatation is utilized because the inner stiffener of the drainage catheter is not used with this method.
5. *Optional*: Additional side holes are cut as needed to ensure drainage holes on either side of the stricture.
6. External to the patient, the back end of the Amplatz wire is threaded through the end hole and brought through the hub. The back end of the Glidewire is then placed through one of the more proximal side holes and then threaded through the hub as well.
7. The primary outer drainage catheter (typically a 14 Fr biliary drainage catheter) is then advanced over both wires while they are pinned. The outer drainage catheter is positioned with side holes positioned proximal and distal to the stricture. Of note, the side hole through which the Glidewire exits must be positioned proximal to the stricture.

8. The inner drainage catheter is chosen based on the desired increase in scaffolding. Typically, the chosen catheter ranges between a 5 Fr hockey stick to an 8.5 Fr biliary drain.
9. Over the Glidewire, the inner drainage catheter is advanced through a Tuohy–Borst adapter (Cook Medical) or Check-Flo valve (Cook Medical) attached to the hub of the outer drainage catheter and similarly placed with the side holes positioned proximal and distal to the stricture (8.5 Fr drain).
10. The outer drainage catheter is secured to the skin, with a sterile dressing ± suture.
11. Hub configuration: This varies depending on the desired scaffolding and hence the inner drainage catheter chosen.
    a. If a 5 Fr hockey stick catheter is selected, we typically pass the catheter through the Tuohy–Borst adapter of the Check-Flo valve attached to the hub of the outer drainage catheter. The Tuohy–Borst is then attached to the outer drainage catheter. The 5 Fr catheter is capped because it provides no drainage function and its tip sits in the duodenum. The 5 Fr catheter is secured to the outer drainage catheter by tightening the Tuohy–Borst or suturing it if a Check-Flo valve is used. The side arm of the Tuohy–Borst is connected to a drainage bag or is clamped depending on the desire for external or internal drainage, respectively.
    b. If an 8.5 Fr biliary drainage catheter is chosen, the catheter is similarly passed through a Tuohy–Borst or Check-Flow valve, and both drainage catheters are either capped or connected to a drainage bag depending on the desire for internal or external drainage, respectively.

Post-cannulation

1. After performing the PTC and obtaining appropriate imaging, an Amplatz wire is placed across the stricture.
2. The tract is dilated to the desired diameter of the outer drainage catheter (typically 14 Fr).
3. *Optional*: Additional side holes are cut as needed to ensure drainage holes on either side of the stricture.
4. With the inner stiffener, the chosen outer drainage catheter (typically 14 Fr biliary catheter) is placed across the stricture with side holes located proximal and distal to the stricture.
5. The Amplatz wire is removed.
6. If the 5 Fr hockey stick catheter provides the desired extra scaffolding, a Tuohy–Borst or Check-Flo valve is secured to the hub of the outer drainage catheter, and the hockey stick catheter is inserted through it.
7. Together with a Glidewire, the hockey stick catheter is steered out one of the proximal side holes of the outer drainage catheter. Note that the side hole selected must be proximal to the biliary stricture.

8. The 5 Fr hockey stick catheter and Glidewire are then advanced beyond the stricture and typically into the duodenum.

9. If the 5 Fr hockey stick catheter is chosen as the final added scaffolding, it is secured to the Tuohy–Borst by tightening it or by suturing it if a Check-Flo valve is used. The hockey stick catheter is capped, and the side arm of the Tuohy–Borst is attached to gravity drainage or capped depending on the desire for internal or external drainage, respectively.

10. If greater scaffolding across the stricture is desired, the hockey stick catheter is exchanged over the wire for a larger inner drainage catheter, typically an 8.5 Fr biliary drainage catheter. The 8.5 Fr inner catheter is positioned such that the side holes are located distal and proximal to the stricture. The catheters are capped or connected to drainage bags depending on the desire for internal or external drainage, respectively. The outer catheter is secured to the skin with a sterile dressing ± suture, and the inner drainage catheter is secured either by tightening the Tuohy–Borst or by suturing it if a Check-Flo valve is used.

Example

See Figures 85.1–85.3.

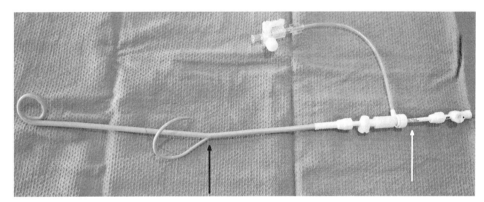

Figure 85.1 Bench model demonstrating the scaffolding technique. An 8 Fr drain exits a proximal side hole of an outer 14 Fr drain. Taken together, this increases the outer diameter to 22 Fr where both drains are together across a biliary stenosis. The 8 Fr drain has been inserted through the hub (white arrow) of a Check-Flo valve that is attached to the hub of the 14 Fr drain. The 14 Fr drain is able to drain externally via the side port of the Check-Flo valve, whereas the 8 Fr drain can be drained externally through its hub in standard fashion.

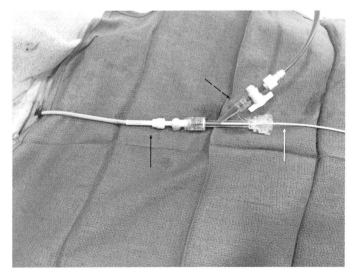

Figure 85.2 Rear assembly of the scaffolding technique utilized on a patient with a benign biliary stricture. An outer 12 Fr drain (solid black arrow) traverses the biliary stenosis. A Touhy–Borst adapter has been attached to the hub of the 12 Fr drain. To obtain additional scaffolding, a 5 Fr hockey stick catheter (solid white arrow) has been advanced through the Tuohy–Borst and terminates in the duodenum (total scaffolding diameter of 17 Fr). Bile from the outer drain can be seen draining through the side arm of the Tuohy–Borst adapter (dashed arrow).

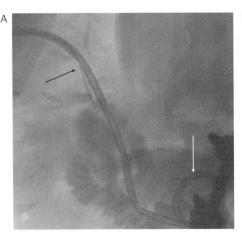
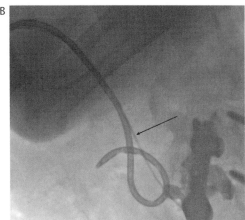

Figure 85.3 (A) A 5 Fr hockey stick catheter and Glidewire (black arrow) are seen exiting a proximal side hole of the outer 12 Fr drain, proximal to a known biliary stenosis. Note that the outer drain (white arrow) terminates in the duodenum. (B) The 5 Fr hockey stick catheter (arrow) is seen traversing the biliary stricture adjacent to the outer 12 Fr drain, yielding a total scaffolding diameter of 17 Fr. As an end-hole catheter, the hockey stick catheter provides no drainage function and terminates in the duodenum as well.

References and Suggested Readings

1. Fidelman N. Benign biliary strictures: Diagnostic evaluation and approaches to percutaneous treatment. *Tech Vasc Interv Radiol.* 2015;18(4):210–217.
2. Kocher M, Cerna M, Havlik R, et al. Percutaneous treatment of benign bile duct strictures. *Eur J Radiol.* 2007;62:170–174.
3. Cantwell CP, Pena CS, Gervais DA, et al. Thirty years' experience with balloon dilation of benign postoperative biliary strictures: Long-term outcomes. *Radiology.* 2008;249:1050–1057.
4. Janssen JJ, van Delden OM, van Lienden KP, et al. Percutaneous balloon dilatation and long-term drainage as treatment of anastomotic and non-anastomotic benign biliary strictures. *Cardiovasc Intervent Radiol.* 2014;37:1559–1567.
5. Zajko AB, Sheng R, Zetti GM, et al. Transhepatic balloon dilation of biliary strictures in liver transplant patients: A 10-year experience. *J Vasc Interv Radiol.* 1995;6:79–83.
6. Weber A, Rosca B, Neu B, et al. Long-term follow-up of percutaneous transhepatic biliary drainage (PTBD) in patients with benign bilioenterostomy stricture. *Endoscopy.* 2009;41:323–328.
7. Ramos-De la Medina A, Misra S, Leroy AJ, et al. Management of benign biliary strictures by percutaneous interventional radiologic techniques (PIRT). *HPB (Oxford).* 2008;10:428–432.
8. Ring EJ, Husted JW, Oleaga JA, et al. A multihole catheter for maintaining long-term percutaneous antegrade biliary drainage. *Radiology.* 1979;132:752–754.
9. Gwon DI, Sung KB, Ko GY, Lee SG. Dual catheter placement technique for treatment of biliary anastomotic strictures after liver transplantation. *Liver Transpl.* 2011;17(2):159–166.

CHAPTER 86

Use of a Fogarty Balloon Catheter to Create Backwall Support and Facilitate Intrahepatic Bile Duct Access During Antegrade Stone Extraction

George Carberry and Orhan Ozkan

Brief Description

Intrahepatic bile duct stones may form upstream from biliary strictures and result in ductal obstruction, cholangitis, or even cholangiocarcinoma.[1] In patients with upper gastrointestinal anatomy unfavorable for endoscopic retrograde cholangiopancreatography, percutaneous transhepatic stone removal may be indicated.[2–4] When biliary calculi are located in a segmental or branch duct adjacent to the cannulated duct, obtaining wire and catheter access into the target duct may be difficult due to the acute angles formed between the ducts. One method to access these ducts that has proven effective in our practice involves inflating a balloon catheter downstream from the origin of the target duct to deflect a wire into the target duct and to provide backwall support at the apex of the wire for advancement of the stiff balloon catheter. With target duct access, sweeps of the calculi can be performed with a balloon catheter.

Applications of the Technique

1. Intrahepatic bile duct stone extraction in patients with surgically altered upper gastrointestinal anatomy, such as following liver transplantation or gastric bypass.
2. Unfavorable angles for balloon catheter access formed between the cannulated bile duct and an adjacent, stone-containing branch or segmental duct.

Challenges of the Procedure

1. The tip of a guidewire must deflect back off the inflated downstream Fogarty occlusion balloon (Edwards Lifesciences, Irvine, CA) in order to access the target duct. This requires gentle but deliberate wire advances until the wire cannulates the targeted duct.
2. Despite repeat attempts, sometimes the wire will not deflect off the inflated Fogarty balloon into the target duct. A reverse curve catheter such as the SOS Omni (AngioDynamics, Latham, NY) or a Bankart catheter can also be used to achieve wire access in the target duct.

Potential Pitfalls/Complications

1. Intra- and extrahepatic biliary strictures may first need to be dilated with an angioplasty balloon prior to sweeping the calculi distally into the small bowel.
2. Insufflate the Fogarty balloon catheter with enough air to provide adequate duct occlusion but not so much as to cause overdistention and possible damage to the bile duct. If the Fogarty balloon is not well visualized, it can be inflated with dilute iodinated contrast.
3. If the patient initially presents with cholangitis due to obstruction, placing a drainage catheter and bringing the patient back for intrahepatic stone extraction is recommended to avoid biliary sepsis from wire manipulation.

Steps of the Procedure

1. Obtain peripheral intrahepatic bile duct access in standard fashion and place at least a 10 Fr vascular introducer sheath. Perform percutaneous transhepatic cholangiography to identify the location and size of intrahepatic stones.
2. Ensure adequate wire purchase by advancing a 0.038-in. wire such as an Amplatz or Glidewire (Terumo, Somerset, NJ) through the papilla of Vater or bilioenteric anastomosis into the duodenum or jejunum, depending on upper gastrointestinal anatomy.
3. Advance a Fogarty occlusion balloon catheter over the wire and position it just downstream of the target hepatic duct origin. A 5 Fr model inflates to a maximum balloon diameter of 11 mm and usually suffices in the intrahepatic biliary tree. Insufflate the balloon to a diameter at which biliary occlusion is present but without overdistention of the hepatic duct.
4. Insert a second Guidewire through the sheath. Using gentle but deliberate motions, deflect the tip of the wire off the inflated balloon catheter and through the origin of the target duct. Once access

into the duct is achieved, advance additional wire to ensure adequate wire purchase.

5. Advance a second Fogarty balloon catheter over the Glidewire in the target duct. The wire and stiff balloon catheter will be supported by the inflated downstream Fogarty balloon, preventing wire dislodgement from the target duct.

6. Deflate the downstream Fogarty balloon catheter and remove it over the biliary-enteric wire. Insufflate the target duct Fogarty balloon.

7. Perform balloon sweeps to "pull" the calculi into the main duct, prior to pushing the calculi out through the distal common duct.

Example
See Figures 86.1 and 86.2.

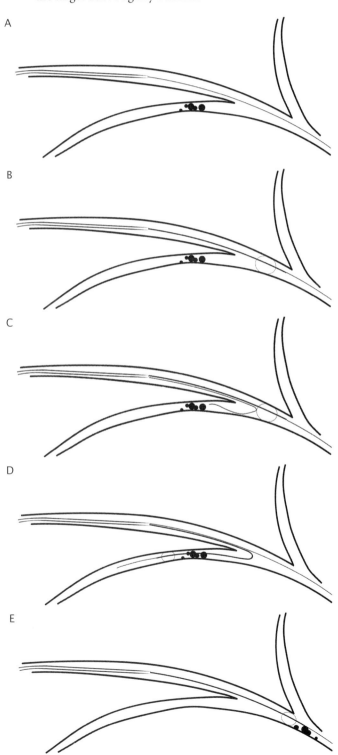

A

B

C

D

E

Figure 86.1 (A) Diagram of a right hepatic duct branch containing the introducer sheath and guidewire. An adjacent duct that contains biliary stones forms an acute angle with the cannulated duct, making direct wire cannulation and stiff catheter advancement over the wire difficult. (B) Inflation of the over-the-wire Fogarty balloon catheter just distal to the origin of the target duct. (C) Deflection of the tip of a guidewire off the inflated balloon often results in cannulation of the target duct without the need for a reverse curve catheter. The downstream Fogarty balloon also provides support at the apex of the wire for advancement of a stiff balloon catheter into the target duct. (D) Once inflated in the target duct, the second Fogarty balloon catheter can be used to sweep the calculi out of the duct. (E) The Fogarty balloon has swept the remaining stones out of the adjacent hepatic duct and is preparing to push the stone debris through the distal common duct.

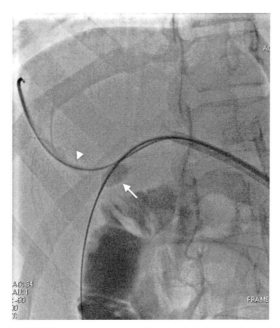

Figure 86.2 Fluoroscopic image showing inflation of the Fogarty balloon that contains dilute iodinated contrast (arrow) just distal to a branch point of the intrahepatic biliary tree. From this position, the balloon provides backwall support for advancement of a second Fogarty balloon catheter over the Glidewire located in the adjacent target duct (arrowhead).

References and Suggested Readings

1. Sakpal SV, Babel N, Chamberlain RS. Surgical management of hepatolithiasis. *HPB (Oxford)*. 2009;11(3):194–202.
2. Stokes KR, Clouse ME. Biliary duct stones: Percutaneous transhepatic removal. *Carciovasc Intervent Radiol*. 1990;13(4):240–244.
3. Garcia-Garcia L, Lanciego C. Percutaneous treatment of biliary stones: Spincteroplasty and occlusion balloon for the clearance of bile duct calculi. *AJR Am J Roentgenol*. 2004;182(3):663–670.
4. Ozcan N, Kahriman G, Mavili E. Percutaneous transhepatic removal of bile duct stones: Results of 261 patients. *Cardiovasc Intervent Radiol*. 2012;35:621–627.

CHAPTER 87

Portal Vein Tract Embolization After Percutaneous Transhepatic Biliary Interventions

Kazim Narsinh, Steven C. Rose, and Thomas Kinney

Brief Description

Bleeding that occurs immediately after percutaneous biliary intervention is usually attributable to a blood vessel that was crossed during drain placement. If a side hole of the catheter is within the tract, advancing the catheter can sometimes effectively tamponade the bleeding vessel, especially if it originates from a hepatic vein branch. However, if tract tamponade is unsuccessful, bleeding may be originating from a hepatic artery or portal vein branch. If bleeding originating from a hepatic artery branch is suspected, hepatic arteriography should be performed with and without the drainage catheter in place over a wire, and subselective embolization can be performed if a suitable target is identified. If a bleeding hepatic artery branch is not identified, bleeding from a portal vein branch, such as in a portal vein-to-biliary tract communication, is suspected. Treatment of portal vein injuries is challenging in this situation because obtaining direct percutaneous portal vein access is ill-advised. This chapter describes a technique to identify the portal vein-to-biliary tract communication via cholangiography and subsequently embolize the transhepatic tract in order to control bleeding originating from the portal vein branch.

Applications of the Technique

1. Bleeding patients who have undergone recent percutaneous transhepatic biliary intervention and are suspected to have a portal vein-to-biliary communication on abdominal computed tomography scan.
2. Bleeding patients who have undergone recent percutaneous transhepatic biliary intervention and have subsequently undergone hepatic arteriography (with the biliary drainage catheter withdrawn over a wire) without identification of a bleeding source.
3. Hemodynamically unstable patients who have recently undergone percutaneous transhepatic biliary intervention.

Challenges of the Procedure

1. Identification of the portal vein-to-biliary tract fistula can be difficult on cholangiography, requiring forceful injection of large volumes of contrast material.
2. A vascular access sheath is used as the conduit to deliver embolic coils or Gelfoam (Pfizer, New York, NY) and must be appropriately sized for the embolic material being used. If the peel-away sheath is too large relative to the coils being used, the coils can partially form within the sheath, making coil advancement difficult. The coils can be deployed through a 5 Fr end-hole catheter to avoid this, if needed.

Potential Pitfalls/Complications

1. Portal vein embolization: If embolic material, such as coils or Gelfoam, is pushed too far into a transhepatic tract containing a portal vein-to-biliary tract fistula, inadvertent embolization of the parent portal vein may occur.
2. Incomplete embolization of the transhepatic tract: In patients with portal hypertension, embolic material can be pushed out of the tract before it is thrombosed in place, causing incomplete tract embolization.
3. Risks of second percutaneous transhepatic biliary intervention: If biliary obstruction is persistent, a second biliary drainage procedure along a new tract will need to be performed after embolization of the first tract. Standard risks apply to the second attempt at percutaneous transhepatic biliary intervention, including risks of bleeding, infection, or bile leak.

Steps of the Procedure

1. Cholangiogram: The existing percutaneous transhepatic biliary drainage (PTBD) catheter

can be injected with 20 ml of a dilution of 70% Omnipaque 300 (GE Healthcare, Chicago, IL) and 30% saline to identify the portal vein-to-biliary tree communication. Opacification of the entire biliary tree is preferred, with particular attention to the transhepatic catheter tract. If tract embolization will be pursued and an indication for biliary drainage persists, a new percutaneous transhepatic biliary access tract can be sought and placed using fluoroscopic or ultrasonographic guidance, using the existing cholangiogram.

2. Sheath placement: Once the portal vein-to-biliary tree communication is identified, the drain is withdrawn over the guidewire, and a peel-away sheath or vascular access sheath with side arm is placed such that the tip of the sheath is just beyond the site of the portal vein-to-biliary tree communication.

3. Preparation of embolic material and pusher: A variety of embolization materials have been used to occlude transhepatic tracts, including Gelfoam, coils, and *n*-butyl cyanoacrylate (*n*-BCA) glue.

   a. Use of Gelfoam with or without coils: The sheath is left in place, and absorbable gelatin sponge (Gelfoam) is prepared in rolls of 3-mm diameter × 4-cm length, commonly referred to as Gelfoam torpedoes or pledgets. A pusher is prepared by cutting the tip off of the inner dilator that is supplied with the sheath. The Gelfoam pledgets are then introduced through the sheath and pushed out of the sheath as it is withdrawn along the length of the tract. Introduction of Gelfoam pledgets can be alternated with placement of 0.035-in. coils, usually between 6 and 8 mm in diameter, depending on the size of the sheath and tract. If there is concern that the coils may partially form within the sheath and thereby make advancement difficult, a 5 Fr end-hole catheter can be used to introduce the coils.

   b. Use of *n*-BCA glue: *n*-BCA (TruFill, Cordis, Miami Lakes, FL) is a liquid embolic agent that solidifies by polymerization upon contact with ionic solutions such as blood. Polymerization of *n*-BCA/lipiodol mixtures can occur in 0.2–5.0 seconds depending on the percentage of *n*-BCA in the mixture. We advise using a 1:1 mixture of *n*-BCA and lipiodol to produce a 50% *n*-BCA mixture totaling 2–4 ml. The sheath is filled with 5% dextrose solution, with a straight-tip access wire in place to maintain access. Then, 2 ml of the *n*-BCA/lipiodol solution is injected into the sheath very slowly until it reaches the tip of the sheath. The glue mixture is chased with 5% dextrose solution, and the glue is slowly deposited along the tract while the sheath is withdrawn. After the glue mixture is deposited, the access guidewire is removed with slow, steady pressure, being careful not to fracture or fragment the glue plug.

4. Sheath withdrawal: The sheath is then withdrawn from the patient, being careful to not disturb the embolic material just placed.

Example
See Figures 87.1–87.9.

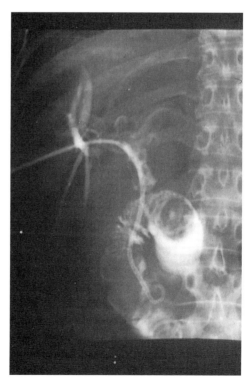

Figure 87.1 Early phase image from initial cholangiogram demonstrating communication between a right hepatic duct branch and a right portal vein branch.

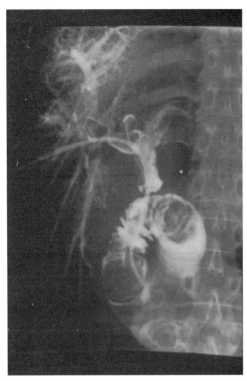

Figure 87.2 Later phase image of cholangiogram demonstrating opacification of peripheral portal vein branches via biliary tract-to-portal vein communication.

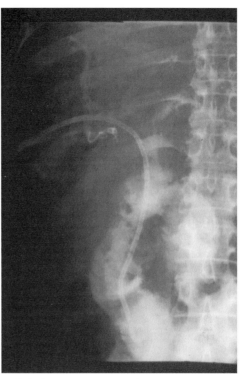

Figure 87.3 Embolization coils and Gelfoam pledgets were placed along the tract, and a second PTBD catheter was placed.

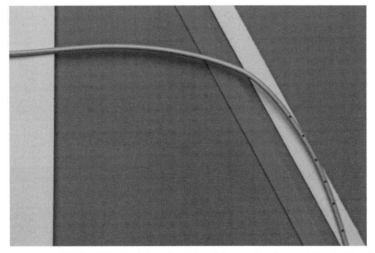

Figure 87.4 Representative depiction of PTBD within the biliary tract (white), crossing the portal vein (Gray).

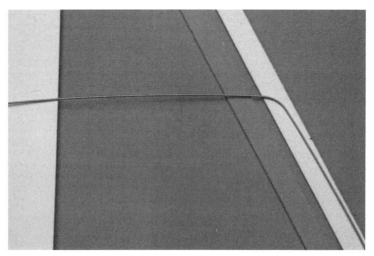

Figure 87.5 Withdraw the PTBD over a guidewire.

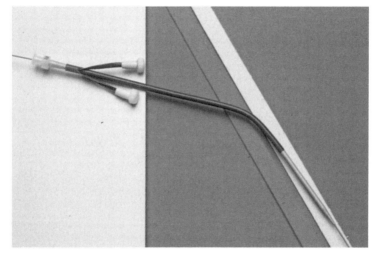

Figure 87.6 Place a peel-away sheath with tip just beyond the portal vein-to-biliary tract communication.

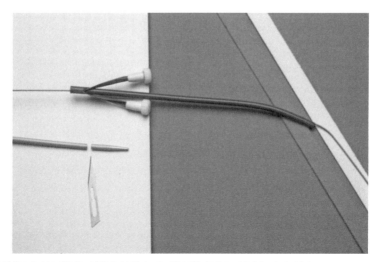

Figure 87.7 Cut the tip off of the inner dilator of the peel-away sheath to be used as a pusher.

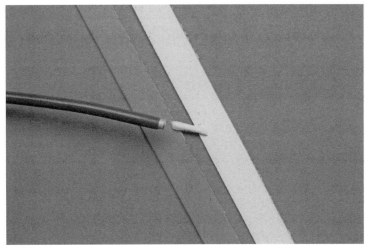

Figure 87.8 Advance gelatin sponge pledgets out of the sheath using the pusher.

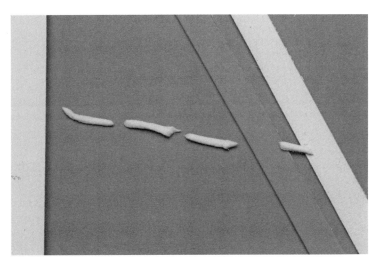

Figure 87.9 Deposit multiple gelatin sponge pledgets along the transhepatic tract as the sheath is withdrawn.

CHAPTER 88

Use of an Elongated Radiopaque Gelatin Sponge Plug for Tract Occlusion After Hepatic Interventions

Sam McCabe, Christopher Harnain, and Grigory Rozenblit

Brief Description

This chapter describes a technique for plugging the hepatic parenchymal tract after percutaneous biliary, portal venous, or hepatic venous access or intervention. Often, embolization coils or a gelatin sponge "slurry" is sufficient for hemostasis following liver intervention.[1] The described technique involves placement of a contrast-soaked gelatin sponge "plug," which offers several advantages: It is inexpensive, commonly available, substantial, radiopaque, and temporary.

After completion of the procedure, a standard 10 Fr vascular sheath should be placed at the access, unless it is already in position. The sheath is then retracted while injecting contrast until the sheath tip is just peripheral to the point of entry into the vessel or duct. A gelatin sponge soaked in angiographic contrast medium is loaded into a delivery cylinder (described later). The delivery cylinder is then advanced into the access sheath, and the plug is positioned using fluoroscopy. The makeshift "pusher" (described later) is then advanced up to the trailing end of the plug, and the delivery cylinder is removed. The plug is deployed by withdrawing the sheath under fluoroscopic guidance while holding the pusher in place, ensuring accurate plug placement.

Applications of the Technique

1. Percutaneous hepatobiliary interventions with concern for bile leak along the access tract.
2. Portal or hepatic vein access or intervention.

Challenges of the Procedure

1. The procedure requires back-table preparation and additional procedural time. Additional radiation exposure should be negligible.
2. Successfully loading the gelatin sponge into the delivery cylinder requires minimal experience.

Potential Pitfalls/Complications

1. Inadvertent deployment of the plug within a vein/duct or outside of the liver. Care must be taken to correctly position the access sheath and constrained plug prior to deployment.

Steps of the Procedure

1. Positioning the sheath: After completion of the procedure, a 10 Fr vascular sheath is positioned in the liver access. Angiographic contrast medium is gently injected through the side arm as the sheath is retracted until its tip lies within the liver parenchyma approximately 2 cm peripheral to the point of entry into the vessel or duct.
2. Preparing and loading the plug: A Gelfoam sponge (Pfizer, New York, NY; 2 cm × 6 cm × 7 mm) is soaked with angiographic contrast medium. The sponge is then loaded into a delivery cylinder (i.e., the sterile safety packaging cylinder from a 7-cm 19 gauge vascular access needle; Cook Medical, Bloomington, IN, or similar). Loading the sponge is facilitated by suction applied to the delivery cylinder with a standard syringe. The syringe Luer connector fits on the end of the delivery cylinder, creating an airtight seal.
3. Positioning the plug: The delivery cylinder loaded with the plug is inserted into the sheath and advanced into position using fluoroscopy. The delivery cylinder may not fit into a sheath smaller than 10 Fr. The makeshift "pusher" is created by cutting off the tip of the 10 Fr sheath inner dilator. This blunt-tipped pusher is then inserted into the delivery cylinder, expelling the plug into the access sheath. The pusher and delivery cylinder are then removed.
4. Deploying the plug: Under fluoroscopic guidance, the pusher is reintroduced into the sheath and advanced to abut the trailing end of the plug. While

holding the pusher in place, the sheath is retracted under fluoroscopy to accurately release the plug. The sheath and pusher are then removed.

Example
See Figures 88.1–88.4.

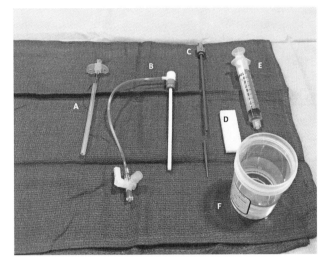

Figure 88.1 Equipment used. (A) Packaging cylinder from a 7-cm 19 gauge thin-wall percutaneous entry needle (Cook; or similar). The needle itself is not used. (B) A 10 Fr sheath (Boston Scientific; Marlborough, MA; or similar). (C) Inner dilator from 10 Fr sheath. The dilator has been cut so it can be used as a blunt pusher (see Figure 88.3). (D) Gelfoam absorbable gelatin sponge 2 cm × 6 cm × 7 mm (Pfizer). (E) A 10-ml Luer lock syringe. (F) Angiographic contrast material.

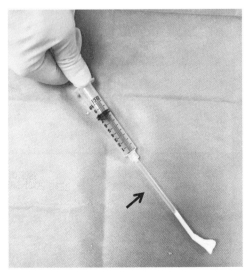

Figure 88.2 Loading the gelatin sponge into the delivery cylinder. A standard 10-ml Luer lock syringe fits onto the delivery cylinder (arrow) to create an airtight seal. The syringe can then be used to aspirate the sponge into the delivery cylinder. Presoaking the sponge in angiographic contrast material (not shown) facilitates this step and also allows fluoroscopic visualization of the plug (see Figure 88.4).

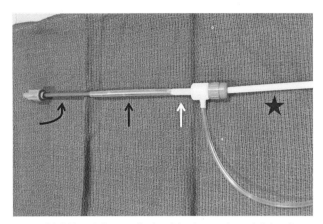

Figure 88.3 The delivery cylinder (black arrow) containing the gelatin sponge soaked in angiographic contrast (white arrow) is loaded into the 10 Fr sheath (black star). The blunt-tipped "pusher" (curved arrow) is used to advance the plug into the sheath.

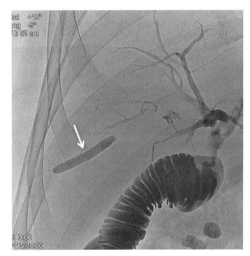

Figure 88.4 Completion image. The deployed plug lies within the liver parenchyma along the access tract, peripheral to the point of duct entry (arrow).

Reference and Suggested Reading
1. Saad WEA, Madoff DC. Percutaneous portal vein access and transhepatic tract hemostasis. *Semin Intervent Radiol.* 2012;29(2):71–80.

Gastroenterology and Genitourinary Interventions

CHAPTER 89

The Air Technique to Determine Appropriate Posterior Calyx for Puncture

Kazim Narsinh and Thomas Kinney

Brief Description

During percutaneous nephrostomy procedures, the preferred access tract typically proceeds along Brödel's avascular plane between the anterior and posterior divisions of the renal artery into a posterior calyx. This route of traversal minimizes risk of injury to arteries that could result in development of a perinephric hematoma, a renal pseudoaneurysm, or a renal arteriovenous fistula. Entry through the infundibulum into an anterior calyx may increase the risk of urinary leak complicating nephrostomy placement. The angles of entry into the anterior calyx may make drainage catheter or ureteral interventions difficult to perform as well. Image-guided access of a posterior calyx is typically facilitated by real-time ultrasound guidance, but in some patients, acoustic penetration is limited due to body habitus. In obese patients, in whom the length of the tract from the skin to the renal collecting system may exceed 15 cm, computed tomography (CT) guidance may be useful, but it is often not easily available. In this setting, air or carbon dioxide can be introduced into the prone patient's collecting system in order to fluoroscopically guide a confident puncture of the posterior calyx of the renal collecting system.

Applications of the Technique

1. Obese patients in whom the tract extends >15 cm from skin to renal collecting system.
2. Access of nondilated collecting systems when ultrasound guidance is not feasible.

Challenges of the Procedure

1. Initial puncture of the renal collecting system must be achieved relatively swiftly under fluoroscopic guidance after the administration of intravenous contrast, before the renal pelvis empties of contrast material.
2. Carbon dioxide can be used as a contrast agent, but room air is easier to handle. Care is required to ensure that air does not enter the venous system.
3. A hydrophilic wire can be advanced within the perirenal fat alongside the calyces toward the renal

sinus, giving the appearance of wire placement within the urinary tract.

Potential Pitfalls/Complications

1. Gas embolism: Needle position within the collecting system must be confirmed by aspiration of urine prior to the injection of air to ensure the absence of arterial or venous gas embolism. The preliminary injection of contrast should be scrutinized to ensure no veins opacify before injecting gas.
2. Urinary leak: Two punctures of the urinary collecting system are performed: The first is performed to inject gas into the urinary collecting system, and the second puncture targets a posterior calyx for definitive nephrostomy insertion. Puncturing the urinary collecting system twice theoretically increases the risk of urinary leak.
3. Vascular injury at the renal hilum: The initial puncture of the renal pelvis occurs in close proximity to large arterial and venous branches at the renal hilum, and it is devoid of renal parenchyma and capsule that can effectively tamponade significant bleeding. Use of a 22 gauge needle and strict anteroposterior orientation during the initial puncture mitigates this risk.
4. Confirming access to the urinary collecting system: Advancement of a guidewire into the ureter and bladder is the best indicator of successful access of a posterior calyx because advancement of a guidewire in the perirenal fat alongside the calyces can mimic access to the urinary collecting system.

Steps of the Procedure

1. Opacification of the urinary collecting system: The patient is placed prone on the interventional table, and 50 ml of iodixanol 320 (Visipaque, GE Healthcare, Chicago, IL) is administered intravenously. After 5 minutes, the renal pelvis is seen and centered within the field of view in anteroposterior orientation. If the patient cannot receive intravenous contrast, ultrasound guidance can be used to

access any visible calyx, any infundibulum, or the renal pelvis.

2. Initial access to the urinary collecting system: The skin overlying the center of the renal pelvis is anesthetized, and with intermittent fluoroscopic guidance, a 22 gauge Chiba needle (Cook Medical, Bloomington, IN) is advanced vertically toward the renal pelvis. When the needle tip is in contact with the kidney, the needle will begin to move with respiration. The texture of the kidney during advancement of the needle differs from that of the softer retroperitoneum. Fluoroscopy will often demonstrate respiratory variation in needle position that follows the renal shadow, thereby confirming needle tip position within the kidney. Then, for left kidney access, the C-arm is rotated to a 20-degree right posterior-oblique angulation (or a 20-degree left posterior-oblique angulation for access to the right kidney). The needle tip is then advanced into the renal pelvis under continuous fluoroscopic guidance. This maneuver must be accomplished swiftly before the renal pelvis empties of contrast material. Aspiration of urine confirms needle tip position.

3. Distention of nondependent posterior-facing calyces: Once needle position has been confirmed, an additional 5–10 ml of iodinated contrast can be injected until all calyces are filled, again checking for any vascular opacification. If no vascular structures are seen, then 5–10 ml of air or carbon dioxide is injected slowly under continuous fluoroscopy. Slow injection is advised because of the expected expansion of gas when warmed to body temperature. Gentle injection also minimizes the risk of intravascular injection, and absence of gas embolism in the renal veins and inferior vena cava should be confirmed fluoroscopically. Gas behaves as a negative contrast material and preferentially distends and fills the nondependent infundibula and calyces.

4. Definitive nephrostomy insertion: The double-contrast pyelogram is used to select a gas-filled nondependent calyx for the nephrostomy insertion site. The skin overlying the center of the chosen calyx is anesthetized, and an access set (Aprima Nonvascular Introducer, Cook Medical) is directed into the selected calyx under intermittent fluoroscopic guidance. Gas in the nondependent calyx drains slowly because of its buoyancy, so the chosen calyx can be accessed without haste. After access, the needle is removed, and a 0.035-in. curved-tip hydrophilic guidewire (Terumo, Somerset, NJ) is inserted through the sheath into the calyx. One should advance the wire into the renal pelvis and

ureter to confirm positioning because advancement of the wire within the renal sinus fat alongside the calyces can mimic appropriate wire position. Watching for gas return from the access needle is not a reliable sign of appropriate needle position within the collecting system. The hydrophilic guidewire is then exchanged for a 0.035-in. stiff guidewire (Superstiff Amplatz, Boston Scientific, Marlborough, MA). The tract is then dilated, and a nephrostomy catheter of choice is placed.

Example

See Figures 89.1–89.4.

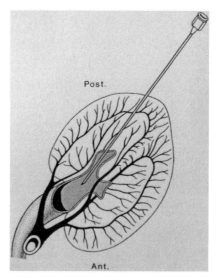

Figure 89.1 Schematic drawing of the left kidney in axial plane demonstrating desired needle tract traversing Brödel's avascular plane.

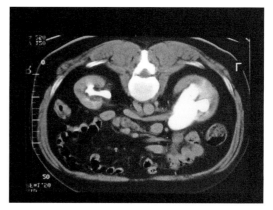

Figure 89.2 Axial CT scan of the left kidney during the excretory phase demonstrating anterior and posterior calyces.

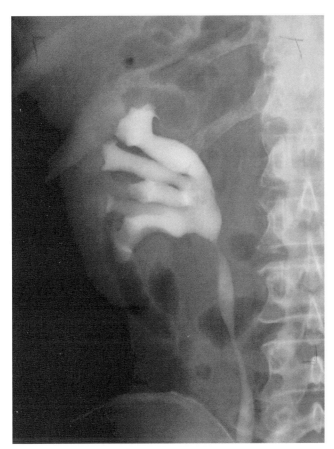

Figure 89.3 Anteroposterior spot fluoroscopic image of the left kidney obtained during the excretory phase demonstrating difficulty discerning anterior and posterior calyces.

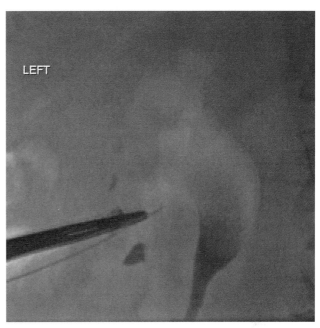

Figure 89.4 Anteroposterior spot fluoroscopic image of the left kidney obtained after instillation of air that preferentially distends and fills the anterior calyces.

CHAPTER 90

Permanent Ureteral Occlusion

Almamoon I. Justaniah

Brief Description

Distal ureteral injuries are uncommon. When present, urine leakage may ensue. Common etiologies are gynecologic surgeries (75%),[1] trauma, pelvic malignancy, and radiation therapy. Clinical presentation varies according to the location of leakage or fistula. For example, patients with ureterovaginal fistula may present with vaginal discharge. Patients with intra-abdominal leakage may develop urinoma or abscess. Diagnosis can be made with cystogram, antegrade or retrograde ureterogram, renal scintigraphy, or delayed-phase contrast-enhanced computed tomography (CT).

Unfortunately, most of these patients are poor surgical candidates due to prior surgery and/or radiation. Therefore, operative repair can be challenging and at times not a valid option. Transrenal ureteral occlusion may provide the best available option for such patients. A trial of urine diversion via percutaneous nephrostomy (PCN) catheter may allow spontaneous healing. If this fails, ureteral occlusion proximal to the leak/fistula can be attempted with a success rate up to 100%.[1] Occlusion techniques include ureteral clipping, radiofrequency cauterization, embolization coils, Amplatzer vascular plugs (St. Jude Medical, St. Paul, MN), detachable balloons, absolute alcohol, Onyx (Medtronic, Minneapolis, MN), and isobutyl-2-cyanoacrylate (glue).

Application of the Technique

1. Ureteral occlusion is indicated in nonsurgical patients with distal urinary leak refractory to conservative management and temporary urinary diversion.
2. It can be used in patients with limited life expectancy to improve their quality of life.
3. It can be used temporarily in patients who are planned for surgical repair/diversion.

Challenges of the Procedure

1. Finding a combination of mechanical and liquid embolics that will permanently occlude the ureter.
2. Keeping the PCN catheter in place and unkinked so that pressure does not build up in the collecting system and cause recanalization.

Potential Pitfalls/Complications

1. Using Amplatzer plugs or coils alone without Gelfoam (Pfizer, New York, NY) or liquid embolics may affect the longevity of the occlusion because urine has no clotting factors.
2. Oversizing the Amplatzer plugs and coils in relation to the ureteral diameter is necessary. Undersizing may lead to migration.
3. Embolizing the ureter just proximal to the site of fistula/leak is optimal. Mid-ureteral embolization may limit further addition of more proximal embolic material when recanalization occurs.
4. Nephrostomy tube kinking or dislodgement may cause increased renal pelvis pressure and make the embolized ureter more prone to recanalization.
5. Complications associated with the PCN catheter include bleeding, infection, catheter leakage, kinking, or displacement.
6. Coil migration to the bladder or to the renal pelvis has been reported.

Steps of the Procedure

1. Place a PCN catheter using standard technique. *Tip*: The catheter is used as a diversion trial to allow for spontaneous healing of the leak/fistula. If this fails and the patient is not a surgical candidate, ureteral embolization should be considered.
2. Remove the PCN catheter over a guidewire and place a sheath into the renal pelvis.
3. Advance a soft-tipped guidewire and a 5 Fr catheter through the sheath into the distal ureter just proximal to the site of the leak. *Tip*: Mid- or proximal ureteral occlusion increases the risk of migration and limits further embolization if recanalization occurs.
4. Remove the guidewire and use as many 0.038-in. embolization coils as needed to form a tight nest of coils in the distal ureter. *Tip*: The coils need to be oversized relative to the ureteral diameter to provide adequate occlusion, fixation, and prevent migration.
5. Place gelatin sponge pledgets (Gelfoam) (3 mm × 1 cm) in a 3-cc syringe with saline.
6. Inject the Gelfoam into and on top of the coil nest. *Tip*: Gelfoam and liquid embolics improve the longevity of ureteral occlusion and prevent future recanalization.

7. Add another nest of tightly packed coils on top of the Gelfoam and the previous coil nest.

8. Perform multiple ureterograms and add coils as needed until complete occlusion is accomplished.

9. Make sure to sandwich smaller coils and the Gelfoam between larger nests of coils on either side.

10. Alternatively, use coils containing Dacron fibers and inject a few drops of absolute alcohol with each coil to induce urothelial sloughing and scarring.

11. Another alternative method: use an 8- to 12-mm type I or type II Amplatzer vascular plug, followed by 0.8–1.5 cc of *n*-butyl cynoacrylate (TruFill, Cordis, Miami Lakes, FL), followed by a second Amplatzer vascular plug.[2]

12. Insert a PCN catheter and leave it to gravity drainage.

13. Obtain a 48- to 72-hour nephrostogram to ensure complete occlusion.

14. Exchange the PCN catheter every 8 weeks.

Example

See Figures 90.1 and 90.2.

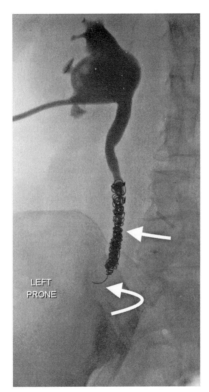

Figure 90.1 A 69-year-old female with a history of cervical carcinoma presented with dark (feculent) urine. The cervical carcinoma had been treated with total hysterectomy, bilateral salpingo-oophorectomy, and radiation therapy 32 years earlier. The feculent urine was secondary to enterovesical fistula as a sequela of radiation-induced cystitis. The fistula was treated surgically with urinary diversion, ileal loop neobladder formation, and fistula repair. The patient developed an intraperitoneal urine leakage at the left ureteral anastomosis that was not able to be repaired surgically. Urine diversion using a PCN catheter was unsuccessful at stopping the leak. The left ureter was successfully embolized using 12 tightly packed coils (3 Tornado 6 cm × 3 mm, 5 Nester 14 cm × 4 mm, 3 Nester 14 cm × 6 mm, and 1 Nester 14 cm × 8 mm [Cook Medical, Bloomington, IN]) (arrow). A few drops of absolute alcohol were injected with each coil to help induce urothelial sloughing and scarring. Left nephrostogram post coils and absolute alcohol embolization demonstrates successful occlusion of the distal ureter with no contrast passing through the embolization point (curved arrow). The ureter has remained occluded for the past 2 years.

Source: Courtesy Christopher Molgaard, MD.

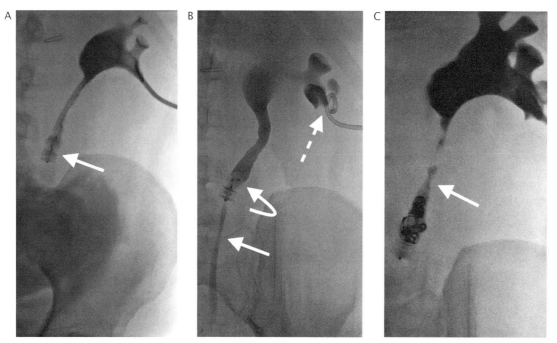

Figure 90.2 A 53-year-old male with a history of fulminant Crohn's colitis presented with dark (feculent) urine. The feculent urine was secondary to a rectovesical fistula as a sequela of rectal adenocarcinoma and Crohn's proctitis. The rectal carcinoma had been treated with abdominoperineal resection of the rectum with pelvic exenteration, neobladder formation, and radiation therapy. The patient developed leakage from both ureteroneocystostomy anastomoses that was complicated by pelvic abscesses requiring multiple drainages. The left ureter was successfully ligated intraoperatively to eliminate further leakage. The right ureter was difficult to access intraoperatively due to hostile abdomen; it continued to leak and fill the pelvic abscess. Urine diversion using a PCN catheter was unsuccessful at stopping the leak. (A) The right ureter was embolized using two 10-mm Amplatzer plugs placed at the mid ureter (arrow). (B) Five weeks later, the patient presented with recurrent output from the pelvic abscess catheter and was found to have recanalization of the ureter (arrow). The superior Amplatzer plug slightly migrated superiorly and changed its orientation (curved arrow) with PCN partial dislodgement (dashed arrow). The ureter was re-embolized using 8 Tornado coils and Gelfoam pledgets. (C) Ten months later, the ureter recanalized and was re-embolized using 0.5 cc of glue (2 cc ethidoil/1 cc histacryl mixture) (arrow).

Source: Courtesy Sebastian Flacke, MD, and Shams Iqbal, MD.

References and Suggested Readings

1. Avritscher R, Madoff DC, Ramirez PT, et al. Fistulas of the lower urinary tract: Percutaneous approaches for the management of a difficult clinical entity. *Radiographics* 2004;24(Suppl 1):S217–S236.

2. Saad WE, Kalagher S, Turba UC, et al. Ureteric embolization for lower urinary tract fistulae: Use of two Amplatzer vascular plugs and *N*-butyl cyanoacrylate employing the "sandwich" technique. *Cardiovasc Intervent Radiol.* 2013;36:1068–1072.

CHAPTER 91

Exchange of Retrograde Occluded Nephroureteral Catheter Through Ileal Conduits Without Losing Access

Jayesh M. Soni

Brief Description

A retrograde nephroureteral catheter is placed in patients who have undergone cystectomy with ileal conduit formation. The catheter exits from the conduit and extends retrograde to the renal pelvis. It is important to understand the anatomy of patients with noncontinent urinary diversion for urinary bladder cancer or other conditions of dysfunctional or nonfunctioning urinary bladders. An ileal conduit connects the ureters to a loop of bowel that is then secured to the anterior abdominal wall to allow for ostomy bag drainage.[1] Up to 15% of patients develop complications in the form of stricture at the ureteroenteric junction causing obstruction. These patients may need temporary diversion of urine through a nephrostomy catheter. The retrograde nephroureteral catheter is a better option because it provides a less invasive and safer approach. Unlike the routine exchange of a nephroureteral catheter over the wire through the ileal conduit, if the catheter is occluded, wire access through the catheter to the renal pelvis is sometimes difficult or impossible.

The major causes of difficulty in advancing the wire through the catheter are encrustation with calcium deposition, catheter fracture, and catheter migration. In these cases, an alternative approach is required such as the use of parallel glidewire, a larger sheath over the catheter, or a larger sheath over the catheter. These techniques can reduce procedure time. If all these attempts fail, then the ureter can be accessed through ileal condutoscopy or percutaneous nephrostomy as a last approach.

Applications of the Technique and Steps of the Procedure/Technique

There are three different methods for exchange:

1. Exchange over the stiff end of the glidewire
2. Coaxial exchange through the sheath and parallel guidewire placement
3. Pericatheter snare technique

Exchange Over the Stiff End of Glidewire

When the catheter is severely encrusted, it is difficult to advanced 0.035-in. regular wire through the catheter to the renal pelvis. One option is to carefully negotiate the stiff end of the wire through the occluded segment and exchange the stiff end over the 5 Fr catheter with the regular floppy end of the wire. Another option is to advance an 0.018-in. wire, which is smaller in diameter, thus increasing the chance of negotiating through the narrowed encrusted catheter. Once the occlusion is crossed successfully, then the wire can be exchanged over the 5 Fr catheter to regular 0.035-in. wire. However, in some cases, the catheter is completely occluded and wire cannot negotiate through the occlusion, thus requiring another option to maintain access.

Coaxial Exchange Through the Sheath and Parallel Wire

The catheter is cut near the hub, and the sheath is advanced over the catheter. Suturing of the catheter with Prolene or Nylon suture may be required, and the suture must be negotiated through the sheath to maintain hold of the catheter through the sheath. Once the sheath is advanced over the catheter to the ileal conduit, the sheath is positioned at the uretero-conduit junction. Next, a buddy wire is advanced through the sheath on the side of the catheter, into the ureter to the renal pelvis. The sheath over the catheter will allow the position of the sheath to be maintained at the uretero-conduit anastomosis and increase the chance of successfully gain access to the ureter and renal pelvis.

Pericatheter Snare Technique

Another approach is to use a pericatheter snare. A snare is placed over the existing catheter and advanced over the scaffolding of the catheter to the ureter and renal pelvis to maintain renal access. Smooth passage of the snare along the occluded catheter allows for negotiation of the dilated ileal conduit, redundancy in catheter, or sharply angled ureteroileal anastomosis.

Example
See Figures 91.1–91.6.

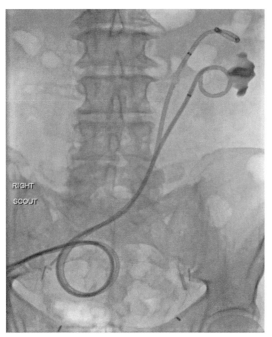

Figure 91.1 A 70-year-old male with a history of bladder carcinoma status post cystectomy with ileal conduit and left nephroureteral catheter placement for duplication collecting system. The patient presented to interventional radiology service for nephrostomogram with nephroureteral tube exchange due to nonflushing catheter. The patient had been unable to flush the catheter since he and his son attempted to "force it" by applying heavy pressure to saline flush. He subsequently heard a "popping" noise and felt transient suprapubic pain. Initial nephrostomogram through catheters shows occluded upper moiety with damage and ballooning of catheter. The lower moiety catheter is patent.

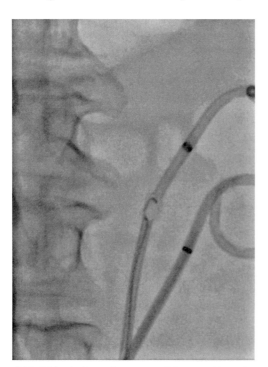

Figure 91.2 Glidewire through upper moiety cannot be advanced and loop into the damaged ballooning area of the catheter.

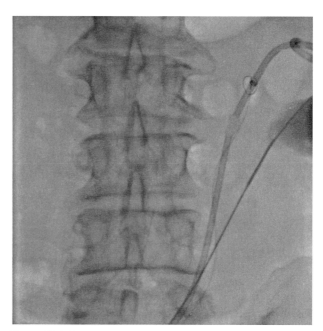

Figure 91.3 A snare was advanced and looped to the pelvicalyceal system.

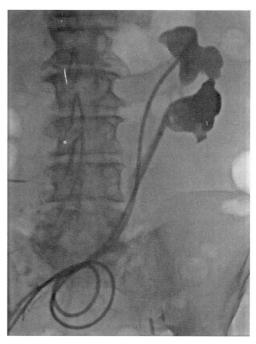

Figure 91.4 Successful placement of new nephroureterostomy catheter.

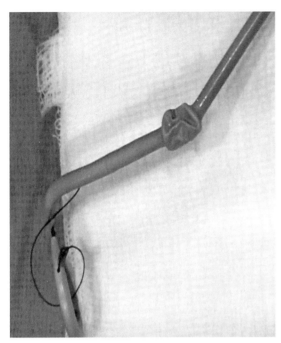

Figure 91.5 Image of catheter with ballooning due to excessive force applied during flush.

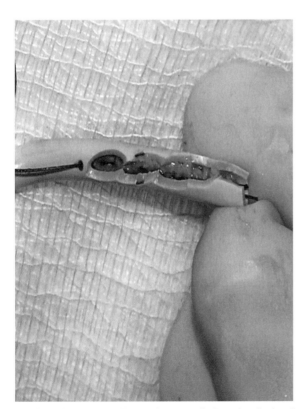

Figure 91.6 Cut open catheter shows occlusion of catheter due to extensive encrustation.

References and Suggested Readings

1. Bodner L, Nosher JL, Siegel R, Russer T, Cummings K, Kraus S. The role of interventional radiology in the management of intra- and extra-peritoneal leakage in patients who have undergone continent urinary diversion. *Cardiovasc Intervent Radiol.* 1997;20(4):274–279.
2. Drake MJ, Cowan NC. Fluoroscopy guided retrograde ureteral stent insertion in patients with a ureteroileal urinary conduit: Method and results. *J Urol.* 2002;167:2049–2051.
3. Tal R, Bachar GN, Baniel J, Belenky A. External–internal nephro-uretero-ileal stents in patients with an ileal conduit: Long-term results. *Urology.* 2004;63(3):438–441.

CHAPTER 92

Use of a Mushroom-Retained Gastrostomy Tube for Stenting Benign Esophageal Stricture

Sam McCabe, Christopher Harnain, and Grigory Rozenblit

Brief Discussion

A standard mushroom-retained gastrostomy (MRG) tube (G22636 PEG-24-PULL-S, Cook Medical, Bloomington, IN) can be used as a replaceable stent in the treatment of benign esophageal strictures (BES). Esophageal stricture is a well-known consequence of caustic ingestion and may also occur after esophagectomy.[1] Dilation with either balloon or bougie is a common treatment for BES; however, dilation alone often cannot achieve prolonged esophageal patency sufficient for oral feeding. Intraluminal stenting, although theoretically attractive, is not commonly used for treatment of BES due to the inherent serious adverse effects. Early adverse effects include chest pain, fever, bleeding, perforation, and migration. Delayed adverse effects include occlusion, esophageal fistula, migration, and stricture recurrence.[2] Bare self-expanding metal stents (SEMS) result in granulation tissue overgrowth and are difficult to remove or exchange. In addition, bleeding, fistulae, recurrent strictures, and erosion have been reported with SEMS.[3] Covered metal stents may cause pain, are prone to migration, and are cumbersome to retrieve or exchange. Self-expanding plastic stents are prone to migration, reported in up to 81.8% of patients.[4]

For effective long-term management, an esophageal stent should be easily placed, repositioned, and retrieved and also resistant to migration. An MRG tube can be effectively used as a replaceable esophageal stent. It is readily available; easy to adjust, remove, or exchange; well tolerated; and functions adequately. The strictured esophagus is first cannulated using standard angiographic techniques, and the stricture is dilated using an angioplasty balloon. After dilation, the MRG tube is cut to size to span the stricture and deployed over a guidewire with the mushroom bumper at the trailing end. The tube spans the stricture, and the mushroom bumper is seated in the hypopharynx.

Applications of the Technique

1. Stenting benign esophageal strictures to allow oral feeding.

Challenges of the Procedure

1. Cannulating the esophagus and crossing the stricture requires standard interventional skill set.
2. Cutting the MRG tube to length requires only an estimation of stricture length, with generous oversizing of the MRG tube well tolerated.

Potential Pitfalls/Complications

1. The MRG tube may be dislodged or inadvertently coughed up by the patient after placement. Replacement is technically simple.
2. Aspiration of angiographic contrast and/or refluxed gastric contents during the procedure can be prevented with use of a meticulous technique. In addition, the patient should be intubated using an endotracheal tube with an inflatable cuff.

Steps of the Procedure

1. General anesthesia: The patient is placed under general anesthesia with an endotracheal tube, which prevents aspiration of contrast media (Iodixanol 320; GE Healthcare, Pittsburgh, PA) during the procedure.
2. Cannulation of esophagus: The esophagus is cannulated and the stricture is crossed using standard interventional techniques. A stiff guidewire (Amplatz Super Stiff, Boston Scientific, Marlborough, MA) is left in place spanning the stricture.
3. Dilation of stricture: The strictured segment is dilated with a 10-mm angioplasty balloon. If the stricture is very tight, serial dilation starting with a smaller appropriately sized balloon should be considered.
4. Sizing the MRG tube: The length of the stricture is measured, and a 24 Fr MRG tube is sized and cut for generous coverage. The remnant piece of the gastrostomy tube is used as a pusher during stent placement

and is loaded onto an angioplasty balloon catheter. The MRG tube is then loaded onto the balloon catheter.

5. Introducing the MRG tube: The assembly is introduced over a stiff guidewire with the partially inflated balloon as a tapered lead point and the trailing gastrostomy tube segment as a pusher.

6. Positioning the MRG tube: The MRG tube is positioned with the trailing mushroom resting at

the esophageal origin, precluding downward stent migration.

7. Verification of patency: Once positioned, the patency of the MRG tube is verified by injection and passage of contrast material.

Example

See Figures 92.1–92.4.

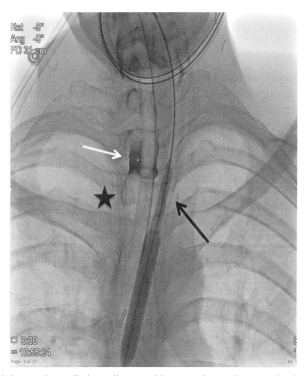

Figure 92.1 A 27-year-old patient status post caustic ingestion requiring esophagectomy and colonic interposition. An upper anastomotic stricture led to intolerance of oral intake. The strictured segment is dilated with a balloon catheter (black arrow). Note contrast material in the trachea (white arrow). Aspiration is prevented by the inflated ET tube cuff (star).

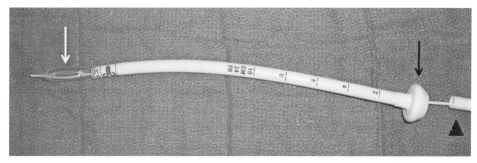

Figure 92.2 A 24-Fr MRG loaded onto a 10 mm × 2-cm angioplasty balloon catheter. The partially inflated balloon (white arrow) serves as a tapered lead point during delivery. The mushroom bumper (black arrow) prevents downward stent migration after placement. The remnant piece of the cut gastrostomy tube (triangle) is used as a pusher during stent placement.

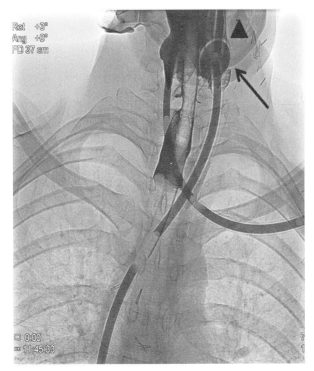

Figure 92.3 The MRG has been positioned spanning the strictured segment with the mushroom seated at the esophageal origin (arrow). The remnant piece of the cut gastrostomy tube is used as a pusher (triangle).

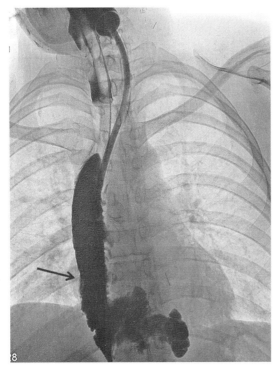

Figure 92.4 Completion esophagram through the MRG demonstrates good position with brisk contrast passage into the widely patent colonic interposition (arrow). The patient was extubated and sent home the same day.

References and Suggested Readings

1. Contini S, Scarpignato C. Caustic injury of the upper gastrointestinal tract: A comprehensive review. *World J Gastroenterol.* 2013;19(25):3918–3930.
2. Hindy P, Hong J, Lam-Tsai Y, Gress F. A comprehensive review of esophageal stents. *Gastroenterol Hepatol.* 2012;8(8):526–534.
3. Holm AN, de la Mora Levy JG, Gostout CJ, Topazian MD, Baron TH. Self-expanding plastic stents in treatment of benign esophageal conditions. *Gastrointest Endosc.* 2008;67:20–25.
4. Sharma P, Kozarek R. Role of esophageal stents in benign and malignant disease. *Am J Gastroenterol.* 2010;105:258–273.

CHAPTER 93

Balloon-Assisted, Fluoroscopically Guided Percutaneous Gastrostomy Tube Placement

Joseph Farnam, Jason Iannuccilli, and Gregory Soares

Brief Description

Fluoroscopic placement of gastrostomy tubes requires creation and dilation of a percutaneous tract through which the tube is placed. Given the relatively large caliber of these tubes, aggressive dilation of the percutaneous tract is necessary prior to their insertion. Tract dilation is most commonly performed via the use of several sequential dilators or a single telescoping serial dilator. We have found these methods to be cumbersome and relatively time-consuming, and as a result, this portion of the procedure can result in considerable patient discomfort as well as technical complications. Fascial dilatation requires substantial axial force in order to generate enough radial force for tissue dilatation. This force can kink or dislodge the guidewire from the gastric lumen, preventing subsequent passage of the gastrostomy tube over the wire or possible tube insertion outside of the stomach within the peritoneum. Excessive damage to the stomach or inadvertent injury to the duodenum can result. In addition, gastropexy T-fasteners can become dislodged during forceful serial dilation, further increasing the chance of extragastric tube placement and leakage of enteric contents into the peritoneum. We recently began using a simple technique that allows rapid dilation of the percutaneous tract using a balloon catheter and subsequent insertion of the gastrostomy tube in a single step, which reduces procedural time and minimizes patient discomfort. The use of balloon catheter dilatation eliminates axial force by applying a direct radial force that can be accomplished with one or two insufflations. In our experience, this technique is better tolerated by patients under conscious sedation and results in fewer technical complications.

Applications of the Technique

1. Any patient requiring percutaneous gastrostomy or gastrojejunostomy tube placement.

2. Patients with excessive or fibrotic soft tissues, such as obese patients and/or those with a history of prior abdominal surgeries.
3. Patients with a narrow window for gastric access, where there is greater risk for collateral damage to adjacent structures.

Challenges of the Procedure

1. Removal of the balloon catheter from the lumen of the gastrostomy tube can be difficult if the balloon is not completely deflated.
2. Advancement of the gastrostomy tube through the tract will be difficult if the balloon catheter is not sized appropriately.
3. Adequate dilation of the access tract may be impossible if skin nick is too small.

Potential Pitfalls/Complications

1. If the tract is not adequately dilated and sized appropriately and appropriate guidewire access is not maintained to the gastric lumen, the gastrostomy tube may be inadvertently placed outside of the stomach. The balloon must be inflated throughout the entire course of the gastrostomy tract.
2. If the entire tract length is not dilated, the gastrostomy tube will not pass.
3. Risk of hemorrhage: This should be no different than with the conventional technique for tract dilation using serial dilators.
4. Risk of infection: This should be no different than with the conventional technique for tract dilation using serial dilators. Administration of prophylactic antibiotics is standard in our practice during this procedure.

Steps of the Procedure

1. Pre-procedure workup: A specific indication is established, patient history is reviewed, a brief physical examination is performed, and pertinent laboratory data are reviewed.
2. Pre-procedure imaging: Cross-sectional imaging is obtained and reviewed to assess the position of the stomach with respect to the solid organs and transverse colon to determine whether a feasible window exists for safe creation of a percutaneous tract through which the tube will be placed.
3. Positioning and patient preparation: The patient is placed on the fluoroscopy table in supine position. Ultrasound is used to identify the liver margin, which is physically marked on the overlying skin surface with indelible marker. A nasogastric tube is inserted, and the stomach is insufflated with air.
4. Pexy placement: Under fluoroscopic guidance, the stomach is punctured below the liver edge and costal margin, and two to four gastropexy T-fasteners are placed.
5. Wire access: A small skin incision is made (approximately 8 mm) centrally through which the pexied gastric wall is again punctured with an 18 gauge needle to introduce a 0.035-in. guidewire into the gastric lumen.
6. Catheter selection: A noncompliant balloon catheter is selected with a maximum diameter that is approximately 2 mm larger than the gastrostomy tube (to accommodate an 18 Fr gastrostomy tube, we utilize an 8-mm balloon). Balloon length should be selected such that the entire tract is dilated on a single inflation—generally 4 cm is sufficient.
7. Gastrostomy tube loading: The gastrostomy tube is preloaded onto the shaft of the balloon catheter, which allows balloon dilation of the tissue tract over the wire and subsequent rapid insertion of the tube through the tract by forward advancement as the balloon is simultaneously deflated.
8. Balloon catheter placement: The preloaded apparatus is advanced over the guidewire into the stomach and then positioned to place the balloon portion in the soft tissue tract. The proximal margin of the balloon should be visualized just outside of the skin.
9. Tract dilation: The balloon is inflated to completely cover the entire length of the percutaneous tract, from distal to proximal. The balloon is sufficiently inflated within the tissues until any visible "waist" is eliminated.
10. Gastrostomy tube advancement: As the balloon is deflated, the gastrostomy catheter and balloon catheter are rapidly advanced in unison over the wire into the stomach lumen. The anchoring balloon on the gastrostomy tube is inflated and pulled snugly to the gastric wall. Both the guidewire and the balloon catheter are removed from the gastrostomy tube lumen, leaving the tube in place within the stomach.

Example

See Figures 93.1–93.3.

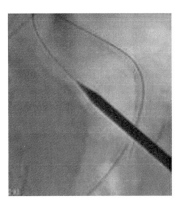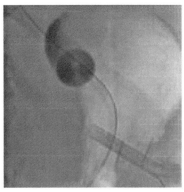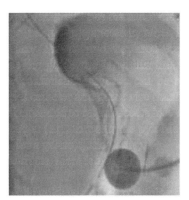

Figure 93.1 An 18 Fr gastrostomy tube placement is demonstrated by progressive dilatation using a 22 Fr telescoping serial dilator and an 18 Fr peel-away sheath (Kimberly-Clark, Irving, TX).

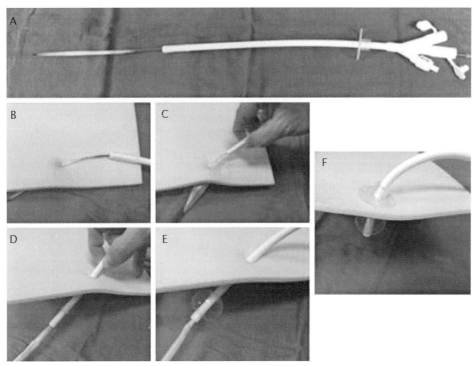

Figure 93.2 (A) Device apparatus: Balloon catheter is shown on 0.035-in. guidewire, preloaded with a gastrostomy tube. Insertion technique is demonstrated with placement of the balloon portion into the intended gastrostomy tract (B), subsequent inflation of the balloon catheter with gastrostomy tube hubbed to the margin of the inflated (C), followed by simultaneous deflation and advancement of the entire device (D). (E) The gastrostomy tube is inflated. (F) Both the balloon catheter and the guidewire are removed, and the gastrostomy tube is secured to skin.

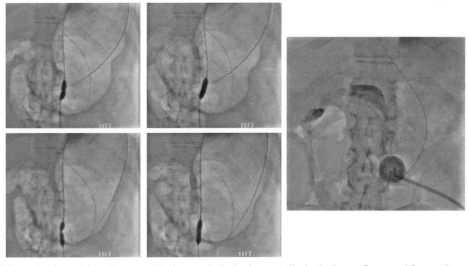

Figure 93.3 An 18 Fr gastrostomy tube placement is demonstrated using a catheter balloon (Conquest 8-mm diameter × 4-cm length [Bard, Tempe, AZ]), requiring two balloon inflations for tract dilatation.

Reference and Suggested Reading

1. Itkin M, DeLegge MH, Fang JC, et al. Multidisciplinary practical guidelines for gastrointestinal access for enteral nutrition and decompression from the Society of Interventional Radiology and American Gastroenterological Association (AGA) Institute, with endorsement by Canadian Interventional Radiological Association (CIRA) and Cardiovascular and Interventional Radiological Society of Europe (CIRSE). *J Vasc Interv Radiol.* 2011;22:1089–2011.

Drainage Procedures

CHAPTER 94

Maximizing Visualization of the Needle During Ultrasound Procedures

Ki Jinn Chin

Brief Description

Safe and successful ultrasound (US)-guided interventional procedures depend on the ability to visualize both anatomical structures of interest and the advancing needle.[1] Although the identification of relevant anatomical structures can become relatively easy with practice and development of a trained eye, accurate and consistent visualization of the needle tip can be more difficult to achieve. Various mechanical and technological innovations continue to be developed to assist with this, including needle guides[2,3] and electromagnetic needle tracking equipment,[4,5] but their advantages have yet to be definitively established in clinical practice. Freehand needle guidance remains the most commonly used technique in US-guided percutaneous needle procedures and affords the greatest degree of flexibility and accuracy in skilled hands.

Applications of the Technique

This chapter focuses on strategies to improve needle visualization and tip localization during any US-guided interventional procedure involving freehand guidance of a needle to a tissue target. The in-plane (IP) approach refers to needle insertion in the same plane as the US beam, and the needle should theoretically appear as a bright hyperechoic line on the US screen. The out-of-plane (OOP) approach refers to needle insertion perpendicular to the plane of the US beam, and the needle will be visualized in cross-section as a bright hyperechoic dot. The needle may also be advanced, inadvertently or deliberately, at an oblique angle to the plane of the US beam, in which case only part of the needle shaft will be visible. This is acceptable as long as the most distal portion of the shaft and tip are kept in view.

Challenges of the Procedure

1. Needles are poorly echogenic on US at insertion angles steeper than 30–45 degrees to the horizontal (needle–beam angles less than 45–60 degrees).[6,7] This is because the smooth metallic surface of a standard needle is a specular (mirror-like) reflector of US waves, and hence fewer echoes will return to the transducer at smaller needle–beam angles. In addition, soft tissue is a heterogeneous mix of fluid, fat, muscle, and connective tissue, each with different acoustic impedances. Reflection of sound waves occurs at each of these tissue interfaces, giving soft tissue a speckled echogenic appearance. The reduced visual contrast between needle and the background of soft tissue makes it difficult to distinguish between the two. The multiple acoustic interfaces also cause refraction (scatter) and attenuation of returning echoes,[8] further reducing needle visibility.

2. Alignment of the needle and US beam is essential for visualization. However, when one considers that the width of an US beam is as little as 1 mm at the focal zone of high-frequency transducers and that the diameters of 16 and 22 gauge needles are 1.6 and 0.7 mm, respectively, it is not surprising that achieving and maintaining alignment in the IP approach is more difficult than it sounds. In the OOP approach, the problem is slightly different. Only the cross-sectional area of the needle is imaged, and the main issue is determining whether the beam is intersecting the needle tip or the shaft, both of which can have similar ultrasonographic appearances. The shaft usually casts a denser acoustic shadow, and this helps distinguish it from the tip.

3. Manipulation of the needle and transducer occurs while looking away from one's hands at the US screen. This requires a good sense of spatial awareness. In addition, US imaging provides only two-dimensional visual information, whereas needle and transducer manipulation are occurring in three dimensions. The effective operator must therefore learn to construct a three-dimensional mental image from the series of two-dimensional images obtained during the scanning process and to correlate this with his or her hand movements.

Potential Pitfalls/Complications

1. Failure to achieve the desired outcome—for example, vessel puncture, accurate biopsy of a lesion,

and effective deposition of local anesthetic around a nerve.

2. Inadvertent mechanical trauma to the target structure or other anatomical structures in its vicinity.

Steps of the Procedure

1. Ensure good ergonomics when performing the procedure. Attention to ergonomics reduces operator fatigue, improves control of needle and transducer, and facilitates the ability to manipulate them effectively while looking away from one's hands at the ultrasound screen. The operator should not have to turn his or her head or body; hands, procedural site, and ultrasound machine should all be within the line of sight. The height of the working surface should allow the operator to be in a comfortable upright position with relaxed shoulders and elbows comfortably by his or her side. The transducer should be held low for maximal control, and both hands should always be braced on the patient to minimize unintentional transducer or needle movement.

2. Increasing needle echogenicity
   a. Optimize needle–beam angle where possible. Needle echogenicity is most easily maximized by using a shallow insertion angle in the IP approach and keeping the needle–beam angle as close to 90 degrees as possible. However, this is not always feasible, particularly for deeper targets, because it may involve an excessively long needle path. Many modern ultrasound machines have a beam steering function that allows the US beam to be angled relative to the transducer, thus increasing the needle–beam angle of incidence toward 90 degrees and helping to increase needle echogenicity.[9] Conversely, in the OOP approach, needle tip visibility is better at smaller needle–beam angles,[6] with the additional advantage that less of the shaft is likely to be mistaken for the tip. Another technique involves inserting the needle at a distance from the transducer equivalent to the depth of the target, such that the tip will eventually intersect the US beam and target at a trajectory angle of approximately 45 degrees. Note that the needle tip should nevertheless be tracked throughout its insertion and approach to the target with the appropriate transducer motions.
   b. Always orientate the needle bevel opening toward the US beam and transducer. Visualization of the tip is better when the bevel opening is oriented either to directly face the US beam (0 degrees) or to face 180 degrees away from the beam. The former is recommended in the IP approach because it produces a characteristic double-echo appearance that prevents the operator from mistaking part of the needle shaft for the tip.
   c. Consider using echogenic needles. Another option is to use commercially available echogenic needles that have etching or dimpling along their shaft to increase ultrasound reflection back to the transducer.[10] These are most useful for deep target lesions (>4 or 5 cm) or when a steep angle of insertion is required. A crude form of etching can be produced by scraping the needle with a sterile metal object (e.g., scalpel blade), with the caveat that this may also produce a jagged surface that will potentially be more traumatic to tissues.

3. Make small, controlled, and appropriate transducer movements to achieve and maintain optimal needle–beam alignment. Needle visualization is predicated on the alignment of two millimeter-wide structures: the needle and the US beam. The beam, and by extension the transducer, must therefore be manipulated in millimeter increments when trying to locate the needle and its tip. The principal motion for this is sliding because it affords the most precise control. Tilting, on the other hand, should be avoided because sweeping the beam through an arc can lead to excessively large lateral displacement, particularly as depth increases. Note, however, that tilting is a useful maneuver for improving the echogenicity of anisotropic tissue targets; the optimal degree of tilt should be determined during the pre-needling scanning phase and maintained thereafter. Rotation is generally only employed to correct inadvertent obliquity of the needle to the beam in an IP approach. In the IP approach, once the needle tip has been located and visualized, only very small sliding transducer motions are generally necessary to maintain alignment as the needle is advanced to the target. In the OOP approach, the transducer must be slid away from the needle over a much larger distance to track the needle tip as it is advanced; this is best achieved in a stepwise fashion of "locate tip–advance needle–slide transducer," repeated as necessary. Note that the needle shaft can be most readily distinguished from the needle tip in the OOP approach by the acoustic shadow it casts.

4. Use indirect cues of needle tip location. The location of the needle tip can be determined with a high degree of precision using various indirect cues even when it is not clearly visible.
   a. Generate needle and tissue motion: Tissue motion is readily visible on ultrasound, and it is often possible to appreciate the approximate location of the needle just by the tissue motion it generates as it is advanced. However, the tip can be located with more precision using certain specific movements and without causing unintentional tissue damage. Jiggling the needle in a vibratory in–out motion is a common maneuver that can be employed in

both IP and OOP approaches. Note, however, that the generated motion can be transmitted beyond the needle tip and can occasionally be misleading. Another useful movement in the IP approach is "seesawing," in which the hub of the needle is lifted and lowered while keeping the needle parallel to the plane of the beam. This will produce a corresponding lifting and lowering motion of the tissues at the needle tip and is more precise for needle tip location than jiggling. In the OOP approach, a "waggling" movement can be employed in which the hub is moved from side to side in a plane parallel to the transducer and beam. As with seesawing, this produces a corresponding magnitude of tissue motion at the needle tip, allowing it to be located and distinguished from the shaft. None of these motions, if performed gently and correctly, should cause significant tissue injury.

b. Pay attention to tactile feedback: Guidance of the needle to the intended target generally involves puncturing skin and various other layers of fascia (including vessel walls). Depending on the sharpness of the needle tip and the thickness of the fascia being pierced, a degree of tissue tenting can be expected before penetration occurs. This can lead to the needle tip appearing to be deeper than its actual depth. Attention should be given in this case to the tactile "pop" that occurs as the fascial layer is pierced, and this is often accompanied by a visual "pop" as the tissues spring back to their original position. These tactile and visual "pops" are most easily appreciated when the needle is advanced in a slow, controlled manner rather than in rapid, jabbing movements (which should be avoided at all times).

c. Hydrolocation: Needle tip location may also be determined by hydrolocation, which involves injecting a small amount of fluid (0.2–0.5 ml is sufficient) and observing the hypoechoic "pocket" that forms.[11] It is also possible to inject air or microbubbles, which are highly echogenic and have been employed as a US contrast agent in many settings. However, the disadvantage of injecting air into soft tissue is deterioration of image quality. Microbubbles can cause acoustic shadowing that can persistently obscure the target area for up to 2 minutes or more and should be avoided if further repositioning of the needle tip is anticipated.

Example

See Figures 94.1–94.9.

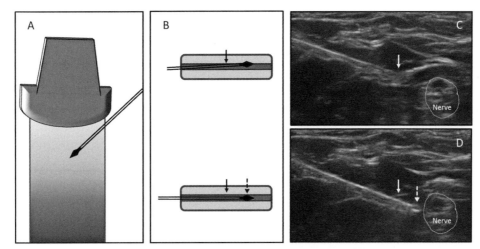

Figure 94.1 The in-plane approach involves needle insertion in the same plane as the US beam. Precise alignment of the needle–beam is essential for needle visualization. (A) Diagrammatic side view of probe–beam–needle. (B) Diagrammatic plan view of probe–beam–needle. The top diagram illustrates a slight obliquity of the needle with respect to the US beam, such that part of the shaft (arrow) is visualized instead of the tip. This results in the US image illustrated in part C, in which the arrow indicates the most distal visible portion of the needle. To avoid mistaking this for the tip, the needle bevel opening should always be oriented toward the transducer. As seen in the US image in part D, this creates a characteristic "double-echo" appearance of the tip (dashed arrow).

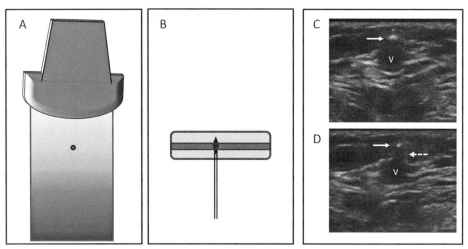

Figure 94.2 The out-of-plane approach involves needle insertion perpendicular to the plane of the US beam. The main issues here are distinguishing the cross-sectional image of the needle tip from the needle shaft (this casts a pronounced acoustic shadow) and the fact that the transducer will have to be advanced with the needle to keep the tip in the plane of the US beam. (A) Diagrammatic side view of probe–beam–needle. (B) Diagrammatic plan view of probe–beam–needle. (C) US image of hyperechoic needle tip (arrow) just adjacent to the wall of a vein (V). (D) In this US image, the hyperechoic dot (solid arrow) represents the needle shaft rather than the tip; this is indicated by the vertical acoustic shadowing (dashed arrow).

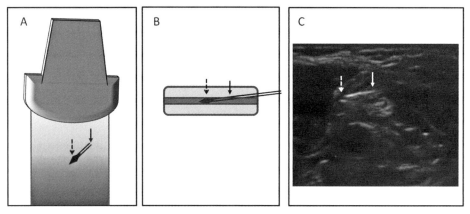

Figure 94.3 (A and B) Imperfect in-plane alignment, such that the needle is inadvertently (a common occurrence) or deliberately inserted oblique to the US beam, is acceptable as long as the distal portion of the shaft (solid arrow) and tip (dashed arrow) are aligned with the beam. (C) Keeping the needle bevel opening oriented toward the transducer produces the characteristic double-echo appearance that allows the tip to be clearly recognized.

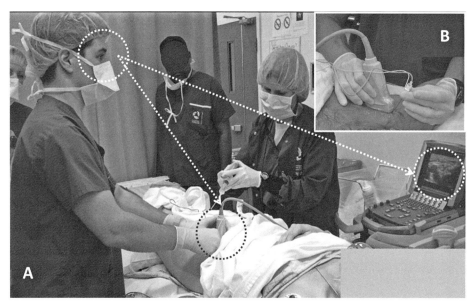

Figure 94.4 (A) The operator should be standing in an upright, relaxed posture, and the operator's hands, the patient, and the US machine should be positioned to keep everything in the operator's line of sight without having to turn one's head or body. (B) The transducer should be held low, and the medial edge and/or fingers of the operator's hand should be resting on the patient to minimize inadvertent movement.

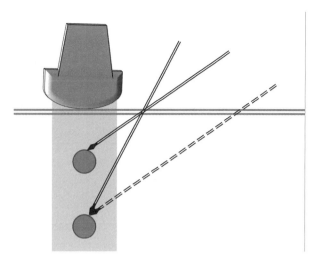

Figure 94.5 In the in-plane approach, there is a trade-off between angle of insertion and needle path length. Shallow angles of needle insertion offer superior needle visibility but are generally not practical for deep targets.

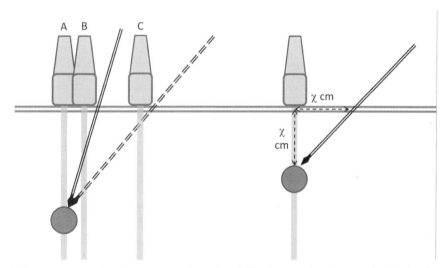

Figure 94.6 In the out-of-plane approach, a steep angle of insertion (left) minimizes the chance of mistaking the shaft for the tip. The transducer only has to track/identify the needle tip between point A and point B. At shallower angles of insertion, the transducer has to be moved to track/identify the needle tip over a much larger distance between point A and point C. An alternative approach is to use a 45-degree angle of insertion and begin insertion at a distance from the transducer equivalent to the depth of the target so that the tip will enter the US beam and become visible when it reaches the target (right). However, this may not be practical for deeper targets due to the excessively long needle path.

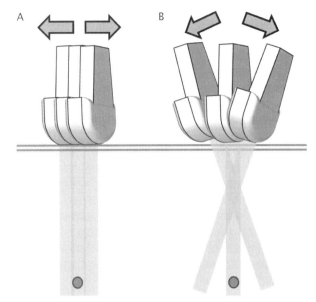

Figure 94.7 (A) Sliding motions of the transducer are used to produce needle–beam alignment because they offer the most precision and control over beam movement. (B) It is very difficult to achieve the millimeter-wide changes in beam position required for alignment by tilting the transducer. Tilting should only be used to optimize tissue target echogenicity or if sliding is not possible due to a physical obstruction.

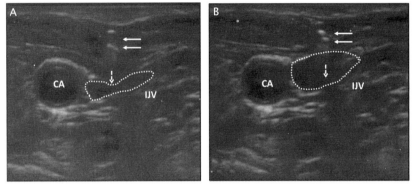

Figure 94.8 An out-of-plane needle approach to internal jugular vein (IJV) cannulation demonstrating the concept of tenting and "springback" of tissue layers as an indicator of needle tip progression and location. (A) The IJV is compressed, and the tissues are tented downward as the needle is advanced with constant forward pressure toward the vein. The shaft and its acoustic shadow are indicated by the solid arrows and the approximate location of the tip by the dashed arrow. (B) Once the vein wall is pierced, the tissue layers and vein wall spring back to their original position. This visual "pop" is accompanied by a tactile "pop." Note that these signs will be lost if the needle is advanced in short jabbing motions. CA, carotid artery.

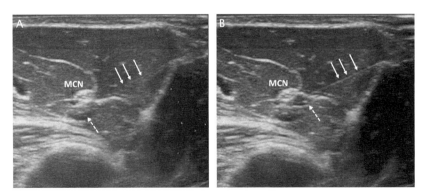

Figure 94.9 Hydrolocation is a useful way of localizing needle tip position in both the in-plane and the out-of-plane approach. (A) In this in-plane approach to the musculocutaneous nerve (MCN), the needle shaft (solid arrows) is poorly visible. Injection of approximately 0.5 ml of fluid produces a hypoechoic "pocket" (dashed arrow) at the tip of the needle, indicating that it is lying within muscle. (B) Following slight withdrawal of the needle, further injection creates a pocket of fluid within the fascial sheath enveloping the nerve (dashed arrow), indicating that the needle tip is now in the correct position to achieve local anesthetic blockade of the MCN.

References and Suggested Readings

1. Chin KJ, Perlas A, Chan VWS, Brull R. Needle visualization in ultrasound-guided regional anesthesia: Challenges and solutions. *Reg Anesth Pain Med*. 2008;33(6):532–544.
2. van Geffen GJ, Mulder J, Gielen M, van Egmond J, Scheffer GJ, Bruhn J. A needle guidance device compared to free hand technique in an ultrasound-guided interventional task using a phantom. *Anaesthesia*. 2008;63(9):986–990.
3. Bluvol N, Kornecki A, Shaikh A, Del Rey Fernandez D, Taves DH, Fenster A. Freehand versus guided breast biopsy: Comparison of accuracy, needle motion, and biopsy time in a tissue model. *AJR Am J Roentgenol*. 2009;192(6):1720–1725.
4. Li R, Li T, Qian X, Qi J, Wu D, Liu J. Real-time ultrasonography-guided percutaneous nephrolithotomy using SonixGPS navigation: Clinical experience and practice in a single center in China. *J Endourol Endourol Soc*. 2015;29(2):158–161.
5. März K, Franz AM, Seitel A, et al. Interventional real-time ultrasound imaging with an integrated electromagnetic field generator. *Int J Comput Assist Radiol Surg*. 2014;9(5):759–768.
6. Maecken T, Zenz M, Grau T. Ultrasound characteristics of needles for regional anesthesia. *Reg Anesth Pain Med*. 2007;32(5):440–447.
7. Nichols K, Wright LB, Spencer T, Culp WC. Changes in ultrasonographic echogenicity and visibility of needles with changes in angles of insonation. *J Vasc Interv Radiol*. 2003;14(12):1553–1557.
8. Sites BD, Brull R, Chan VWS, et al. Artifacts and pitfall errors associated with ultrasound-guided regional anesthesia: Part I. Understanding the basic principles of ultrasound physics and machine operations. *Reg Anesth Pain Med*. 2007;32(5):412–418.
9. Uppal V, Sondekoppam RV, Ganapathy S. Effect of beam steering on the visibility of echogenic and non-echogenic needles: A laboratory study. *Can J Anaesth J Can Anesth*. 2014;61(10):909–915.
10. Hocking G, Mitchell CH. Optimizing the safety and practice of ultrasound-guided regional anesthesia: The role of echogenic technology. *Curr Opin Anaesthesiol*. 2012;25(5):603–609.
11. Bloc S, Mercadal L, Dessieux T, et al. The learning process of the hydrolocalization technique performed during ultrasound-guided regional anesthesia. *Acta Anaesthesiol Scand*. 2010;54(4):421–425.

CHAPTER 95

Method for Optimal Tract Anesthesia During Biopsies, Drainage Catheter Placement, Nephrostomies, and Percutaneous Transhepatic Cholangiography

Robert Evans Heithaus, Almas Syed, and Chet R. Rees

Brief Description

Transrectal and transvaginal approaches for abscess drainage can be safer than other approaches but may cause greater patient discomfort at the time of placement. This method of local anesthetic application can reduce pain and permit more procedures to be done using moderate sedation rather than general anesthesia. This technique is similar to the technique described in Chapter 96 but with modifications that make it more suitable for this purpose. This technique can also be used to obtain tract anesthesia during biopsies, nephrostomy tube placement, and percutaneous transhepatic cholangiograms.

In essence, for the technique of tract anesthesia, a side port adaptor and high-quality 3-cc syringe are used to provide high-pressure injections of lidocaine through the needle and/or dilator, around the wire, whose position is always maintained. Careful attention to copious lidocaine injection is made when the access needle is precisely inside tissues that are difficult to anesthetize (e.g., the tissues of the vaginal cuff) when the resistance to injection may be at its highest.

Applications of the Technique

1. Percutaneous drainage catheter placement.
2. Transrectal drain placement or biopsy/aspiration.
3. Transvaginal drain placement or biopsy/aspiration.
4. Percutaneous transhepatic cholangiogram.
5. Percutaneous nephrostomy tube placement.

Challenges of the Procedure

1. Achieving optimal anesthesia is sometimes difficult depending on the procedure performed, particularly when using the transvaginal or transrectal approach.

2. When drainage catheters are placed in which a large amount of soft tissue must be traversed, obtaining anesthesia deep in the tract may be difficult.

Potential Pitfalls/Complications

1. No specific complications are noted with this procedure. However, as with all local anesthesia administration, aspiration of the syringe along the planned tract prior to injection is recommended to ensure that the local anesthetic is not injected directly into a blood vessel.
2. When this technique is used to anesthetize deeper tracks, the risk of inadvertent vessel traversal increases.

Steps of the Procedure

1. If possible, obtain superficial anesthesia at the point of entry.
2. Advance a guide needle into the target area.
3. Advance a guidewire into the collection or target area.
4. Attach a side port adapter to the needle hub.
5. Fill a high-quality 3-cc syringe with lidocaine (or anesthetic of choice) and insert into the side port adapter.
6. Apply copious amounts of anesthetic while withdrawing the needle.
7. When placing a drain transvaginially, ensure a large amount of anesthetic is injected into the vaginal wall at the point of greatest resistance.

Example

See Figures 95.1–95.5.

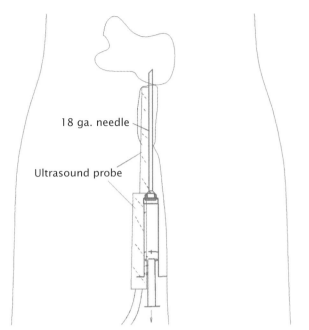

Figure 95.1 Transvaginal abscess drainage. Under sonographic guidance, an 18 or 19 gauge needle is inserted into the collection. A syringe can be placed on the needle to aspirate a sample.

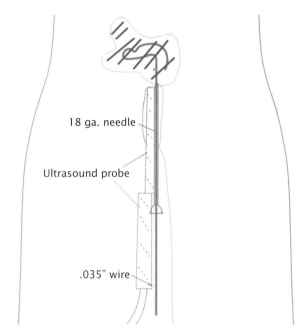

Figure 95.3 A 0.035-in. guidewire is advanced into the collection.

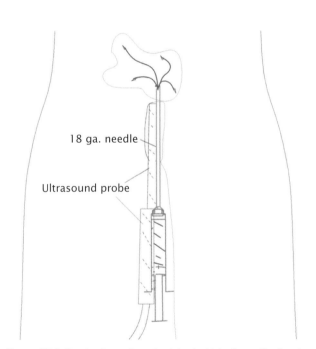

Figure 95.2 Contrast can then be injected into the collection to confirm location and further evaluate the extent of the cavity.

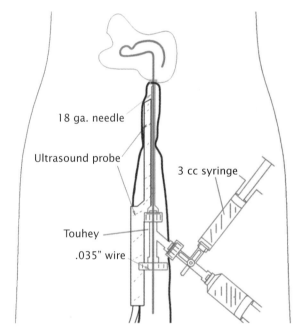

Figure 95.4 A side port is attached to the needle, and a high-pressure, high-quality 3-cc syringe is used to instill local anesthetic while withdrawing the needle. Careful attention is given to copious administration into the tissues of the vaginal cuff, when the resistance to injection may be at its highest.

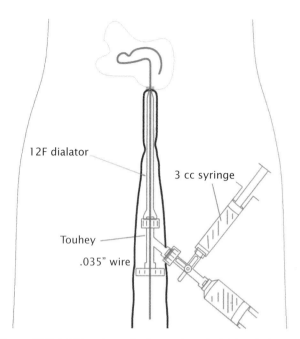

12F dialator

3 cc syringe

Touhey

.035" wire

Figure 95.5 Additional anesthetic can be administered while advancing a dilator using a similar technique. Subsequently, less pain occurs during advancement of the drainage catheter (not shown).

CHAPTER 96

Tract-o-gram to Reduce the Risk of Non-Target Catheterization During Placement of a Drainage Tube

Almas Syed, Robert Evans Heithaus, and Chet R. Rees

Brief Description

Certain abscesses, fluid collections, and other targets have a poor window for percutaneous access, and one of the most severe complications is non-target catheterization. Inadvertent involvement of bowel, spleen, and liver have all been reported.[1] Similarly, the risk of traversing a blood vessel with consequent hemorrhage is inherent with these procedures. Risk factors include an obese body habitus, surrounding bowel, and the inability to optimally position critically ill patients. Bowel transgression by drainage catheters may later become evident by signs and symptoms of peritonitis, copious catheter output, sepsis, or fistula formation. Complications of small needle transgression alone, without tube transgression, are far less significant. The methods described in this chapter, with performance of a tract-o-gram, can identify critical transgressed structures when only a small needle has been passed. This permits a re-attempt and repeat safety check. Employment of a tract-o-gram allows interventionalists to safely perform more aggressive drainage procedures. In this chapter, various iterations of the technique are discussed, which differ by the choice of needle, dilator, and syringe utilized. As demonstrated, use of a larger needle or a modified triaxial dilator allows for an easier contrast injection but does so at the expense of a modestly larger access. Regardless of the method chosen, each is easy to perform and readily accomplished with standard equipment available in virtually all angiography suites.

Applications of the Technique

1. Percutaneous drainage tube placement when there is a small window of access with an increased risk of transgression of visceral or vascular structures.
2. Critically ill patients with limited mobility and reduced ability for optimal positioning.

Challenges of the Procedure

1. Generating high pressure through a 21 gauge needle while withdrawing it can be challenging. This is ameliorated by the added use of a modified triaxial

dilator and side port adapter, as discussed later as an alternative technique.
2. An inadequate tract-o-gram may result from insufficient contrast injection or withdrawing the needle too quickly.

Potential Pitfalls/Complications

1. Repeated non-target catheterization may result in an increased risk of complications despite the use of a small catheterization needle.
2. Free spillage of contrast could be misinterpreted as intraluminal contrast, yielding a false-positive interpretation. Alternatively, an inadequate injection of contrast may not adequately identify and opacify traversed bowel.

Steps of the Procedure

Standard Technique

1. A 21 gauge needle is inserted under image guidance to the target.
2. A 0.018-in. wire is inserted through the needle and coiled within the cavity.
3. A side port adapter (Passage hemostasis valve, Merit Medical, South Jordan, UT) with a three-way stopcock is attached to the needle hub over the wire.
4. Using a high-quality 3-cc syringe (Medallion, Merit Medical), contrast is injected through the side port attached to the needle as it is slowly withdrawn, maintaining wire position in the cavity.
5. Contrast will dribble out slowly but sufficiently to perform an excellent tract-o-gram. If no critical structures have been traversed, the procedure is completed in standard fashion.

Alternative Technique with 19 Gauge Needle

1. A 19 gauge needle is inserted under imaging guidance to the target.

2. A 0.018-in. wire is inserted through the needle and coiled within the cavity.

3. A side port adaptor is attached to the needle hub, and contrast is easily injected along the tract using low pressure while the 19 gauge needle is slowly retracted over the wire.

4. After confirming that no critical structures were transgressed, the procedure is completed over the wire in a standard fashion.

Alternative Technique with Modified Triaxial Dilator

1. A 21 gauge needle is inserted as usual into the target under image guidance.

2. A 0.018-in. wire is inserted through the needle and coiled within the cavity.

3. The needle is removed over the wire.

4. A triaxial dilator from a standard 21 gauge needle/ 0.018-in. wire access kit is modified by removal of the outer dilator, leaving only the metal stiffener and surrounding inner dilator (approximately equivalent to an 18 gauge needle in diameter). The metal stiffener and inner dilator are advanced as a unit over the wire until the tip is in the cavity.

5. The metal stiffener is removed, leaving the inner dilator and the wire in place.

6. A side port adaptor is then attached, and contrast is easily injected along the tract using low pressure while the inner dilator is slowly retracted over the wire.

7. After confirming that no critical structures were transgressed, the procedure is completed over the wire in a standard fashion.

Example

See Figures 96.1–96.5.

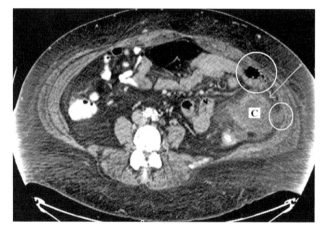

Figure 96.1 Computed tomography image of the abdomen demonstrates a cavitary lesion (C) surrounded by colon (white circles) in a slightly obese patient. The proposed trajectory (gray arrow) indicates a narrow window that is free of bowel. Drainage was performed using ultrasound and fluoroscopic guidance with the aid of the tract-o-gram technique.

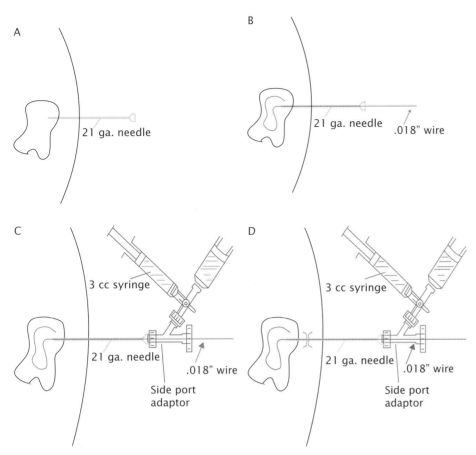

Figure 96.2 A 21 gauge needle is inserted into the cavitary lesion (A), followed by passage of a 0.018-in. wire that is coiled within the cavity (B). (C) A side port adapter (with a three-way stopcock) is attached to the needle hub. (D) Contrast is injected under high pressure through the needle as it is slowly withdrawn, maintaining wire position in the cavity, until the needle is completely removed. A high-pressure injection is necessary to generate an adequate tract-o-gram through a 21 gauge needle containing a wire. We therefore recommend use of a high-quality 3-cc syringe. The larger syringe attached to the three-way stopcock serves as a contrast reservoir to refill the 3-cc syringe as needed. The contrast will dribble out slowly, but sufficiently, to perform a tract-o-gram if the needle is withdrawn slowly.

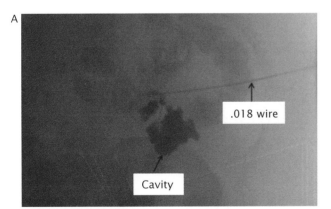

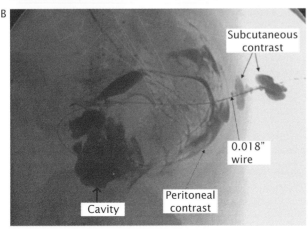

Figure 96.3 (A) Radiographic image demonstrates contrast opacification of the cavity obtained before the needle is withdrawn. (B) After withdrawal of the needle and injection of contrast into the tract, the tract-o-gram demonstrates free spillage of contrast into the peritoneum with no contrast identified in the colon, confirming a safe tract for drainage tube placement. The wire remains in place for subsequent steps.

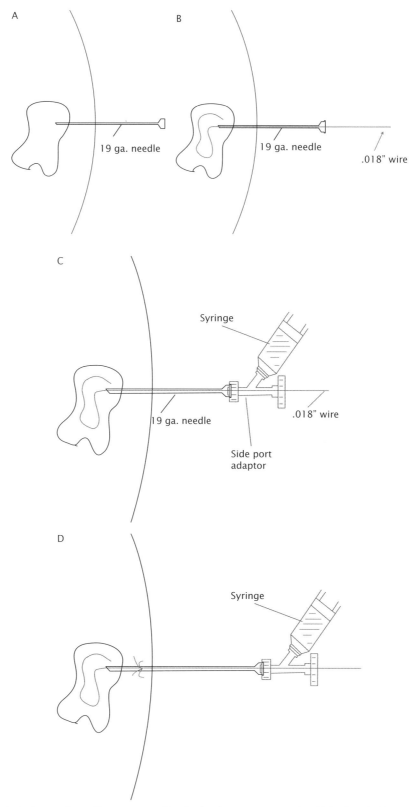

Figure 96.4 Alternative technique using a 19 gauge needle allowing low-pressure contrast injection. A 19 gauge needle is advanced into the cavity (A), and a 0.018-in. wire is inserted (B), leaving plenty of space inside the needle for a low-pressure contrast injection. (C) A side port adaptor with contrast is attached. (D) Contrast is easily injected to perform the tract-o-gram. The procedure is subsequently completed in the usual manner over the 0.018-in. wire using a standard access kit designed for use with a 21 gauge needle and 0.018-in. wire.

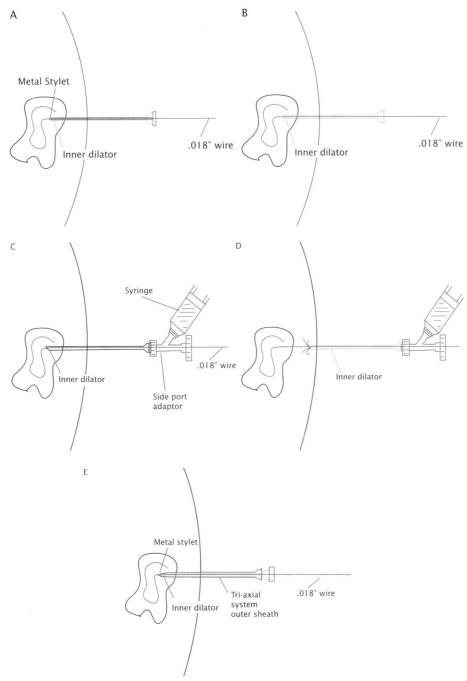

Figure 96.5 Alternative technique using a 21 gauge access needle allowing low-pressure contrast injection. As with the technique outlined in Figure 96.4, this allows an easy, low-pressure injection but does require modest upsizing with a modified triaxial dilator. A 21 gauge needle and 0.018-in. wire are passed into the cavity using standard technique (as shown in Figures 96.1A and B). The needle is removed, leaving only the wire in the patient. (A) Subsequently, a triaxial dilator (from a standard 21 gauge needle/0.018-in. wire access kit) is modified by removal of the outer dilator, leaving only the metal stiffener and surrounding inner dilator (approximately equivalent to an 18 gauge needle in diameter), which are advanced as a unit over the wire until the tip is in the cavity. (B) The metal stiffener is removed, leaving the inner dilator and the wire in place. (D) A side port adaptor is then attached, and contrast is easily injected along the tract using a low-pressure, controlled injection while the dilator is retracted over the wire. (E) Upon confirmation of the absence of non-target transgression, the triaxial system is reassembled and advanced over the wire, allowing the procedure to be completed in a standard fashion.

Reference and Suggested Reading

1. Lorenz J, Thomas JL. Complications of percutaneous fluid drainage. *Semin Intervent Radiol.* 2006;23(2):194–204.

CHAPTER 97

Advancing the Difficult Drainage Catheter

Robert Evans Heithaus, Almas Syed, and Chet R. Rees

Brief Description

Advancing a percutaneous nephrostomy, biliary, or abscess drainage catheter can be difficult in certain situations, particularly when the catheter "accordions" on itself and stalls as it is advanced. The solution can be found through applying the majority of the advancing force at the hub of the metal stiffener rather than along the midportion of the catheter, thereby exerting force at the tip of the catheter via the internal metal stiffener, which is lodged against a small "shelf" inside the catheter.

Biliary, percutaneous nephrostomy, or abscess drainage catheters typically include an inner metal stiffener. The typical tendency is to apply forward force to the shaft of the catheter during advancement; however, this may cause buckling of the distal catheter and prevent its progress. Much better results are achieved by applying the force to the hub where the metal stiffener and flexible catheter are locked, together thereby transmitting most of the force to the catheter tip. The operator steadies the shaft of the catheter with the other hand but consciously avoids applying forward force on the shaft. The overall effect is somewhat like "pulling" the catheter through the tissues by its tip, which prevents buckling.

When curved anatomy is encountered, the catheter is paid off over the metal stiffener; however, buckling may now occur in some cases. Changing to the flexible stiffener at this point may facilitate completion.

Applications of the Technique

1. Nephrostomy drainage catheter placement.
2. Percutaneous biliary catheter placement.
3. Abscess drainage catheter placement.

Challenges of the Procedure

1. Soft drainage catheters tend to accordion when an inner stiffener is not in place.

2. Even with a stiffener/inner cannula in place, the catheter may accordion when the operator applies forward force along the shaft of the catheter.

Potential Pitfalls/Complications

1. Inappropriate torque placed on a long catheter by applying force at the hub if care is not taken to advance the device in line with the guidewire.

Steps of the Procedure

1. Gain wire access to the area of interest.
2. Dilate the tract to the appropriate diameter.
3. Insert the stiffener/inner cannula into the catheter.
4. Use the nondominant hand to guide the proximal end of the catheter.
5. With the dominant hand, apply force at the hub of the catheter.
6. The catheter should not accordion on itself if a majority of the forward force is applied at the hub of the metal stiffener rather than the shaft.
7. When tortuous anatomy is encountered, the catheter is paid off from the metal stiffener (i.e., the metal stiffener is held in place while the catheter is advanced).
8. If the catheter continues to buckle, insertion of the soft plastic inner stiffener may allow the operator to advance the catheter through an area of tortuosity.

Example

See Figures 97.1–97.3.

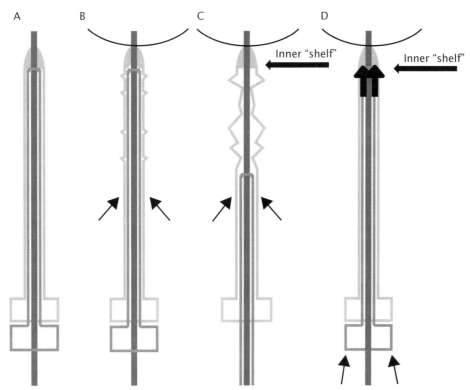

Figure 97.1 (A) Drainage catheters (outer structure) often include an inner metal stiffener (middle structure) through which a wire can be passed (inner structure). (B and C) If force (arrows) is applied to the catheter shaft, the catheter can "accordion" on itself. (D) If force is applied at the metal stiffener, then the force is transmitted to the "shelf" at the proximal end of the catheter, resulting in the rest of catheter being "pulled" through the tissues.

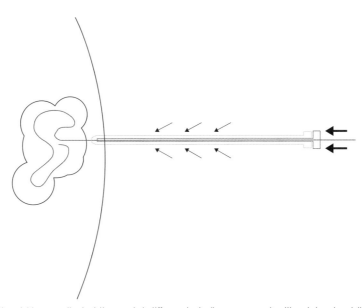

Figure 97.2 Maximal force should be applied at the metal stiffener hub (large arrows) with minimal guiding force along the catheter shafts (small arrows).

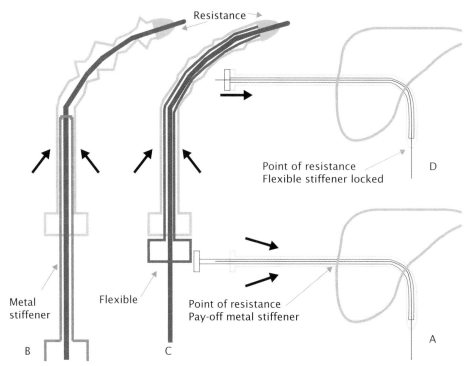

Figure 97.3 When the catheter reaches curved anatomy, the catheter should be paid off the metal stiffener (middle structure in figure A). If the catheter accordions, then the flexible stiffener (middle structure in figure B) should be inserted to aid in advancing the catheter through the curved anatomy.

CHAPTER 98

Creation of a Steerable Coaxial Needle System for Indirect Line-of-Site Computed Tomography-Guided Procedures

S. Lowell Kahn

Brief Description

A standard computed tomography (CT)-guided biopsy, aspiration, injection, or drainage procedure typically requires a direct line of access from the skin to the target lesion or collection. Although safe traversal of the bowel is described for biopsies, this method is typically avoided by most operators. Safe performance of these procedures is ideally performed without violation of vascular structures or solid or hollow viscous. When a direct pathway to the target is absent, patients are commonly denied the procedure and instead referred to surgery.

Recently, the Morrison Steerable Needle (AprioMed, Londonderry, NH)[1] became the first commercially available needle designed to be steered around critical structures during biopsy, aspiration, or injection. There is no doubt that this device has significant utility, but currently there is little market penetrance, with availability limited to a few institutions. Moreover, cost considerations should be made when other viable alternatives exist.

This chapter describes a solution for CT-guided procedures when a direct line of access to the intended target is unavailable. The technique involves a coaxial needle system with simple modification (curving) of the inner needle, which readily allows access to a structure when a non-target structure lies between the surface and the intended site. With proper employment, this is an efficient, cost-effective method to steer around critical structures and obviates the need for surgery.

Applications of the Technique

1. Access for percutaneous biopsy, aspiration, or injection when critical structures lie in the access trajectory.
2. Access for percutaneous drainage when critical structures lie in the access trajectory.
3. Access to the nidus of an endoleak for symptomatic or enlarging type II endoleaks.

Challenges of the Procedure

1. Appropriate curving of the inner needle is imperative. A certain degree of straightening occurs when the curved inner needle is inserted into the straight outer needle of the coaxial system.
   a. Too gentle of a curve results in inadequate directional control of the inner needle.
   b. Too much curving of the inner needle carries the following risks:
      i. Kinking, which can cause failure of the biopsy needle or compromise of the lumen. That might impede aspiration, injection, or passage of a guidewire, depending on the intended procedure.
      ii. Too much friction of the system, which can impede passage of the inner needle.
2. During drainage procedures, a guidewire must be passed through the lumen of the inner needle. As noted previously, when the needle is curved, the inner lumen is invariably narrowed, and increased friction will occur between the needle and the guidewire. After successful access to the target, the needle must be removed over the guidewire, and there is a risk of dislodgement of the system if the friction between the guidewire and the needle is excessive.

Potential Pitfalls/Complications

1. Inadequate steerage of the needle resulting in inadvertent injury to the structure that the operator is attempting to avoid.
2. Inability to adequately shape (curve) the needle to reach the intended target. The intended target should be only marginally off course. This method does not work well if accessing the intended target requires a sharp turn after the avoided structure is passed.
3. Failure of the biopsy needle when it is manually curved.

4. Kinking of the inner needle with the complications as listed previously.

Steps of the Procedure

1. Pre-procedural planning for the CT-guided access is performed in the usual fashion. The critical structure that lies in the desired path is identified. A preliminary site (A) is identified immediately adjacent and just beyond the structure to be avoided. The chosen location of preliminary site A should minimize the amount of course deviation required to reach the intended target (B) of the procedure.
2. A 17 or 18 gauge outer needle is selected that is of adequate length to reach preliminary site A.
3. The straight outer needle is directed under CT guidance to preliminary site A.
4. A second inner needle is chosen. Depending on the needle manufacturer, typically a needle that is two or more sizes below the gauge of the outer needle will allow passage of the inner needle. For example, for most needles, a 20 gauge needle will pass coaxially within the lumen of an 18 gauge needle.
   a. The greater the difference in needle sizes, the less friction will be present upon passage of the modified (curved) inner needle. Therefore, the smaller the inner needle, the easier it is to actuate through the outer needle. However, the inner needle must have an adequate lumen for the intended intervention (e.g., passage of a 0.018-in. wire for drainage procedures), and use of a smaller inner needle has the disadvantage of decreased longitudinal strength and rigidity. At our institution, we typically select an 18 gauge outer needle with a 21 gauge inner needle.
   b. The inner needle should be 5 cm or greater in length than the outer needle.
5. The inner needle is manually shaped at its tip, typically over a distance of approximately 5 cm.
   a. The degree of curvature depends on how much course deviation is required from point A to point B. We have found that for most cases, 30 degrees of curvature is sufficient, recognizing that a degree of straightening will occur when the inner needle passes through the straight outer needle.
   b. Recall that too much curvature can cause kinking, device failure, or unacceptable friction.
   c. If the inner needle has a bevel, the curve should be made such that the inner curve is consistent with the long side of the bevel. The bevel will enhance steerage of the needle toward the direction of the curve.
6. The inner needle is inserted into the outer needle with the curve of the needle maintained toward the direction of the intended target (B). When the tip of the inner needle reaches the tip of the outer needle, the inner needle is carefully advanced toward the intended target (B) under CT guidance.
7. Upon reaching the intended target, the procedure is completed (e.g., injection, aspiration, biopsy, or passage of a wire [prior to placement of a drainage catheter]) with removal of the inner and outer needle as necessary.

Example

See Figure 98.1.

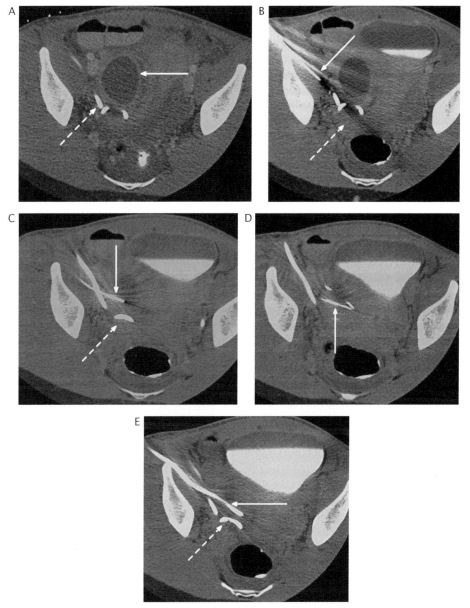

Figure 98.1 An 18-year-old female with pelvic pain. The first CT (not shown) demonstrated a pelvic abscess, which was successfully drained. (A) She failed to improve, and a repeat CT demonstrated a new adjacent abscess (solid arrow) that was not in communication with the first abscess (dashed arrow) located posteriorly. A direct line of site for safe percutaneous access to the new abscess was not present secondary to overlying bowel as well as osseous and vascular structures. A steerable coaxial system was created. (B) A straight 17 gauge needle (solid arrow) was advanced immediately anterior to the pelvis in a line as close as possible toward the abscess without crossing critical vessels or bowel. The existing drain (dashed arrow) is again noted posteriorly. (C) A 21 gauge Chiba needle (Cook Medical, Bloomington, IN) is manually curved and then inserted into the 17 gauge needle after the stylet of the 17 gauge needle is removed. The inner 21 gauge needle (solid arrow) is seen curving toward and entering the abscess cavity. The existing drain (dashed arrow) is evident posteriorly. (D) After the stylet of the 21 gauge needle is removed, a 0.018-in. wire is advanced through the end of the Chiba needle (arrow) and coils within the abscess cavity. (E) Final CT now demonstrates the new drain (solid arrow) in the pelvic abscess adjacent to the original drain (dashed arrow), with complete decompression of both abscesses.

References and Suggested Readings

1. AprioMed. Morrison steerable needle. http://apriomed.com/products/morrison-steerable-needle.

2. Sears P, Dupont PE. Inverse kinematics of concentric tube steerable needles. *IEE Int Conf Robot Autom*. 2007 April: 1887–1892.

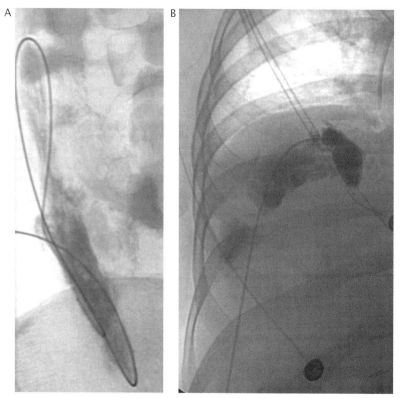

Figure 99.2 (A) Fluoroscopic image of the abdomen: A 0.035-in. guidewire is looped within the multiloculated collection. (B) Fluoroscopic image of the abdomen: A 0.035-in. guidewire is advanced through the septations of the multiloculated collection and into the perihepatic component (filled with a small amount of injected contrast).

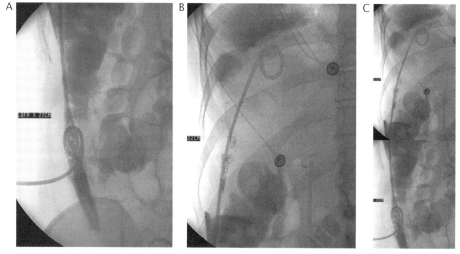

Figures 99.3 Fluoroscopic image of the abdomen: An 8 Fr double-pigtail nephroureterostomy catheter is placed such that the proximal loop is within the caudal component of the collection (A), the distal loop is within the perihepatic component of the collection (B), and the multiloculated collection is drained through a single percutaneous access route (C).

References and Suggested Readings

1. Charles HW. Abscess drainage. *Semin Intervent Radiol.* 2012;29:325–336.

2. Liu CH, Gervais DA, Hahn PF. Percutaneous hepatic abscess drainage: Do multiple abscesses or multiloculated abscesses preclude drainage or affect outcome? *J Vasc Interv Radiol.* 2009;20:1059–1065.

CHAPTER 100

Transurethral Retrograde Approach to Pelvic Abscess Drainage in Post-cystectomy Patients

George Carberry and Orhan Ozkan

Brief Description

Transurethral drainage has been described for the treatment of prostatic abscesses,[1,2] but we have found it to be particularly well tolerated in patients for whom pelvic fluid drainage is needed following radical cystectomy. This technique has been described only once in the literature[3]; it provides pelvic fluid drainage through a fully epithelialized tract as opposed to percutaneous, transrectal, or transvaginal approaches to pelvic abscess drainage. Furthermore, if the posterior urethra has not been oversewn at the time of surgery, the guidewire will often easily slide into the fluid collection, requiring no needle puncture. Although blind Foley catheter placement could potentially be used for transurethral drainage in these patients, urologic surgeons have preferred fluoroscopically guided drain placement to ensure atraumatic placement and optimal drain positioning. This chapter describes our experience with the technique.

Application of the Technique

1. Drainage of pelvic fluid collections in patients who have previously undergone radical cystectomy.

Challenges of the Procedure

1. If the transurethral guidewire does not initially access the pelvic fluid collection, guidance with computed tomography (CT) or transabdominal or transrectal ultrasound may be helpful to ensure positioning of the wire inside the fluid collection.
2. If the guidewire is having difficulty passing through the posterior urethra, try applying gentle upward traction on the penis, which straightens the path that the wire must take and facilitates passage of the wire.

Potential Pitfalls/Complications

1. Our experience with the technique has involved only those patients in whom the posterior urethra

had not been oversewn at the time of surgery; therefore, we cannot recommend any particular method for recanalization of the posterior urethra if it is not patent. Referral to the surgeon's operative notes may help to determine if the posterior urethra was closed at the time of surgery.

Steps of the Procedure

1. Review prior cross-sectional imaging to verify absence of urinary bladder and proximity of pelvic fluid collection to posterior urethra.
2. Position patient prone on fluoroscopy table. Cleanse urethral meatus with betadine solution in a fashion similar to preparation of Foley catheter placement.
3. Advance a short Berenstein catheter (Angio-Dynamics, Latham, NY) over an angled Glidewire (Terumo, Somerset, NJ) into the anterior urethra.
4. Perform retrograde urethrogram to delineate urethral anatomy and determine if contrast communicates with pelvic fluid collection.
5. Advance the Berenstein catheter through the posterior urethra into the pelvis over the Glidewire.
6. Repeat contrast injection to confirm catheter is located within the fluid collection.
7. Exchange Glidewire for a short Amplatz wire (Boston Scientific, Marlborough, MA).
8. Over the Amplatz wire, deploy an 8 Fr pigtail drainage catheter in standard fashion.
9. Attach drainage catheter to additional tubing and connect to a leg bag if the patient is ambulatory or to a standard abscess drainage bag.
10. Prescribe routine drain flushing instructions and patient follow-up for abscess drainage.

Example

See Figures 100.1–100.5.

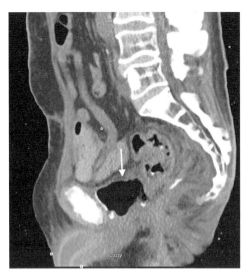

Figure 100.1 Sagittal CT image of the pelvis shows a gas and fluid collection in the pelvis (arrow) following cystectomy and partial colectomy for rectal cancer.

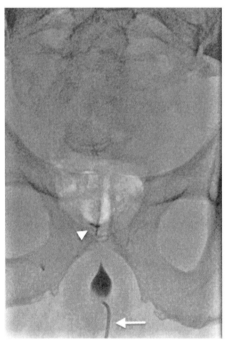

Figure 100.2 Anteroposterior (AP) projection fluoroscopic image demonstrates distal end of Berenstein catheter in the anterior urethra (arrow) with injection of a small amount of contrast filling the gas-filled abscess (arrowhead).

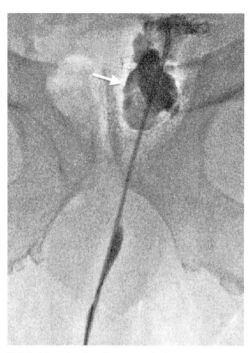

Figure 100.3 AP projection fluoroscopic image showing catheter extending through the urethra into the pelvic abscess. Its position has been verified with contrast injection (arrow).

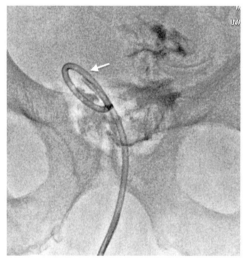

Figure 100.4 Fluoroscopic image showing pigtail end of drain (arrow) formed within the abscess.

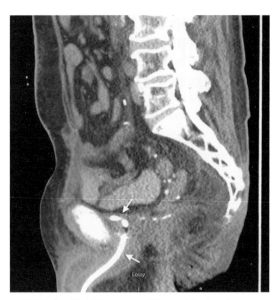

Figure 100.5 Sagittal CT image of the pelvis showing transurethral drain in place (arrow) with no residual pelvic abscess.

References and Suggested Readings

1. El-Shazly M, El-Enzy N, El-Enzy K, Yordanov E, Hathout B, Allam A. Transurethral drainage of prostatic abscess: Points of technique. *Nephrourol Mon.* 2012;4(2):458–461.
2. Jang K, Lee DH, Lee SH, Chung BH. Treatment of prostatic abscess: Case collection and comparison of treatment methods. *Korean J Urol.* 2012;53(12):860–864.
3. Place C, Nolan RL, Nickel JC. Alternate approaches to pelvic abscess drainage after cystectomy. *Urol Radiol.* 1989;11:161–164.

CHAPTER 101

Creation of an Additional Side Hole as a Method to Exchange Obstructed Percutaneous Drainage Catheters

Jessica M. Ho and Michael D. Katz

Brief Description

Percutaneous drainage catheter placement is a frequently performed interventional radiology procedure. One of the common management complications of such catheters is obstruction or clogging of the catheter. Occluded drainage catheters are routinely exchanged over a guidewire under fluoroscopic guidance. At times, however, a guidewire cannot be passed through the catheter obstruction, and exchanging the catheter over a guidewire may become difficult or even impossible without losing access. To prevent loss of access when exchanging a completely obstructed catheter, the creation of an additional side hole is a technique that may be useful. By creating an extra side hole that allows the guidewire to exit the catheter rather than stop at the point of catheter occlusion, the guidewire can be passed into the target organ, maintaining access. Once the guidewire is passed into the target structure, successful catheter exchange in the typical fashion can be performed.

Applications of the Technique

1. Exchanging clogged abscess drainage catheters.
2. Exchanging clogged feeding tubes.
3. Exchanging clogged nephrostomy catheters.
4. Exchanging clogged biliary drains.
5. Exchanging any other obstructed/clogged catheters in which a wire cannot be advanced.

Challenges of the Procedure

1. It can be difficult to readvance the catheter after cutting a large side hole, particularly if the tract is very immature.
2. If there is little wire length within the catheter due to extensive catheter occlusion, it can be difficult to readvance the catheter after partial withdrawal even after an extra side hole is created.
3. If the catheter is obstructed all the way to the hub, there may be no room to cut a side hole. The hub can be cut off, and debris can then be milked backward to make a portion of the catheter patent.

4. The guidewire may not exit the newly cut side hole. An angled guidewire should be used. If it still cannot be made to exit the side hole, the procedure can be attempted with the guidewire already slightly out through the side hole.
5. Care should be taken that the catheter is not transected when cutting the side hole. A large hole makes guidewire exit easier, but it makes the catheter more floppy when readvancing.

Potential Pitfalls/Complications

1. This technique requires that the catheter be sufficiently long to be partially withdrawn and then readvanced without losing access. This could be problematic with short catheters and long subcutaneous tracts (e.g., short nephrostomy catheters in obese patients).
2. This method ensures preservation of access into the organ of interest while the nonfunctioning tube is removed; however, it will not maintain distal access for long tubes (i.e., gastrojejunostomy tubes, internal–external biliary drains, and nephroureterostomy tubes). Once the guidewire is within the organ of interest, the nonfunctioning tube can be removed, and additional catheter and guidewire manipulation would then be needed to regain access into the more distal final target (e.g., through the pylorus into the small bowel for a gastrojejunostomy).
3. In immature tracts, there is a small risk of creating a false tract.
4. Stiff hydrophilic guidewires facilitate this procedure, but inadvertent recoil of these catheters can make loss of access more frequent. Choice of guidewire is left to the operator.

Steps of the Procedure

1. The existing catheter is retracted slightly without loss of access into the target organ. The length of retraction will depend on patient body habitus as

well as catheter and subcutaneous tract length. It may be advantageous to cut the hub off the catheter.

2. A large extra side hole is cut into the side of the existing catheter by folding it backwards and cutting one edge.

3. An angled steerable stiff guidewire is inserted through the catheter and positioned so that the guidewire tip is directly pointing at the newly created side hole.

4. The catheter and wire are then readvanced as a unit to maintain access through the existing tract until it is expected that the newly created side hole is within the target organ.

5. Once the catheter–wire combination is within the target organ, the wire is advanced out the extra

side hole of the catheter so that the tip is within the target organ.

6. The guidewire is then advanced adequately to maintain access during an over-the-guidewire exchange without losing access.

7. The existing clogged/obstructed catheter is removed over the guidewire and routine catheter exchange performed.

Example

In Figures 101.1–101.7, the vertical black line represents the skin. The occlusion within the catheter—in this case, a jejunostomy tube—is indicated by the black area on the catheter.

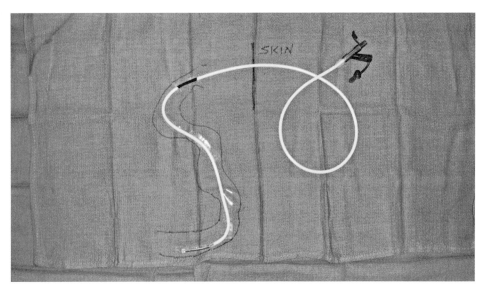

Figure 101.1 An occluded jejunostomy catheter is shown diagrammatically within the jejunum. A guidewire will not pass across the occluded segment (black area).

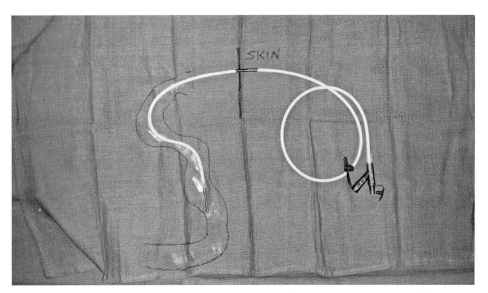

Figure 101.2 The catheter has been partially withdrawn through the tract, but the blockage remains. There is adequate catheter remaining within the target organ (jejunum) to preserve access.

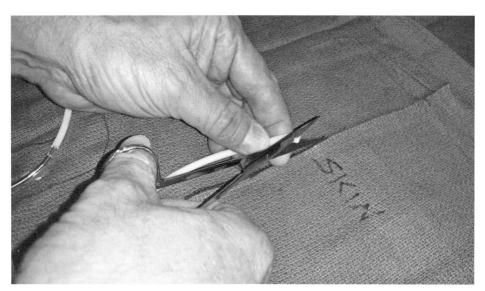

Figure 101.3 A large side hole is cut by bending the catheter, outside the patient, and cutting one edge. Care should be taken to not transect the catheter.

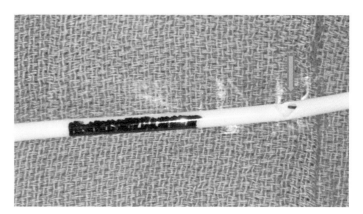

Figure 101.4 A large side hole has been cut outside the patient, but the blockage remains. A hydrophilic angled stiff guidewire is passed through the catheter lumen, and its tip is seen pointing toward the newly cut side hole (arrow).

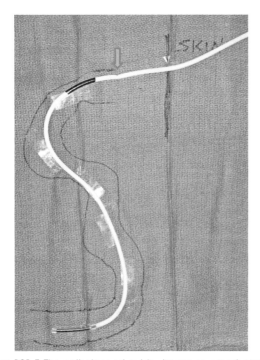

Figure 101.5 The catheter and guidewire are now readvanced as a unit through the existing tract until the side hole is back into the bowel or target organ. The arrow indicates the side hole pushed back into jejunum.

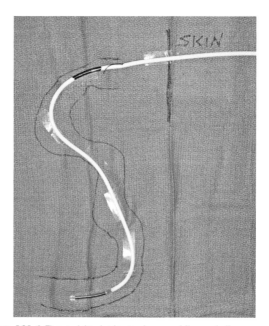

Figure 101.6 The guidewire is readvanced through the pre-existing catheter and out the newly created side hole into bowel or other target organ. Once a large amount of guidewire is advanced, the catheter can be safely exchanged.

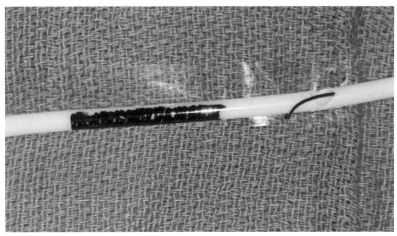

Figure 101.7 In cases in which the steerable guidewire will not exit the side hole, which can occur with tight tracts, the catheter can be partially withdrawn again and the wire placed so it is already slightly out the side hole. Then, the catheter and guidewire can be readvanced as a unit. It may be more uncomfortable for the patient to have the guidewire tip drag through the subcutaneous tract.

References and Suggested Readings

1. Cope C. Replacement of obstructed loop and pigtail nephrostomy and biliary drains. *Am J Radiol*. 1982;139: 1022–1023.

2. Lee AS, vanSonnenberg E, Wittich GR, Casola G. Exchange of occluded catheters with transcatheter and pericatheter maneuvers. *Radiology*. 1987;163(1):273–274.

CHAPTER 102

Use of a Peel-Away Sheath as a Method to Exchange a Clogged Drainage Tube

Harsha R. Jonna and Michael D. Katz

Brief Description

There are many methods of exchanging occluded or clogged percutaneous catheters. Typically, catheter exchange is simply performed over a guidewire. When debris occluding the lumen is compact, chronic, or extensive, such exchanges are difficult. Occasionally, hydrophilic stiff wires can be used to re-establish access through the lumen of the catheter by slipping through cleavage planes of the obstructing debris. In the setting of chronic and hard occlusions or multifocal or long segments of occlusion, this may be tedious or impossible. Instead, methods to preserve the tract while removing the nonfunctioning tube may need to be employed. Advancing a coaxial telescoping peel-away sheath over a drainage catheter is one such technique to preserve the tract and provide a conduit for any further intervention.

Applications of the Procedure

1. Exchanging clogged feeding tubes.
2. Exchanging clogged nephrostomy catheters: Precipitated debris surrounding and within the catheter may prevent loosening of the retention string, but advancing a coaxial telescoping outer sheath may loosen the pigtail and the string.
3. Exchanging clogged biliary drains.
4. Exchanging clogged abscess drainage catheters.
5. Exchanging nonfunctioning or damaged vascular access catheters or sheaths where flushing/aspiration or wire manipulation may not be safe.

Challenges of the Procedure

1. Occluded nephrostomy catheters may have radiolucent precipitated debris on the extraluminal outside surface of their distal retention pigtail occluding the side holes and tip. This may make removing the catheter through the peel-away sheath difficult or impossible, depending on their bulk and chronicity. Removal may require significant force, and when possible, the debris may be sheared off the surface of the catheter and remain in the collecting system.
2. Exchanging vascular access catheters by this method can lead to significant blood loss due to back bleeding

if exchange is not rapid. A second operator to compress around the catheter can minimize this problem.
3. Tubes made of silicone are more difficult to exchange in this manner because there is greater friction between them and the outer plastic sheaths. This can be circumvented by using sheaths that are at least 4 Fr larger than the tube, which would dilate the tract, or by instilling lubricant into the sheath before advancing.
4. The sheath should be large enough to accommodate removal of distal retention balloons such as those in some gastrostomy tubes. In these situations, the retention disk on the skin should be removed and the catheter should be advanced into the stomach for greater "purchase" prior to deflating the balloon and advancing the sheath. Where there is great respiratory excursion, this is the point when the catheter could be "breathed out" by the patient, and the operator should be careful to not withdraw the catheter until the peel-away sheath is advanced securely into the stomach.
5. Some sheaths are not radiopaque and may not be definitively seen on fluoroscopy when advancing. Judgment and estimation of the tract length will be needed to know when the sheath has been advanced far enough.

Potential Pitfalls/Complications

1. For safe and controlled exchange, this technique requires a peel-away sheath that is shorter than the length of the tube that is exposed but longer than the length of the tract. This ensures that the operator will always have a grasp of the clogged tube while advancing the outer sheath. This is of particular importance when exchanging vascular catheters because there is risk of "losing" the catheter inside the patient. Sheaths with such dimensions may not be readily available and may require back table adjustments prior to exchange. These include trimming the catheter by cutting it with scissors to reduce length or simply partially peeling back the peel-away sheath (partially peeling can reduce the pushabillity of peel-away sheaths). Occasionally, depending on the patient's body habitus and the tube in question, the

tract may be longer than the exposed tube, precluding the use of this method (e.g., large patients with short nephrostomy or gastrostomy tubes).

2. This method ensures preservation of access into the organ of interest while the nonfunctioning tube is removed; however, it will not maintain distal access for long tubes, (i.e., internal–external biliary drains, gastro-jejunostomy tubes, and nephroureterostomy tubes). Once the sheath is across the tract and into the organ of interest, the nonfunctioning tube can be removed. Then, the sheath can be used as a conduit for additional wire and catheter manipulation needed to regain access into the distal area of interest (e.g., through the pylorus into the small bowel for a gastrojejunostomy). The sheath can summarily be removed, and the new catheter can be replaced over a wire.

Steps of the Procedure

1. Choose a peel-away sheath that is 1.5–2 Fr larger than the occluded catheter for easier manipulation (e.g., for an 8.5 Fr pigtail catheter, chose a 10 F peel-away).
2. Remove the inner dilator from the peel-away sheath.
3. Cut the occluded catheter's hub off as close to the hub as possible so the remaining catheter is as long as possible.
4. Ideally, the peel-away sheath should be shorter than the exposed portion of the drainage tube but longer than the tract. If it is in fact too long, cut the sheath to size on the back table. Alternatively, for tubes that are shorter than the sheath available, the drainage tube can be "lengthened" by placing a suture through the proximal portion and slipping the sheath over both the suture and the catheter.

5. Advance the peel-away over the cut drainage catheter and into the tract while holding onto the catheter at all times with strong back tension. If more support/stiffness is needed, a stiff guidewire or even a stiff guidewire and small catheter (if it can be passed part way down the occluded catheter) can be used in some applications to straighten and firm the obstructed catheter to ease advancement of the peel-away sheath. Some peel-away sheaths are not radiopaque, and operator judgment will be necessary to determine when the peel-away is securely in the organ of interest.
6. Withdraw the occluded catheter through the peel-away while maintaining forward tension on the sheath to preserve access.
7. Once the occluded catheter is removed, a new guidewire can be introduced through the peel-away. Once guidewire access is achieved, further manipulation for proper positioning can be performed for final catheter positioning with steerable catheters and/or guidewires.
8. The peel-away sheath is removed and the exchange completed as per routine.

Example
See Figure 102.1.

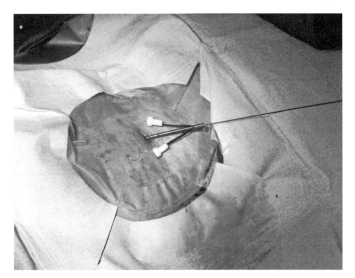

Figure 102.1 Exchange of an occluded nephrostomy. A guidewire could only be passed a short distance into the catheter due to debris, thus preventing controlled catheter exchange. A 10 Fr peel-away sheath has been placed over the nephrostomy. If there is little remaining catheter length to hold onto, as in this case, the peel-away can be partially peeled down to expose more of the catheter.

References and Suggested Readings

1. Cope C. Replacement of obstructed loop and pigtail nephro-stomy and biliary drains. *Am J Radiol.* 1982;139: 1022–1023.

2. Lee AS, vanSonnenberg E, Wittich GR, Casola G. Exchange of occluded catheters with transcatheter and pericatheter maneuvers. *Radiology.* 1987;163(1):273–274.

Imaging and Pharmacology Techniques

CHAPTER 103

Optimizing Carbon Dioxide Peripheral Arteriography

Mikin V. Patel and Steven Zangan

Brief Description

Carbon dioxide (CO_2) angiography is a useful alternative to iodinated agents in providing intravascular contrast during angiography. The fundamental principle of CO_2 angiography is reduction in X-ray attenuation of a blood vessel relative to the adjacent soft tissue and fat by displacement of blood with CO_2 gas. Typically, angiographic images are inverted and can also be stacked to improve image quality. In certain situations, such as placement of transjugular intrahepatic portosystemic shunts, CO_2 has distinct advantages over iodinated contrast. CO_2 is also an inexpensive and safe option for peripheral arteriography and intervention in patients with renal impairment or severe iodinated contrast allergy. However, there are a number of challenges and complications unique to this technique that should be considered. CO_2 is relatively buoyant, so incomplete filling of vessels leads to incomplete displacement of blood and, thus, poor contrast. In addition, the CO_2 bolus begins to dissolve and fragment in blood upon injection, so vessels with slow flow or areas near vessel bifurcations may not be adequately visualized, creating pseudostenoses. When planning intervention, the expansile properties of CO_2 within an elastic vessel can lead to overestimation of vessel size. Although CO_2 angiography is relatively safe, operators should be aware of the possible hazards reported. The most notorious complication is the "vapor lock" phenomenon (more likely in patients receiving nitrous oxide anesthetic), but other reported complications include transient ischemia of peripheral or visceral tissues, alterations of blood chemistry, and neurotoxicity. A number of techniques can be employed to improve imaging quality and mitigate the risks of CO_2 angiography. To improve imaging of distal lower extremity arteries, the volume of CO_2 can be increased while maintaining the same rate. Additional postural maneuvers can be attempted, such as elevating the patient's legs to facilitate gas entry into nondependent anatomy. When possible, the vessels of interest can be selectively catheterized to direct the CO_2 bolus. In difficult cases, small doses of vasodilator can be used to improve imaging of peripheral arteries. To mitigate the risk of complication, special considerations apply to patients with right-to-left shunt or chronic obstructive pulmonary disease.

Applications of the Technique

1. Patients with renal impairment requiring diagnostic and therapeutic peripheral arteriography.
2. Peripheral arteriography in patients with severe allergy to iodinated contrast agents.

Challenges of the Procedure

1. CO_2 angiography depends on the displacement of blood by CO_2 gas causing differences in X-ray attenuation between the vessel and adjacent soft tissue and fat. Because CO_2 is buoyant on the column of blood, an insufficient volume of CO_2 leads to inadequate displacement of the blood and, thus, inadequate contrast. This tends to be an issue in CO_2 angiography of larger vessels.
2. An injected CO_2 gas bolus can break up into discrete bubbles, particularly at vessel bifurcations, and cause the appearance of artifacts that can be perceived as stenoses.
3. CO_2 dissolves within the blood, so in areas of slow flow, the volume of intravascular gas may be insufficient to provide the contrast needed to outline the vessel.
4. In elastic vessels completely distended with CO_2, diameter can be overestimated. This should factor into sizing of therapeutic devices such as stents.

Potential Pitfalls/Complications

1. Large volumes of CO_2 gas trapped in the heart can obstruct normal blood flow and cause hemodynamic changes. This vapor lock phenomenon is classically reported in venography with CO_2 gas becoming trapped in the heart, preventing normal venous return. Similarly, injection of CO_2 during peripheral arteriography can produce symptoms of leg pain or paresthesias.
2. In patients receiving nitrous oxide anesthesia, the nitrous oxide can diffuse into the CO_2 bubbles and decrease their solubility. This, in turn, increases the potential for vapor lock. Thus, CO_2 angiography is

not recommended in patients receiving nitrous oxide for anesthesia.

3. CO_2 injection into the carotid arteries can lead to ischemic cerebral damage, so CO2 angiography is not used above the diaphragm and is contraindicated in upper limb angiography.

4. Likewise, CO_2 angiography is not used in the presence of a right-to-left cardiac shunt to mitigate the risk of ischemic cerebral damage.

5. In patients with chronic respiratory failure, the increased CO_2 load can overwhelm the ventilatory capacity of the lungs. Injected CO_2 of 50 ml/min is equivalent to an estimated 20% increase in basal CO_2 production, and the likelihood of clinically significant CO_2 retention is low. Nevertheless, a decreased injection volume with increased time interval between injections is routine practice.

Steps of the Procedure

1. The CO_2 delivery system is prepared with particular attention paid to eliminating room air and purging the catheter of blood to prevent "explosive" delivery of CO_2 during angiography. The system must be closed to room air.

2. The catheter is positioned for selective arteriogram, always below the level of the diaphragm.

3. The patient is positioned supine with elevation of the legs for optimal evaluation of the calves and feet. This position allows the injected, buoyant CO_2 to rise and fill the arteries.

4. Angiographic runs are performed at 2–6 frames/sec with image inversion using digital subtraction. Image stacking can also be employed to improve imaging quality.

5. An appropriate volume of CO_2 is injected to provide necessary contrast: 30–50 ml is typical for aortograms, less for selective arteriography. Typically, an injection rate of 20–30 ml/sec will adequately fill the lumen of a vessel that is less than 10 mm in diameter.

6. Multiple runs can be performed but should be done so at 2- to 3-minute intervals, allowing time for the injected CO_2 bubbles to dissolve.

7. If needed, the total volume of CO_2 injected (rather than the rate of injection) can be increased to fully displace blood from the vessel and improve visualization.

8. Nitroglycerine can be administered intra-arterially in 100-µg aliquots to enhance gas filling of the distal arteries. Blood pressure is monitored carefully during and after nitroglycerine administration.

Example

See Figures 103.1 and 103.2.

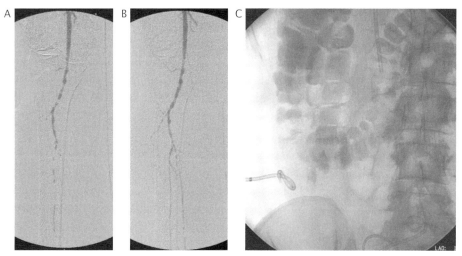

Figure 103.1 (A) Digital subtraction angiography (DSA) image of right lower extremity three-vessel runoff performed with CO_2, suboptimal technique. Note that the arteries do not fill well, and the bolus of CO_2 is fragmented. This produces a number of pseudostenoses and, ultimately, a nondiagnostic image. (B) DSA image of right lower extremity three-vessel runoff performed with CO_2, optimized technique. CO_2 adequately displaces the blood from the arteries, and the tibioperoneal trunk, peroneal artery, and posterior tibial artery are well-defined. (C) DSA image of right lower extremity three-vessel runoff performed with dilute visipaque. Similar to the optimized CO_2, irregular stenoses are seen in the distal popliteal artery. Tibioperoneal trunk, peroneal artery, and posterior tibial artery are well-defined.

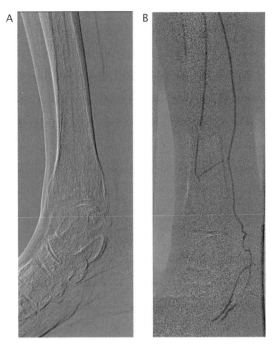

Figure 103.2 (A) DSA image of right lower extremity angiography with CO_2, suboptimal technique. Note that the arteries are not opacified, producing a nondiagnostic image. (B) DSA image of right lower extremity angiography with CO_2. After increasing volume of CO_2 and elevating the legs, the posterior tibial artery is well opacified to the level of the forefoot.

References and Suggested Readings

1. Funaki B. Carbon dioxide angiography. *Semin Intervent Radiol.* 2008;25(1):65–70.
2. Shaw DR, Kessel DO. The current status of the use of carbon dioxide in diagnostic and interventional angiographic procedures. *Cardiovasc Intervent Radiol.* 2006;29(3):323–331.
3. Patel BN, Kapoor BS, Borghei P, et al. Carbon dioxide as an intravascular imaging agent: Review. *Curr Probl Diagn Radiol.* 2011;40(5):208–217.
4. Spinosa DJ, Maysumoto AH, Angle JF, et al. Transient mesenteric ischemia: A complication of carbon dioxide angiography. *J Vasc Interv Radiol* 1998;9:561–564.
5. Lang EV, Gossler AA, Fick LJ, et al. Carbon dioxide angiography: Effect of injection parameters on bolus configuration. *J Vasc Interv Radiol.* 1999;10(1):41–49.

CHAPTER 104

Local Administration of Fresh Frozen Plasma and Platelets in the Critically Ill Patient

Salim E. Abboud, Dean A. Nakamoto, and John R. Haaga

Brief Description

Intraprocedural computed tomography (CT) and ultra-sound guidance allow precise localization of the needle tip and visualization of vascular structures, which contribute immensely to the safety profile of image-guided microsurgery. Despite this and various other innovations in technique, imaging equipment, and instrumentation, life-threatening periprocedural hemorrhage can occur. Prudent evaluation and correction of spontaneous or medication-induced coagulopathy prior to a planned procedure per Society of Interventional Radiology guidelines are therefore necessary.[1,2]

Systemic administration of blood products can be very effective, but many clinical circumstances (discussed later) may limit its use or efficacy. The locally injected blood elements (LIBE) technique was first employed to allow safe percutaneous drainage of a hemothorax in a leukemic patient with a platelet count less than 100/μ and refractory to systemic platelet administration due to preformed antibodies.[3] The efficacy of LIBE to reduce blood loss after solid organ biopsy in the setting of coagulopathy has since been demonstrated in an animal model.[4] The physiologic rationale of LIBE is based on the "seroma" of blood product that is created along the needle tract and target site. When an instrument is introduced through the path, it encounters markedly elevated "local" levels of platelets and/or platelets and clotting factors so that a high-quality blood clot will form.[5-7]

Our group has employed the LIBE technique for hundreds of coagulopathic patients during approximately the past 15 years with good results and no adverse reactions. An ongoing prospective study has demonstrated no side effects and equal efficacy compared to systemic administration of blood products (J. R. Haaga et al., personal communication, unpublished data). Note that although LIBE is not a US Food and Drug Administration (FDA)-approved use of platelets or fresh frozen plasma (FFP), it is permitted under current statutes that permit the off-label use of an FDA-approved product (blood products) for clinical care of patients and approved research protocols (*Belmont Report*).[8,9]

Applications of the Technique

Indications for LIBE include and expand on those for systemic administration of blood products to reverse pre-procedural coagulopathy.[1,2] LIBE is particularly useful in situations in which systemic blood product administration is ineffective or contraindicated, including various scenarios encountered in the critically ill patient. These include the following:

1. Contraindications to systemic reversal of pharmacologic anticoagulation.
2. Precarious fluid volume status, where the additional volume of systemic blood products is contraindicated.
3. Severe coagulopathy that would otherwise require large amounts of systemic blood products to normalize.
4. Minimization of risk of pulmonary edema in patients with low pulmonary reserve.
5. Patient has a history of adverse reaction or other intolerance to desired blood product.
6. A history of failed response to prior systemic administration of blood products (i.e., preformed antibodies, hypersplenism, etc.).
7. Limited availability of desired blood product: Cost, safety, and ethical considerations demand judicious use of blood products whenever possible. Because LIBE usually requires only up to 20 ml of blood product, a single unit of any desired blood product will almost always be sufficient for any application of LIBE. In fact, there is often a significant amount of unused blood product after LIBE, and this portion must be discarded post-procedure or alternatively may be systemically administered if indicated. In the future, wider adoption of LIBE and distribution of blood products in smaller volumes than current standard units may limit waste of precious blood products.

Challenges of the Procedure

1. Alternating the injection between blood product and lidocaine is somewhat of a challenge, and this may be facilitated with use of stopcock if desirable.

Potential Pitfalls/Complications

1. Minimize coagulopathies prior to the procedure: If not clinically contraindicated, effort should be made to minimize bleeding diathesis prior to the procedure, including withholding common medications such as aspirin, nonsteroidal anti-inflammatory drugs, and anticoagulants per consensus guidelines.[1,2]

2. Ensure that LIBE is truly administered locally: Inadvertent intravascular administration of blood products, although constituting the usual route for blood products and therefore safe in most instances, will prevent formation of the blood product seroma required for potent local effects. Injection of products into a fluid-filled cavity adjacent to the intended tract or target will similarly prevent effective seroma formation. Gentle aspiration of the needle during LIBE will help ensure the needle tip is not intravascular or in a fluid-filled cavity. The seroma is seldom visualized after injection with CT or during injection with ultrasound guidance.

3. Consider additional techniques to minimize bleeding in very vascular lesions: If lesion to be biopsied or accessed demonstrates extreme vascularity on a diagnostic study (perfusion CT or Doppler ultrasound), consider altering the procedure (e.g., switching to noncutting or smaller caliber needle) or halting the planned procedure altogether. Alternatively, an occlusive hemostatic technique using angiographic coils or gelfoam pledgets might be used.

Steps of the Procedure

1. Select target and skin entrance site.
2. Use usual sterile technique and antiseptic preparation of entrance site.
3. The skin entrance site is anesthetized by creating a small wheel with 1% or 2% lidocaine, and a small stab wound is made. Bleeding time of the stab wound is assessed; if bleeding time is excessive, it is prudent to defer the procedure until repeat coagulation tests can be made.
4. The entire planned access tract from skin surface to the target organ surface or lesion is injected with lidocaine and the blood product (platelets or FFP). This may be accomplished by alternating injections with separate lidocaine and blood product syringes via a single needle or through a stopcock. The FDA does not permit mixing blood products with other drugs during administration. It is known that lidocaine inhibits platelet function.[10-12]
5. After the needle is fully inserted, reinjection of 10 cc of 100% blood product should be made as the needle is withdrawn.
6. If a coaxial technique is used for biopsy, additional blood product may be injected into the biopsy tracts through the guidance cannula as it is withdrawn.

Example

See Figure 104.1.

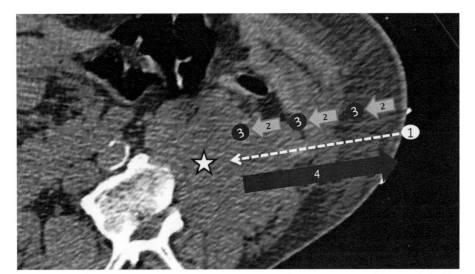

Figure 104.1 Local injection of blood elements (LIBE) during percutaneous needle biopsy of left retroperitoneal mass (white star). (1) The needle access tract (dashed arrow) is planned, and the skin surface lidocaine wheel is made. (2) The needle is inserted a short distance while injecting lidocaine (gray arrow). (3) Needle advancement is halted, and a volume of blood product equivalent to that of the lidocaine just administered is injected at this site (black circles). Lidocaine and blood product are injected via separate syringes (a stopcock may facilitate this process). This process of alternating between lidocaine and blood product injections is repeated until the target is reached. (4) While withdrawing the needle, approximately 10 cc of pure blood product is injected along the needle pathway (black arrow).

References and Suggested Readings

1. Patel IJ, Davidson JC, Nikolic B, et al; Standards of Practice Committee, with Cardiovascular and Interventional Radiological Society of Europe (CIRSE) Endorsement. Consensus guidelines for periprocedural management of coagulation status and hemostasis risk in percutaneous image-guided interventions. *J Vasc Interv Radiol.* 2012;23(6):727–736.

2. Patel IJ, Davidson JC, Nikolic B, et al; Standards of Practice Committee, with Cardiovascular and Interventional Radiological Society of Europe (CIRSE) Endorsement; Standards of Practice Committee of the Society of Interventional Radiology. Addendum of newer anticoagulants to the SIR consensus guideline. *J Vasc Interv Radiol.* 2013;24(5):641–645.

3. Haaga JR, Timothy L. Haaga TL, Wu H. Image-guided intervention and basic science. In: Haaga JR, Dogra VS, Forsting M, Gilkeson RC, Ha HK, Sundaram M, eds. *CT and MRI of the Whole Body.* 5th ed. St. Louis: Mosby; 2008.

4. Nakamoto DA, Wilkins LR, Haaga JR. Hemostasis effects of direct intraparenchymal injection of platelets and fresh frozen plasma before cutting needle biopsy in an animal model. *J Vasc Interv Radiol.* 2011;22(11):1601–1605.

5. Shams Hakimi C, Fagerberg Blixter I, Hansson EC, Hesse C, Wallén H, Jeppsson A. Effects of fibrinogen and platelet supplementation on clot formation and platelet aggregation in blood samples from cardiac surgery patients. *Thromb Res.* 2014;134(4):895–900.

6. Kornblith LZ, Kutcher ME, Redick BJ, Calfee CS, Vilardi RF, Cohen MJ. Fibrinogen and platelet contributions to clot formation: Implications for trauma resuscitation and thromboprophylaxis. *J Trauma Acute Care Surg.* 2014;76(2):255–256; discussion 262–263.

7. Harr JN, Moore EE, Ghasabyan A, et al. Functional fibrinogen assay indicates that fibrinogen is critical in correcting abnormal clot strength following trauma. *Shock.* 2013;39(1):45–49.

8. US Food and Drug Administration. "Off-label" and investigational use of marketed drugs, biologics, and medical devices: Information sheet. http://www.fda.gov/RegulatoryInformation/Guidances/ucm126486.htm. Accessed December 20, 2014.

9. National Commission for the Protection of Human Subjects of Biomedical and Behavioral Research. *The Belmont Report.* Washington, DC: US Department of Health, Education, and Welfare; 1979.

10. Feinstein MB, Fiekers J, Fraser C. An analysis of the mechanism of local anesthetic inhibition of platelet aggregation and secretion. *J Pharmacol Exp Ther.* 1976;197:215–228.

11. Borg T, Modig J. Potential anti-thrombotic effects of local anaesthetics due to their inhibition of platelet aggregation. *Acta Anaesthesiol Stand.* 1985;29:739–742.

12. Huang GS, Lin TC, Wang JY, Ku CH, Ho ST, Li CY. Lidocaine priming reduces ADP-induced P-selectin expression and platelet–leukocyte aggregation. *Acta Anaesthesiol Taiwan.* 2009;47(2):56–61.

CHAPTER 105

Reducing Operator Exposure Using Suspended Radiation Protection System

Almas Syed, Robert Evans Heithaus, and Chet R. Rees

Introduction

Increasing utilization of radiation for diagnostic and therapeutic procedures has provided impetus for improved strategies of radiation protection for interventionalists. A suspended radiation protection system (SPRPS) employs the use of a "weightless" shield resembling a thick, large lead apron with head shield and arm shields. The shield moves with the operator like a garment, providing extensive protection without orthopedic strain or discomfort while maintaining full user functionality.

Technique

The scientific community is working to improve its understanding of the growing use of medical radiation, the stochastic risks for cancer, and ways to limit exposure. There has been an increase in the average effective dose to individuals exposed to radiation from medical imaging from approximately 4.8 mSv in 1996 to 7.8 mSv in 2010.[1] In addition, the obesity epidemic in the United States and most of the developing world has resulted in larger doses of radiation to both patient and operator.[2] A striking increase in operator dose is noted with increasing patient abdominal thickness. One study confirmed that exposure to the operator at the waist level almost doubled with each additional 5 cm (1.97 in) of phantom (patient) thickness and that an increase in phantom (patient) thickness of 10 cm (from 24 to 34 cm) caused dramatic increases in entrance air kerma by a factor of 8.4.[3]

The need for improved operator protection from radiation and potentially career-shortening orthopedic injuries has been voiced by many, including a multidisciplinary task force.[4] The SPRPS addresses both the exposure and the orthopedic issues. It consists of a lead–acrylic head shield (0.5 mm Pb equiv) and protective flexible apron (1.0 mm Pb equiv), which are attached to a skeletal frame that is suspended from a motion apparatus that allows smooth motion in all three spatial planes with little effort and the sensation of weightlessness to the operator. This allows for abundant shielding reaching several times the mass of a conventional apron because it has a much higher attenuation profile and more expansive coverage of the body.[5,6] The operator may "slip" in and out of the shield quickly and with maintenance of full sterility through use of a magnetic system that includes a small metal disc worn on the operator in combination with a sterile drape around the shield. The device can be set aside and parked when not in use, and it can be brought back in for use at any time.

The commercially available device extends farther down the calves than conventional aprons and includes arm flaps to cover the shoulder, axilla, and proximal arms (CFI Medical Solutions, Fenton, MI). Using electronic dosimeters, exposure reductions of 99% for head and eye were detected compared to those of conventional lead aprons, thyroid shield, table shields, and hanging shields.[5,6] In addition, exposure reductions of 88–98% for humerus, tibia, and head regions were seen using conventional optically stimulated luminescence dosimeter badges.[5] Due to the enhanced area of coverage and the substantially greater attenuation power of 1 mm Pb compared to wearable garments, total body exposures are presumed to be considerably lower.

Example

See Figures 105.1–105.5.

Figure 105.1 Increasing radiation effects of increasing abdominal thickness from 24 cm (A) to 34 cm (B).

Source: From Schueler BA, et al. An investigation of operator exposure in interventional radiology. *Radiographics* 2006;26:1533–1541. Reproduced with permission from RSNA.

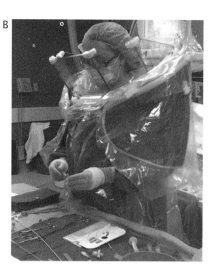

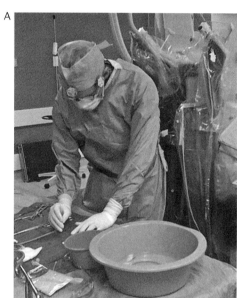

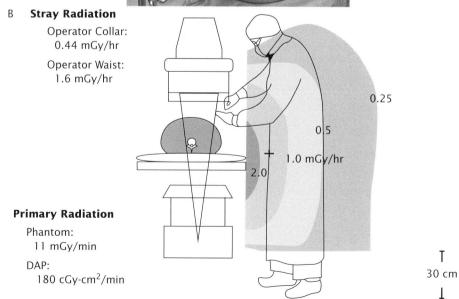

B   **Stray Radiation**
       Operator Collar:
         0.44 mGy/hr

       Operator Waist:
         1.6 mGy/hr

       0.25
       0.5
       1.0 mGy/hr
       2.0

       30 cm

Primary Radiation
   Phantom:
     11 mGy/min

   DAP:
     180 cGy-cm²/min

Figure 105.2 (A) Operator using suspended personal radiation protection system (CFI Medical Solutions). The system moves with the operator (B) and may be disengaged and re-engaged while the device and operator remain sterile (C).

Source: Reproduced from Savage C, et al. Evaluation of a suspended personal radiation protection system vs. conventional apron and shields in clinical interventional procedures. *Open J Radiol.* 2013;3(3):143–151.

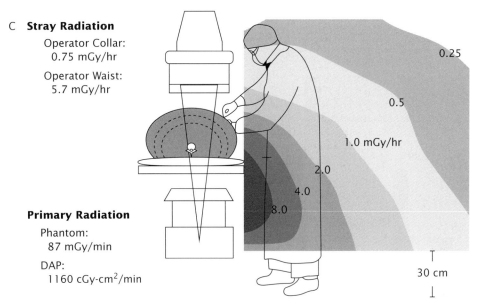

C   **Stray Radiation**

Operator Collar:
0.75 mGy/hr

Operator Waist:
5.7 mGy/hr

Primary Radiation

Phantom:
87 mGy/min

DAP:
1160 cGy-cm^2/min

Figure 105.2 Continued

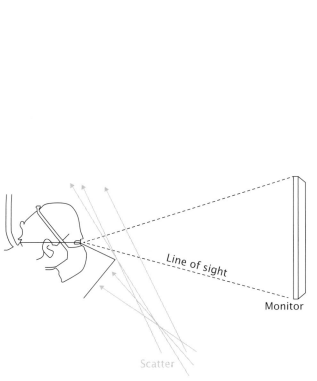

Figure 105.3 The head shield is positioned to obstruct scatter from the field while remaining out of the operator's line of sight to the monitor.

Source: Reproduced from Savage C, et al. Evaluation of a suspended personal radiation protection system vs. conventional apron and shields in clinical interventional procedures. *Open J Radiol.* 2013;3(3):143–151.

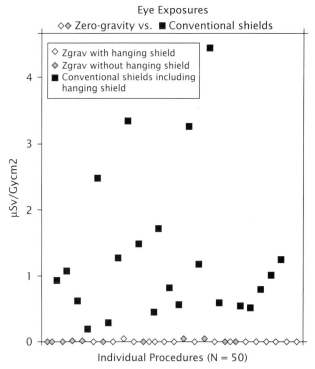

Figure 105.4 Operator eye exposures for 50 procedures using a suspended personal radiation protection system (SPRPS) versus apron and shields including mobile hanging shield, under-table shield, and side table shield. The degree of eye exposures was higher for all conventional-shield cases compared to all SPRPS cases. Individual case exposures (μSv) were measured with electronic direct dosimeter and standardized to patient dose area product (Gycm^2).

Source: Reproduced Savage C, et al. Evaluation of a suspended personal radiation protection system vs. conventional apron and shields in clinical interventional procedures. *Open J Radiol.* 2013;3(3):143–151.

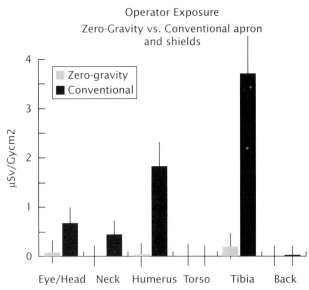

Operator Exposure
Zero-Gravity vs. Conventional apron and shields

Figure 105.5 Operator exposures using a suspended personal radiation protection system versus conventional apron, thyroid shield, mobile hanging shield, under table shield, and side table shield.[5] Optically stimulated luminescence dosimeter badges worn at the locations indicated provided readings. Operator exposures (μSv) were standardized to patient dose area product (Gycm^2).

Source: Reproduced from Savage C, et al. Evaluation of a suspended personal radiation protection system vs. conventional apron and shields in clinical interventional procedures. *Open J Radiol.* 2013;3(3):143–151.

References and Suggested Readings

1. Smith-Bindman R, Miglioretti DL, Johnson E, et al. Use of diagnostic imaging studies and associated radiation exposure for patients enrolled in large integrated health care systems, 1996–2010. *JAMA.* 2012;307:2400–2409.

2. World Health Organization. Obesity and overweight. http://www.who.int/mediacentre/factsheets/fs311/en. Accessed September 24, 2014.

3. Schueler BA, Vrieze TJ, Bjarnason H, Stanson AW. An investigation of operator exposure in interventional radiology. *Radiographics* 2006;26:1533–1541.

4. Klein LW, Miller DL, Balter S, et al. Occupational health hazards in the interventional laboratory: Time for a safer environment. *Radiology.* 2009;250(2):538–544.

5. Savage C, Seale TM IV, Shaw CJ, Angela BP, Marichal D, Rees CR. Evaluation of a suspended personal radiation protection system vs. conventional apron and shields in clinical interventional procedures. *Open J Radiol.* 2013;3(3):143–151.

6. Ray JM, Mohammad F, Taylor WB, Cura M, Savage C. Comparison of operator eye exposures when working from femoral region, side, or head of patient. *Proc (Baylor Univ Med Cent)* 2013;26(3):243–246.

Index

Page references for figures are indicated by *f* and for tables by *t*.

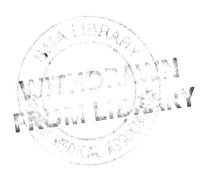